Essential Bioimaging Methods

Reliable Lab Solutions

Essential Bioimaging Methods

Reliable Lab Solutions

Edited by

P. Michael Conn

Director, Office of Research Advocacy (OHSU)
Senior Scientist, Divisions of Reproductive Sciences
and Neuroscience (ONPRC)

Professor, Departments of Pharmacology and Physiology,
Cell and Developmental Biology, and Obstetrics and Gynecology (OHSU)
Beaverton, Oregon

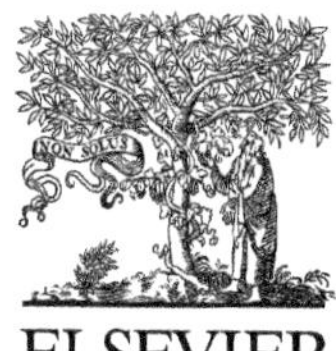

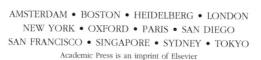

AMSTERDAM • BOSTON • HEIDELBERG • LONDON
NEW YORK • OXFORD • PARIS • SAN DIEGO
SAN FRANCISCO • SINGAPORE • SYDNEY • TOKYO
Academic Press is an imprint of Elsevier

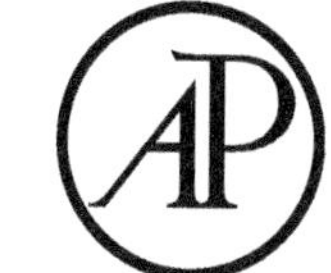

Academic Press is an imprint of Elsevier
Linacre House, Jordan Hill, Oxford OX2 8DP, UK
30 Corporate Drive, Suite 400, Burlington, MA 01803, USA
525 B Street, Suite 1900, San Diego, CA 92101-4495, USA
32 Jamestown Road, London NW1 7BY, UK

First edition 2009

Material in the work originally appeared in Volume 385 (Elsevier Inc., 2004) and Volume 386 (Elsevier Inc., 2004) of *Methods in Enzymology*

ISBN: 978-0-12-375043-3

For information on all Academic Press publications
visit our website at elsevierdirect.com

Printed and bound by CPI Group (UK) Ltd, Croydon, CR0 4YY
Transferred to Digital Printing, 2013

CONTENTS

Contributors xi

Preface xv

PART I Imaging in Animal and Human Models

1. Positron Emission Tomography (PET): Research to Clinical Practice
Rakesh Kumar and Suman Jana

I. Introduction 4
II. Tracers 4
III. Drug Evaluation 5
IV. Biological Function Evaluation 7
V. Clinical Applications 8
VI. Future Perspectives 16
VII. Conclusions 18
References 18

2. Biophysical Basis of Magnetic Resonance Imaging of Small Animals
Bruce M. Damon and John C. Gore

I. Introduction 27
II. Spin Relaxation 28
III. Effects of Exchange and Compartmentation 31
IV. Paramagnetic Relaxation 33
V. Susceptibility Contrast and BOLD Effects 33
VI. Effects of Spin Motion 34
VII. An Illustrative Example: MRI of Exercising Skeletal Muscle 35
References 45

3. Functional Magnetic Resonance Imaging of Macaque Monkeys
Kiyoshi Nakahara

I. Introduction 47
II. Potential of Functional MRI in Macaque Monkeys 48

III. Brief History of fMRI in Macaque Monkeys 49
IV. Experimental Procedures 50
V. Conclusion 52
References 52

4. Atlas Template Images for Nonhuman Primate Neuroimaging: Baboon and Macaque
Kevin J. Black, Jonathan M. Koller, Abraham Z. Snyder, and Joel S. Perlmutter

I. Introduction 56
II. Methods 57
III. Discussion 64
References 65

5. Magnetic Resonance Imaging of Brain Function
Stuart Clare

I. Update 67
II. Introduction 68
III. Experimental Procedures 69
IV. An Application of Functional MRI 80
V. Discussion and Conclusion 81
References 81

PART II Imaging of Receptors, Small Molecules, and Protein-Protein Interactions

6. Positron Emission Tomography Receptor Assay with Multiple Ligand Concentrations: An Equilibrium Approach
Doris J. Doudet and James E. Holden

I. Update 86
II. Introduction 88
III. Overview of *In Vivo* Receptor Assay 89
IV. Methods 93
V. Example Applications 98
VI. Conclusions 101
References 101

7. Estimation of Local Receptor Density, B'_{max}, and Other Parameters via Multiple-Injection Positron Emission Tomography Experiments

Evan D. Morris, Bradley T. Christian, Karmen K. Yoder, and Raymond F. Muzic, Jr.

I. Update 106
II. Introduction 107
III. Theory 109
IV. Experimental Protocol and Considerations 115
V. Models and Data Fitting 120
VI. Results and Interpretation 125
VII. Understanding and Designing M-I Experiments 128
VIII. Conclusion 131
References 132

8. Magnetic Resonance Imaging in Biomedical Research: Imaging of Drugs and Drug Effects

Markus Rudin, Nicolau Beckmann, and Martin Rausch

I. Introduction 135
II. Drug Imaging and PK Studies 136
III. Noninvasive Assessment of Drug Efficacy/Pharmacodynamic Studies 138
IV. Disease and Efficacy Biomarkers as Bridge Between Preclinical and Clinical Drug Evaluation 145
V. Conclusion and Outlook 147
References 148

9. Imaging Myocardium Enzymatic Pathways with Carbon-11 Radiotracers

Carmen S. Dence, Pilar Herrero, Sally W. Schwarz, Robert H. Mach, Robert J. Gropler, and Michael J. Welch

I. Introduction 152
II. Overview of the Production of Carbon-11 153
III. Overview of the Quality Assurance of C-11 Radiopharmaceuticals 163
IV. Dosimetry Calculations 165
V. Conduct of GAP Studies 166
VI. Conclusion 177
References 178

PART III Disease Models

10. Molecular and Functional Imaging of Cancer: Advances in MRI and MRS

Arvind P. Pathak, Barjor Gimi, Kristine Glunde, Ellen Ackerstaff, Dmitri Artemov, and Zaver M. Bhujwalla

I. Update 184
II. Introduction 185
III. Vascular Imaging of Tumors with MRI 186
IV. Cellular and Molecular Imaging 200
V. Metabolic and Physiologic Spectroscopy and Spectroscopic Imaging with MRS and MRSI 214
VI. Examples of Integrated Imaging and Spectroscopy Approaches to Studying Cancer 222
References 229

11. A Modified Transorbital Baboon Model of Reperfused Stroke

Anthony L. D'Ambrosio, Michael E. Sughrue, J. Mocco, William J. Mack, Ryan G. King, Shivani Agarwal, and E. Sander Connolly, Jr.

I. Update 238
II. Introduction 238
III. Preoperative Care 240
IV. Operative Technique 243
V. Postoperative Care 246
VI. Data Collection and Analysis 246
VII. Model Application: HuEP5C7 249
VIII. Conclusion 249
References 250

12. Structural and Functional Optical Imaging of Angiogenesis in Animal Models

Richard L. Roberts and Pengnian Charles Lin

I. Introduction 251
II. Intravital Microscopy and Animal Window Models 252
III. Imaging of Tumor-Host Interaction and Angiogenesis Initiation Using Fluorescent Protein-Labeled Tumor Cells 256
IV. Vascular Reporter Transgenic Mouse Model 260
V. Conclusions 266
References 267

13. MRI of Animal Models of Brain Disease

Rob Nabuurs, David L. Thomas, John S. Thornton, Mark F. Lythgoe, and Louise van der Weerd

How to Avoid Pittfalls: Tips and Tricks 270
I. Introduction 270
II. Biophysical Background and Methods 271
III. Applications of MRI to Experimental Neuropathology 284
IV. Conclusion 294
References 295

14. Magnetic Resonance Imaging in Animal Models of Pathologies

Pasquina Marzola, Stefano Tambalo, and Andrea Sbarbati

I. Update 301
II. Introduction 302
III. Bacterial Infections 303
IV. Ischemic Pathologies 309
V. Neoplastic Pathologies 311
VI. Lipid Accumulation in Metabolic-Degenerative Disorders 316
VII. Conclusions 320
References 320

15. Application of Combined Magnetic Resonance Imaging and Histopathologic and Functional Studies for Evaluation of Aminoguanidine Following Traumatic Brain Injury in Rats

Jia Lu and Shabbir Moochhala

I. Introduction 325
II. Materials and Methods 326
III. Results and Discussion 334
References 335

PART IV Preparation of Materials

16. Vascular-Targeted Nanoparticles for Molecular Imaging and Therapy

Samira Guccione, King C.P. Li, and Mark D. Bednarski

I. Introduction 339
II. Rationale Behind Choosing a Vascular Target for Molecular Imaging 341
III. Design and Preclinical Studies of a Vascular-Targeted Molecular Imaging Agent 344

IV. Molecular Imaging and Vascular-Targeted Therapeutics 351
V. Summary 354
References 355

17. Generation of DOTA-Conjugated Antibody Fragments for Radioimmunoimaging

Peter M. Smith-Jones and David B. Solit

I. Introduction 358
II. Selection of a Radionuclide and Chelating Agent 359
III. Generation of Antibody Fragments 364
IV. Conjugation of DOTA to Intact Antibodies or Fragments 365
V. Radiolabeling of DOTA Conjugates 366
VI. Characterization of DOTA-F(ab′)$_2$ Conjugates 367
VII. PET Imaging 369
VIII. Conclusion 369
References 370

PART V General Methods

18. The Application of Magnetic Resonance Imaging and Spectroscopy to Gene Therapy

Po-Wah So, Kishore K. Bhakoo, I. Jane Cox, Simon D. Taylor-Robinson, and Jimmy D. Bell

I. Introduction 374
II. Magnetic Resonance Techniques 376
III. MR Overview 377
IV. MR Imaging (MRI) 377
V. MR Spectroscopy (MRS) 380
VI. Role of Magnetic Resonance Methods in GT 380
VII. MRI-Based Systems 383
VIII. MRS-Based Systems 387
IX. Conclusions 389
References 390

19. Voxelation Methods for Genome Scale Imaging of Brain Gene Expression

Daniel M. Sforza and Desmond J. Smith

I. Update 399
II. Introduction 400
III. Methods 401
IV. Data Analysis 405
References 408

Index 411

CONTRIBUTORS

Numbers in parentheses indicate the pages on which the authors' contributions begin.

Ellen Ackerstaff (183), JHU ICMIC Program, Russell H. Morgan Department of Radiology and Radiological Science, The Johns Hopkins University School of Medicine, Baltimore, Maryland 21205

Shivani Agarwal (237), Department of Neurological Surgery, Columbia University, New York, New York 10032-2699

Dmitri Artemov (183), JHU ICMIC Program, Russell H. Morgan Department of Radiology and Radiological Science, The Johns Hopkins University School of Medicine, Baltimore, Maryland 21205

Nicolau Beckmann (135), Novartis Institute for Biomedical Research, Analytical and Imaging Sciences Unit, CH-4002 Basel, Switzerland

Mark D. Bednarski (339), Department of Radiology, Lucas MRI Research Center, Stanford University, Stanford, California 94305-5488

Jimmy D. Bell (373), Metabolic and Molecular Imaging Group, MRC Clinical Sciences Centre, Imperial College London, Hammersmith Hospital, London W12 0HS, United Kingdom

Kishore K. Bhakoo (373), Translational Molecular Imaging Group, Singapore Bioimaging Consortium, Agency for Science Technology and Research (ASTAR), #02–02 Helios, Singapore 138667, Singapore

Zaver M. Bhujwalla (183), JHU ICMIC Program, Russell H. Morgan Department of Radiology and Radiological Science, The Johns Hopkins University School of Medicine, Baltimore, Maryland 21205

Kevin J. Black (55), Departments of Psychiatry, Neurology, and Radiology, Washington University School of Medicine, St. Louis, Missouri 63110-1093

Bradley T. Christian (105), PET Physics, Waisman Laboratory for Brain imaging and Behavior, Departments of Medical Physics and Psychiatry, University of Wisconsin-Madison, Madison

Stuart Clare (67), Department of Clinical Neurology, Centre for Functional Magnetic Resonance Imaging of the Brain, John Radcliffe Hospital, University of Oxford, Headington, Oxford OX39DU, United Kingdom

E. Sander Connolly, Jr. (237), Department of Neurological Surgery, Columbia University, New York, New York 10032-2699

I. Jane Cox (373), Imaging Sciences Department, Division of Clinical Sciences, Imperial College London, London W12 0HS, United Kingdom

Anthony L. D'Ambrosio (237), Department of Neurological Surgery, Columbia University, New York, New York 10032-2699

Bruce M. Damon (27), Department of Radiology and Radiological Sciences, Vanderbilt University Institute of Imaging Science, Nashville, Tennessee 37232

Carmen S. Dence (151), Department of Radiology, School of Medicine, Washington University, St. Louis, Missouri 63110

Doris J. Doudet (85), Department of Medicine, Division of Neurology, and TRIUMF, University of British Columbia, Vancouver, British Columbia V6T 2A3, Canada

Barjor Gimi (183), JHU ICMIC Program, Russell H. Morgan Department of Radiology and Radiological Science, The Johns Hopkins University School of Medicine, Baltimore, Maryland 21205

Kristine Glunde (183), JHU ICMIC Program, Russell H. Morgan Department of Radiology and Radiological Science, The Johns Hopkins University School of Medicine, Baltimore, Maryland 21205

John C. Gore (27), Department of Radiology and Radiological Sciences, Vanderbilt University Institute of Imaging Science, Nashville, Tennessee 37232

Robert J. Gropler (151), Department of Radiology, School of Medicine, Washington University, St. Louis, Missouri 63110

Samira Guccione (339), Department of Radiology, Lucas MRI Research Center, Stanford University, Stanford, California 94305-5488

Pilar Herrero (151), Department of Radiology, School of Medicine, Washington University, St. Louis, Missouri 63110

James E. Holden (85), Department of Medical Physics, University of Wisconsin, Madison, Wisconsin 53705

Suman Jana (3), Cardiovascular Research Center, University of Kentucky, Lexington, Kentucky 40536-0200

Ryan G. King (237), Department of Neurological Surgery, Columbia University, New York, New York 10032-2699

Jonathan M. Koller (55), Department of Psychiatry, Washington University School of Medicine, St. Louis, Missouri 63110-1093

Rakesh Kumar (3), Department of Nuclear Medicine and PET, All India Institute of Medical Sciences, New Delhi 110029, India

King C.P. Li (339), Department of Radiology, Stanford University, Stanford, California 94305-5488

Pengnian Charles Lin (251), Department of Pathology, Vanderbilt-Ingram Cancer Center, Vanderbilt University Medical Center, Nashville, Tennessee 37232

Jia Lu (325), Defence Medical Research Institute, Singapore 117510, Singapore

Mark F. Lythgoe (269), Department of Medicine and Institute of Child Health, Centre for Advanced Biomedical Imaging, University College London, London, United Kingdom

Robert H. Mach (151), Department of Radiology, School of Medicine, Washington University, St. Louis, Missouri 63110

William J. Mack (237), Department of Neurological Surgery, Columbia University, New York, New York 10032-2699

Pasquina Marzola (301), Department of Morphological and Biomedical Sciences, Section of Anatomy, University of Verona, Verona, Italy

J. Mocco (237), University of Florida, Gainesville, FL 32610-0261

Shabbir Moochhala (325), Defence Medical Research Institute, Singapore 117510, Singapore

Evan D. Morris (105), Departments of Diagnostic Radiology and Biomedical Engineering, Yale PET Center, Yale School of Medicine, New Haven, Connecticut 06510

Raymond F. Muzic, Jr. (105), Departments of Radiology, Biomedical Engineering, and Oncology, Case Western Reserve University, Cleveland, Ohio

Rob Nabuurs (269), Department of Radiology, Molecular Imaging Laboratories Leiden, Leiden University Medical Center, Leiden, The Netherlands

Kiyoshi Nakahara (47), Department of Physiology, The University of Tokyo School of Medicine, Tokyo 113-0033, Japan

Arvind P. Pathak (183), JHU ICMIC Program, Russell H. Morgan Department of Radiology and Radiological Science, The Johns Hopkins University School of Medicine, Baltimore, Maryland 21205

Joel S. Perlmutter (55), Departments of Neurology, Radiology, Anatomy and Neurobiology, and the Program in Physical Therapy, Washington University School of Medicine, St. Louis, Missouri 63110-1093

Martin Rausch (135), Novartis Institute for Biomedical Research, Analytical and Imaging Sciences Unit, CH-4002 Basel, Switzerland

Richard L. Roberts (251), Department of Pathology, Vanderbilt-Ingram Cancer Center, Vanderbilt University Medical Center, Nashville, Tennessee 37232

Markus Rudin (135), Novartis Institute for Biomedical Research, Analytical and Imaging Sciences Unit, CH-4002 Basel, Switzerland

Andrea Sbarbati (301), Department of Morphological and Biomedical Sciences, Section of Anatomy, University of Verona, Verona, Italy

Sally W. Schwarz (151), Department of Radiology, School of Medicine, Washington University, St. Louis, Missouri 63110

Daniel M. Sforza (399), Department of Molecular and Medical Pharmacology, Geffen School of Medicine, UCLA, 23-120 CHS, Box 951735, Los Angeles, California 90095-1735

Desmond J. Smith (399), Department of Molecular and Medical Pharmacology, Geffen School of Medicine, UCLA, 23-120 CHS, Box 951735, Los Angeles, California 90095-1735

Peter M. Smith-Jones (357), Nuclear Medicine Service, Department of Radiology, Memorial Sloan-Kettering Cancer Center, New York, New York 10021

Abraham Z. Snyder (55), Departments of Radiology and Neurology, Washington University School of Medicine, St. Louis, Missouri 63110-1093

Po-Wah So (373), Preclinical Imaging Unit, Department of Clinical Neuroscience, King's College London, Institute of Psychiatry, James Black Centre, London SE4 9NU, United Kingdom

David B. Solit (357), Department of Medicine, Memorial Sloan-Kettering Cancer Center, New York, New York 10021

Michael E. Sughrue (237), Department of Neurological Surgery, Columbia University, New York, New York 10032-2699

Stefano Tambalo (301), Department of Morphological and Biomedical Sciences, Section of Anatomy, University of Verona, Verona, Italy

Simon D. Taylor-Robinson (373), Department of Hepatology and Gastroenterology, Division of Medicine, Faculty of Medicine, Imperial College London, St Mary's Hospital, London W2 1NY, United Kingdom

David L. Thomas (269), Department of Medical Physics and Bioengineering, University College London, London, United Kingdom

John S. Thornton (269), Lysholm Department of Neuroradiology, National Hospital for Neurology and Neurosurgery, London, United Kingdom

Louise van der Weerd (269), Department of Anatomy and Embryology, Molecular Imaging Laboratories Leiden, Leiden University Medical Center, Leiden, The Netherlands and Department of Radiology, Molecular Imaging Laboratories Leiden, Leiden University Medical Center, Leiden, The Netherlands

Michael J. Welch (151), Department of Radiology, School of Medicine, Washington University, St. Louis, Missouri 63110

Karmen K. Yoder (105), Center for Neuroimaging, Stark Neurosciences Research Institute, and Department of Radiology, Indiana University School of Medicine, Indianapolis, Indiana

PREFACE

At the time that the *Methods in Enzymology* volumes from which this book was taken were going to press, American Paul C. Lauterbur and Briton Sir Peter Mansfield have just been selected for the Nobel Prize in Medicine and Physiology for their discoveries leading to the development of the MRI.

The *Washington Post* ran a story on October 6, 2003, announcing the accolade and noted. "Magnetic resonance imaging, or MRI, has become a routine method for medical diagnosis and treatment. It is used to examine almost all organs without the need for surgery, but is especially valuable for detailed examination of the brain and spinal cord." The article would have been farsighted, had it mentioned the additional role of this technique in basic research, but it did not.

The usefulness of this technology in both clinical and basic science is reflected in tens of thousands of articles on PUBMED—and more than tens of thousands of people helped both in the clinics and by the new technologies that basic scientists have developed.

MRI and other imaging methods have made it possible to glance inside living systems and, for some, obviated the need for surgery. Because of the great value and continuing utility of these approaches, we are pleased that Academic Press has chosen to feature these methods in this new volume.

The authors were selected based on research contributions and their ability to describe their methodological contributions in a clear and understandable way. They have been encouraged to make use of graphics and comparisons to other methods, and to provide insight into the tracks and approaches that make it possible to adapt methods to other systems.

The editor expresses thanks to the contributors, and especially to Tara Hoey and the staff at Academic Press, for facilitation of the book.

P. Michael Conn

PART I

Imaging in Animal and Human Models

CHAPTER 1

Positron Emission Tomography (PET): Research to Clinical Practice

Rakesh Kumar* and Suman Jana†

*Department of Nuclear Medicine and PET
All India Institute of Medical Sciences
New Delhi 110029, India

†Cardiovascular Research Center
University of Kentucky
Lexington, Kentucky 40536-0200

I. Introduction
II. Tracers
III. Drug Evaluation
    A. Small Animal PET Imaging (Micro-PET)
IV. Biological Function Evaluation
V. Clinical Applications
    A. PET in Oncology
    B. PET in Neurology
    C. PET in Cardiology
    D. PET in Infectious and Inflammatory Diseases
VI. Future Perspectives
    A. Assessment of Multidrug Resistance
    B. Quantitation of Angiogenesis
    C. Tumor Hypoxia
    D. Apoptosis
    E. Gene Expression
VII. Conclusions
    References

DOI: 10.1016/B978-0-12-375043-3.00001-9

I. Introduction

Positron emission tomography (PET) is an advanced diagnostic imaging technique, which cannot only detect and localize but also quantify physiological and biochemical processes in the body noninvasively. The ability of PET to study various biological processes opens up new possibilities for both fundamental research and day-to-day clinical use. PET imaging utilizes β-emitting radionuclides such as ^{11}C, ^{13}N, ^{15}O, and ^{18}F, which can replace their respective stable nuclei in biologically active molecules. These radionuclides decay by positron emission. After being emitted from the nucleus, a positron will combine with a nearby electron through a process known as annihilation. Annihilation converts the mass of both particles into energy in the form of two antiparallel 511-keV γ-rays. The PET detectors are arranged in a ring in order to detect these γ-rays.

At present, 2-deoxy-2-[^{18}F] fluoro-D-glucose (^{18}F-FDG) is the most commonly used positron-emitting radiopharmaceutical used for PET imaging. ^{18}F-FDG is a radioactive analog of glucose and is able to detect altered glucose metabolism in pathological processes. Like glucose, FDG is transported into cells by means of a glucose transporter protein and begins to follow the glycolytic pathway. FDG is subsequently phosphorylated by an enzyme known as hexokinase to form FDG-6-phosphate (McGowan *et al.*, 1995; Wahl, 1996). However, FDG-6-phosphate cannot continue through glycolysis because it is not a substrate for glucose-6-phosphate isomerase. As a result, FDG-6-phosphate is trapped biochemically within the cell. This process of metabolic trapping constitutes the basis of PET imaging of the biodistribution of FDG. Because there can be a manyfold increase or decrease in the glucose metabolism of diseased tissue as compared to normal tissue, it is easy to detect such differences in metabolism using PET. This chapter discusses general aspects of PET, including drug evaluation, biological functions evaluation, clinical applications, and future directions of PET imaging.

Initially, PET was used alone without any computed tomography (CT) or magnetic resonance imaging (MRI) hybridization. Since there are few limitations associated with PET alone, a novel combined PET/CT system has recently been built that improves the ability to correctly localize and interpret radiotracer uptake. Hybrid PET/CT scanners provide both the anatomical and functional aspects of the tissue. Now for clinical uses PET alone machines are not available in the market. Integrated PET-CT using various radiotracers has shown encouraging results for the management of various cancers.

II. Tracers

PET uses radioisotopes of naturally occurring elements, such as ^{11}C, ^{13}N, and ^{15}O, in order to perform *in vivo* imaging of biologically active molecules. Although there is no radioisotope of H that can be used for PET, many molecules can replace a hydrogen or hydroxyl group with ^{18}F without changing its biological properties.

Table I
Positron-Emitter Radiotracers

Radioisotope	Half-life (min)
Carbon-11	20.4
Fluorine-18	109.8
Nitrogen-13	10
Oxygen-15	2.03
Copper-62	9.7
Rubidium-82	1.25
Yttrium-86	14.7

Fluorine-18 can also be used as a substitute in fluorine-containing compounds such as 5-fluorouresil (5-FU), as demonstrated by Mintun *et al.* (1988).

Most PET tracers utilize a radioisotope that has a short half-life and can be produced by a cyclotron (see Table I for a list of important tracers). However, there are some radiotracers, such as copper-62, that can be manufactured in a nuclear generator. Radiopharmaceuticals are produced after the radioisotope has been generated and substituted into the compound of interest. Because of the short half-lives of most PET tracers, sequential scanning on the same day is not usually possible.

III. Drug Evaluation

The development of new drugs presents many questions that must be addressed: Is the drug sufficiently delivered to target of interest? How is normal tissue affected? At what dose is toxicity produced? How much drug is eliminated from both target tissue and normal tissue in relation to time? Does the drug affect target tissue in the predicted way? All of these questions can be answered by labeling the drug of interest with an appropriate radionuclide for PET imaging.

In addition, mathematical kinetic modeling is necessary for all aspects of drug pharmacology and to measure physiological functions, such as tissue perfusion, metabolic rate, and elimination. Dynamic data can be collected in a specific biological organ or tissue by defining the region of interest and recording the radioactivity over time. Input functions can be calculated by measuring tracer concentration in arterial blood. By comparing the input functions and time activity curves over the organ or tissue of interest with theoretical models, it is possible to calculate the metabolism of the applied drugs. When these drugs are not metabolized in the tissue, the calculation of drug concentration is very simple. However, most drugs will undergo some degree of metabolism to produce metabolites. If these metabolites do not include the original radionuclide, there is no problem regarding the calculation of drug metabolism. However, if these metabolites also contain a radionuclide it can be difficult for PET to distinguish signals from the parent radiopharmaceutical and those from its metabolite. Blasberg *et al.* (2000) and Salem *et al.* (2000) have suggested a number of mathematical calculations in order to determine the parent contribution from total measured radiotracer activity.

Pharmacokinetic studies of new pharmaceuticals are greatly simplified by labeling these compounds with a PET tracer. It is possible to measure the time-dependent, *in vivo* biodistribution of a new drug labeled with PET tracer in one experiment, which can be subsequently compared to many animal experiments. Furthermore, the various effects of a drug on different biological processes, such as blood flow, tissue metabolism, and receptor activation, can also be demonstrated *in vivo* through PET imaging.

A. Small Animal PET Imaging (Micro-PET)

Animal models have been used in biomedical research for the study of mechanisms of biological process, aging, transduction of signals, different diseases, and possible cures of human disease, for validation of gene therapies and for new drug development (Blasberg *et al.*, 2000; Del Guerra *et al.*, 2002; McGowan *et al.*, 1995; Salem *et al.*, 2000; Sossi *et al.*, 2005; Wang *et al.*, 2005). Due to recent biogenetic innovations, transgenic animals showing particular anomalies obtained by genetic modification are now available. The genetic likelihood of transgenic rodents with humans, its short reproductive cycle and its simple breeding made mice and rats to be used widely as experimental models (Del Guerra *et al.*, 2002; Sossi *et al.*, 2005; Wang *et al.*, 2005). For years researchers have used small animal models of human disease to address questions by using radiotracers and autoradiography. While providing high spatial resolution, these techniques suffer from two major shortcomings: data can only be collected postmortem and might not provide a true representation of *in vivo* processes (Sossi *et al.*, 2005). Therefore, noninvasive imaging modalities like PET, CT, MRI, and optical imaging are being increasingly used (Sossi *et al.*, 2005; Wang *et al.*, 2005).

1. Applications of Micro-PET in Research

Studies using micro-PET have been used for functional and molecular imaging in cardiology, oncology, and neurology. The focus of these studies contribute to advancements in one of the following areas: disease mechanism and diagnosis, identification of drug target, assessment of treatment efficacy, and drug development (Sossi *et al.*, 2005; Wang *et al.*, 2005). In cardiology micro-PET has been used for perfusion imaging, metabolic imaging, receptor-binding imaging, and gene expression imaging (Inubushi *et al.*, 2003; Patel *et al.*, 2006; Wang *et al.*, 2005). Micro-PET imaging is perfectly suited for the functional imaging of cancer with its ability to image metabolism, proliferation, abnormal receptor density, hypoxia, angiogenesis, success of gene and stem cell therapy (Ray *et al.*, 2007; Wang *et al.*, 2005). In addition to measuring the PD of cancer therapies, the cancer drug itself can be labeled and the PK of the drug can be evaluated, providing information on biodistribution, toxicity, mechanism of action, and potential efficacy (Gangloff *et al.*, 2005; Gupta *et al.*, 2002; Wang *et al.*, 2005). Advantages of PET in preclinical animal studies of cancer are the ability to perform multiple longitudinal studies in the same animal and the reduction in the number of expensive transgenic animals needed to obtain statistical data (Aboagye *et al.*, 2005; Wang *et al.*, 2005). Utilized in this manner, PET has the potential to reduce the time and money required to develop a new cancer drug. However, micro-PET contributed most extensively in neurology research to study brain function, addiction, and a number of central nervous system (CNS) diseases. Basic neuroscience inquiries on location, density, and kinetics of receptors can be used to uncover the cause of disease, identify drug targets, and define PD (Wang *et al.*, 2005). Studies that investigate ways to diagnose disease and monitor its progression accurately and noninvasively can help assess efficacy of a drug candidate in both small animals and human (Wang *et al.*, 2005).

2. Limitations and Future Directions

The limitations of micro-PET are low resolution, poor anatomic detail and requirement of anesthesia to image an animal (anesthesia can potentially alter the metabolism). The resolution of micro-PET has increased over the years, from 2 to 3 to 1.3 mm in the newest micro-PET scanners. A micro-PET scanner with a resolution less than 1 mm is currently in development (Kim *et al.*, 2007; Sossi *et al.*, 2005; Wang *et al.*, 2005). There is presently a strong trend toward the development of PET scanners with even higher sensitivity and resolution and toward an integrated, multi-imaging modality approach to the investigation of biochemistry and anatomy in small animals (Sossi *et al.*, 2005). Combined PET and MRI, CT, SPECT, US, or optical scanners are being investigated (Davis *et al.*, 2002; Sossi *et al.*, 2005) as well as methods to combine information from structural and functional imaging (Sossi *et al.*, 2005; Wang *et al.*, 2005; Zhang *et al.*, 2008). Two methods have been developed to avoid use of anesthesia. On one hand, the animal can be trained to remain still during imaging. Alternatively, a small PET camera that can be attached to the animal head to allow scanning in the awakened state is in development (Sossi *et al.*, 2005; Wang *et al.*, 2005).

IV. Biological Function Evaluation

Theoretically, any biological function can be studied *in vivo* using an appropriately labeled PET tracer molecule. However, at present, PET tracers, which are utilized most commonly, are small molecules, which can be labeled by well-defined methods. Another important consideration is that the concentration of any PET tracer molecule should be significantly higher at the target sites than in the background. This allows biological function to be measured by determining tracer concentration over a specified time interval and by drawing a region of interest over the specified target tissue or organ region. Physiological processes such as oxygen consumption, blood flow, and tissue metabolism can also be demonstrated *in vivo* using PET tracers.

In the body, binding of an activating molecule (agonist) to a biochemical structure (receptor) can activate many biological functions. The same process can be blocked by an antagonist, which may have a higher affinity for receptors as compared to the agonist. Receptors can be visualized and quantified by labeling receptor-binding substances (ligands) with PET tracers. Most receptors have several biochemically similar subtypes and are composed of multiple subunits. Identification of these subtypes and subunits requires specific ligands. The details of *in vivo* research of receptors and their clinical applications in the diagnosis of neurodegenerative and heart diseases are discussed later.

V. Clinical Applications

The resolution of CT and MRI is excellent for the visualization of both normal and diseased tissues. However, all disease processes start with molecular and cellular abnormalities. Most disease processes take a long time to progress to a stage where they can be detected by these structural imaging techniques. In fact, many diseases may already be in advanced stages by the time they are detected by MRI or CT. However, the principle of PET is to detect the altered metabolism of disease processes and not the altered anatomy, such as CT and MRI. PET, as a functional molecular imaging technique, can also provide highly accurate quantitative results and, therefore, can be used for various research and clinical applications.

Kumar *et al.* (2003a) discussed the role of ^{18}F-FDG PET in the management of cancer patients. For these patients, PET has become important in diagnosis, staging, monitoring the response to treatment, and detecting recurrence. However, PET has also played an important role for both diagnostic and therapeutic purposes in patients with neurological and craniological infections and inflammations, vasculitis, and other autoimmune diseases (Schirmer *et al.*, 2003).

A. PET in Oncology

^{18}F-FDG is the most widely used radiotracer in oncology. Because glucose metabolism is increased manyfold in malignant tumors as compared to normal cells, PET has high sensitivity and a high negative predictive value. It has a well-established role in initial staging, monitoring response to the therapy, and management of many types of cancer, including lung cancer, colon cancer, lymphoma, melanoma, esophageal cancer, head and neck cancer, and breast cancer (Table II).

Table II
Important Indications of ^{18}F-FDG PET in Oncology

Clinical application	Tumor
Differentiation of benign	Solitary pulmonary nodules from malignant
Diagnosis and initial staging	Lung cancer
	Colorectal cancer
	Lymphoma
	Esophageal cancer
	Breast cancer
	Head and neck cancer
	Melanoma
Evaluation response to chemotherapy	Lymphoma
	Breast cancer
	Lung cancer
	Head and neck cancer
	Brain tumors
	Bone tumors
Recurrence	Lymphoma
	Breast cancer
	Head and neck cancer
	Brain tumors
	Colorectal cancer
	Melanoma

1. Differential Diagnosis

Benign versus malignant lesions. FDG PET has been used successfully as a noninvasive diagnostic test for solitary pulmonary nodules (SPN) in order to distinguish benign lesions from malignancies. A meta-analysis by Gould *et al.* (2001) of 40 studies that included 1474 SPNs has reported a sensitivity of 96.9% and specificity of 77.8% for detecting malignancy by PET. Studies by Matthies *et al.* (2002) and Zhuang *et al.* (2001a) have demonstrated the advantages of dual time point imaging in the differentiation of malignant from benign lesions. These authors concluded that malignant nodules have a greater tendency to show an increase in FDG uptake over time, whereas pulmonary nodules of benign origin have a decreasing pattern of uptake over time. FDG PET imaging makes it possible to calculate a specific uptake value that is called a "standardized uptake value" (SUV). A lesion with an SUV greater than 2.5 is considered to have a high probability of malignancy (Knight *et al.*, 1996; Lowe, 1997). Gambhir *et al.* (1998) suggested that biopsy or surgery of PET-positive lesions is also very cost-effective.

2. Cancer of Unknown Origin

Many authors have investigated the diagnostic contribution of PET in patients with unknown primary malignancies (Aassar *et al.*, 1999; Bohuslavizki *et al.*, 2000; Greven *et al.*, 1999; Kole, 1998; Lassen *et al.*, 1999). However, there are very few studies to date that have analyzed the impact of PET results on therapeutic management. Rades *et al.* (2001) detected the primary site in 18 of 42 patients who had localized cancer of unknown origin by using conventional staging procedures. PET was positive for disseminated diseases in 38% of patients. In 69% of patients, PET results influenced selection of the definitive treatment.

3. Diagnosis and Initial Staging

The impact of FDG PET on diagnosis and initial staging has been shown for various tumors. Many PET studies for lung cancer have included nonsmall cell lung cancer (NSLC) patients in whom the regional and distant involvement of disease can change staging and guide the therapeutic approach. Dwamena *et al.* (1999) performed a meta-analysis of staging lung cancer by PET and CT, and concluded that PET was significantly more accurate than CT. They reported a sensitivity and specificity of 79% and 91% for PET and 60% and 77% for CT, respectively. Pieterman (2000) reported sensitivity and specificity for the evaluation of mediastinal nodal involvement, which were 91% and 86% for PET and 75% and 66% for CT, respectively. A whole-body PET scan is able to detect more unknown distant metastases and is more accurate than conventional imaging in staging of patients with lung cancer, as shown by Pieterman (2000) and Laking and Price (2001). Gambhir *et al.* (1996) found PET to be cost-effective by avoiding surgeries that would not benefit the patient. Up to 20% of lung cancer patients are found to have an adrenal mass by CT, without necessarily confirming metastasis. It has been confirmed, however, that FDG PET can eliminate the need for a biopsy of enlarged adrenal glands in lung cancer patients (Bury *et al.*, 1999; Lamki, 1997).

PET also has high sensitivity for the preoperative diagnosis of colorectal carcinoma. However, it has no important role in early-stage patients because they require surgical diagnosis and staging. Abdel-Nabi *et al.* (1998) reported 100% sensitivity of PET imaging in the identification of all primary lesions in 48 patients. PET was found to be superior to CT for the identification of liver metastases, with a sensitivity and specificity of 88% and 100%, respectively, for PET and 38% and 97%, respectively, for CT.

The accuracy of PET is also better than CT-MRI and gallium scintigraphy in the staging of patients with lymphoma, as demonstrated by Sasaki *et al.* (2002) and Even-Sapir and Israel (2003). Moog *et al.* (1997) demonstrated 25 additional lesions using PET in 60 consecutive patients with Hodgkin's disease (HD) and non-Hodgkin's lymphoma (NHL), whereas CT found only six additional lesions, of which three were false positive. Stumpe *et al.* (1998) had a similar experience when the accuracy of FDG PET was compared to CT. There was no significant difference in the sensitivity of PET and CT. However, PET specificity was 96% for HD and 100% for NHL, whereas CT specificity was 41% for HD and 67% for NHL. Sasaki *et al.* (2002) showed a specificity of 99% for combined PET-CT, but sensitivity was 65% for CT alone and 92% for PET alone. These studies show that there is a large variation in sensitivity and specificity of CT, whereas these figures are not as variable for PET. Furthermore, PET results modified therapy in 25% of all lymphoma patients. In one study, 23% of patients were assigned a different stage by FDG PET imaging when compared with conventional imaging (Moog *et al.*, 1997; Partridge *et al.*, 2000; Schoder *et al.*, 2001).

The sensitivity of PET for primary breast cancer varies between 68% and 100% as reported by Bruce *et al.* (1995), Avril *et al.* (2001), and Schirrmeister *et al.* (2001). A study by Schirrmeister *et al.* (2001) showed that a whole-body FDG PET scan is as accurate as a panel of imaging modalities currently employed in detecting disease and is significantly more accurate in detecting multifocal disease, lymph node involvement, and distant metastasis. Metastasis to axillary lymph nodes is one of the most important prognostic factors in breast cancer patients. Kumar *et al.* (2003b) demonstrated that sentinel lymph node sampling has high accuracy even in multifocal and multicentric breast cancer.

The sensitivity of FDG PET in the detection of axillary lymph node metastasis varies from 79% to 100% (Crippa *et al.*, 1998; Greco *et al.*, 2001). However, PET can fail to detect micrometastases in lymph nodes because there are fewer cells, which may have a detectable increase in glucose metabolism.

4. Response to Treatment

FDG PET imaging is metabolically based and is, therefore, a more accurate method to differentiate tumor from scar tissue. CT and other conventional imaging use shrinkage in tumor size. It is often difficult to differentiate recurrence and posttreatment fibrotic masses using CT. Bury *et al.* (1999) demonstrated that PET was more sensitive and equally specific as compared to other imaging modalities for the detection of residual disease or recurrence after surgery or radiotherapy in lung cancer patients. Vitola *et al.* (1996) studied the effects of regional chemoembolization therapy in patients with colon cancer using FDG uptake as a criterion and found that decreased FDG uptake correlated with response, whereas the presence of residual uptake was used to guide further regional therapy. Findlay *et al.* (1996) concluded that PET was accurate for the differentiation of responders from nonresponders, both on lesion-by-lesion or patient-by-patient analysis.

Wahl *et al.* (1993) demonstrated that PET can detect metabolic changes in breast cancer as early as 8 days after the initiation of chemotherapy. Several studies were able to differentiate responders from nonresponders after the first course of therapy using FDG PET imaging (Bassa *et al.*, 1996; Jansson *et al.*, 1995; Schelling *et al.*, 2000). Smith *et al.* (2000) correctly identified responders with a sensitivity of 100% and a specificity of 85% after the first course of chemotherapy. Vranjesevic *et al.* (2002) compared PET and conventional imaging (CT-MRI-USG) to evaluate the response to chemotherapy in breast cancer patients. PET was more accurate than combined conventional imaging modalities, with positive and negative predictive values of 93% and 84%, respectively, for PET versus 85% and 59%, respectively, for conventional imaging modalities. The accuracy was 90% for FDG PET and 75% for conventional imaging modalities.

Jerusalem *et al.* (1999) compared the prognostic role of PET and CT after first-line treatment in 54 NHL-HD patients. PET showed higher diagnostic and prognostic values than CT (positive predictive value 100% vs. 42%).The 1-year progression-free survival (PFS) was 86% in PET-negative patients as compared to 0% in PET-positive patients. Spaepen *et al.* (2001) evaluated 60 patients with HD who had an FDG PET scan at the end of first-line treatment with or without residual mass. The 2-year disease-free survival (DFS) was 4% for the PET-positive compared to 85% for the PET-negative group. Kostakoglu *et al.* (2002) showed that FDG PET can predict a response to chemotherapy as early as after the first cycle of chemotherapy.

5. Recurrence/Restaging

Early surgical intervention or reintervention can cure a significant number of patients with recurrent cancer. The best example in this indication is the treatment of recurrent colorectal cancer. Usually, serial serum carcinoembryonic antigen (CEA) levels are used for recurrence monitoring, but when a high serum level of CEA is encountered, imaging will be necessary to localize the site of possible recurrence. Steele *et al.* (1991) demonstrated that CT is usually incapable of differentiating postsurgical changes from recurrence and that CT commonly misses hepatic and extrahepatic abdominal metastases. However, PET can be used to identify the metabolic characteristics of the lesions that are equivocal or undetected by CT. Valk *et al.* (1999) demonstrated that PET was found to be more sensitive than CT for all metastatic sites except the lung, where both modalities had equivalent sensitivities. They also reported that one-third of PET-positive lesions in the abdomen, pelvis, and retroperitoneum were negative on CT. PET can also differentiate postsurgical changes from recurrence. The accuracy of PET for detection of recurrence varies from 90% to 100%, whereas for CT it is 48–65%.

For patients with breast cancer, 35% will experience locoregional and distant metastases within 10 years of initial surgery, as was demonstrated by van Dongen *et al.* (2000). Gallowitsch *et al.* (2003) reported sensitivity, specificity, PPV, NPV, and accuracy of 97%, 82%, 87%, 96%, and 90%, respectively, for FDG PET and 84%, 60%, 73%, 75%, and 74%, respectively, for conventional imaging. On a lesion basis, significantly more lymph nodes (84 vs. 23) and fewer bone metastases (61 vs. 97) were detected using FDG as compared with conventional imaging. Kamel *et al.* (2003) analyzed the role of FDG PET for 60 patients and demonstrated that overall sensitivity, specificity, and accuracy were 89%, 84%, and 87%, respectively, for locoregional metastasis and 100%, 97%, and 98%, respectively, for distant metastasis. The authors also concluded that FDG PET was more sensitive than serum tumor marker CA 15–3 in detecting breast cancer relapse. Eubank *et al.* (2002) compared FDG PET and CT in 73 recurrent/metastatic breast cancer patients for evaluation of mediastinal and internal mammary lymph nodes metastases. In 33 patients amenable to follow-up CT or biopsy, FDG PET revealed a superior detection rate of 85% compared to CT (54%) (Eubank *et al.*, 2001).

Approximately two-thirds of patients with HD present with a mass lesion in the location of a previous tumor manifestation, but only about 20% of patients ultimately relapse (Canellos, 1988; Lowe and Wiseman, 2002). Similarly, in patients with high-grade NHL, 50% present with mass lesion and only 25% relapse (Hoskin, 2002). Gallium scintigraphy has proved useful in patients with recurrent disease, but has limitations in intraabdominal and low-grade lymphoma (Front *et al.*, 2000). Cremerius *et al.* (1999) reported a sensitivity of 88% and a specificity of 83% for the detection of residual disease by PET. The corresponding values for CT were 84% and 31%, respectively. A study by Mikosch *et al.* (2003) compared PET with CT-US in detecting recurrence and reported a sensitivity of 91%, a specificity of 81%, a PPV of 79%, a NPV of 92%, and an accuracy of 85%. For CT-US, these values were 88%, 35%, 48%, 81%, and 56%, respectively.

B. PET in Neurology

PET allows a noninvasive assessment of physiological, metabolic, and molecular processes of brain functions. PET may become the critical test for selecting the appropriate patients for treatment when the disease process is still at the molecular level. FDG and l-[methyle-11C]methionine (MET) are the most frequently used PET tracers for the evaluation of glucose and amino acid metabolism for various brain disorders. 6-[^{18}F]fluorol-dopa (F-DOPA) binds to dopamine transporter sites and allows for the assessment and imaging of presynaptic dopaminergic neurons.

1. Epilepsy

FDG PET is accepted as a useful and highly sensitive tool for the localization of epileptogenic zones. The sites of glucose hypometabolism at seizure foci as shown by FDG PET correlated strongly with epileptogenic zones at surgery. PET imaging has an accuracy of 85–90% in detecting epileptic focus as shown by Newberg *et al.* (2002), Moran *et al.* (2001), and Kobayashi *et al.* (2003) reported that long-standing seizure episodes eventually lead to significant atrophy, which can be detected by MRI. Therefore, accurate localization of seizure foci can be obtained using a combination of MRI and FDG PET. Kim *et al.* (2003) reported a sensitivity of 89% and a specificity of 91% for PET in the detection of epileptic foci in patients with temporal lobe epilepsy.

2. Alzheimer's Disease and Related Disorders

Alzheimer's disease (AD) is the most common cause of dementia in the elderly. PET imaging can differentiate AD from other forms of dementia. In patients with AD, there is a decrease in glucose metabolism in the temporoparietal lobes that is not evident in patients with other forms of dementia. The basal ganglia, thalamus, and primary sensorimotor cortex are spared in AD. Salmon *et al.* (1994)

demonstrated a sensitivity of 96% and 87% for PET in diagnosing moderate to severe and mild disease, respectively, in 129 cognitively impaired patients.

A new PET tracer, 2-(1-{6-[(2-[^{18}F]fluoroethyle) (methyl)amino]-2-naphthyl} ethylidene)malononitrile (^{18}F-FDDNP), has been developed to target amyloid saline plaques and neurofibrillary tangles in AD. This tracer shows prolonged retention in affected areas of the brain (Agdeppa *et al.*, 2001; Shoghi-Jadid *et al.*, 2002). According to several studies, other brain disorders, such as head injury, frontal lobe dementia, and Huntington's disease, can also be assessed with high accuracy using PET (Kuwert *et al.*, 1989; Mazziotta *et al.*, 1987; Montoya *et al.*, 2006; Newberg *et al.*, 2003; Silverman *et al.*, 2001).

3. Movement Disorders

Several radionuclide-labeled neuroreceptors and neurotransmitters have shown excellent results with PET (Davis *et al.*, 2002; Huang *et al.*, 2003; Vingerhoets *et al.*, 1996). These PET radiopharmaceuticals have great potential for the assessment of movement disorders. 2-Carbomethoxy-3-(4-chlorophenyl)-8-(2-^{18}F-fluoroethyl) nortropane (FECNT) and F-DOPA both allow assessment of the integrity of presynaptic dopaminergic neurons. These compounds are able to diagnose Parkinson's disease and other diseases effectively. Davis *et al.* (2002) demonstrated that FECNT is an excellent candidate as a radioligand for *in vivo* imaging of dopamine transporter density in healthy humans and subjects with Parkinson's disease.

C. PET in Cardiology

The detection of myocardial viability is the most important task of predicting functional recovery after medical or surgical interventions. Myocardial perfusion SPECT scintigraphy has a very high sensitivity, but has lower specificity for detection of viability as shown by Arnese *et al.* (1995), Pasquet *et al.* (1999), and Bax *et al.* (2002). PET is considered the "gold standard" for the detection of myocardial viability. Other indications of PET in cardiology include the evaluation of ischemic heart disease, cardiomyopathies, postcardiac transplant, and cardiac receptors for the regulation of cardiovascular functions.

1. Myocardial Viability

The extent of viable myocardium is an important factor for both prognosis and prediction of outcome after revascularization in patients with ischemic cardiomyopathy and chronic left ventricular dysfunction, as demonstrated by Tillisch *et al.* (1986), Tamaki *et al.* (1995), Pagano *et al.* (1998), and Pasquet *et al.* (1999). PET imaging shows metabolism in viable myocardial segments. Knuesel *et al.* (2003) concluded that most metabolically viable segments on PET imaging recover function after revascularization. ^{13}N ammonia is also being used for PET assessments of myocardial viability, but this compound has limitations due to its short half-life. Another PET tracer, rubidium-82, has shown good results in the detection of myocardial perfusion abnormalities (deKemp *et al.*, 2000; Yoshida *et al.*, 1996).

2. Cardiac Neurotransmission

Many pathophysiological processes take place in the nerve terminals, synaptic clefts, and postsynaptic sites in the heart. These processes are altered in many diseases such as heart failure, diabetic autonomic neuropathy, idiopathic ventricular tachycardia and arrhythmogenic right ventricular cardiomyopathy, heart transplantation, drug-induced cardiotoxicity, and dysautonomias (Dae *et al.*, 1995; Goldstein *et al.*, 1997; Lefroy *et al.*, 1993; Liggett *et al.*, 1998; Wichter *et al.*, 2000). Cardiac neurotransmission imaging can be obtained using PET. The most commonly used PET radiopharmaceuticals for imaging presynaptic activity are ^{18}F-fluorodopamine, ^{11}C-hydroxyphedrine, and ^{11}C-ephidrine. Postsynaptic agents include ^{11}C-(4-(3-*t*-butylamino-2-hydroxypropoxy)benzimidazol-1) CGP, and ^{11}C-carazolol.

D. PET in Infectious and Inflammatory Diseases

FDG has been used in the management of various cancers and in neurological and cardiological diseases (Bar-Shalom *et al.*, 2000; Bax *et al.*, 2000; Salanova *et al.*, 1999). Its ability to image glucose metabolism has been key to the success of PET in various disease settings. FDG PET has been used successfully in oncological imaging. However, FDG is not tumor or disease specific. Increased FDG uptake is seen in any tissue with increased glucose metabolism. Yamada *et al.* (1995) demonstrated that glucose metabolism is also increased in inflammatory tissues.

1. Osteomyelitis

FDG PET can be used for the diagnosis of acute or chronic osteomyelitis as studied by Pauwels *et al.* (2000). De Winter *et al.* (2001) demonstrated a sensitivity of 100%, a specificity of 85%, and an accuracy of 93% for this purpose. Zhuang *et al.* (2000) reported a sensitivity, a specificity, and an accuracy of 100%, 87.5%, and 91%, respectively, in 22 patients of suspected chronic osteomyelitis. Chianelli *et al.* (1997) demonstrated the advantage of FDG PET over labeled leukocyte imaging. Because glucose is smaller than antibodies and leukocytes, it can penetrate faster and more easily at the lesion site.

2. Prosthetic Joint Infections

To detect infection in a prosthetic joint is challenging, as there are no simple modalities for this purpose. Zhuang *et al.* (2001b) evaluated 74 prostheses with FDG PET in order to determine its role in this setting (38 hip and 36 knee prostheses). They reported a sensitivity of 91% and a specificity of 72% for detecting knee prosthesis infections and a sensitivity of 90% and a specificity of 89% for detecting hip prosthesis infections. However, Love *et al.* (2000) reported a very high sensitivity of 100% but a low specificity of 47% in 26 hip and knee prostheses.

3. Fever of Unknown Origin

Localization of an infective focus in patients with fever of unknown origin is a difficult task. Stumpe *et al.* (2000) demonstrated a sensitivity, specificity, and accuracy of 98%, 75%, and 91%, respectively, in patients of fever of unknown origin with suspected infections. On the bases of studies published by Sugawara *et al.* (1998), Meller *et al.* (2000), Blockmans *et al.* (2001), and Lorenzen *et al.* (2001). PET has greater capabilities than conventional imaging in screening 40–70% of patients with fever of unknown origin.

VI. Future Perspectives

PET imaging has the potential to detect almost any physiological, biochemical, and molecular process in the human body and in animals. PET can describe such processes in both normal and diseased tissues. PET can also be used to observe key steps in various disease processes, including carcinogenesis. This section discusses several of these processes, including angiogenesis, apoptosis, and hypoxia.

A. Assessment of Multidrug Resistance

One of the most common factors for chemotherapeutic failure is multidrug resistance (MDR) in cancer patients. Overexpression of P-glycoprotein (Pgp) is responsible for MDR in many tumors, as suggested by Gottesman and Pastan (1993) and Germann *et al.* (1993). Tc99m-labeled sestamibi, tetrofosmin, and furifosmin all act as substrates for Pgp and have been shown with SPECT imaging to predict tumors expressing MDR (Chen *et al.*, 1997). However, these techniques are limited by a lack of quantitative data. However, PET imaging using ^{11}C-verapamil, ^{11}C-daunorubicin, and ^{11}C-colchicine as *in vivo* Pgp probes has been investigated in experimental studies by Elsinga *et al.* (1996), Hendrikse *et al.* (1999), and Levchenko *et al.* (2000). Kurdziel *et al.* (2003) demonstrated that ^{18}F-paclitaxel (FPAC) uptake is an indicator of Pgp function in tissues from rhesus monkeys. These studies may have a potential role in the selection of patients in whom the modulation of Pgp may be beneficial before and during chemotherapy.

B. Quantitation of Angiogenesis

Angiogenesis is one of the most important steps in tumor development. PET imaging is transforming our understanding of angiogenesis and the evolution of drugs that stimulate or inhibit angiogenesis. PET tracers such as ^{11}C- or

^{18}F-labeled thymidine can be used to determine cellular proliferation rates, as demonstrated by Vander Borght *et al.* (1991), van Eijkeren *et al.* (1996), Barthel *et al.* (2002), and Wagner *et al.* (2003). Shields *et al.* (1998) have shown very promising results using 3-deoxy-3-[^{18}F]fluorothymidine (FLT) to detect cell proliferation. Accordingly, FLT may be more specific for the evaluation of response to chemotherapy, as cytotoxic agents affect cell division directly.

C. Tumor Hypoxia

Hypoxia in tumor cells is an important prognostic indicator of chemotherapy or radiation therapy outcome. Hypoxic cells are more resistant to treatment. Therefore, patients with hypoxia in particular tumors may be pretreated with drugs to enhance oxygenation in order to improve therapeutic response. Nitroimidazole-based compounds labeled with technetium-99m, iodine-123, and iodine-131 have been evaluated for this purpose with variable success rates (Ballinger *et al.*, 1996; Cherif *et al.*, 1996; Cook *et al.*, 1998; Linder, 1994). Valk *et al.* (1992) and Rasey (1996, 1999) demonstrated encouraging results in detecting tumor hypoxia using PET imaging with ^{18}F-fluoromisonidazole, although this compound has a relatively low uptake in hypoxic cells. Two newer ^{18}F-labeled compounds, ^{18}F-fluoroerythroimidazole, and ^{18}F-fluoroetanidazole, have overcome some of the nonoxygen-dependent metabolism seen with ^{18}F-fluoromisonidazole (Gronroos, 2001). Another ^{18}F-labeled compound, ^{18}F-EF 5, has shown good results in animal studies and may prove to be effective for noninvasive tumor hypoxia imaging (Ziemer *et al.*, 2003). ^{64}Cu-ATSM has been investigated to detect tumor hypoxia (Lewis, 1999). This compound is reduced in metabolically active mitochondria with oxygen-deficient electron transport chains.

D. Apoptosis

Detection of the process of cell death in both malignant and benign disorders by noninvasive imaging is another interesting area of study. All chemotherapeutic agents and radiation therapies induce programmed cell death in patients with malignant disease. Annexin V, an endogenous protein labeled with technetium-99m, has led the way to detect apoptosis as demonstrated by Blankenberg *et al.* (1999), Yang *et al.* (2001), and Blankenberg and Trauss (2001). The mechanism of Tc99m-annexin uptake is through its binding with phosphatidylserine, which is externalized in the cell membrane following apoptosis, as studied by Blankenberg *et al.* (1998). Labeling annexin V with ^{18}F may further increase the utility of this promising method and may provide greater insight into the therapeutic response in patients with cancer.

E. Gene Expression

Advances in molecular genetic imaging allow the visualization of cellular process in normal and abnormal cells. Current PET molecular imaging studies with radiolabeled probes use HSV1-tk as the reporter gene (Blakey *et al.*, 1995; Weissleder, 1999; Wunderbaldinger *et al.*, 2000).

Several PET tracers, which are analogs of uracil and thymidine, are being developed by Tjuvajev *et al.* (1998) and Gambhir *et al.* (1999). The details of the reporter gene technique are given elsewhere in this volume.

VII. Conclusions

PET is a powerful technique that provides noninvasive, quantitative, *in vivo* assessment of physiological and biological processes. Molecular imaging based on PET tracer kinetics has become a main source of information for both research purposes and patient management. In the near future, PET may become the critical modality both for diagnosing a variety of diseases and for selecting appropriate treatments when disease processes are still at the molecular level.

References

Aassar, O. S., Fischbein, N. J., Caputo, G. R., Kaplan, M. J., Price, D. C., Singer, M. I., Dillon, W. P., and Hawkins, R. A. (1999). Metastatic head and neck cancer: Role and usefulness of FDG PET in locating occult primary tumors. *Radiology* 210(1), 177–181.

Abdel-Nabi, H., Doerr, R. J., Lamonica, D. M., Cronin, V. R., Galantowicz, P. J., Carbone, G. M., and Spaulding, M. B. (1998). Staging of primary colorectal carcinomas with fluorine-18 fluorodeoxyglucose whole-body PET: Correlation with histopathologic and CT findings. *Radiology* 206(3), 755–760.

Aboagye, E. O. (2005). Development. *Mol. Imaging Biol.* 7(1), 53–58.

Agdeppa, E. D., Kepe, V., Liu, J., Flores-Torres, S., Satyamurthy, N., Petric, A., Cole, G. M., Small, G. W., Huang, S. C., and Barrio, J. R. (2001). Binding characteristics of radiofluorinated 6-dialkylamino-2-naphthylethylidene derivatives as positron emission tomography imaging probes for beta-amyloid plaques in Alzheimer's disease. *J. Neurosci.* 21(24), RC189.

Arnese, M., Cornel, J. H., Salustri, A., Maat, A., Elhendy, A., Reijs, A. E., Ten Cate, F. J., Keane, D., Balk, A. H, Roelandt, J. R., *et al.* (1995). Prediction of improvement of regional left ventricular function after surgical revascularization. A comparison of low-dose dobutamine echocardiography with 201Tl single-photon emission computed tomography. *Circulation* 91(11), 2748–2752.

Avril, N., Menzel, M., Dose, J., Schelling, M., Weber, W., Jänicke, F., Nathrath, W., and Schwaiger, M. (2001). Glucose metabolism of breast cancer assessed by 18F-FDG PET: Histologic and immunehistochemical tissue analysis. *J. Nucl. Med.* 42(1), 9–16.

Ballinger, J. R., Kee, J. W., and Rauth, A. M. (1996). *In vitro* and *in vivo* evaluation of a technetium-99m-labeled 2-nitroimidazole (BMS181321) as a marker of tumor hypoxia. *J. Nucl. Med.* 37(6), 1023–1031.

Bar-Shalom, R., Valdivia, A. Y., and Blaufox, M. D. (2000). PET imaging in oncology. *Semin. Nucl. Med.* 30(3), 150–185.

Barthel, H., Cleij, M. C., Collingridge, D. R., Hutchinson, O. C., Sman, S., Qimin, H. E., Luthra, S. K., Brady, F., Price, P. M., and Aboagye, E. O. (2003). 3′-Deoxy-3′-[^{18}F]fluorothymidine as a new marker for monitoring tumor response to antiproliferative therapy *in vivo* with positron emission tomography. *Cancer Res.* 63, 3791–3798.

Bassa, P., Kim, E. E., Inoue, T., Wong, F. C., Korkmaz, M., Yang, D. J., Wong, W. H., Hicks, K. W., Buzdar, A. U., and Podoloff, D. A. (1996). Evaluation of preoperative chemotherapy using PET with fluorine-18-fluorodeoxyglucose in breast cancer. *J. Nucl. Med.* 37(6), 931–938.

Bax, J. J., Patton, J. A., Poldermans, D., Elhendy, A., and Sandler, M. P. (2000). 18-Fluorodeoxyglucose imaging with positron emission tomography and single photon emission computed tomography: Cardiac applications. *Semin. Nucl. Med.* 30(4), 281–298.

Bax, J. J., Poldermans, D., Schinkel, A. F., Boersma, E., Elhendy, A., Maat, A., Valkema, R., Krenning, E. P., and Roelandt, J. R. (2002). Perfusion and contractile reserve in chronic dysfunctional myocardium: Relation to functional outcome after surgical revascularization. *Circulation* 106 (12 Suppl. 1), I14–I18.

Blakey, D. C., Burke, P. J., Davies, D. H., Dowell, R. I., Melton, R. G., Springer, C. J., and Wright, A. F. (1995). Antibody-directed enzyme prodrug therapy (ADEPT) for treatment of major solid tumour disease. *Biochem. Soc. Trans.* 23(4), 1047–1050.

Blankenberg, F. G., and Strauss, H. W. (2001). Will imaging of apoptosis play a role in clinical care? A tale of mice and men. *Apoptosis* 6(1-2), 117–123.

Blankenberg, F. G., Katsikis, P. D., Tait, J. F., Davis, R. E., Naumovski, L., Ohtsuki, K., Kopiwoda, S., Abrams, M. J., Darkes, M., Robbins, R. C., Maecker, H. T., and Strauss, H. W. (1998). *In vivo* detection and imaging of phosphatidylserine expression during programmed cell death. *Proc. Natl. Acad. Sci. USA* 95(11), 6349–6354.

Blankenberg, F. G., Katsikis, P. D., Tait, J. F., Davis, R. E., Naumovski, L., Ohtsuki, K., Kopiwoda, S., Abrams, M. J., and Strauss, H. W. (1999). Imaging of apoptosis (programmed cell death) with 99mTc annexin V. *J. Nucl. Med.* 40(1), 184–191.

Blasberg, R. G., Roelcke, U., Weinreich, R., Beattie, B., von Ammon, K., Yonekawa, Y., Landolt, H., Guenther, I., Crompton, N. E., Vontobel, P., Missimer, J., Maguire, R. P., *et al.* (2000). Imaging brain tumor proliferative activity with [124I]iododeoxyuridine. *Cancer Res.* 60(3), 624–635.

Blockmans, D., Knockaert, D., Maes, A., De Caestecker, J., Stroobants, S., Bobbaers, H., and Mortelmans, L. (2001). Clinical value of [(18)F]fluoro-deoxyglucose positron emission tomography for patients with fever of unknown origin. *Clin. Infect. Dis.* 32(2), 191–196.

Bohuslavizki, K. H., Klutmann, S., Kröger, S., Sonnemann, U., Buchert, R., Werner, J. A., Mester, J., and Clausen, M. (2000). FDG PET detection of unknown primary tumors. *J. Nucl. Med.* 41(5), 816–822.

Bruce, D. M., Evans, N. T., Heys, S. D., Needham, G., BenYounes, H., Mikecz, P., Smith, F. W., Sharp, F., and Eremin, O. (1995). Positron emission tomography: 2-deoxy-2-[18F]-fluoro-D-glucose uptake in locally advanced breast cancers. *Eur. J. Surg. Oncol.* 21(3), 280–283.

Bury, T., Corhay, J. L., Duysinx, B., Daenen, F., Ghaye, B., Barthelemy, N., Rigo, P., and Bartsch, P. (1999). Value of FDG-PET in detecting residual or recurrent nonsmall cell lung cancer. *Eur. Respir. J.* 14(6), 1376–1380.

Canellos, G. P. (1988). Residual mass in lymphoma may not be residual disease. *J. Clin. Oncol.* 6(6), 931–933.

Chen, C. C., Meadows, B., Regis, J., Kalafsky, G., Fojo, T., Carrasquillo, J. A., and Bates, S. E. (1997). Detection of *in vivo* P-glycoprotein inhibition by PSC 833 using Tc-99m sestamibi. *Clin. Cancer Res.* 3(4), 545–552.

Cherif, A., Wallace, S., Yang, D. J., Newman, R. A., Harrod, V. L., Nornoo, A., Inoue, T., Kim, C. G., Kuang, L. R., Kim, E. E., and Podoloff, D. A. (1996). Development of new markers for hypoxic cells: [131I]Iodomisonidazole and [131I]Iodoerythronitroimidazole. *J. Drug Target* 4(1), 31–39.

Chianelli, M., Mather, S. J., Martin-Comin, J., and Signore, A. (1997). Radiopharmaceuticals for the study of inflammatory processes: A review. *Nucl. Med. Commun.* 18(5), 437–455.

Cook, G. J., Houston, S., Barrington, S. F., and Fogelman, I. (1998). Technetium-99m-labeled HL91 to identify tumor hypoxia: Correlation with fluorine-18-FDG. *J. Nucl. Med.* 39(1), 99–103.

Cremerius, U., Fabry, U., Kröll, U., Zimny, M., Neuerburg, J., Osieka, R., and Büll, U. (1999). Clinical value of FDG PET for therapy monitoring of malignant lymphoma—results of a retrospective study in 72 patients. *Nuklearmedizin* 38(1), 24–30.

Crippa, F., Agresti, R., Seregni, E., Greco, M., Pascali, C., Bogni, A., Chiesa, C., De Sanctis, V., Delledonne, V., Salvadori, B., Leutner, M., and Bombardieri, E. (1998). Prospective evaluation of fluorine-18-FDG PET in presurgical staging of the axilla in breast cancer. *J. Nucl. Med.* 39(1), 4–8.

Dae, M. W., O'Connell, J. W., Botvinick, E. H., and Chin, M. C. (1995). Acute and chronic effects of transient myocardial ischemia on sympathetic nerve activity, density, and norepinephrine content. *Cardiovasc. Res.* 30(2), 270–280.

Davis, M. R., Votaw, J. R., Bremner, J. D., Byas-Smith, M. G., Faber, T. L., Voll, R. J., Hoffman, J. M., Grafton, S. T., Kilts, C. D., and Goodman, M. M. (2003). Initial human PET imaging studies with the dopamine transporter ligand ^{18}F-FECNT. *J. Nucl. Med.* 44, 855–861.

DeKemp, R. A., Ruddy, T. D., Hewitt, T., Dalipaj, M. M., and Beanlands, R. S. (2000). Detection of serial changes in absolute myocardial perfusion with 82Rb PET. *J. Nucl. Med.* 41(8), 1426–1435.

Del Guerra, A., and Belcari, N. (2002). Advances in animal PET scanners. *Q. J. Nucl. Med.* 46(1), 35–47.

De Winter, F., van de Wiele, C., Vogelaers, D., de Smet, K., Verdonk, R., and Dierckx, R. A. (2001). Fluorine-18 fluorodeoxyglucose-position emission tomography: A highly accurate imaging modality for the diagnosis of chronic musculoskeletal infections. *J. Bone Joint Surg. Am.* 83-A(5), 651–660.

Dwamena, B. A., Sonnad, S. S., Angobaldo, J. O., and Wahl, R. L. (1999). Metastases from non-small cell lung cancer: Mediastinal staging in the 1990s—meta-analytic comparison of PET and CT. *Radiology* 213(2), 530–536.

Elsinga, P. H., Franssen, E. J., Hendrikse, N. H., Fluks, L., Weemaes, A. M., van der Graaf, W. T., de Vries, E. G., Visser, G. M., and Vaalburg, W. (1996). Carbon-11-labeled daunorubicin and verapamil for probing P-glycoprotein in tumors with PET. *J. Nucl. Med.* 37(9), 1571–1575.

Eubank, W. B., Mankoff, D. A., Takasugi, J., Vesselle, H., Eary, J. F., Shanley, T. J., Gralow, J. R., Charlop, A., Ellis, G. K., Lindsley, K. L., Austin-Seymour, M. M. Funkhouser, C. P., *et al.* (2001). 18fluorodeoxyglucose positron emission tomography to detect mediastinal or internal mammary metastases in breast cancer. *J. Clin. Oncol.* 19(15), 3516–3523.

Eubank, W. B., Mankoff, D. A., Vesselle, H. J., Eary, J. F., Schubert, E. K., Dunnwald, L. K., Lindsley, S. K., Gralow, J. R., Austin-Seymour, M. M., Ellis, G. K., and Livingston, R. B.(2002). Detection of locoregional and distant recurrences in breast cancer patients by using FDG PET. *Radiographics* 22(1), 5–17.

Even-Sapir, E, and Israel, O. (2003). Gallium-67 scintigraphy: A cornerstone in functional imaging of lymphoma. *Eur. J. Nucl. Med. Mol. Imaging* 30(Suppl. 1), S65–S81.

Findlay, M., Young, H., Cunningham, D., Iveson, A., Cronin, B., Hickish, T., Pratt, B., Husband, J., Flower, M., and Ott, R. (1996). Noninvasive monitoring of tumor metabolism using fluorodeoxyglucose and positron emission tomography in colorectal cancer liver metastases: Correlation with tumor response to fluorouracil. *J. Clin. Oncol.* 14(3), 700–708.

Front, D., Bar-Shalom, R., Mor, M., Haim, N., Epelbaum, R., Frenkel, A., Gaitini, D., Kolodny, G. M., and Israel, O. (2000). Aggressive non-Hodgkin lymphoma: Early prediction of outcome with 67Ga scintigraphy. *Radiology* 214(1), 253–257.

Gallowitsch, H. J., Kresnik, E., Gasser, J., Kumnig, G., Igerc, I., Mikosch, P., and Lind, P. (2003). F-18 fluorodeoxyglucose positron-emission tomography in the diagnosis of tumor recurrence and metastases in the follow-up of patients with breast carcinoma: A comparison to conventional imaging. *Invest. Radiol.* 38(5), 250–256.

Gambhir, S. S., Hoh, C. K., Phelps, M. E., Madar, I., and Maddahi, J. (1996). Decision tree sensitivity analysis for cost-effectiveness of FDG-PET in the staging and management of non-small-cell lung carcinoma. *J. Nucl. Med.* 37(9), 1428–1436.

Gambhir, S. S., Shepherd, J. E., Shah, B. D., Hart, E., Hoh, C. K., Valk, P. E., Emi, T., and Phelps, M. E. (1998). Analytical decision model for the cost-effective management of solitary pulmonary nodules. *J. Clin. Oncol.* 16(6), 2113–2125.

Gambhir, S. S., Barrio, J. R., Phelps, M. E., Iyer, M., Namavari, M., Satyamurthy, N., Wu, L., Green, L. A., Bauer, E., MacLaren, D. C., Nguyen, K., Berk, A. J., *et al.* (1999). Imaging adenoviral-directed reporter gene expression in living animals with positron emission tomography. *Proc. Natl. Acad. Sci. USA* 96(5), 2333–2338.

Gangloff, A., Hsueh, W. A., Kesner, A. L., Kiesewetter, D. O., Pio, B. S., Pegram, M. D., Beryt, M., Townsend, A., Czernin, J., Phelps, M. E., and Silverman, D. H. (2005). Estimation of paclitaxel biodistribution and uptake in human-derived xenografts *in vivo* with (18)F-fluoropaclitaxel. *J. Nucl. Med.* 46(11), 1866–1871.

Germann, U. A., Pastan, I., and Gottesman, M. M. (1993). P-glycoproteins: Mediators of multidrug resistance. *Semin. Cell Biol.* 4(1), 63–76.

Goldstein, D. S., Holmes, C., Cannon, R. O., 3rd, Eisenhofer, G., and Kopin, I. J. (1997). Sympathetic cardioneuropathy in dysautonomias. *N. Engl. J. Med.* 336(10), 696–702.

Gottesman, M. M., and Pastan, I. (1993). Biochemistry of multidrug resistance mediated by the multidrug transporter. *Annu. Rev. Biochem.* 62, 385–427.

Gould, M. K., Maclean, C. C., Kuschner, W. G., Rydzak, C. E., and Owens, D. K. (2001). Accuracy of positron emission tomography for diagnosis of pulmonary nodules and mass lesions: A meta-analysis. *JAMA* 285(7), 914–924.

Greco, M., Crippa, F., Agresti, R., Seregni, E., Gerali, A., Giovanazzi, R., Micheli, A., Asero, S., Ferraris, C., Gennaro, M., Bombardieri, E., and Cascinelli, N. (2001). Axillary lymph node staging in breast cancer by 2-fluoro-2-deoxy-D-glucose-positron emission tomography: Clinical evaluation and alternative management. *J. Natl. Cancer Inst.* 93(8), 630–635.

Greven, K. M., Keyes, J. W., Jr., Williams, D. W., 3rd, McGuirt, W. F., and Joyce, W. T. (1999). Occult primary tumors of the head and neck: Lack of benefit from positron emission tomography imaging with 2-[F-18]fluoro-2-deoxy-D-glucose. *3rd. Cancer* 86(1), 114–118.

Grönroos, T., Eskola, O., Lehtiö, K., Minn, H., Marjamäki, P., Bergman, J., Haaparanta, M., Forsback, S., and Solin, O. (2001). Pharmacokinetics of [18F]FETNIM: A potential marker for PET. *J. Nucl. Med.* 42(9), 1397–1404.

Gupta, N., Price, P. M., and Aboagye, E. O. (2002). PET for *in vivo* pharmacokinetic and pharmacodynamic measurements. *Eur. J. Cancer* 38(16), 2094–2107.

Hendrikse, N. H., Franssen, E. J., van der Graaf, W. T., Vaalburg, W., and de Vries, E. G. (1999). Visualization of multidrug resistance *in vivo*. *Eur. J. Nucl. Med.* 26(3), 283–293.

Hoskin, P. J. (2002). FDG PET in the management of lymphoma: A clinical perspective. *Eur. J. Nucl. Med. Mol. Imaging* 29(4), 449–451.

Huang, W. S., Chiang, Y. H., Lin, J. C., Chou, Y. H., Cheng, C. Y., and Liu, R. S. (2003). Crossover study of (99m)Tc-TRODAT-1 SPECT and (18)F-FDOPA PET in Parkinson's disease patients. *J. Nucl. Med.* 44(7), 999–1005.

Inubushi, M., Wu, J. C., Gambhir, S. S., Sundaresan, G., Satyamurthy, N., Namavari, M., Yee, S., Barrio, J. R., Stout, D., Chatziioannou, A. F., Wu, L., and Schelbert, H. R., *et al.* (2003). Positron-emission tomography reporter gene expression imaging in rat myocardium. *Circulation* 107(2), 326–332.

Jansson, T., Westlin, J. E., Ahlström, H., Lilja, A., Långström, B., and Bergh, J. (1995). Positron emission tomography studies in patients with locally advanced and/or metastatic breast cancer: A method for early therapy evaluation? *J. Clin. Oncol.* 13(6), 1470–1477.

Jerusalem, G., Beguin, Y., Fassotte, M. F., Najjar, F., Paulus, P., Rigo, P., and Fillet, G. (1999). Whole-body positron emission tomography using 18F-fluorodeoxyglucose for posttreatment evaluation in Hodgkin's disease and non-Hodgkin's lymphoma has higher diagnostic and prognostic value than classical computed tomography scan imaging. *Blood* 94(2), 429–433.

Kamel, E. M., Wyss, M. T., Fehr, M. K., von Schulthess, G. K., and Goerres, G. W. (2003). [18F]-Fluorodeoxyglucose positron emission tomography in patients with suspected recurrence of breast cancer. *J. Cancer Res. Clin. Oncol.* 129(3), 147–153.

Kim, Y. K., Lee, D. S., Lee, S. K., Kim, S. K., Chung, C. K., Chang, K. H., Choi, K. Y., Chung, J. K., and Lee, M. C. (2003). Differential features of metabolic abnormalities between medial and lateral temporal lobe epilepsy: Quantitative analysis of (18)F-FDG PET using SPM. *J. Nucl. Med.* 44(7), 1006–1012.

Kim, J. S., Lee, J. S., Im, K. C., Kim, S. J., Kim, S. Y., Lee, D. S., and Moon, D. H. (2007). Performance measurement of the micropet focus 120 scanner. *J. Nucl. Med.* 48(9), 1527–1535.

Knight, S. B., Delbeke, D., Stewart, J. R., and Sandler, M. P. (1996). Evaluation of pulmonary lesions with FDG-PET. Comparison of findings in patients with and without a history of prior malignancy. *Chest* 109(4), 982–988.

Knuesel, P. R., Nanz, D., Wyss, C., Buechi, M., Kaufmann, P. A., von Schulthess, G. K., Lüscher, T. F., and Schwitter, J. (2003). Characterization of dysfunctional myocardium by positron emission tomography and magnetic resonance: Relation to functional outcome after revascularization. *Circulation* 108(9), 1095–1100.

Kobayashi, E., D'Agostino, M. D., Lopes-Cendes, I., Berkovic, S. F., Li, M. L., Andermann, E., Andermann, F., and Cendes, F. (2003). Hippocampal atrophy and T2-weighted signal changes in familial mesial temporal lobe epilepsy. *Neurology* 60(3), 405–409.

Kole, A. C., Nieweg, O. E., Pruim, J., Hoekstra, H. J., Koops, H. S., Roodenburg, J. L., Vaalburg, W., and Vermey, A. (1998). Detection of unknown occult primary tumors using positron emission tomography. *Cancer* 82(6), 1160–1166.

Kostakoglu, L., Coleman, M., Leonard, J. P., Kuji, I., Zoe, H., and Goldsmith, S. J. (2002). PET predicts prognosis after 1 cycle of chemotherapy in aggressive lymphoma and Hodgkin's disease. *J. Nucl. Med.* 43(8), 1018–1027.

Kumar, R., Bhargava, P., Bozkurt, M. F., Zhuang, H., Potenta, S., and Alavi, A. (2003a). Positron emission tomography imaging in evaluation of cancer patients. *Indian J. Cancer* 40(3), 87–100.

Kumar, R., Jana, S., Heiba, S. I., Dakhel, M., Axelrod, D., Siegel, B., Bernik, S., Mills, C., Wallack, M., and Abdel-Dayem, H. M. (2003b). Retrospective analysis of sentinel node localization in multifocal, multicentric, palpable, or nonpalpable breast cancer. *J. Nucl. Med.* 44(1), 7–10.

Kurdziel, K. A., Kiesewetter, D. O., Carson, R. E., Eckelman, W. C., and Herscovitch, P. (2003). Biodistribution, radiation dose estimates, and *in vivo* Pgp modulation studies of 18F-paclitaxel in nonhuman primates. *J. Nucl. Med.* 44(8), 1330–1339.

Laking, G., and Price, P. (2001). 18-Fluorodeoxyglucose positron emission tomography (FDG-PET) and the staging of early lung cancer. *Thorax* 56(Suppl. 2), ii38–ii44.

Lamki, L. M. (1997). Positron emission tomography, bronchogenic carcinoma, and the adrenals. *AJR Am. J. Roentgenol.* 168(5), 1361–1362.

Lassen, U., Daugaard, G., Eigtved, A., Damgaard, K., and Friberg, L. (1999). 18F-FDG whole body positron emission tomography (PET) in patients with unknown primary tumours (UPT). *Eur. J. Cancer* 35(7), 1076–1082.

Lefroy, D. C., de Silva, R., Choudhury, L., Uren, N. G., Crake, T., Rhodes, C. G., Lammertsma, A. A., Boyd, H., Patsalos, P. N., Nihoyannopoulos, P., *et al.* (1993). Diffuse reduction of myocardial beta-adrenoceptors in hypertrophic cardiomyopathy: A study with positron emission tomography. *J. Am. Coll. Cardiol.* 22(6), 1653–1660.

Levchenko, A., Mehta, B. M., Lee, J. B., Humm, J. L., Augensen, F., Squire, O., Kothari, P. J., Finn, R. D., Leonard, E. F., and Larson, S. M. (2000). Evaluation of 11C-colchicine for PET imaging of multiple drug resistance. *J. Nucl. Med.* 41(3), 493–501.

Lewis, J. S., McCarthy, D. W., McCarthy, T. J., Fujibayashi, Y., and Welch, M. J. (1999). Evaluation of 64Cu-ATSM *in vitro* and *in vivo* in a hypoxic tumor model. *J. Nucl. Med.* 40(1), 177–183.

Liggett, S. B., Wagoner, L. E., Craft, L. L., Hornung, R. W., Hoit, B. D., McIntosh, T. C., and Walsh, R. A. (1998). The Ile164 beta2-adrenergic receptor polymorphism adversely affects the outcome of congestive heart failure. *J. Clin. Invest.* 102(8), 1534–1539.

Linder, K. E., Chan, Y. W., Cyr, J. E., Malley, M. F., Nowotnik, D. P., and Nunn, A. D. (1994). TcO (PnA-O-1-(2-nitroimidazole)) [BMS-181321], a new technetium-containing nitroimidazole complex for imaging hypoxia: Synthesis, characterization, and xanthine oxidase-catalyzed reduction. *J. Med. Chem.* 37(1), 9–17.

Lorenzen, J., Buchert, R., Bohuslavizki, K. H. (2001). Value of FDG PET in patients with fever of unknown origin. *Nucl. Med. Commun.* 22(7), 779–783.

Love, C., Pugliese, P. V., Afriyie, M. O., Tomas, M. B., Marwin, S. E., and Palestro, C. J. (2000). Utility of F-18 FDG imaging for diagnosing the infected joint replacement. *Clin. Positron Imaging* 3(4), 159.

Lowe, V. J., and Wiseman, G. A. (2002). Assessment of lymphoma therapy using (18)F-FDG PET. *J. Nucl. Med.* 43(8), 1028–1030.

Lowe, V. J., Duhaylongsod, F. G., Patz, E. F., Delong, D. M., Hoffman, J. M., Wolfe, W. G., and Coleman, R. E. (1997). Pulmonary abnormalities and PET data analysis: A retrospective study. *Radiology* 202(2), 435–439.

Matthies, A., Hickeson, M., Cuchiara, A., and Alavi, A. (2002). Dual time point 18F-FDG PET for the evaluation of pulmonary nodules. *J. Nucl. Med.* 43(7), 871–875.

Mazziotta, J. C., Phelps, M. E., Pahl, J. J., Huang, S. C., Baxter, L. R., Riege, W. H., Hoffman, J. M., Kuhl, D. E., Lanto, A. B., Wapenski, J. A., *et al.* (1987). Reduced cerebral glucose metabolism in asymptomatic subjects at risk for Huntington's disease. *N. Engl. J. Med.* 316(7), 357–362.

McGowan, K. M., Long, S. D., and Pekala, P. H. (1995). Glucose transporter gene expression: Regulation of transcription and mRNA stability. *Pharmacol. Ther.* 66(3), 465–505.

Meller, J., Altenvoerde, G., Munzel, U., Jauho, A., Behe, M., Gratz, S., Luig, H., and Becker, W. (2000). Fever of unknown origin: Prospective comparison of [18F]FDG imaging with a double-head coincidence camera and gallium-67 citrate SPET. *Eur. J. Nucl. Med.* 27(11), 1617–1625.

Mikosch, P., Gallowitsch, H. J., Zinke-Cerwenka, W., Heinisch, M., Pipam, W., Eibl, M., Kresnik, E., Unterweger, O., Linkesch, W., and Lind, P. (2003). Accuracy of whole-body 18F-FDP-PET for restaging malignant lymphoma. *Acta Med. Austriaca* 30(2), 41–47.

Mintun, M. A., Welch, M. J., Siegel, B. A., Mathias, C. J., Brodack, J. W., McGuire, A. H., and Katzenellenbogen, J. A. (1988). Breast cancer: PET imaging of estrogen receptors. *Radiology* 169(1), 45–48.

Montoya, A., Price, B. H., Menear, M., and Lepage, M. (2006). Brain imaging and cognitive dysfunctions in Huntington's disease. *J. Psychiatry Neurosci.* 31(1), 21–29.

Moog, F., Bangerter, M., Diederichs, C. G., Guhlmann, A., Kotzerke, J., Merkle, E., Kolokythas, O., Herrmann, F., and Reske, S. N. (1997). Lymphoma: Role of whole-body 2-deoxy-2-[F-18]fluoro-D-glucose (FDG) PET in nodal staging. *Radiology* 203(3), 795–800.

Moran, N. F., Lemieux, L., Kitchen, N. D., Fish, D. R., and Shorvon, S. D. (2001). Extrahippocampal temporal lobe atrophy in temporal lobe epilepsy and mesial temporal sclerosis. *Brain* 124(Pt. 1), 167–175.

Newberg, A. B., and Alavi, A. (2003). Neuro imaging in patients with head injury. *Semin. Nucl. Med.* 33(2), 136–147.

Newberg, A., Alavi, A., and Reivich, M. (2002). Determination of regional cerebral function with FDG-PET imaging in neuropsychiatric disorders. *Semin. Nucl. Med.* 32(1), 13–34.

Pagano, D., Townend, J. N., Littler, W. A., Horton, R., Camici, P. G., and Bonser, R. S. (1998). Coronary artery bypass surgery as treatment for ischemic heart failure: The predictive value of viability assessment with quantitative positron emission tomography for symptomatic and functional outcome. *J. Thorac. Cardiovasc. Surg.* 115(4), 791–799.

Partridge, S., Timothy, A., O'Doherty, M. J., Hain, S. F., Rankin, S., and Mikhaeel, G. (2000). 2-Fluorine-18-fluoro-2-deoxy-D glucose positron emission tomography in the pretreatment staging of Hodgkin's disease: Influence on patient management in a single institution. *Ann. Oncol.* 11(10), 1273–1279.

Pasquet, A., Robert, A., D'Hondt, A. M., Dion, R., Melin, J. A., and Vanoverschelde, J. L. (1999). Prognostic value of myocardial ischemia and viability in patients with chronic left ventricular ischemic dysfunction. *Circulation* 100(2), 141–148.

Patel, M. K., Factor, S. M., Wang, J., Jana, S., and Strauch, B. (2006). Limited myocardial muscle necrosis model allowing for evaluation of angiogenic treatment modalities. *J. Reconstr. Microsurg.* 22(8), 611–615.

Pauwels, E. K., Sturm, E. J., Bombardieri, E., Cleton, F. J., and Stokkel, M. P. (2000). Positron-emission tomography with [18F]fluorodeoxyglucose. Part I. Biochemical uptake mechanism and its implication for clinical studies. *J. Cancer Res. Clin. Oncol.* 126(10), 549–559.

Pieterman, R. M., van Putten, J. W., Meuzelaar, J. J., Mooyaart, E. L., Vaalburg, W., Koëter, G. H., Fidler, V., Pruim, J., and Groen, H. J. (2000). Preoperative staging of non-small-cell lung cancer with positron-emission tomography. *N. Engl. J. Med.* 343(4), 254–261.

Rades, D., Kühnel, G., Wildfang, I., Börner, A. R., Schmoll, H. J., and Knapp, W. (2001). Localised disease in cancer of unknown primary (CUP): The value of positron emission tomography (PET) for individual therapeutic management. *Ann. Oncol.* 12(11), 1605–1609.

Rasey, J. S., Koh, W. J., Evans, M. L., Peterson, L. M., Lewellen, T. K., Graham, M. M., and Krohn, K. A. (1996). Quantifying regional hypoxia in human tumors with positron emission tomography of [18F]fluoromisonidazole: A pretherapy study of 37 patients. *Int. J. Radiat. Oncol. Biol. Phys.* 36(2), 417–428.

Rasey, J. S., Hofstrand, P. D., Chin, L. K., and Tewson, T. J. (1999). Characterization of [18F] fluoroetanidazole, a new radiopharmaceutical for detecting tumor hypoxia. *J. Nucl. Med.* 40(6), 1072–1079.

Ray, P., Tsien, R., and Gambhir, S. S. (2007). Construction and validation of improved triple fusion reporter gene vectors for molecular imaging of living subjects. *Cancer Res.* 67(7), 3085–3093.

Salanova, V., Markand, O., and Worth, R. (1999). Longitudinal follow-up in 145 patients with medically refractory temporal lobe epilepsy treated surgically between 1984 and 1995. *Epilepsia* 40(10), 1417–1423.

Salem, A., Yap, J., Osman, S., Brady, F., Lucas, S. V., Jones, T., Price, P. M., and Aboagye, E. O. (2000). Modulation of fluorouracil tissue pharmacokinetics by eniluracil: *In-vivo* imaging of drug action. *Lancet* 355(9221), 2119–2124.

Salmon, E., Sadzot, B., Maquet, P., Degueldre, C., Lemaire, C., Rigo, P., Comar, D., and Franck, G. (1994). Differential diagnosis of Alzheimer's disease with PET. *J. Nucl. Med.* 35(3), 391–398.

Sasaki, M., Kuwabara, Y., Koga, H., Nakagawa, M., Chen, T., Kaneko, K., Hayashi, K., Nakamura, K., and Masuda, K. (2002). Clinical impact of whole body FDG-PET on the staging and therapeutic decision making for malignant lymphoma. *Ann. Nucl. Med.* 16(5), 337–345.

Schelling, M., Avril, N., Nährig, J., Kuhn, W., Römer, W., Sattler, D., Werner, M., Dose, J., Jänicke, F., Graeff, H., and Schwaiger, M. (2000). Positron emission tomography using [(18)F]fluorodeoxyglucose for monitoring primary chemotherapy in breast cancer. *J. Clin. Oncol.* 18(8), 1689–1695.

Schirmer, M., Calamia, K. T., Wenger, M., Klauser, A., Salvarani, C., and Moncayo, R. (2003). 18F-fluorodeoxyglucose-positron emission tomography: A new explorative perspective. *Exp. Gerontol.* 38(4), 463–470.

Schirrmeister, H., Kühn, T., Guhlmann, A., Santjohanser, C., Hörster, T., Nüssle, K., Koretz, K., Glatting, G., Rieber, A., Kreienberg, R., Buck, A. C., and Reske, S. N., *et al.* (2001). Fluorine-18 2-deoxy-2-fluoro-D-glucose PET in the preoperative staging of breast cancer: Comparison with the standard staging procedures. *Eur. J. Nucl. Med.* 28(3), 351–358.

Schöder, H., Meta, J., Yap, C., Ariannejad, M., Rao, J., Phelps, M. E., Valk, P. E., Sayre, J., and Czernin, J. (2001). Effect of whole-body (18)F-FDG PET imaging on clinical staging and management of patients with malignant lymphoma. *J. Nucl. Med.* 42(8), 1139–1143.

Shields, A. F., Grierson, J. R., Dohmen, B. M., Machulla, H. J., Stayanoff, J. C., Lawhorn-Crews, J. M., Obradovich, J. E., Muzik, O., and Mangner, T. J. (1998). Imaging proliferation in vivo with [F-18]FLT and positron emission tomography. *Nat. Med.* 4(11), 1334–1336.

Shoghi-Jadid, K., Small, G. W., Agdeppa, E. D., Kepe, V., Ercoli, L. M., Siddarth, P., Read, S., Satyamurthy, N., Petric, A., Huang, S. C., and Barrio, J. R. (2002). Localization of neurofibrillary tangles and beta-amyloid plaques in the brains of living patients with Alzheimer disease. *Am. J. Geriatr. Psychiatry* 10(1), 24–35.

Silverman, D. H., Small, G. W., Chang, C. Y., Lu, C. S., Kung De Aburto, M. A., Chen, W., Czernin, J., Rapoport, S. I., Pietrini, P., Alexander, G. E., Schapiro, M. B., Jagust, W. J., *et al.* (2001). Positron emission tomography in evaluation of dementia: Regional brain metabolism and long-term outcome. *JAMA* 286(17), 2120–2127.

Smith, I. C., Welch, A. E., Hutcheon, A. W., Miller, I. D., Payne, S., Chilcott, F., Waikar, S., Whitaker, T., Ah-See, A. K., Eremin, O., Heys, S. D., Gilbert, F. J., *et al.* (2000). Positron emission tomography using [(18)F]-fluorodeoxy-D-glucose to predict the pathologic response of breast cancer to primary chemotherapy. *J. Clin. Oncol.* 18(8), 1676–1688.

Sossi, V., and Ruth, T. J. (2005). Micropet imaging: *In vivo* biochemistry in small animals. *J. Neural. Transm.* 112(3), 319–330.

Spaepen, K., Stroobants, S., Dupont, P., Thomas, J., Vandenberghe, P., Balzarini, J., De Wolf-Peeters, C., Mortelmans, L., and Verhoef, G. (2001). Can positron emission tomography with [(18)F]-fluorodeoxyglucose after first-line treatment distinguish Hodgkin's disease patients who need additional therapy from others in whom additional therapy would mean avoidable toxicity? *Br. J. Haematol.* 115(2), 272–278.

Steele, G., Jr., Bleday, R., Mayer, R. J., Lindblad, A., Petrelli, N., and Weaver, D. A. (1991). Prospective evaluation of hepatic resection for colorectal carcinoma metastases to the liver: Gastrointestinal tumor study group protocol 6584. *J. Clin. Oncol.* 9(7), 1105–1112.

Stumpe, K. D., Urbinelli, M., Steinert, H. C., Glanzmann, C., Buck, A., and von Schulthess, G. K. (1998). Whole-body positron emission tomography using fluorodeoxyglucose for staging of lymphoma: Effectiveness and comparison with computed tomography. *Eur. J. Nucl. Med.* 25(7), 721–728.

Stumpe, K. D., Dazzi, H., Schaffner, A., and von Schulthess, G. K. (2000). Infection imaging using whole-body FDG-PET. *Eur. J. Nucl. Med.* 27(7), 822–832.

Sugawara, Y., Braun, D. K., Kison, P. V., Russo, J. E., Zasadny, K. R., and Wahl, R. L. (1998). Rapid detection of human infections with fluorine-18 fluorodeoxyglucose and positron emission tomography: Preliminary results. *Eur. J. Nucl. Med.* 25(9), 1238–1243.

Tamaki, N., Kawamoto, M., Tadamura, E., Magata, Y., Yonekura, Y., Nohara, R., Sasayama, S., Nishimura, K., Ban, T., and Konishi, J. (1995). Prediction of reversible ischemia after revascularization. Perfusion and metabolic studies with positron emission tomography. *Circulation* 91(6), 1697–1705.

Tillisch, J., Brunken, R., Marshall, R., Schwaiger, M., Mandelkern, M., Phelps, M., and Schelbert, H. (1986). Reversibility of cardiac wall-motion abnormalities predicted by positron tomography. *N. Engl. J. Med.* 314(14), 884–888.

Tjuvajev, J. G., Avril, N., Oku, T., Sasajima, T., Miyagawa, T., Joshi, R., Safer, M., Beattie, B., DiResta, G., Daghighian, F., Augensen, F., Koutcher, J., *et al.* (1998). Imaging herpes virus thymidine kinase gene transfer and expression by positron emission tomography. *Cancer Res.* 58 (19), 4333–4341.

Valk, P. E., Mathis, C. A., Prados, M. D., Gilbert, J. C., and Budinger, T. F. (1992). Hypoxia in human gliomas: Demonstration by PET with fluorine-18-fluoromisonidazole. *J. Nuc. Med.* 33(12), 2133–2137.

Valk, P. E., Abella-Columna, E., Haseman, M. K., Pounds, T. R., Tesar, R. D., Myers, R. W., Greiss, H. B., and Hofer, G. A. (1999). Whole-body PET imaging with [18F]fluorodeoxyglucose in management of recurrent colorectal cancer. *Arch. Surg.* 134(5), 503–511, (discussion 511-513).

Vander Borght, T., Labar, D., Pauwels, S., and Lambotte, L. (1991). Production of [2-11C]thymidine for quantification of cellular proliferation with PET. *Int. J. Rad. Appl. Instrum. A* 42(1), 103–104.

van Dongen, J. A., Voogd, A. C., Fentiman, I. S., Legrand, C., Sylvester, R. J., Tong, D., van der Schueren, E., Helle, P. A., van Zijl, K., and Bartelink, H. (2000). Long-term results of a randomized trial comparing breast-conserving therapy with mastectomy. European organization for research and treatment of cancer 10801 trial. *J. Natl. Cancer Inst.* 92(14), 1143–1150.

van Eijkeren, M. E., Thierens, H., Seuntjens, J., Goethals, P., Lemahieu, I., and Strijckmans, K. (1996). Kinetics of [methyl-11C]thymidine in patients with squamous cell carcinoma of the head and neck. *Acta Oncol.* 35(6), 737–741.

Vingerhoets, F. J., Schulzer, M., Ruth, T. J., Holden, J. E., and Snow, B. J. (1996). Reproducibility and discriminating ability of fluorine-18-6-fluoro-L-Dopa PET in Parkinson's disease. *J. Nucl. Med.* 37(3), 421–426.

Vitola, J. V., Delbeke, D., Meranze, S. G., Mazer, M. J., and Pinson, C. W. (1996). Positron emission tomography with F-18-fluorodeoxyglucose to evaluate the results of hepatic chemoembolization. *Cancer* 78(10), 2216–2222.

Vranjesevic, D., Filmont, J. E., Meta, J., Silverman, D. H., Phelps, M. E., Rao, J., Valk, P. E., and Czernin, J. (2002). Whole-body (18)F-FDG PET and conventional imaging for predicting outcome in previously treated breast cancer patients. *J. Nucl. Med.* 43(3), 325–329.

Wagner, M., Seitz, U., Buck, A., Neumaier, B., Schultheiss, S., Bangerter, M., Bommer, M., Leithäuser, F., Wawra, E., Munzert, G., and Reske, S. N. (2003). 3′-[18F]fluoro-3′-deoxythymidine ([18F]-FLT) as positron emission tomography tracer for imaging proliferation in a murine B-Cell lymphoma model and in the human disease. *Cancer Res.* 63(10), 2681–2687.

Wahl, R. L. (1996). Targeting glucose transporters for tumor imaging: "Sweet" idea, "sour" result. *J. Nucl. Med.* 37(6), 1038–1041.

Wahl, R. L., Zasadny, K., Helvie, M., Hutchins, G. D., Weber, B., and Cody, R. (1993). Metabolic monitoring of breast cancer chemohormonotherapy using positron emission tomography: Initial evaluation. *J. Clin. Oncol.* 11(11), 2101–2111.

Wang, J., and Maurer, L. (2005). Positron emission tomography: Applications in drug discovery and drug development. *Curr. Top. Med. Chem.* 5(11), 1053–1075.

Weissleder, R. (1999). Molecular imaging: Exploring the next frontier. *Radiology* 212(3), 609–614.

Wichter, T., Schäfers, M., Rhodes, C. G., Borggrefe, M., Lerch, H., Lammertsma, A. A., Hermansen, F., Schober, O., Breithardt, G., and Camici, P. G. (2000). Abnormalities of cardiac sympathetic innervation in arrhythmogenic right ventricular cardiomyopathy: Quantitative assessment of presynaptic norepinephrine reuptake and postsynaptic beta-adrenergic receptor density with positron emission tomography. *Circulation* 101(13), 1552–1558.

Wunderbaldinger, P., Bogdanov, A., and Weissleder, R. (2000). New approaches for imaging in gene therapy. *Eur. J. Radiol.* 34(3), 156–165.

Yamada, S., Kubota, K., Kubota, R., Ido, T., and Tamahashi, N. (1995). High accumulation of fluorine-18-fluorodeoxyglucose in turpentine-induced inflammatory tissue. *J. Nucl. Med.* 36(7), 1301–1306.

Yang, D. J., Azhdarinia, A., Wu, P., Yu, D. F., Tansey, W., Kalimi, S. K., Kim, E. E., and Podoloff, D. A. (2001). *In vivo* and *in vitro* measurement of apoptosis in breast cancer cells using 99mtc-EC-annexin V. *Cancer Biother. Radiopharm.* 16(1), 73–83.

Yoshida, K., Mullani, N., and Gould, K. L. (1996). Coronary flow and flow reserve by PET simplified for clinical applications using rubidium-82 or nitrogen-13-ammonia. *J. Nucl. Med.* 37(10), 1701–1712.

Zhang, M., Huang, M., Le, C., Zanzonico, P. B., Claus, F., Kolbert, K. S., Martin, K., Ling, C. C., Koutcher, J. A., and Humm, J. L. (2008). Accuracy and reproducibility of tumor positioning during prolonged and multi-modality animal imaging studies. *Phys. Med. Biol.* 53(20), 5867–5882, (Epub 2008 Sep 30).

Zhuang, H., Duarte, P. S., Pourdehand, M., Shnier, D., and Alavi, A. (2000). Exclusion of chronic osteomyelitis with F-18 fluorodeoxyglucose positron emission tomographic imaging. *Clin. Nucl. Med.* 25(4), 281–284.

Zhuang, H., Duarte, P. S., Pourdehnad, M., Maes, A., Van Acker, F., Shnier, D., Garino, J. P., Fitzgerald, R. H., and Alavi, A. (2001a). The promising role of 18F-FDG PET in detecting infected lower limb prosthesis implants. *J. Nucl. Med.* 42(1), 44–48.

Zhuang, H., Pourdehnad, M., Lambright, E. S., Yamamoto, A. J., Lanuti, M., Li, P., Mozley, P. D., Rossman, M. D., Albelda, S. M., and Alavi, A. (2001b). Dual time point 18F-FDG PET imaging for differentiating malignant from inflammatory processes. *J. Nucl. Med.* 42(9), 1412–1417.

Ziemer, L. S., Evans, S. M., Kachur, A. V., Shuman, A. L., Cardi, C. A., Jenkins, W. T., Karp, J. S., Alavi, A., Dolbier, W. R., Jr., and Koch, C. J. (2003). Noninvasive imaging of tumor hypoxia in rats using the 2-nitroimidazole 18F-EF5. *Eur. J. Nucl. Med. Mol. Imaging* 30(2), 259–266.

CHAPTER 2

Biophysical Basis of Magnetic Resonance Imaging of Small Animals

Bruce M. Damon and John C. Gore

Department of Radiology and Radiological Sciences
Vanderbilt University Institute of Imaging Science
Nashville, Tennessee 37232

I. Introduction
II. Spin Relaxation
III. Effects of Exchange and Compartmentation
IV. Paramagnetic Relaxation
V. Susceptibility Contrast and BOLD Effects
VI. Effects of Spin Motion
VII. An Illustrative Example: MRI of Exercising Skeletal Muscle
   A. Effects of Exercise on Muscle T_2: Introduction
   B. Transverse Relaxation Studies of Water Compartmentation
   C. Physiological Influences on NMR Relaxation in the Intracellular Space
   D. Physiological Influences on NMR Relaxation in the Interstitial Space
   E. Physiological Influences on NMR Relaxation in the Vascular Space
   F. Conclusion: How Can We Use Transverse Relaxation Measurements to Learn about Exercising Muscle?
References

I. Introduction

Magnetic resonance (MR) images of small animals can be acquired routinely in reasonable times to portray anatomic features and functional characteristics with spatial resolution nearing true microscopic imaging. The methods available for mapping information about tissues spatially, and the various trade-offs that may be made for specific purposes in terms of image quality, resolution, and imaging strategies, are described elsewhere in this volume. This chapter provides an overview of the nature of the underlying information that may be obtained from the most

ESSENTIAL BIOIMAGING METHODS
Reprinted from *Methods in Enzymology*, Volume 385 (Academic Press, 2004).

DOI: 10.1016/B978-0-12-375043-3.00002-0

common types of images and explains the physical origins of the contrast obtainable. It should be emphasized that there are many qualitatively different types of MR images, and the signals acquired and mapped into images may be manipulated to portray or accentuate different tissue properties. The specific method used for image acquisition (i.e., the pattern of radio frequency and gradient waveforms used) determines the manner in which the image depends on different underlying characteristics, which may be regarded as analogous to the stains used in conventional microscopy. This chapter describes only those mechanisms commonly available to modulate images based on so-called proton (^{1}H) nuclear magnetic resonance (NMR). While NMR signals from other nuclei (notably sodium) may, in principle, be used to create images, the high natural abundance and favorable nuclear properties of protons (hydrogen nuclei) make them by far the most suitable for producing high-quality images. The large majority of imaging studies of small animals rely on acquiring images of mobile hydrogen nuclei that are contained mainly in water molecules. Water comprises approximately 80% of most soft tissues, which therefore contain roughly 90 M water protons. Most images portray an NMR property of the water within tissues, which indirectly reveals information on tissue structure or function. As we will show, many physiological or pathological processes of interest modify the properties of the water in an "MRI-visible" manner, albeit often in a nonspecific fashion. A second important type of contrast is also available from mobile nonwater protons contained mainly within lipids, which forms the basis of separate fat and water imaging.

The primary properties of tissues (or any other medium) that modify the NMR signal are the density of nuclei, the relaxation times of the nuclear magnetization (which, as we shall see, describe the times for recovery of the nuclear magnetization back to equilibrium after disturbance by applied radiofrequency (RF) pulses), the magnetic homogeneity of the environment, and the rate of transport of molecules (whether due to flow or via Brownian motion) within the medium. Each of these may in turn be affected by subtle changes in the properties of the tissue, such as the confinement of water with compartments, restrictions to water molecular diffusion, or physicochemical effects such as tissue pH and the presence of certain trace elements. Although in principle of effects of many of these influences are understood, it is often not straightforward to interpret changes in NMR signals in terms of any single or simple underlying causes. Tissue is an extremely heterogeneous medium, and the NMR signal in an image voxel represents the summed behavior of a large number of molecules undergoing a wide variety of interactions, so there is often no direct or specific interpretation of the variations within tissues depicted in MR images.

II. Spin Relaxation

It may be recalled that each hydrogen nucleus (proton) may be considered to possess spin, which in turn gives rise to a magnetic dipole moment. When a large number of such magnetic nuclei are placed in an external and static magnetic field, the majority tend to align themselves in the direction of the field, giving rise to a measurable macroscopic magnetization. MRI involves disturbing this magnetization using oscillating magnetic fields that alternate at a specific resonant RF, the Larmor frequency, that is proportional to the strength of the applied static magnetic field (=42.6 MHz/T applied field). The disturbed magnetization induces small electrical signals in coils of wire tuned to this same frequency as it recovers back to equilibrium. At any instant during this recovery there may exist components of the magnetization along the applied field direction (by convention the z direction) and orthogonal to this direction (the xy plane). The latter are responsible for signals measured during any acquisition. The relaxation times T_1 and T_2 and their corresponding rates R_1 ($=1/T_1$) and R_2 ($=1/T_2$) denote the characteristic time constants of the recovery back toward equilibrium of the z (longitudinal) and xy (transverse) components, respectively. When there are variations in the applied magnetic field within the sample or intrinsic magnetic inhomogeneities (such as occur within some tissues, as described later), the transverse component decays at an accelerated rate denoted as R_2^* ($=1/T_2^*$).

After being disturbed, the nuclear magnetization does not spontaneously recover very fast, but relies almost entirely on interactions of hydrogen nuclei with the surrounding material to reequilibrate. R_1 is called the spin-lattice relaxation rate. The "lattice" denotes the molecular environment surrounding a hydrogen nucleus and includes the remainder of the host molecule, as well as other solute and solvent molecules. Spin-lattice relaxation occurs because of magnetic interactions between nuclear spin dipoles and the local, randomly fluctuating, magnetic fields that exist on an atomic scale inside any medium. These originate mainly from neighboring magnetic nuclei, such as other hydrogen protons (e.g., within a water molecule, each hydrogen affects the neighbor) and are modulated by the motion of other surrounding dipoles in the lattice, which have components fluctuating with the same frequency as the resonance frequency. The recovery is very efficient when there is a local fluctuating field that can provide a magnetic perturbation at the Larmor frequency. For example, each proton in a water molecule has a neighboring proton that is also a magnetic dipole, which generates a magnetic field at the neighboring proton of about 5 g (0.5 mT). This field is constantly changing in amplitude and direction as the water molecule rotates rapidly and moves about in the liquid. It also changes as a result of intermolecular collision, translation, or chemical dissociation and exchange. The magnetic field experienced by any nucleus will fluctuate with a frequency spectrum that is dependent on the molecular tumbling due to the random thermal motion of the host and surrounding molecules. The mean strength of the local field is determined by the strength of the magnetic dipoles in the medium and how close they approach to the hydrogen nuclei. The component of the frequency spectrum, which is equal to the resonance frequency (or, for reasons beyond our discussion, twice as high), is effective in stimulating an energy exchange to induce recovery back toward equilibrium (i.e., spin-lattice relaxation). In liquids, the characteristic frequencies of thermal motion are of the order of 10^{11} Hz or higher, much greater than NMR frequencies

10^7–10^8 Hz. Consequently, the component of the frequency spectrum from molecular motion that can induce spin-lattice relaxation is small and the process is slow. As the molecular motion becomes slower, either due to a lower temperature or an increased molecular size, the intensity of the fluctuations of the magnetic field at the resonance frequency increases, reaches a maximum, and then decreases again as the energy of the motion becomes increasingly concentrated in frequencies lower than the NMR range. Thus, R_1 passes through a maximum value when the molecular tumbling rate matches the Larmor frequency as the molecular motion becomes slower. It may be noted from this that relaxation rates depend on the frequency of the NMR measurement, and thus are usually shorter at low field strengths. The effect of the molecular motion is usually expressed by a correlation time, T, characteristic of the time of rotation of a molecule or of the time of its translation into a neighboring position. Relaxation rates in simple liquids are affected, for example, by viscosity, temperature, and the presence of dissolved ions and molecules, which alter the correlation times of molecular motion or the amplitudes of the dipolar interactions.

Whereas T_1 is sensitive to RF components of the local field, T_2 is also sensitive to low-frequency components. R_2 ($=1/T_2$) is called the spin-spin relaxation rate. When an ensemble of nuclei is excited with RF, a transverse component of magnetization, orthogonal to the applied field direction, may develop, and it is this component that then rotates and induces the MRI signal in a receiver coil. T_2 reflects the time it takes for the ensemble to become disorganized and for the transverse component to decay. Since any growth of magnetization back toward equilibrium must correspond to a loss of transverse magnetization, all contributions to T_1 relaxation affect T_2 at least as much. In addition, components of the local dipolar fields that oscillate slowly, at low frequency, may be directed along the main field direction and thus can modulate the precessional frequency of a neighboring nucleus. Such frequency perturbations within an ensemble of nuclei result in rapid loss of the transverse magnetization and accelerated spin-spin relaxation. Because the low-frequency content of the local dipolar field increases monotonically as molecular motion progressively slows, although T_1 passes through a minimum value, T_2 continues to decrease and then levels off so that T_1 and T_2 then take on quite different values.

In the picture just developed, relaxation results from the action on fluctuating local magnetic fields experienced by protons, which accelerate the return to equilibrium. In pure water the dominant source of such effects is return to equilibrium. In pure water the dominant source of such effects is the dipole-dipole interaction between neighboring hydrogen nuclei in the same water molecule. The tumbling of each water molecule then causes the weak magnetic field produced by each proton to fluctuate randomly, and at the site of a neighboring proton these random alterations in the net field produce relaxation. The timescale characteristic of the dipolar interaction reflects molecular motion and clearly is expected to influence the efficacy of relaxation. Qualitatively, when there is a concentration of kinetic motion in the appropriate frequency range, relaxation will be efficient. We can envisage other types of motion that will be too rapid or too slow to be effective. The key important descriptor is the correlation time, T, which measures the time over which the local fluctuating field appears continuous and deterministic. It represents the time it takes on average for the field to change significantly.

In simple liquids such as water the molecular motion is rapid and, on average, is isotropic. The motions are so fast that relaxation is not very efficient—the dipolar fields fluctuate too rapidly to be very efficient and the motion averages out any net effects of the local fields (so-called motional averaging). In pure water, T_1 is several seconds long, whereas in water relaxation times are shorter than in pure water because of the presence of large macromolecules and chemical species that promote relaxation. Proteins and other macromolecular structures produce, via protons on their surfaces, dipolar fields that fluctuate relatively slowly and do not average out on the NMR timescale, and these are efficient sites for relaxation. Water molecules or single protons may exchange between these sites and the rest of tissue water, thereby spreading the effect. Proteins are often considered to contain one or more layers of hydration, which if often loosely termed the "bound water" fraction, and this plays an important role in mediating interactions between the bulk aqueous medium and the macromolecular surface. Although some specific chemical side groups, notably hydroxyl and amide moieties, are known to be efficient conduits for relaxation, the large array of environments and chemical species within tissue usually make it impossible to identify specific interactions that dominate.

Solutions of macromolecules and biological tissues are chemically heterogeneous, and thus water in such media may experience a wide variety of different environments and chemical species with which to interact. Even in simple protein solutions, there may be different ranges and distributions of correlation time, coupling strengths, and molecular dynamics, that affect of correlation time, coupling strengths, and molecular dynamics, that affect the local dipolar fields experienced by water protons. An even greater variety of different scales and types of constituents occur within cells and whole tissues. Tissues contain diverse, freely tumbling solute ions and molecules, such as small proteins and lipids, as well as relatively immobilized or even rigid macromolecular assemblies, such as membranes and mitochondria. Tissues are also spatially inhomogeneous, containing many different types of cells or structures, and there may exist multiple compartments that are not connected or in which water transport is restricted. Nonetheless, although tissues are markedly heterogeneous at the cellular level, NMR relaxation will still reflect the average character of local dipolar fields experienced by water protons.

III. Effects of Exchange and Compartmentation

At any time only a small proportion of water protons may be in close juxtaposition to efficient relaxation sites. Then the average water proton relaxation rate (which is what is measured) will depend on how effectively, and at what rate, these effects are spread through the rest of the water population. Such exchange processes have profound effects on the observable NMR relaxation phenomena. In a time of 50 ms, water molecules diffuse distances of the order of 20 μm so that they sample many different environments on the cellular level within the timescale of relaxation. In many (although by no means all) situations, very rapid exchange may occur between bulk water and bound and interfacial water in biological systems. Suppose, for example, there are two types of environment in exchange; fraction f of water at any instant occupies sites with relaxation rate R_a, while the remaining fraction $1 - f$ is bulk solvent with relaxation rate R_b. If the exchange is very rapid, then the average relaxation rate is R:

$$R = fR_a + (1 - f)R_b \tag{1}$$

so that

$$R = R_b + f(R_a - R_b).$$

If $R_a >> R_b$, then R is very sensitive to small changes in f, which in turn increases with protein content in tissues. This is believed to be the origin for many increases in T_1 or T_2 in various pathologies, such as edematous changes following insults to tissue, or in rapidly dividing cells that have higher water fractions. Changes in tissue water and protein content in general will affect relaxation.

Note that the existence of water in separate compartments that are only slowly exchanging gives rise to more complex behavior that is not described adequately by a single relaxation rate. For example, the transverse decay may be measured as a sum of exponential terms, but by appropriate analysis of the decay curve some inferences may be made about the sizes of the contributing compartments and the rate of water exchange between them.

An additional contribution to R_2 can arise when there are protons present in different chemical species for whom the resonance frequencies are slightly different. Several surface groups (e.g., amides on proteins), may exchange protons with water, and they start with slightly different resonance frequencies. This mixing causes a further increase in the transverse relaxation rate, and so R_2 is sensitive to pH and other factors that affect the rate of such mixing.

We have suggested that relaxation in tissues is affected by interactions that occur between water protons and protons at or near the surface of macromolecules. Longitudinal proton magnetization can be exchanged between water and neighboring nuclei (whether interfacial water that is hydrogen bonded to the surface or protons within other chemical groups that are part of the macromolecule) by direct through-space dipolar couplings, as well as by the so-called chemical exchange of protons. Chemical dissociation of protons occurs at rates that are pH dependent, providing possible interchanges between water and surface sites (hydroxyls, amides, and so forth) as intact water molecules move constantly in and out of the hydration layers of macromolecular surfaces and exchange protons. These mechanisms give rise to so-called *magnetization transfer* between pools of water in different environments, and images may be produced that are sensitized to these processes.

IV. Paramagnetic Relaxation

Paramagnetic agents may be administered to animals or they may arise naturally in some conditions, and they reduce the relaxation times of tissue water. Paramagnetic agents such as manganese, gadolinium, and several other transition and rare-earth metal ions are materials that, on the atomic scale, generate extremely strong local magnetic fields. The origin of their strong local fields lies in the fact that they contain unpaired electrons that have not been "matched" (paired off) in a chemical bond with spins of opposite character so that there is a net residual magnetic dipole is 658 times greater than the proton essentially because it has a smaller radius but the same charge so any water molecules that approach close to an unpaired electron will experience an intense interaction that can promote relaxation. For example, a 1 mM solution of gadolinium, even when chelated with diethylenetriamine pentaacetic acid (DTPA), reduces the T_1 of water to under 250 ms.

V. Susceptibility Contrast and BOLD Effects

Another important factor that may modulate the MRI signal intensity is the magnetic homogeneity of the local environment in which water molecules reside. In particular, if there are variations in the magnetic susceptibility within the sample, then the transverse magnetization, and therefore the measured signal, decays more rapidly. Variations in the susceptibility arise, for example, at interfaces between air and tissue. Within tissues there may also be small-scale variations in susceptibility due to the presence of metals within tissues, such as iron-containing proteins such as hemosiderin and hemoglobin. MRI may be usefully employed for the noninvasive detection of iron deposition in animal models.

A specific example of susceptibility variations arises from the vasculature within tissues because of the presence of hemoglobin in the circulation. This particular variation leads to the so-called blood oxygenation level-dependent (BOLD) effect, which has been found very useful for studies of brain activation and tissue oxygenation. In the brain, the physical origins of BOLD signals are reasonably well understood, although their precise connections to the underlying metabolic and electrophysiological activity need to be clarified further. It is well established that increasing neural activity in a region of the cortex stimulates an increase in the local blood flow in order to meet the increased demand for oxygen and other substrates. At the capillary level, there is a net increase in the balance of oxygenated arterial blood to deoxygenated venous blood. Essentially, the change in tissue perfusion exceeds the additional metabolic demand so the concentration of deoxyhemoglobin within tissues decreases. This decrease has a direct effect on the signals used to produce MR images. While blood containing oxyhemoglobin is not very different in terms of its magnetic susceptibility to the rest of tissues or water, it transpires that dexoyhemoglobin is significantly paramagnetic, and thus deoxygenated blood differs substantially in its magnetic properties from surrounding tissues. When oxygen is not bound to hemoglobin, the difference between the magnetic field applied by the MRI machine and that experienced close to a molecule of the blood protein is much greater than when the oxygen is bound. On a microscopic scale, replacing deoxygenated blood by oxygenated blood makes the local magnetic environment more uniform. The longevity of the signals used to produce MR images depends directly on the uniformity of the magnetic field experienced by water molecules—the less uniform the field, the greater the mixture of different signal frequencies that arise from the sample, and therefore the quicker the overall signal decays. The result of having lower levels of deoxyhemoglobin present in blood in a region of brain tissue is therefore that the MRI signal from that region decays less rapidly and so is stronger when it is recorded in a typical MR image acquisition. This small signal increase is the BOLD signal recorded in functional MRI and is typically around 1% or less, although this varies depending on the applied field strength (one of the reasons why higher field MRI systems are being developed). As can be predicted from the aforementioned explanation, the magnitude of the signal depends on the changes in blood flow and volume within tissue, as well as the change in local oxygen tension, so there is no simple relation between the signal change and any single physiological parameter. Furthermore, as neurons become more active, there is a time delay before the necessary vasodilation can occur to increase flow and for the washout of deoxyhemoglobin from the region. Thus the so-called hemodynamic response detected by BOLD has a delay and a duration of several seconds following a stimulating event. BOLD effects also occur in other tissues and may be manipulated, for example, by alterations in the oxygen content of the inspired gas of the animal.

VI. Effects of Spin Motion

Water molecules are in constant motion, and there are various ways in which their movements may affect the signals used to produce MR images. For example, the Brownian motion of molecules is random and gives rise to the self-diffusion of water within an aqueous compartment. In the presence of applied magnetic field gradients, Brownian motion causes the net signal from water to attenuate to a degree that depends on the rate of diffusion. Experimental measurements typically involve a specific timescale over which the effects of diffusion affect the signal: in small animal imaging, this is typically a few milliseconds. MR measurements of diffusion rely on the fact that the net distance that a molecule moves away from a starting position increases with time-in free diffusion, the mean squared distance moved is proportional to time and the self-diffusion coefficient D. If, during the time of the measurement, water that is initially freely diffusing encounters an obstructing boundary (such as a membrane that is not permeable), then its ability to move away from the original position is reduced and thus the *apparent diffusion coefficient* (ADC) is reduced. The manner in which ADC falls below the intrinsic value of D is a measure of the sizes and permeabilities of the cellular compartments in which water resides. Theory and experiments have shown that ADC in the brain is affected by the sizes of the intra- and extracellular water spaces, and it alters when fluid shifts between them, as in ischemia, seizure, and other conditions. Images can be acquired that depict areas of higher ADC as darker than areas of lower ADC, and such images are very sensitive to physiological and pathological perturbations. Moreover, some tissues are markedly anisotropic, and diffusion is faster in some directions than in others. For example, muscle fibers and neuronal tracts in white matter contain structures that permit water to move more freely along their length than orthogonally. The distances between restricting boundaries are much greater along a fiber or tract than across them, so the ADC is anisotropic and is properly described by a tensor. By measuring diffusion in different directions and noting how the tensor in adjacent pixels changes from point to point, it is possible to trace the principal direction of diffusion and thereby assess the direction of the corresponding fibers or tracts.

There are additional methods for sensitizing the MRI signal to other types of spin motion. In particular, a variety of methods have been devised in which the bulk motion of blood within vessels can modulate the signal within an MR image in such a way that flow velocity can be quantified. Others are sensitive to the variation of flow directions and speeds within a small volume element, which is more typical of microvascular perfusion than large vessel laminar flow. An additional and important dynamic effect in images may come from the transient passage of a bolus of paramagnetic contrast material, such as occurs following an intravenous injection. Images taken at frequent intervals can be used to record the transient signal changes caused by the temporary changes in relaxation times that occur as the material passes through the vasculature and tissue. This time course reflects the kinetic behavior of the agent, and appropriate analysis of the concentration-time curve can be used to derive measurements of flow and transit time. In some circumstances, such as occur when capillary epithelium is damaged, the rate of extravasation of the agent from the blood and into the interstitial space can be measured and quantities such as the permeability-surface area product of the vasculature can be derived.

VII. An Illustrative Example: MRI of Exercising Skeletal Muscle

T_2-weighted imaging of exercising skeletal muscle is an excellent example of how biophysical influences on NMR signal can introduce physiological significance into an image. Isolated skeletal muscle has long been a preferred tissue for studying fundamental biophysical NMR properties because it is accessed easily by dissection, has a well-understood physiology, and, in the case of muscles from poikilotherms, can be maintained easily in good physiological condition *ex vivo*. Isolated muscle preparations allow well-controlled manipulations of basic physiological properties (such as temperature, PH, and water content), creation of exercise conditions that validly model the intramuscular changes that occur during exercise *in vivo*, and access to NMR methods that allow the detailed evaluation of the effects of such manipulations on water compartmentation, relaxation times, and diffusive and chemical exchange of magnetization. Within limits, the results of isolated tissue studies can be extended theoretically and experimentally to the more complex *in vivo* condition.

A. Effects of Exercise on Muscle T_2: Introduction

For almost 40 years, it has been recognized that the T_2 of muscle water increases during and following exercise (Bratton *et al.*, 1945). Some of the earliest imaging studies reported similar changes in T_1 (Hutchison and Smith, 1983), and Fleckenstein *et al.* (1988) reported signal intensity increases from exercises muscles in T_2-weighted images (those designed to provide contrast on the basis of T_2 differences between structures). Since that time, investigation of the mechanism of exercise-induced increases in T_2 has led to considerable insight into how physiological variables influence NMR relaxation. In addition, measuring T_2 changes during exercise has been proposed as an indicator of the extent and spatial pattern of neural activation in human studies because the image intensity changes are localized spatially and relate directly to both exercise intensity (Adams *et al.*, 1992; Fisher *et al.*, 1990; Jenner *et al.*, 1994; Price *et al.*, 1998) and electromyographic measures of neural activation (Fisher *et al.*, 1990; Price *et al.*, 2003). In order to understand more specifically what these changes may indicate about the physiology of exercising muscle, this chapter explores four critical concepts: water compartmentation and its evaluation using transverse relaxation and the effects of physiological changes in the intracellular, interstitial, and vascular spaces on NMR relaxation.

B. Transverse Relaxation Studies of Water Compartmentation

Since the early 1970s, it has become well established that transverse relaxation measurements of muscle water protons can be used to study the compartmentation of muscle water. The basis of such measurements is that the transverse relaxation of muscle water protons is multiexponential (Belton *et al.*, 1972). In studies of isolated frog muscle performed at 25 °C, Belton *et al.* (1972) identified three components to the proton NMR signal of water: 18% of the signal had a very short T_2 (10 ms), 67% of the signal had an intermediate T_2 ($\approx$40 ms), and the remaining 15% of the signal had a long T_2 ($\approx$170 ms). Many other studies of isolated muscle have since demonstrated similar relaxation times and relative volume fractions (Belton and Packer, 1974; Belton *et al.*, 1972; Cole *et al.*, 1993; Damon *et al.*, 2002a; Fung and Puon, 1981; Hazlewood *et al.*, 1974; Polak *et al.*, 1988). Substantial effort has been placed into unidentifying the origins of these signals.

It is now generally accepted that the source of signals in the short T_2 component is the water bound to macromolecules (so-called hydration water), discussed earlier (Belton and Packer, 1974; Belton *et al.*, 1972; Cole *et al.*, 1993; Fung and Puon, 1981; Hazlewood *et al.*, 1974; Saab *et al.*, 1999, 2000, 2001). To demonstrate this, Belton *et al.* (1972) froze the tissue; this caused 80% of the signal to disappear. This signal loss probably corresponded to the freezing of free water; as a solid, ice has an extremely short T_2, rendering it unobservable in typical data acquisitions. The remaining 20% did not freeze, even at temperatures al low as $-30\,°C$. Because water does not freeze when it is absorbed to surfaces (such as proteins or phospholipids), Belton *et al.* (1972) speculated that the short T_2 component is composed of macromolecular hydration water. This water has a short T_2 because the macromolecules in skeletal muscle undergo slow, anisotropic motion; as discussed earlier, low-frequency molecular motion results in static magnetic field inhomogeneties and causes transverse relaxation very effectively. Water bound to the macromolecule adopts this motion and so relaxes efficiently as well.

Likewise, a consensus has emerged concerning the other T_2 components, with most authors accepting an anatomical compartmentation theory in which the intermediate and long components represent intracellular and interstitial water, respectively. This was originally proposed by Belton *et al.* (1972) who based this conclusion on the similarity between the relative volume fractions of the intermediate and long T_2 components and the space determinations made using inulin and other sugars (Law and Phelps, 1966). Direct experimental support for this proposition was provided in subsequent studies. Belton and Packer (1974) showed that dessicating the muscle progressively caused first the loss of signal from the putative interstitial T_2 component and next from the putative intracellular component. Finally, the bound water component shrank in absolute size over time, but did not completely dehydrate. Overall, these data are consistent with a unidirectional flow of water from the "innermost" to "outermost" of three compartments connected in series to the atmosphere (intracellular-bound water $\rightarrow$ free intracellular water $\rightarrow$ interstitial water $\rightarrow$ atmosphere). The volume fractions in multicomponent T_2 analysis also correspond to the relative compartment sizes implied by the analysis of sodium and chloride ion efflux curves (Neville and White, 1979). In addition, Cole *et al.* (1993) showed that tissue maceration eliminates T_2 compartmentation. The reasons for the different T_2 values for the intracellular and interstitial spaces ($\sim$40 ms vs. $\sim$150 ms) are considered later.

It is noteworthy that other models of anatomical compartmentation have also been proposed. First, Le Rumeur *et al.* (1987), Noseworthy *et al.* (1999), and Stainsby and Wright (2001) each proposed that intermediate T_2 component represents all of the tissue parenchyma (i.e., intracellular and interstitial water together), whereas the long T_2 component represents blood. The evidence for these conclusions is that changes in venous volume affect the apparent volume fraction of the long component and the changes in blood oxygen content affect its T_2. Conversely, in *vivo* transverse relaxation data reported by Saab *et al.* (1999, 2000, 2001) obtained using high signal-to-noise ratio (SNR) acquisition methods suggest the existence of two water compartments with T_2 values grater than 100 ms, which they proposed to be interstitial and vascular water; these were resolvable from the intracellular water components. In attempting to reconcile these observations with each other and the compartmentation model presented earlier, we note that the volume fraction associated with the long T_2 component was as much as 10% in the studies by Le Rumeur *et al.* (1987), Noseworthy *et al.* (1999), and Stainsby and Wright (2001). This is much larger than the capillary volume fraction (~1.5%) calculated from optical measurements Kindig *et al.* (1998) and Porter *et al.* (2002) or the total vascular volume fraction (2–4%) implied by application of the intra-voxel incoherent motion model of Le Bihan *et al.* (1988) to skeletal muscle by Morvan (1995). The inclusion of all of the tissue parenchyma into a single relaxation component is also not consistent with work by Landis *et al.* (1999) indicating an *in vivo* intracellular residence time for skeletal muscle water of 1.1 s. This result indicates that the trans-sarcolemmal water exchange is sufficiently slow that distinct intracellular and interstitial T_2 components *must* exist. It is therefore possible that in attempting the difficult task of making multiexponential transverse relaxation measurements in skeletal muscle *in vivo*, the methods used by Wright and colleagues provided too few data points (48) and/or too low of a SNR (670) to distinguish the interstitial and vascular components, and the long T_2 component that they measured in fact represented the entire extracellular space (interstitial + vascular water). We also note that Saab *et al.* (1999, 2000, 2001) have suggested that there may in fact be an additional intracellular T_2 component, but a definitive identification of such a water compartment has not been demonstrated experimentally.

We will therefore continue with a model for transverse relaxation of muscle water that includes four components: water bound to macromolecules (which is not typically observed in most transverse relaxation measurements), free intracellular water, free interstitial water, and vascular water. In order to discuss them unambiguously, we will refer to them as $T_{2,\mathrm{Bound}}$, $T_{2,\mathrm{Intra}}$, $T_{2,\mathrm{Inter}}$, and $T_{2,\mathrm{Blood}}$. As shown later, the latter three are subject to considerable variation as a result of normal physiological changes in the muscle. This has taught us much about the biological influences on NMR relaxation and how in the future we might use NMR relaxation measurements to make inferences about the underlying tissue biology.

C. Physiological Influences on NMR Relaxation in the Intracellular Space

The two variables that have the most important effects on NMR relaxation in the intracellular space of skeletal muscle under physiological conditions are free intracellular water content and intracellular pH. The most likely mechanism through which free intracellular water content effects T_1 and T_2 is through a dilution of the intracellular protein content. As discussed previously, the protein concentration is among the most important influences on relaxation times in all cells. This is particularly true in muscle because it has a very high protein content (~20% by weight; Wilkie, 1976) and in order to function appropriately, the contractile proteins are oriented parallel to the long axis of the cell at all times. As discussed earlier, the slow anisotropic motion of a large amount of cellular protein leads to very effective transverse relaxation of both the protein itself and the water bound to it. Because rapid exchange exists between free intracellular water and hydration water and/or between free intracellular water and titratable protons on the protein (Civan *et al.*, 1978; Hazlewood *et al.*, 1974), relaxation of the free intracellular water is also affected. This shortens $T_{2,\mathrm{Intra}}$ considerably relative to $T_{1,\mathrm{Intra}}$ ($T_{1,\mathrm{Intra}} \approx 40$ ms; $T_{1,\mathrm{Intra}} \approx 1000$ ms; aforementioned discussion and Landis *et al.* (1999). Consistent with this high protein content, there is also a significant magnetization transfer effect in muscle (Balaban and Ceckler, 1992; Yoshioka *et al.*, 1994; Zhu *et al.*, 1992) that originates primarily from the intracellular space (Harrison *et al.*, 1995).

A number of studies have demonstrated outright the effect of free intracellular water content on $T_{2,\mathrm{Intra}}$. First, although not the principal purpose of their study, the tissue dessication studies of Belton and Packer (1974) demonstrated the importance of water content in determining the $T_{2,\mathrm{Intra}}$. As the time of dessication progressed and the absolute volume of water in the intracellular space decreased, the $T_{2,\mathrm{Intra}}$ did as well. The results are plotted in Fig. 1. Note that data have been plotted as the transverse relaxation rate (R_2) because concentration effects are expected to be linear with R_2 but not T_2. For all conditions in which dessication did not affect the amount of macromolecular hydration water (intracellular volume $\geq$8% of initial volume), the relationship between $R_{2,\mathrm{Intra}}$ and intracellular volume of highly linear. Damon *et al.* (2002a) tested this hypothesis explicitly as well by manipulating the osmolarity of the bathing solution. By modifying the Ringer's solution around frog sartorius muscles to be hypotonic, we the solution to make it

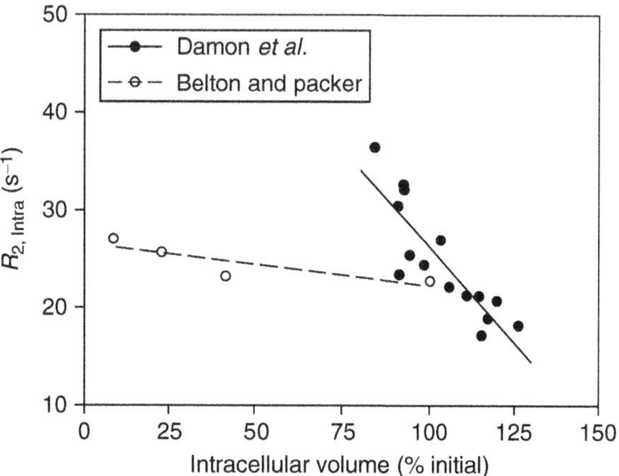

Fig. 1 Relationship between intracellular volume changes and $R_{2,\mathrm{Intra}}$ in skeletal muscle. Data shown have been replotted from studies by Damon *et al.* (2002b) (filled circles and solid line) and from Belton and Packer (1974) (open circles and dashed line). The more robust relationship reported by Damon *et al.* (2002b) may result from a greater magnetic field strength used in this study.

hypertonic, we caused water to leave the cell and decrease $T_{2,\text{Intra}}$. Figure 1 includes data from this study. The slope of the relationship is greater in our study than in the Belton and Packer study, probably because of the different magnetic field strengths employed; this point is expanded upon later.

The importance of osmotically induced water shifts in determining muscle T_2 has been shown in *in vivo* imaging studies as well. Among the most creative demonstrations of this was a study performed by Meyer *et al.* (2001) in which muscle contractions were stimulated electrically in the tail muscles of lobsters (which are osmoconformers with an intracellular osmolarity of ~1 Osm) and freshwater crayfish (which are osmoregulators with an intracellular osmolarity of 340 mOsm). Thus an accumulation of osmolytes during exercise would be expected to have an approximately threefold smaller effect in osmoconformers than in osmoregulators, and the T_2 change should be smaller as a result. This is exactly what was observed.

Several studies have also shown that intracellular pH may be an important influence on $T_{2,\text{Intra}}$ as well. In isolated strips of rabbit psoas muscle permeabilized by incubation with glycerin (Fung and Puon, 1981), showed that decreases in intracellular pH cause $T_{2,\text{Intra}}$ to decrease. This has also been shown in intact isolated frog sartorius muscles made acidic by exposure to NH_4^+ and subsequent washout of NH_3 (Damon *et al.*, 2002a). The results of both studies are shown in Fig. 2, again plotting the relaxation data as $R_{2,\text{Intra}}$. Again, a more robust relationship is observed at the higher magnetic field strength used in the Damon *et al.* (2002a) study (7.05 T) than in the Fung and Puon (1981) study (~0.5 T). Conversely, other studies (Meyer

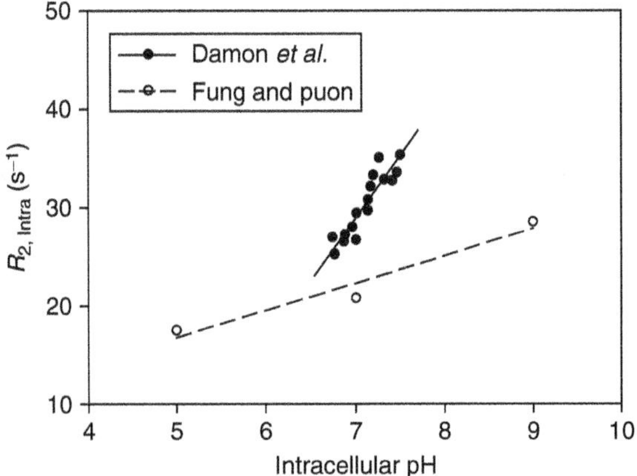

Fig. 2 Relationship between intracellular pH changes and $R_{2,\text{Intra}}$ in skeletal muscle. Data shown have been replotted from studies by Damon *et al.* (2002b) (filled circles and solid line) and from Fung and Puon (1981) (open circles and dashed line). The more robust relationship reported by Damon *et al.* (2002a) may result from a greater magnetic field strength used in this study.

et al., 2001; Prior *et al.*, 2001) have provided evidence that intracellular pH changes do not influence the whole muscle T_2, as measured in images.

The field strength dependences of $T_{2,\text{Intra}}$ on intracellular pH and volume are important clues to the specific relaxation mechanism that is active, as well as to why these studies have reported different conclusion concerning the role of intracellular pH in helping determine the $T_{2,\text{Intra}}$. A field strength dependence of T_2 could, in principle, result from either chemical exchange between sites that differ in Larmor frequency or diffusion through magnetic field gradients. Diffusion though intracellular magnetic field gradients is unlikely to depend on pH changes and has also been ruled experimentally (Damon *et al.*, 2002a). In addition, Damon *et al.* (2002b) and others (Moser *et al.*, 1995) have provided direct experimental evidence that chemical exchange between sites differing in Larmor frequency is important to at least the pH effect. Because the quantitative importance of exchange processes on $T_{2,\text{Intra}}$ lessens when the transverse relaxation decay is sampled at low frequencies, such as those used during imaging (Luz and Meiboom, 1963), this may explain the absent or very small effects of pH on $T_{2,\text{Intra}}$ reported by some investigators (Meyer *et al.*, 2001; Prior *et al.*, 2001). It is also likely that the effect of intracellular volume changes also acts through the chemical exchange mechanism, as changing the relative amount of free and macromolecular hydration water or exchangeable protons would affect the kinetics of the exchange. This mechanism would therefore also explain the field strength dependence of the effect of intracellular volume on $T_{2,\text{Intra}}$ depicted in Fig. 1.

A working interpretation of the aforementioned results is that both intracellular free water content and intracellular pH affect the $T_{2,\text{Intra}}$, but in each case the actual quantitative importance depends on magnetic field strength and data acquisition conditions. Given this, one would anticipate that glycolysis would be a major contributor to T_2 changes during exercise because it results in both a substantial accumulation of osmolytes (lactate and sugar phosphates) and a severe acidosis (up to one pH unit). The importance of glycolysis to the T_2 change was first demonstrated by Fleckenstein *et al.* (1991) in their study of myophosphorylase deficiency patients, who do not undergo a T_2 change following exercise. In principle, the lack of T_2 change in these patients could also relate to an absence of glycogen metabolism (glycogen binds ~4 g of water for each 1 g of glucose, and so the release of this water with glycogenolysis might be expected to increase $T_{2,\text{Intra}}$). However, Price and Gore (1998) showed that glycogen depletion affects neither the resting T_2 nor the T_2 change of exercise. In subsequent studies of isolated frog muscle, the principle reason for the smaller change in $T_{2,\text{Intra}}$ in muscles poisoned with iodoacetic acid (a glycolytic inhibitor) than in those poisoned with NaCN (an oxidative phosphorylation inhibitor) was the greater lactate and hydrogen ion accumulation in the latter metabolic condition. Thus, at exercise durations long enough for glycolysis to be activated significantly, the primary cause of the increase in the $T_{2,\text{Intra}}$ appears to be the end products of anaerobic metabolism.

D. Physiological Influences on NMR Relaxation in the Interstitial Space

As discussed earlier, $T_{2,\text{Inter}}$ is lengthened relative to $T_{2,\text{Intra}}$; this and a relatively slow exchange of water across the sarcolemma allow the resolution of these two T_2 components using appropriate data acquisition and analysis methods. Both the relatively longer value for T_2 and the finding that there is less magnetization transfer in this T_2 component than in the intracellular space are consistent with the lower protein concentration in the interstitium (Karatzas and Zarkadas, 1989). It is known that $T_{2,\text{Inter}}$ increases during exercise *ex vivo* (Damon *et al.*, 2002a); this may be due to osmotically induced water entry into the interstitium secondary to lactate accumulation (Sjogaard and Saltin, 1982). Apart from this, there has been little investigation of the physiological influences on $T_{2,\text{Inter}}$.

During exercise conditions, the positive contribution of changes in the interstitial space to T_2-weighted signal intensity is likely to be quite small because of its low volume fraction. In fact, the application of negative pressure to the leg increases the appearance of the interstitial T_2 component in multiexponential T_2 analyses dramatically, but causes only a modest increase in signal intensity in T_2-weighted images (Ploutz-Snyder *et al.*, 1997). However, after severe exercise in which muscles lengthen under load (so-called "eccentric" contractions), T_2 can remain elevated for almost 2 months (Foley *et al.*, 1999; Nosaka and Clarkson, 1996). These latter changes appear to reflect increases in interstitial volume brought about by muscle damage.

E. Physiological Influences on NMR Relaxation in the Vascular Space

As revealed by near-infrared spectroscopy studies and a long history of arterial and venous oxygen content measurements, blood oxygen extraction increases during exercise. There are two possible ways through which blood oxygenation changes could affect image signal intensity. The first is through an effect on the transverse relaxation of the blood itself (the intravascular BOLD effect). A number of authors (Meyer *et al.*, 1995; Spees *et al.*, 2001; Thulborn *et al.*, 1982) have shown that the $T_{2,\text{Blood}}$ decreases with decreasing values of oxyhemoglobin saturation. This results from a change in the magnetic susceptibility of the hemoglobin molecule when oxygen is released (Pauling and Coryell, 1936); the difference in magnetic susceptibility between water in the red cell and in the plasma, which exchange rapidly, accelerates transverse relaxation. As the transcapillary exchange is slow in skeletal muscle capillaries, a decrease in $T_{2,\text{Blood}}$, such as that caused by increased oxygen extraction, would attenuate the signal in a T_2-weighted image by a factor directly proportional to the blood volume fraction.

Second, the mismatch in magnetic susceptibility between blood and tissue parenchyma caused by increased oxygen extraction would promote the dephasing of spins in the tissue parenchyma (the extravascular BOLD effect). As discussed previously, a number of authors have investigated this phenomenon theoretically, including our own group (Kennan *et al.*, 1994; Stables *et al.*, 1998). The magnitude of the magnetic susceptibility difference between vasculature and tissue parenchyma depends on a number of tissue physiological and architectural parameters, including capillary size, spacing, and geometry; the hematocrit of the blood; oxyhemoglobin saturation; and the diffusion coefficient for water.

Using reasonable values for each of these parameters (listed in Table I), we can estimate the extravascular BOLD effect in three muscles; the biceps brachii, a fusiform muscle in which the fibers and capillaries would be oriented essentially parallel to the magnetic field in typical imaging experiments; the anterior tibialis, in which the fiber and capillary orientations would be slightly oblique to the field; and the soleus, in which the fibers and capillary orientation would be slightly oblique to the field; and the soleus, in which the fibers and capillary orientation would be significantly different from the magnetic field. In each case, the relative blood volumes can be assumed to be similar because each muscle is composed of predominantly slow, oxidative fibers. The results of these calculations are shown in Fig. 3. For the biceps brachii, the predominant orientation of the capillaries parallel to the field causes us to predict that there would be no extravascular effect of blood oxygenation changes. Conversely, for the soleus muscle, in which the fibers and capillaries are oriented ~40° to the field, there is a strong extravascular effect that is predicted. The effect diminishes in magnitude at low oxygen tensions because myoglobin, an oxygen-binding protein in muscle cells, abruptly deoxygenates at ~4 mm Hg, causing a better magnetic susceptibility match between vasculature and tissue parenchyma. For the anterior tibialis, an intermediate effect is predicted. Clearly, full interpretation of these effects *in vivo* requires an understanding of tissue architecture.

Table I
Model Parameters Used in Predicting Extravascular Bold Effects in Skeletal Muscle (Footnotes Represent the References Used in Assuming These Values)

	Muscle		
Parameter	Soleus	Anterior tibialis	Biceps brachii
Blood volume (%)[a]	1.5	1.5	1.5
Capillary diameter (μm)[a]	5.4	5.4	5.4
Capillary orientation (°)[b]	40	15	0
Transverse diffusion coefficient ($cm^2\ s^{-1}$)[c]	1.0×10^{-5}	1.0×10^{-5}	1.0×10^{-5}
Capillary hematocrit[d]	0.22	0.22	0.22

[a]Kindig *et al.* (1998) and Porter *et al.* (2002).
[b]Kawakami *et al.* (1998) and Maganaris and Baltzopoulos (1999).
[c]Damon *et al.* (2002c).
[d]Kindig *et al.* (1998).

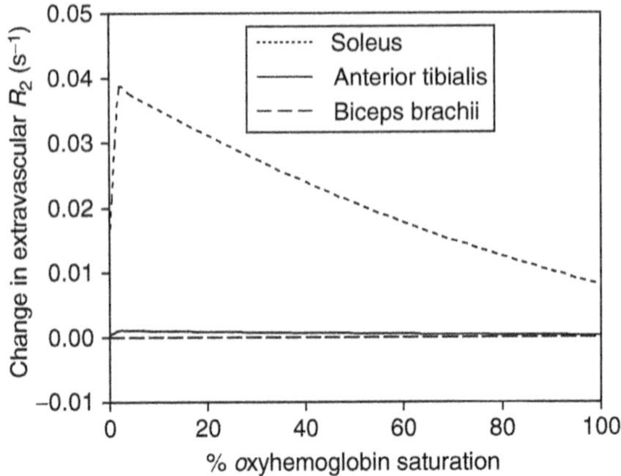

Fig. 3 Predicted contribution to extravascular R_2 due to changes in blood oxygenation. Data are based on theoretical models of Kennan *et al.* (1994) and Stables *et al.* (1998) and are shown for the soleus, anterior tibialis, and biceps brachii muscles. Model parameters are given in Table I.

F. Conclusion: How Can We Use Transverse Relaxation Measurements to Learn About Exercising Muscle?

An overall conclusion to be drawn from the aforementioned discussion is that changes in T_2-weighted signal intensity in MR images of exercising skeletal muscle primarily reflect the metabolic and hemodynamic responses to exercise. Moreover, it is likely that the relative contributions of these events change as functions of exercise during and intensity. Because a sufficient theoretical understanding of the exact contributions of different physiological and biochemical responses to exercise does not yet exist, specific conclusions about the intensity of the metabolic or hemodynamic responses (or the neural output to the muscle that is ultimately responsible for them) cannot be made, However, end-exercise T_2 measurements can certainly be used in human studies to detect muscles that have been activated during a given exercise task.

For small animal MRI experiments, there is not yet an overly compelling reason to measure T_2 changes during stimulated exercise tasks. While these changes could also be used to detect the spatial pattern of muscle activation during stimulated exercise protocols, it is likely that the stimulation pattern would already be known on the basis of the placement of stimulating electrodes over a muscle (in cases of direct muscle stimulation) or by the anatomical distribution of the motor nerve (in cases of indirect muscle stimulation via the nerve). In addition, many of the fundamental contributions to T_2-weighted signal intensity, such as metabolite accumulation, pH, and blood flow, can be measured more directly and with similar time resolution through other means.

Why, then, might we measure T_2 in skeletal muscles during small animal experiments? The answer to this question lies in the prediction that by developing a comprehensive understanding of the biophysical influences on NMR relaxation in muscle, we will be able to image parameters not otherwise accessible through noninvasive methods. For example, changes in capillary geometry, distribution, and size that occur in diabetes (Kindig *et al.*, 1998) would be expected to influence the magnitude of the extravascular BOLD effect (and therefore the ratio of R_2 to R_2*). Such measurements might therefore serve as a marker of capillary morphologic changes in animal models of this disease. Additionally, measurements of sarcolemma water permeability, as well as an understanding of how this parameter affects the overall T_2 of the muscle, would be useful in experimental models of muscular dystrophy and muscle damage. Such measurements will require continued efforts to develop a comprehensive understanding of the biological influences on NMR relaxation in skeletal muscle.

References

Adams, G. R., Duvoisin, M. R., and Dudley, G. A.(1992). *J. Appl. Physiol.* **73,** 1578.

Balaban, R. S., and Ceckler, T. L.(1992). *Magn. Reson. Q.* **8,** 116.

Belton, P. S., and Packer, K. J.(1974). *Biochim. Biochim. Biophys. Acta* **354,** 305.

Belton, P. S., Jackson, R. R., and Packer, K. J.(1972). *Biochim. Biophys. Acta* **286,** 16.

Bratton, C. B., Hopkins, A. L., and Weinberg, J. W.(1945). *Science* **147,** 738.

Civan, M. M., Achlama, A. M., and Shporer, M.(1978). *Biophys. J.* **21,** 127.

Cole, W. C., LeBlanc, A. D., and Jhingran, S. G.(1993). *Magn. Reson. Med.* **29,** 19.

Damon, B. M., Freyer, A. S., and Gore, J. C.(2002a). *In* "Proceedings of International Society for Magnetic Resonance in Medicine 10th Scientific Meeting and Exbihition," p. 619.

Damon, B. M., Ding, Z., Anderson, A. W., Freyer, A. S., and Gore, J. C.(2002b). *Magn. Reson. Med.* **48,** 97.

Damon, B. M., Gregory, C. D., Hall, K. L., Stark, H. J., Gulani, V., and Dawson, M. J.(2002c). *Magn. Reson. Med.* **47,** 14.

Fisher, M. J., Meyer, R. A., Adams, G. R., Foley, J. M., and Potchen, E. J.(1990). *Invest. Radiol.* **25,** 480.

Fleckenstein, J. L., Candy, R. C., Parkey, R. W., and Peshock, R. M.(1988). *AJR Am. J. Roentgenol.* **151,** 231.

Fleckenstein, J. L., Haller, R. G., Lewis, S. F., Archer, B. T., Barker, B. R., Payne, J., Parkey, R. W., and Peshock, R. M.(1991). *J. Appl. Physiol.* **71,** 961.

Foley, J. M., Jayaraman, R. C., Prior, B. M., Pivarnik, J. M., and Meyer, R. A.(1999). *J. Appl. Physiol.* **87,** 2311.

Fung, B. M., and Puon, P. S.(1981). *Biophys. J.* **33,** 27.

Harrison, R., Bronskill, M. J., and Henkelman, R. M.(1995). *Magn. Reson. Med.* **33,** 490.

Hazlewood, C. F., Chang, D. C., Nichols, B. L., and Woessner, D. E.(1974). *Biophys. J.* **14,** 583.

Hutchison, J. M. S., and Smith, F. W.(1983). *In* "Nuclear Magnetic Resonance (NMR) Imaging" (C. L. Partain, A. E. James, F. D. Rollo, and R. R. Price, eds.), p. 231. Saunders, Philadelphia.

Jenner, G., Foley, J. M., Cooper, T. G., Potchen, E. J., and Meyer, R. A.(1994). *J. Appl. Physiol.* **76,** 2119.

Karatzas, C. N., and Zarkadas, C. G.(1989). *Poult. Sci.* **68,** 811.

Kawakami, Y., Ichinose, Y., and Fukunaga, T.(1998). *J. Appl. Physiol.* **85,** 398.

Kennan, R. P., Zhong, J., and Gore, J. C.(1994). *Magn. Reson. Med.* **31,** 9.

Kindig, C. A., Sexton, W. L., Fedde, M. R., and Poole, D. C.(1998). *Respir. Physiol.* **111,** 163.

Landis, C. S., Li, X., Telang, F. W., Molina, P. E., Palyka, I., Vetek, G., and Springer, C. S.(1999). *Magn. Reson. Med.* **42,** 467.

Law, R. O., and Phelps, C. F.(1966). *J. Physiol.* **186,** 547.

Le Bihan, D., Breton, E., Lallemand, D., Aubin, M. L., Vignaud, J., and Laval-Jeantet, M.(1988). *Radiology* **168,** 497.

Le Rumeur, E., De Certaines, J., Toulouse, P., and Rochcongar, P.(1987). *Magn. Reson. Imaging* **5,** 267.

Luz, Z., and Meiboom, S.(1963). *J. Chem. Phys.* **39,** 366.

Maganaris, C. N., and Baltzopoulos, V.(1999). *Eur. J. Appl. Physiol. Occup. Physiol.* **79,** 294.

Meyer, M. E., Yu, O., Eclancher, B., Grucker, D., and Chambron, J.(1995). *Magn. Reson. Med.* **34,** 234.

Meyer, R. A., Prior, B. M., Siles, R. I., and Wiseman, R. W.(2001). *NMR Biomed.* **14,** 199.

Morvan, D.(1995). *Magn. Reson. Imaging* **13,** 193.

Moser, E., Winklmayr, E., Holzmuller, P., and Krssak, M.(1995). *Magn. Reson. Imaging* **13,** 429.

Neville, M. C., and White, S.(1979). *J. Physiol.* **288,** 71.

Nosaka, K., and Clarkson, P. M.(1996). *Med. Sci. Sports Exerc.* **28,** 953.

Noseworthy, M. D., Kim, J. K., Stainsby, J. A., Stanisz, G. J., and Wright, G. A.(1999). *Magn. Reson. Imaging* **9,** 814.

Pauling, L., and Coryell, C.(1936). *Proc. Natl. Acad. Sci. USA* **19,** 349.

Ploutz-Snyder, L. L., Nyren, S., Cooper, T. G., Potchen, E. J., and Meyer, R. A.(1997). *Magn. Reson. Med.* **37,** 676.

Polak, J. F., Jolesz, F. A., and Adams, D. F.(1988). *Invest. Radiol.* **23,** 107.

Porter, M. M., Stuart, S., Boij, M., and Lexell, J.(2002). *J. Appl. Physiol.* **92,** 1451.

Price, T. B., and Gore, J. C.(1998). *J. Appl. Physiol.* **84,** 1178.

Price, T. B., Kennan, R. P., and Gore, J. C.(1998). *Med. Sci. Sports Exerc.* **30,** 1374.

Price, T. B., Kamen, G., Damon, B. M., Knight, C. A., Applegate, B., Gore, J. C., Eward, K., and Signorile, J. F.(2003). *Magn. Reson. Imaging* **21,** 853–861.

Prior, B. M., Ploutz-Snyder, L. L., Cooper, T. G., and Meyer, R. A.(2001). *J. Appl. Physiol.* **90,** 615.

Saab, G., Thompson, R. T., and Marsh, G. D.(1999). *Magn. Reson. Med.* **42,** 150.

Saab, G., Thompson, R. T., and Marsh, G. D.(2000). *J. Appl. Physiol.* **88,** 226.

Saab, G., Thompson, R. T., Marsh, G. D., Picot, P. A., and Moran, G. R.(2001). *Magn. Reson. Med.* **46,** 1093.

Sjogaard, G., and Saltin, B.(1982). *Am. J. Physiol.* **243,** R271.

Spees, W. M., Yablonskiy, D. A., Oswood, M. C., and Ackerman, J. J.(2001). *Magn. Reson. Med.* **45,** 533.

Stables, L. A., Kennan, R. P., and Gore, J. C.(1998). *Magn. Reson. Med.* **40,** 432.

Stainsby, J. A., and Wright, G. A.(2001). *Magn. Reson. Med.* **45,** 662.

Thulborn, K. R., Waterton, J. C., Matthews, P. M., and Radda, G. K.(1982). *Biochim. Biophys. Acta* **714,** 265.

Wilkie, D. R.(1976). "Muscle," Edward Arnold, London.

Yoshioka, H., Takahashi, H., Onaya, H., Anno, I., Niitsu, M., and Itai, Y.(1994). *Magn. Reson. Imaging* **12,** 991.

Zhu, X. P., Zhao, S., and Isherwood, I.(1992). *Br. J. Radiol.* **65,** 39.

CHAPTER 3

Functional Magnetic Resonance Imaging of Macaque Monkeys

Kiyoshi Nakahara

Department of Physiology
The University of Tokyo School of Medicine
Tokyo 113-0033, Japan

I. Introduction
II. Potential of Functional MRI in Macaque Monkeys
III. Brief History of fMRI in Macaque Monkeys
IV. Experimental Procedures
    A. Animal Experiments
    B. fMRI in Anesthetized Monkeys: Anesthetic Procedures
    C. fMRI in Awake Monkeys
    D. Some Apparatus
    E. Scan Procedures
    F. Data Analyses
V. Conclusion
References

I. Introduction

Functional magnetic resonance imaging (fMRI) is a noninvasive functional brain-imaging method that utilizes blood oxygenation level-dependent (BOLD) signals as a measure of brain activation (Ogawa *et al.*, 1990, 1992). This method can be applied to human subjects while they perform certain cognitive tasks and can be used to visualize a map of regional brain activation correlated with the cognitive functions required to perform the task across the whole brain. Although not much time has passed since the discovery of the BOLD signal, this method has been used in thousands of researches on a wide variety of human brain functions, from perception to high-level cognitive functions, and has become a major tool in cognitive neuroscience (Courtney and Ungerleider, 1997; Frackowiak *et al.*, 1997;

ESSENTIAL BIOIMAGING METHODS
Reprinted from *Methods in Enzymology*, Volume 385 (Academic Press, 2004)

DOI: 10.1016/B978-0-12-375043-3.00003-2

Raichle, 1998). In the late-1990s, some laboratories began to apply fMRI to macaque monkeys (Dubowitz *et al.*, 1998; Hayashi *et al.*, 1999; Logothetis *et al.*, 1999; Stefanacci *et al.*, 1998; Vanduffel *et al.*, 2001). Why should monkey fMRI be developed in addition to human fMRI? What are the advantages?

II. Potential of Functional MRI in Macaque Monkeys

First, this method offers opportunities to make direct comparisons of the functional architectures of the brains of humans and monkeys. Macaque monkeys have been used over the past half-century as a major experimental model for humans, and a vast amount of physiological and anatomical knowledge of brain function has been accumulated using invasive but informative methods, such as microelectrode recordings, tracer injections, microstimulation, inactivation, and experimental lesions. Obviously, comparisons and integration of results from human studies with fMRI and monkey studies with these methods are very important for obtaining a more precise view of our brain mechanisms. However, such attempts have been hampered by species and methodological differences. A straightforward solution is to apply the same physiological method under the same experimental design to both monkey and human subjects. fMRI of macaque monkeys is an ideal tool for such investigations and could provide a bridge between humans and monkeys (Nakahara *et al.*, 2002; Tootell *et al.*, 2003).

Second, this method could be used to clarify the relationships between the BOLD signals and the electrical activities of neurons. Thousands of studies on human cognitive function using fMRI have already been reported. However, the physiological origin and the nature of the BOLD signal are largely unknown. Measuring the electrical activities and the BOLD signal simultaneously in macaque monkeys will be a promising approach to this issue. One such study reported that the BOLD signal showed a greater correlation with the local field potential compared with multi- or single-unit activity (Logothetis *et al.*, 2001). Further experiments in line with this kind of approach will clarify a precise interpretation of the observed BOLD signal, which seems to be essential for bringing fMRI to completion as a "physiological" tool (Kim, 2003).

Third, this method can be strong complement to traditional microelectrode recordings. Microelectrode recordings provide microscopic information about electrical activities from the level of single neuron to local neuronal circuits. However, cognitive functions are executed by the coordinated activities of distributed neuronal networks across several cortical areas, and the use of microelectrode recordings alone presents difficulties in seeing how local neuronal activities participate in the global networks. fMRI in monkeys can depict a macroscopic activation map across the whole brain, which could complement the microscopic information obtained by microelectrode recordings (Leopold *et al.*, 2003). Moreover, this method can serve as a guide for choosing brain areas for microelectrode recordings. When researchers want to start research using microelectrode recordings, and if the responsive brain regions are unknown, the choice of recording sites usually relies on previous information from anatomical and lesion studies, which often give only an estimation. Using fMRI, researchers can identify multiple responsive brain regions rapidly and obtain a navigation map for the appropriate choice of electrode penetration sites.

Finally, other than these inherent potential benefits, fMRI in monkeys would be of unexpected value to researchers in cognitive neuroscience (Miyashita and Hayashi, 2000). Its potential seems to be even greater when it is combined with other invasive methods, such as experimentally placed lesions, microstimulation, reversible inactivation, and labeling of fiber projection using contrast agents (Saleem *et al.*, 2002).

III. Brief History of fMRI in Macaque Monkeys

The earliest applications of fMRI to macaque monkeys were reported independently by Dubowitz *et al.* (1998) and Stefanacci *et al.* (1998). They scanned awake macaque monkeys with conventional clinical 1.5-T MR scanners while the subjects observed visual stimuli passively and demonstrated the stimulus-related BOLD signal in the visual cortex of the monkey. Some laboratories made efforts to develop MR systems specially adapted to monkey experiments. Logothetis's group developed a customized MR system equipped with a high-field (4.7 T) vertical magnet specially designed for monkey studies and achieved much progress in several aspects of imaging techniques, including simultaneous fMRI microelectrode recordings and ultra high-resolution fMRI (voxel size = 0.0113 μl) using implantable radiofrequency (RF) coils (Logothetis *et al.*, 1999, 2001, 2007; Saleem *et al.*, 2002). Orban's group took a different approach to improving fMRI sensitivity in a normal magnetic field (1.5–3 T) rather than using a high-field magnet (Leite *et al.*, 2002; Vanduffel *et al.*, 2001). They injected an MR contrast agent [dextran-coated monocrystalline iron oxide nanoparticles (MION)] intravenously into monkey subjects and achieved increments of signal sensitivity and more precise signal localization relative to the conventional BOLD technique. Our laboratory also started fMRI of macaque monkeys at an early stage. Our first monkey fMRI experiment was reported in 1999, where we mapped somatosensory activation in anesthetized monkeys using a conventional 1.5-T machine and demonstrated the ability to discriminate topographical organization in two adjacent functional areas: hand and face representations in primary and secondary somatosensory cortices (Hayashi *et al.*, 1999). In the next study, we succeeded in using fMRI of conscious monkeys performing a high-level cognitive task and made a direct comparisons of the functional organization of the prefrontal cortex of humans and monkeys (Nakahara *et al.*, 2002). Section IV introduces current experimental procedures using a 1.5-T scanner with anesthetized and awake, task-performing monkeys (Fig. 1).

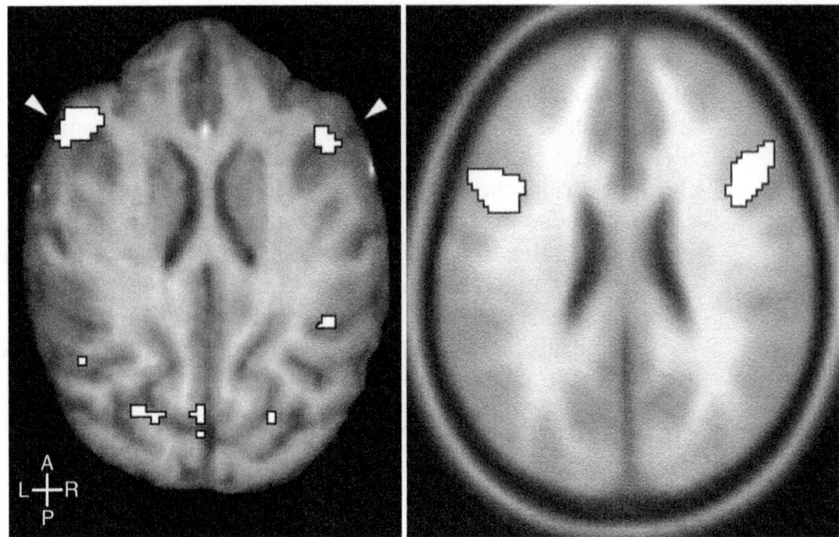

Fig. 1 Comparative fMRI of macaque monkeys and humans. During the fMRI scans, both the monkey and the human subjects performed the Wisconsin card-sorting task, which required congnitive set shifting, a characteristic function of the prefrontal cortex. Event-related BOLD activation correlated with the cognitive set shifting was analyzed with SPM99 software, and cortical areas that showed significant activation were superimposed on transverse sections of the anatomical images (white pixels). Prominent prefrontal activation is observed in the bilateral bank of the arcuate sulcus in monkeys (left) and in the bilateral inferior frontal sulcus in humans (right) (Nakahara *et al.*, 2002). The statistical threshold was set at $p < 0.001$ (uncorrected) with conjunction analysis in humans. A, anterior; P, posterior; R, right; L, left. Arrowheads, arcuate sulcus.

IV. Experimental Procedures

A. Animal Experiments

All of our experimental procedures are carried out in full compliance with the NIH guidelines for the care and use of laboratory animals and the regulations of the University of Tokyo School of Medicine.

B. fMRI in Anesthetized Monkeys: Anesthetic Procedures

Because some anesthetic agents can influence cerebral blood flow or oxygen consumption, special care is needed in the selection of the anesthetic procedures for monkey fMRI. As a matter of fact, in our pilot studies, we failed to acquire BOLD signals in monkeys anesthetic agents, we found that the BOLD signal can be obtained reproducibly in monkeys anesthetized with droperidol or propofol. Droperidol was reported to show no significant effect on cerebral blood flow and oxygen consumption in humans (Cottrell and Smith, 1994; Sari *et al.*, 1972). Although propofol was reported to decrease both cerebral blood flow and oxygen consumption, it preserved vascular reactivity in humans and was feasible in fMRI of rats (Scanley *et al.*, 1997; Stephan *et al.*, 1987). A careful use of gas anesthesia together with muscle relaxant was also reported to be successful in high-field monkey fMRI (Logothetis *et al.*, 1999). In our current protocol, monkeys are anesthetize with either intravenous droperidol (0.5–1.5 mg/kg/h; Sankyo, Tokyo, Japan) or intravenous propofol (3–7.5 mg/kg/h; Zeneca, Tokyo, Japan) during fMRI scans.

C. fMRI in Awake Monkeys

For fMRI in awake monkeys, a major concern is how to make the subjects behave cooperatively in the noisy and small space of the bore of the MR machine. The animals must not only keep still, but also perform a cognitive task during fMRI scans. To realize this, monkeys are trained in three steps. In the first step, monkey subjects are trained on a cognitive task of interest while sitting vertically in a standard primate chair. After they achieve good performances (>90%) on the task, they go to the second step, where the subjects are habituated in performing the task in the posture and noise of MR scans. In this stage, the monkeys are laid in a custom-built horizontal monkey container, which is also used in the actual scans, and trained to perform the task in it. The sound of recorded MR noise is sometimes played back during the second step training. Use of a mock-up MR bore at this stage makes habituation training more effective. Finally, the subjects are trained to perform the task in a real MR machine. With these habituation procedures, monkeys can adapt easily to performing the cognitive tasks quietly in the MR bore without showing considerable additional body movements.

D. Some Apparatus

All of the apparatus used in MR bore must be made of nonferrous materials and should be preexamined for effects on image quality using a control MB phantom. We usually use acarylic, ceramic, polysulphone, or Delrin (DuPont) according to the purpose. During scans, monkeys lie in a custom-made acrylic monkey container, which is anchored to the bed of the MR machine. The monkey container can be equipped with fiber-optic-based MR-compatible buttons (Omron, Kyoto, Japan), which are used for the responses of the subjects. Prior to MR scans, custom-made head posts (polysulphone) are implanted in the skull of the monkey using ceramic screws (zirconium oxide; Kyocera, Kyoto, Japan) under general anesthesia in aseptic conditions. With these head posts, the head of the monkey is fixed to a custom-built head holder (acrylic), which is anchored to the bed and makes the head position constant relative to the magnet. Usually, the observed head movements are less than 0.5 mm throughout each scan session (about 10 min). A custom-built acrylic bite bar is used to minimize licking movements. A liquid reward can be delivered through this bite bar. Visual stimuli are back projected from an LCD projector (Sony, Tokyo, Japan).

E. Scan Procedures

Functional imaging of monkeys is performed on a clinical 1.5-T scanner (Stratis II; Hitachi Medical Corp., Tokyo, Japan). A knee coil (quadrature, with an inner diameter of 190 mm) is used as a RF probe. Scan parameters should be optimized carefully for each MR system and each experimental design to obtain the best images. Usually, we use four-segmented gradient-echo echo-planar imaging, where FOV is 128×128 mm, Tr is 750 ms, Te is 18.4 or 20 ms, flip angle is 64°, matrix is 64×64, slice thickness is 2 mm, and the interslice gap is 0.5 mm, with nine transverse slices. These parameters can be used for both anesthetized and conscious monkeys.

F. Data Analyses

Functional images are analyzed with SPM99 software package (http://www.fil.ion.ucl.ac.uk/spm/) running on MATLAB (Math Words, MA) with a Pentium-based PC. Functional images are first realigned, normalized spatially to a template with interpolation to a $1 \times 1 \times 1$-mm space and then smoothed with a Gaussian kernel (FWHM 4–6 mm). The template is made from fine three-dimensional structural images of one monkey's whole brain (voxel size is $1 \times 1 \times 1$ mm) according to the standard procedure implemented in SPM99. The template is arranged in a bicommissural coordinate system where the origin is placed at the anterior commissure. This normalization procedure allows us to perform group analyses. In monkey experiments, because it is difficult to correct data from enough subjects for random effect analysis, conjunction analysis (Friston *et al.*, 1999) is used for group analyses is our laboratory. Functional brain activation is modeled and analyzed statistically using a general liner model implemented in SPM99 software in both blocked and event-related designs.

V. Conclusion

fMRI in macaque monkeys is one of the most exciting tools for current and future neuroscience studies. We cannot only use this method alone, but we can also use it with other invasive methods in macaques. Moreover, we are now able to perform "parallel" researches into the mechanisms of primate brains using human and monkey fMRI. In conclusion, fMRI of macaque monkeys will open up new perspectives to cognitive neuroscience researchers and will provide insights into the brain mechanisms of human and nonhuman primates.

References

Cottrell, J. E., and Smith, D. S. (1994). "Anesthesia and Neurosurgery." Mosby, St. Louis.

Courtney, S. M., and Ungerleider, L. G. (1997). *Curr. Opin. Neurobiol.* **7,** 554.

Dubowitz, D. J., Chen, D. Y., Atkinson, D. J., Grieve, K. L., Gillikin, B., Bradley, W. G., Jr., and Andersen, R. A. (1998). *Neuroreport* **9,** 2213.

Frackowiak, R. S. J., Friston, K. J., Frith, C. D., Dolan, R. J., and Mazziotta, J. C. (1997). "Human Brain Function." Academic Press, San Diego.
Friston, K. J., Holmes, A. P., and Worsley, K. J. (1999). *Neuroimage* **10,** 1.
Hayashi, T., Konishi, S., Hasegawa, I., and Miyashita, Y. (1999). *Eur. J. Neurosci.* **11,** 4451.
Kim, S. G. (2003). *Proc. Natl. Acad. Sci. USA* **100,** 3550.
Leite, F. P., Tsao, D., Vanduffel, W., Fize, D., Sasski, Y., Wald, L. L., Dale, A. M., Kwong, K. K., Orban, G. A., Rosen, B. R., Tootell, R. B. H., and Mandeville, J. B. (2002). *Neuroimage* **16,** 283.
Leopold, D. A., Murayama, Y., and Logothetis, N. K. (2003). *Cerebr. Cortext* **13,** 422.
Logothetis, N. K., Guggenberger, H., Peled, S., and Pauls, J. (1999). *Nat. Neurosci.* **2,** 555.
Logothetis, N. K., Pauls, J., Augath, M., Trinath, T., and Oeltermann, A. (2001). *Nature* **412,** 150.
Logothetis, N. K., Merkle, H., Augath, M., Trinath, T., and Ugurbil, K. (2007). *Neuron* **35,** 227.
Miyashita, Y., and Hayashi, T. (2000). *Curr. Opin. Neurobiol.* **10,** 187.
Nakahara, K., Hayashi, T., Konishi, S., and Miyashita, Y. (2002). *Science* **295,** 1532.
Ogawa, S., Lee, T. M., Kay, A. R., and Tank, D. W. (1990). *Proc. Natl. Acad. Sci. USA* **87,** 9868.
Ogawa, S., Tank, D. W., Menon, R., Ellermann, J. M., Kim, S. G., Merkle, H., and Ugurbil, K. (1992). *Proc. Natl. Acad. Sci. USA* **89,** 5951.
Raichle, M. E. (1998). *Proc. Natl. Acad. Sci. USA* **95,** 765.
Saleem, K. S., Pauls, J. M., Augath, M., Trinath, T., Prause, B. A., Hashikawa, T., and Logothetis, N. K. (2002). *Neuron* **34,** 685.
Sari, A., Okuda, Y., and Takeshita, H. (1972). *Br. J. Anaesth.* **44,** 330.
Scanley, B. E., Kennan, R. P., Cannen, S., Skudlarski, P., Innis, R. B., and Gore, J. C. (1997). *Magn. Reson. Med.* **37,** 969.
Stefanacci, L., Reber, P., Costanza, J., Wong, E., Buxton, R., Stuart, Z., Squire, L., and Albright, T. (1998). *Neuron* **20,** 1051.
Stephan, H., Sonntag, H., Schenk, H. D., and Kohlhausen, S. (1987). *Anaesthesist* **36,** 60.
Tootell, R. B. H., Tsao, D., and Vanduffel, W. (2003). *J. Neurosci.* **23,** 3981.
Vanduffel, W., Fize, D., Madeville, J. B., Nelissen, K., Van Hecke, P., Rosen, B. R., Tootell, R. B. H., and Orban, G. A. (2001). *Neuron* **32,** 565.

CHAPTER 4

Atlas Template Images for Nonhuman Primate Neuroimaging: Baboon and Macaque

Kevin J. Black,* Jonathan M. Koller,† Abraham Z. Snyder,‡ and Joel S. Perlmutter§

*Departments of Psychiatry, Neurology, and Radiology
Washington University School of Medicine
St. Louis, Missouri 63110-1093

†Department of Psychiatry
Washington University School of Medicine
St. Louis, Missouri 63110-1093

‡Departments of Radiology and Neurology
Washington University School of Medicine
St. Louis, Missouri 63110-1093

§Departments of Neurology, Radiology
Anatomy and Neurobiology, and the Program in Physical Therapy
Washington University School of Medicine
St. Louis, Missouri 63110-1093

I. Introduction
 A. Multisubject Studies in Atlas Space for Humans
 B. Motivation for Neuroimaging Studies in Nonhuman Subjects
 C. Need for Three-Dimensional Atlas Template Image for Nonhuman Studies
II. Methods
 A. Development of the "b2k" Baboon Atlas
 B. Development of the Baboon Blood Flow Template, "b2kf"
 C. Macaque Template Images: The "n2k" and "n2kf" Templates
 D. Using the Templates in Analyzing Functional Imaging Data
 E. Anatomic Interpretation of Statistical Images

ESSENTIAL BIOIMAGING METHODS
Reprinted from *Methods in Enzymology*, Volume 385 (Academic Press, 2004).

DOI: 10.1016/B978-0-12-375043-3.00004-4

III. Discussion
A. Similar Methods
B. Future Applications
References

I. Introduction

A. Multisubject Studies in Atlas Space for Humans

Coregistration of functional brain images across many subjects is a technique that has been widely used for studies in humans. Some of the advantages to this multisubject approach include the ability to detect signals in regions not known *a priori*, reduced influence of individual anatomic variation, ease of analysis, and increased sensitivity to low-magnitude responses (Fox *et al.*, 1985, 1988; Raichle *et al.*, 1991). Combining data across human subjects is now most often accomplished using computerized, voxel-based image registration algorithms (Strother *et al.*, 1994; Viergever *et al.*, 1995). These programs rely on a high-quality template image that is usually related to a published atlas. Template images are readily available for human studies, but methods have lagged considerably for neuroimaging in other species.

B. Motivation for Neuroimaging Studies in Nonhuman Subjects

Neuroimaging in humans offers many advantages, but nonhuman species may be more appropriate for some studies, such as lesion models of human disease, drug development, pharmacologic investigations, and methods development. Baboons (*Papio* spp.) have been employed frequently in positron emission tomography (PET) studies due to their relatively large brain volume. Macaques of various species have long been used for functional neuroimaging studies (Perlmutter *et al.*, 1991) and have been trained to perform various tasks in the scanner.

C. Need for Three-Dimensional Atlas Template Image for Nonhuman Studies

Until recently, functional imaging studies in nonhuman species were analyzed as case reports or by combining numerical data extracted from functional images by reference to anatomic regions chosen *a priori*. Automated methods for combining nonhuman primate brain images across subjects not only convey an increased value to the images, but also lessen the need for physical restraint in images that can be acquired fast enough to minimize within-scan movement (e.g., [^{15}O] water images or echoplanar [EPI] images). These two advantages are favorable to animal welfare.

This chapter describes the creation of template images for baboon brain using T_1-weighted magnetic resonance imaging (MRI) and PET [^{15}O]water blood flow images (Black *et al.*, 2001a). Similar templates were created for macaque brain

(Black *et al.*, 2001b). Methods for creating the atlas template image have broader application and could be adapted for other species. In fact, similar methods were first used in generating a multisubject human template image conforming to the Talairach and Tournoux atlas (Corbetta *et al.*, 1998; Talairach and Tournoux, 1988).

Our approach to testing our methods could also be applied to future work. Specifically, we examined the accuracy of the template vis-à-vis radiological landmarks and a photomicrographic atlas. Using two approaches to combining functional images across subjects, we confirmed both the accuracy of fit to the atlas and the accuracy of our voxel-based (AIR) software. The various methods are discussed approximately in chronological order of development.

II. Methods

A. Development of the "b2k" Baboon Atlas

1. Subjects

The images used to create the MRI template derive from nine baboons, six male and three female. Ages for the animals ranged from approximately 4.5 to 20 years.

2. Image Acquisition

Using a 1.5-T Siemens scanner, we acquired sagittal magnetization prepared rapid gradient echo (MPRAGE) images with a voxel volume of ~ 1.25 mm^3 in sedated baboons. Higher image resolutions could be obtained by various techniques, but given the magnitude of residual anatomic variability after linear coregistration, the *de facto* resolution of commonly applied functional imaging methods, and the spatial smoothing used for cross-subject analysis, higher image resolution was felt to be superfluous. For some animals, two acquisitions were averaged to reduce noise.

3. Image Registration

Automatic voxel-based registration of the individual images to the template was performed using in-house computer programs implemented on the Solaris operating system environment. Within-modality (individual MRI to template MRI) registration was performed by minimizing the variance of difference images, as described previously (Snyder, 1996). The result of each individual-to-template registration is a linear (12-parameter, or affine) transform of the individual image to the template image. No preparation is needed to run the registration programs unless an image is rotated by a significant amount ($>\sim 30°$) relative to the template. In this case, the user must initialize the transformation manually to approximately account for the rotation before the automatic registration can be performed.

However, it is important to emphasize that other registration methods could be used, including the AIR method (Woods *et al.*, 1992, 1993, 1998) or the approach of Friston and colleagues (Ashburner and Friston, 1999; Friston *et al.*, 1995). Laboratories familiar with one of these methods could use that approach.

4. Template Image Development

We created the template image by a "bootstrap" method that ensured registration of the template with the atlas, followed by iterative refinement of the averaged atlas image (Fig. 1).

The first step in creating the MRI template image is to transform each of the nine individual baboon MPRAGE images to atlas space. This "bootstrap" step is accomplished using a previously validated but labor-intensive method that requires expert identification of certain radiological landmarks (Black *et al.*, 1997a). The images are intensity scaled using a histogram method and averaged together voxelwise to create the initial template image, "template$_0$."

This image (top image in Fig. 2) demonstrates substantial spatial noise due to significant residual uncorrected spatial differences. This is addressed iteratively, with each iteration consisting of three steps. In the first iteration, each individual MPRAGE image is registered to template$_0$ using the within-modality registration

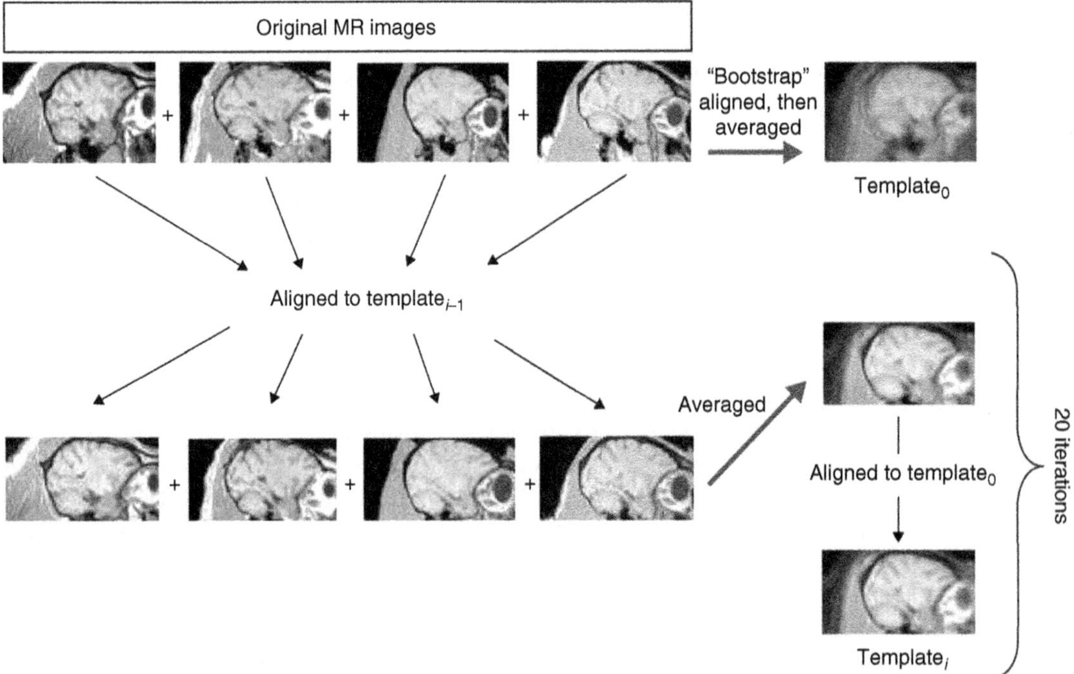

Fig. 1 Schematic diagram of the iterative process used to create b2k and n2k atlas templates.

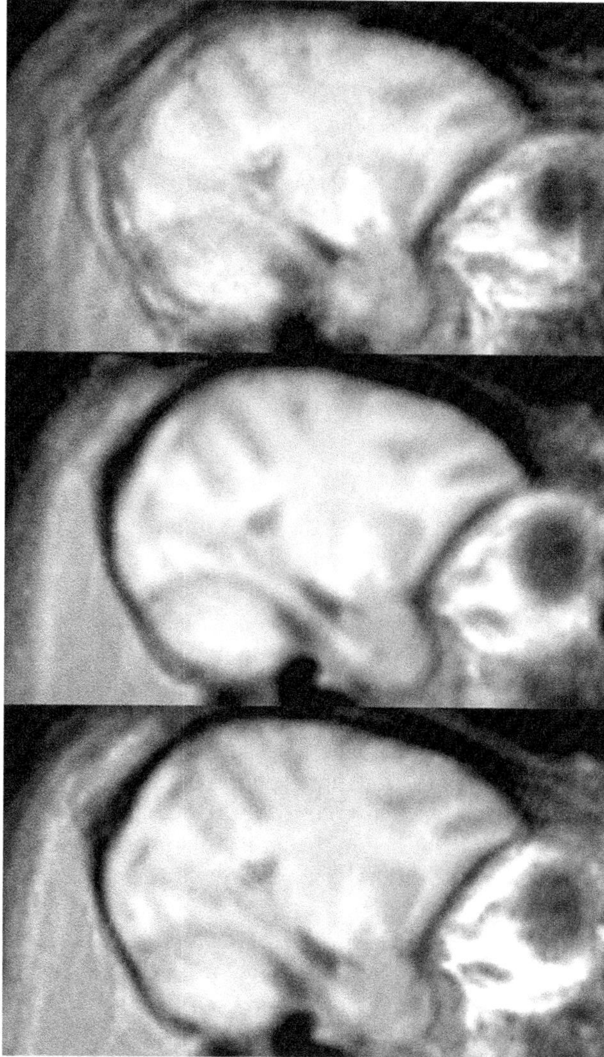

Fig. 2 Sagittal section from an image formed by averaging the transformed MPRAGE from each of nine normal baboons. (Top) Using our 1997 method (template$_0$). (Center) The first iteration using the new method (template$_1$). (Bottom) The final MRI template image (template$_{20}$ = "b2k"). For further details, see text. Note that the improvement in registration of extracranial structures is especially remarkable, as all transformations were computed after explicitly masking out these voxels in the target image.Reprinted from Black *et al.* (2001) with permission.

method described in the previous section. These transformed images are then averaged, producing substantially improved uniformity of registration. This average is then registered to template$_0$ to prevent spatial drift and to ensure backward compatibility, yielding a new image, template$_1$ (center image in Fig. 2).

This process is iterated 20 times to create the final template image. Specifically, for $i = 1\text{–}20$, the individual MR images are registered to template$_{i-1}$, the most recent iteration of the average template image. These transformed individual images are averaged to create a (temporary) new average image. Third, this temporary image is registered to the template$_0$ image to ensure backward compatibility. At each step, template$_{i+1}$ is recreated from the original unfiltered MPRAGE images using matrix multiplication and a single resampling step, thus avoiding the accumulation of smoothing due to repeated interpolation. Because the coregistration algorithm matches the intensity of the image from each baboon, after averaging, each animal contributes approximately equally to the each iteration of the template. After the first few iterations, the transformation matrices describing registration of the individual images to the template image remain consistent. A C-shell script automates this process. The final "b2k" template is template$_{20}$ (bottom image in Fig. 2).

5. Validation

Visual inspection of the new template image shows substantial preservation of the high-spatial-frequency image content (bottom image in Fig. 2).

For quantitative results, we tested absolute three-dimensional error (distance in mm) for 23 subcortical test points and 12 cortical sulcal landmarks. An expert rater identified these points in the published atlas (Davis and Huffman, 1968) (for the subcortical landmarks) or in the final template atlas image (cortical landmarks). Later, the expert rater identified these same points on the individual images registered to the final template. The images were displayed without the atlas coordinates so that the expert rater was unaware of the "correct" answer. The mean error at each point (i.e., the Cartesian distance from the atlas coordinate to the point identified in the individual image, averaged across animals) ranged from 0.99 to 2.43 mm. The mean error averaged across all nine baboons and all subcortical test points was 1.53 mm, compared to a minimum possible mean error of 0.54 mm. The maximum error for any point in any animal was 3.96 mm. The mean error for the cortical test points across all nine baboons was 1.99 mm, with a maximum error of 4.43 mm.

We also tested absolute error in subcortical and cortical test points for four animals that were not used in creating the template atlas image. Testing these images for absolute error provides an estimate for the generalizability of our method. The average subcortical error in these images was 1.85 mm, with a maximum error of 5.24 mm. The average cortical error was 2.63 mm, with a maximum error of 6.61 mm.

B. Development of the Baboon Blood Flow Template, "b2kf"

1. Subjects and Image Acquisition

The PET template image was created using 396 total individual PET images from seven of the nine normal baboons used to create the MRI template. Usually, 12 [^{15}O] water PET blood flow images were obtained from a single animal on a given day. Because the head of the subject was held in a fixed position relative to the scanner for all 12 scans, the 12 individual scans were averaged to form one image for each subject. We had confirmed previously that there was no meaningful movement of the brain among these individual scans (Black *et al.*, 1996).

2. Registration

Within-modality image registration (PET-PET) was performed as described for the MRI template. Cross-modality (PET-MRI) image registration was implemented using a variant of the image intensity gradient correlation method (Andersson *et al.*, 1995; Pluim *et al.*, 2000). Whereas in the original method the intensity gradient vector orientations were ignored, here the cost function depended on the relative orientations of these vector quantities. Again, other voxel-based image registration techniques could have been substituted. All cross-modality registrations were performed within a single subject and therefore were modeled as a rigid-body (six-parameter) transform.

3. Template Image Development

To create the PET template image, each subject's 12-scan average PET image was registered to that same subject's MPRAGE image. That subject's MPRAGE image was then registered to the MRI template image as described previously. The two transformation matrices resulting from these two registration steps were then multiplied to obtain a matrix that transformed the individual PET scans to MRI template atlas space (PET to MRI $\times$ MRI to template $=$ PET to template).

4. Validation

The PET template was created by registering a 12-scan average PET image to that subject's MPRAGE image and then registering that MPRAGE image to the MRI template atlas. Ideally, these atlas-space 12-scan PET images would be identical to a transformation obtained by directly registering the 12-scan PET image to the PET template image. To test this, we compared the rotation, translation, and stretch (also called zoom) parameters computed from the transformation matrices from these two methods. The results were highly similar, thus confirming the accuracy of the two image registration methods, as well as of the two templates.

C. Macaque Template Images: The "n2k" and "n2kf" Templates

Using essentially identical methods, we created macaque template images by iteratively combining MPRAGE and $[^{15}O]$ water PET blood flow images from 12 male, neurologically normal *Macaca nemestrina* monkeys (pigtail macaques) (Black *et al.*, 2001b). Images were created in register with the baboon b2k template given our interest in comparing functional imaging data across species (Hershey *et al.*, 2000; Kaufman *et al.*, 2003). Additionally, we registered the monkey template to a published three-dimensional image set including MRI and labeled cryosection images from a single macaque (Cannestra *et al.*, 1997). The resulting "n2kc" atlas is also available at the n2k web site.

We validated the template accuracy using a subset of the points described earlier. Even when comparing macaque landmarks to the baboon template, the measured accuracy was 1.9 mm (mean error). This error measurement includes not only image registration error but also all of the following: human error in identification of brain landmarks, true nonlinear morphologic differences among the individual macaque brains, morphologic differences between species, and the degree to which the baboon atlas is atypical of living baboon brains. This quite reasonable between-species fit may seem remarkable, but in fact, both we and others had shown previously that a macaque brain image can be aligned linearly to a baboon atlas with fairly good accuracy (Black *et al.*, 1997a; Martin and Bowden, 1996).

D. Using the Templates in Analyzing Functional Imaging Data

1. Registering a PET Image to Atlas Space

The focus of this section is to illustrate some typical uses of the MRI and PET templates in neuroimaging studies based on our functional imaging studies of pharmacologic activation in baboons and macaques (Black *et al.*, 1997b, 2000, 2002a,b; Hershey *et al.*, 2000). We usually had 5–12 [^{15}O] water PET blood flow images on a given day. We use an in-house program that registers each individual PET scan to each other PET scan and computes a best-fit transformation matrix for each scan to every other PET scan. We then create an average scan by transforming each scan to one of the scans (usually the first) and averaging them together. This 12-scan average image then serves as a source image for the rest of the process of transforming the scans to atlas space.

A different program then registers the 12-scan average image to atlas space. This can be done by registering the 12-scan average image directly to the PET template[1] or by registering to atlas space via that particular animal's MPRAGE. In the latter case, the 12-scan average PET image is registered via a rigid body model transformation to the MPRAGE, and the MPRAGE is registered to the MRI template image, as described earlier. The transformation from the 12-scan average image to PET template is then computed by matrix multiplication of the 12-scan to MPRAGE and MPRAGE to the MRI template. As shown in the previous section, either method is sound and produces very similar results. The direct PET to flow

[1] The atlas template images are freely available on the Internet (www.purl.org/net/kbmd/b2k and www.purl.org/net/kbmd/n2k). The template images are available in various formats, including the SPM format with atlas origin labeled; this allows SPM99 to automatically report results in atlas coordinates. Although we have used our own software for image alignment, the templates are suitable for use as targets with other registration methods, including automated image registration (AIR) or the methods included in the SPM suite of tools.

template method minimizes assumptions and is available if a structural MR image from the same time period is not available.

2. Use in SPM Analysis

The aforementioned steps result in functional images from a number of different baboons (or monkeys) registered to a common template with greatly reduced spatial differences between subjects. The images can now be analyzed for differences based on an independent variable of interest. Various approaches could be used, and the images could be analyzed for structural as well as functional images. We apply SPM99 (http://www.fil.ion.ucl.ac.uk/spm/spm99.html) to these images to generate voxelwise statistical maps and to correct for multiple comparisons. In doing so, we currently use the following protocol.

We copy a MATLAB.mat file to each template-registered image included in the analysis; this file identifies image orientation and the origin to SPM99 and facilitates use of our preferred image format in the preceding steps. The SPM99 "Full Monty" option allows explicit identification of a mask image, which we supply (available at: (http://www.purl.org/net/kbmd/b2k and www.purl.org/net/kbmd/n2k). For each image, we compute the average in-brain image intensity over the voxels included in this standard brain mask and include the list of global brain intensities as a linear covariate of no interest. Independent variables are identified for each scan. In several of our studies, this includes Boolean variables identifying each subject (to account for subject-specific effects) and the dose of drug given before each scan. An F image is computed to allow a single primary analysis that identifies either increases or decreases of regional blood flow with any of several independent variables of interest (e.g., drug dose). Subsequent analyses use pairwise contrasts to show unidirectional effects of a single variable. Our convention is to accept as significant clusters of voxels for which SPM99 computes a *corrected* p-value of 0.05 or less. The clusters that enter this analysis are defined by contiguous voxels at which the F (or t) statistic exceeds the value corresponding to $p = 0.001$. To avoid type II error, all such clusters whose peak falls in the brain are reported for heuristic value, without a claim of statistical significance.

E. Anatomic Interpretation of Statistical Images

The final use of the templates is to provide anatomic identification for the results of the statistical analysis. In SPM99, activated clusters can be color coded readily for intensity and superimposed directly onto the gray-scale atlas image for visual inspection (Fig. 3). For activation foci falling within the published atlas(es) (Cannestra *et al.*, 1997; Davis and Huffman, 1968), reference to those works provides quick anatomic identification. In the baboon atlas, cortical points can be displayed on a three-dimensional rendering of the brain; atlas points can be transformed into the coordinates of the display software by simple addition.

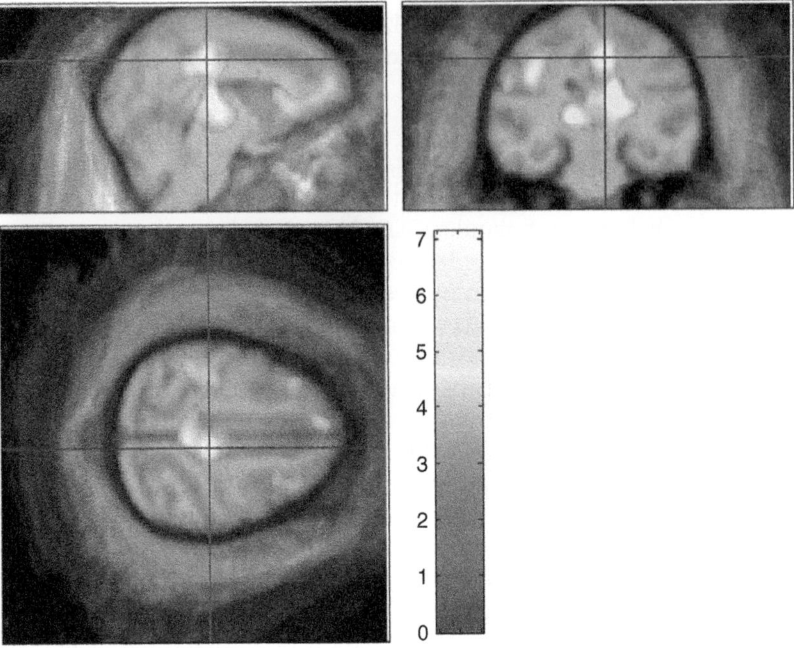

Fig. 3 An image consisting of voxel-by-voxel one-tailed t values (in color) from a comparison of regional cerebral blood flow (rCBF) at rest to rCBF after 0.5 mg/kg pramipexole IV in seven normal baboons (previously unpublished image from the study reported by Black *et al.*, 2002). Prior to statistical analysis, individual positron emission tomographic images of rCBF were aligned to the b2k template, and hence to the Davis and Huffman (1968) atlas of baboon brain. The t image is thresholded at 3.19, the value corresponding to $p = 0.001$ (87 df), and superimposed on slices from the b2k MRI atlas (in gray and white). Crosshairs are centered at atlas coordinate (Black *et al.*, 1997; Perlmutter *et al.*, 1991; Viergever *et al.*, 1995) (posterior cingulate cortex).

We use the Volume Render program of ANALYZE, the template MR image, and the brain mask (loaded as a binary object) for this purpose.

III. Discussion

A. Similar Methods

Greer *et al.* (2002) took a somewhat different approach by creating a baboon template based on a single brain and labeling anatomy based on their template image. Cross *et al.* (2000) created a multisubject macaque template with reference to the bicommissural line. Another approach to data analysis that can provide valuable insights is to transform images to a flat map of the cortex (Van Essen *et al.*, 2001).

B. Future Applications

A surprisingly wide array of nonhuman primate brains can be registered linearly quite reasonably to each other (Black *et al.*, 2001b; Bowden and Dubach, 2000) Therefore, brain images from other macaque species, and perhaps other primate species, can likely be registered to the b2k or n2kc atlases. In order to work with data from species with substantially different brain volumes, however, the first step will likely be to estimate the approximate ratio, R, of the brain volume of the new species to the brain volume of the template (given on the b2k and n2k web pages). Then, before registering images to the template, one will need to initialize the registering software with stretch (zoom) factors of $R^{1/3}$ in each dimension. Alternatively, for some brain atlases in other species, digital images are available that could be useful in the first or "bootstrapping" step of creating a new template corresponding to that atlas.

Acknowledgments

Preparation of this manuscript was supported in part by NINDS Grants NS044598 and NS39913.

References

Andersson, J. L., *et al.* (1995). *J. Nucl. Med.* **36,** 1307.
Ashburner, J., and Friston, K. J. (1999). *Hum. Brain Mapp.* **7,** 254.
Black, K. J., *et al.* (1996). *J. Comput. Assist. Tomogr.* **20,** 855.
Black, K. J., *et al.* (1997a). *J. Comput. Assist. Tomogr.* **21,** 881.
Black, K. J., *et al.* (1997b). *J. Neurosci.* **17,** 3168.
Black, K. J., *et al.* (2000). *J. Neurophysiol.* **84,** 549.
Black, K. J., *et al.* (2001a). *Neuroimage* **14,** 736.
Black, K. J., *et al.* (2001b). *Neuroimage* **14,** 744.
Black, K. J., *et al.* (2002a). *J. Neuropsychiatry Clin. Neurosci.* **14,** 118.
Black, K. J., *et al.* (2002b). *Proc. Natl. Acad. Sci. USA* **99,** 17113.
Bowden, D. M., and Dubach, M. F. (2000). *In* "Primate Brain Maps: Structure of the Macaque Brain" (R. F. Martin, and D. M. Bowden, eds.), p. 38. Elsevier, New York.
Cannestra, A. F., *et al.* (1997). *Brain Res. Bull.* **43,** 141.
Corbetta, M., *et al.* (1998). *Neuron* **21,** 761.
Cross, D. J., *et al.* (2000). *J. Nucl. Med.* **41,** 1879.
Davis, R., and Huffman, R. (1968). "A Stereotaxic Atlas of the Brain of the Baboon." University of Texas Press, Austin, TX.
Fox, P. T., *et al.* (1985). *J. Comput. Assist. Tomogr.* **9,** 141.
Fox, P. T., *et al.* (1988). *J. Cereb. Blood Flow Metab.* **8,** 642.
Friston, K. J., *et al.* (1995). *Hum. Brain Mapp.* **2,** 165.
Greer, P., *et al.* (2002). *Brain Res. Bull.* **58,** 429.
Hershey, T., *et al.* (2000). *Exp. Neurol.* **166,** 342.
Kaufman, J. A., *et al.* (2003). *Am. J. Phys. Anthropol.* **121,** 369.
Martin, R. F., and Bowden, D. M. (1996). *Neuroimage* **4,** 119.
Perlmutter, J. S., *et al.* (1991). *J. Cereb. Blood Flow Metab.* **11,** 229.

Pluim, J. P., *et al.* (2000). *IEEE Trans. Med. Imaging* **19,** 809.
Raichle, M. E., *et al.* (1991). *J. Cereb. Blood Flow Metab.* **11,** S364.
Snyder, A. Z. (1996). *In* "Quantification of Brain Function Using PET" (R. Myers *et al.*, eds.) Academic Press, San Diego.
Strother, S. C., *et al.* (1994). *J. Comput. Assist. Tomogr.* **18,** 954.
Talairach, J., and Tournoux, P. (1988). Co-Planar Stereotaxic Atlas of the Human Brain. Theime Verlag, New York.
Van Essen, D. C., *et al.* (2001). *Vision Res.* **41,** 1359.
Viergever, M. A., *et al.* (1995). *In* "Image Processing" (M. H. Loew, ed.), SPIE Proceedings, **2434,** p. 2.
Woods, R. P., *et al.* (1992). *J. Comput. Assist. Tomogr.* **16,** 620.
Woods, R. P., *et al.* (1993). *J. Comput. Assist. Tomogr.* **14,** 536.
Woods, R. P., *et al.* (1998). *J. Comput. Assist. Tomogr.* **22,** 153.

CHAPTER 5

Magnetic Resonance Imaging of Brain Function

Stuart Clare

Department of Clinical Neurology
Centre for Functional Magnetic Resonance Imaging of the Brain
John Radcliffe Hospital
University of Oxford
Headington, Oxford OX39DU
United Kingdom

I. Update
  A. Hints and Tips for Performing fMRI
II. Introduction
III. Experimental Procedures
  A. Overview of Methods
  B. Blood Oxygenation and MRI
  C. Rapid MRI for fMRI
  D. Experimental Design
  E. Analysis of Images
IV. An Application of Functional MRI
V. Discussion and Conclusion
References

I. Update

The scope of human behavior that has been studied using fMRI and the range of uses to which that information has been put continues to grow and grow. From investigating new drug therapies, to informing marketing executives, many people want to use functional imaging to gain more insight into the brain. However, good experimental design and practice still lies at the heart of producing useful insights rather than just pretty pictures.

MRI systems operating at 3 T, offering increased sensitivity to brain activation, are now increasingly commonplace in hospital radiology departments. There are

DOI: 10.1016/B978-0-12-375043-3.00005-6

also an ever-increasing number of 7 T systems now available. This push to higher field strength, offering the possibility of localizing activations to a very high spatial extent (<1 mm), is also complemented by a number of other hardware developments such as receive RF coils with 32 or more independent channels, boosting sensitivity by factors of 4 or more (Wiggins *et al.*, 2006).

While the basic methods outlined in this chapter remain the same, the desire for a more quantifiable and specific measure of brain activity has lead to an increase in methods for fMRI. The use of MRI-based quantitative cerebral blood flow (CBF) measurements (Liu *et al.*, 2007) and cerebral blood volume measurements (Lu *et al.*, 2003) has increased, giving the ability to tease apart the different components of the hemodynamic response to neural activation. Combining measurements of CBF with traditional BOLD detection of the hemodynamic response allows comparison in activation levels in subjects between scans on different days (Leontiev and Buxton, 2007).

One other area that has seen an increase over the recent years is the development of targeted "molecular" contrast agents. These compounds contain an MR image-enhancing molecule (such as gadolinium or ultra small particles of iron oxide) bound to other molecules that will in turn bind to specific targets in the body (Frank *et al.*, 2004). While use of these compounds in humans to detect brain activity is not yet possible, this area is sure to increase over the coming years.

A. Hints and Tips for Performing fMRI

- Design of the stimulus paradigm is crucial to the success of the experiment: choose baseline and task conditions that tease apart the effect you are interested in.
- Be sure your stimulus presentation equipment is MR compatible and does not introduce radio waves into the MR environment.
- Estimate your effect size, with either literature values or pilot experiments, to ensure that you have enough trials or blocks in your main experiment.
- Understand what the fMRI analysis packages are doing "under the hood": they may offer simple interfaces to get your data analyzed, but you will get much more from your data if you understand the statistics they are computing.
- Analyze your data as you go along, rather than waiting to the end of the study: many flaws in the design can be picked up at an early stage.

II. Introduction

The rapid development of methods for noninvasive brain mapping, particularly over the past decade, has led to exciting advances in our understanding of the human brain. Foremost in these methodologies is the technique of functional magnetic resonance imaging (fMRI). Utilizing the intrinsic magnetic properties of the blood, it is possible to identify the brain region associated with a specific sensory, motor, or even cognitive task to a high spatial precision. Unlike positron emission tomography (PET), MRI does not use radioactively labeled compounds and is essentially noninvasive and safe for repeat studies. Although fMRI does not share the temporal resolution of electroencephalography (EEG) or magnetoencephalography (MEG), it does have a spatial resolution of millimeters, and the most recent experiments suggest that it may be able to detect activations at the level of the cortical layers (Silva and Koretsky, 2002).

While fMRI is a complex methodology, developments in recent years, particularly by the scanner manufacturers and other commercial and academic groups, have meant that the tools for fMRI, while expensive, are more commonly available. In particular, the available software for both fMRI stimulus presentation and image analysis are highly sophisticated and user-friendly. This means that human fMRI is now achievable by research groups without dedicated physics and image analysis support.

III. Experimental Procedures

A. Overview of Methods

Functional MRI relies on detecting the small changes in image brightness on MRI scans, associated with the hemodynamic changes in the brain, in response to a specific external stimulus or "internal" cognitive process (Belliveau *et al.*, 1991). Carrying out an fMRI experiment therefore consists of three primary components: presenting or otherwise cueing the stimulus, scanning the brain rapidly using MRI, and analyzing the MRI scans to detect changes in image intensity.

While the subject is being scanned repeatedly, ideally covering the whole brain every 3 s, a stimulus or cue is presented to them. This could be a simple visual stimulus, such as a flashing light, or a more complex stimulus, such as a list of numbers to remember and recall at some point. This stimulus is repeated a number of times to build up confidence in determining the brain regions that are truly responding to the stimulus, while averaging out other "random" brain processes. The resulting images are then analyzed using computer software to detect those regions in the images that show a significantly time-locked response to the stimulus. These regions are displayed as bright "activations" overlaid on a conventional brain scan or brain atlas, such as shown in Fig. 1.

Human fMRI can be performed using most modern MRI scanners found in radiology departments of many hospitals, operating at a field strength of 1.5 T. However, in recent years, the desire to detect these small hemodynamic changes has led to the successful use of field strengths of 3–4 T in research MRI systems. A small number of research sites worldwide are experimenting with the use of even

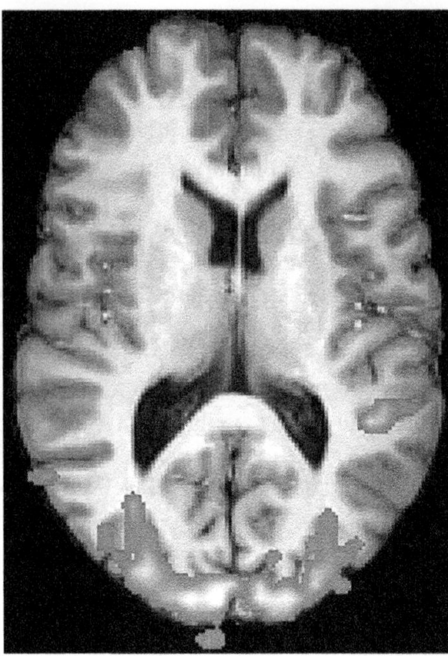

Fig. 1 Example of an fMRI result showing activation in the visual areas resulting from the subject looking at a contrast reversing checkerboard stimulus. (See plate no. 1 in the Color Plate Section.)

higher field strengths for human imaging, the highest currently being 9 T; however, the difficulties with producing high-quality human brain images diminish the benefits in signal detection offered at such high field strengths (Chan, 2002).

Functional MRI of nonhuman primates and rodents is covered in more detail in other chapters in this volume. For the rest of this chapter, the use of human subjects is assumed; however, much of the underlying methodology is the same for human or animal subjects.

B. Blood Oxygenation and MRI

The oxygen carrier in blood, hemoglobin, gets its red color from the iron molecule, which forms the binding site of oxygen. This presence of iron in the molecule makes it magnetically sensitive. In its deoxygenated state, hemoglobin displays paramagnetic properties, meaning that the local magnetic field is increased in the presence of an external magnetic field (Thulborn *et al.*, 1982). In contrast, oxygenated hemoglobin is diamagnetic and has little effect on the local magnetic field. The effect of these local changes in magnetic field can be detected in type of MR scan that is said to be T_2* weighted. On a T_2*-weighted MR image, a pixel that contains predominantly oxygenated hemoglobin will appear brighter than a pixel that contains predominantly oxygenated hemoglobin. This form of image contrast in MRI is termed blood oxygenation level-dependent (BOLD) contrast (Ogawa *et al.*, 1990).

Although it is possible to quantify the change in hemoglobin oxygenation using MRI, it is typical in fMRI to just detect the relative signal changes. The exact link between neuronal firing and the BOLD signal change that is detected is complex and not entirely understood. Upon the metabolic demand that synaptic activity produces, oxygen is removed from the blood and the concentration of deoxyhemoglobin increases. This would result in a small dip in the MR image intensity, which is sometimes observed in fMRI experiments. However, the much stronger effect is the large increase in image intensity that follows, peaking at about 6 s after the neural activity. This represents a large increase in the concentration of oxyhemoglobin, far greater than its resting state level. This results from a large increase in the local blood flow rate and local blood volume due to capillary expansion. While this apparently excessive overcompensation in oxygen delivery was initially a puzzling result, recent physiological models have demonstrated the need for such increases to maintain the necessary oxygen delivery rate to the mitochondria (Buxton *et al.*, 1998).

Following this peak in local oxygenation level, the signal returns back toward its baseline state, but is often observed to decrease still further (known as the undershoot), as the relative contribution of oxygen extraction, blood flow, and blood volume return to their baseline state. Most fMRI "activations" are detected as regions that display the large increase in signal, peaking several seconds after the stimulus. In fact, the presence of either the initial dip in signal or the poststimulus undershoot is not detected in many experiments, as it seems to vary by brain location and can be obscured by image noise, particularly at lower field strengths (Buxton, 2001).

The complex physiological processes that give rise to the signal changes observed in fMRI mean that there are a number of reasons for caution in interpreting the experimental results. First, and most obviously, is that the signal arises from hemodynamic effects and not directly from neural activity. The location of peak BOLD effects could indeed be some distance from the site of the activating neurons. This is particularly the case when imaging using methods that are more sensitive to the signal from the large draining veins, which could be centimeters from the actual activation site (Kim *et al.*, 1994). To guard against this particular problem it is advisable to interpret the spatial location of fMRI activations with reference to a map of veins (as can be acquired easily using MRI or from standard atlases).

Second, thought must be given to the time characteristics of the fMRI response. The timing of peak activation relative to the signal needs to be taken into account when analyzing the images, as it may vary over brain regions. Care must also be exercised in interpreting any differences in signal timing as representing temporal differences in the onset of neural activation. While it is certainly possible to obtain an indication of neural timing from the BOLD response, a lag in signal in one region relative to another does not necessarily mean a difference in neural timing and may just represent a difference in blood supply in those regions (Miezin *et al.*, 2000). The large delay after activation before the signal returns to baseline also has implications for experimental design and is discussed in more detail later.

It should also be noted here that BOLD contrast is not the only way to perform fMRI, although it is by far the easiest and most commonly used method. MR images can also be made sensitive to the blood flow rate alone. Such experiments suffer from low signal-to-noise ratio (SNR) and do not have the same temporal resolution as BOLD fMRI, but are very useful in interpreting the BOLD signal changes and may turn out to be more spatially specific than BOLD (Liu *et al.*, 2002).

C. Rapid MRI for fMRI

MR images are essentially maps of water content in the brain generated by the NMR phenomenon that certain atoms, when placed in a strong magnetic field, will absorb and emit radiofrequency energy at a specific frequency dictated by the strength of that applied magnetic field. However, it is straightforward in MRI to modulate this basic signal such that the intensity in a region of the image is not just dependent on water content but also on the local structural environment or other physiological parameters. Examples of this are the T_1- and T_2-weighted images often used in clinical diagnosis, where, for example, the region of cell damage produced by a stroke can be seen very clearly. Another example of this is the so-called T_2*-weighted image, which is highly sensitive to the local magnetic environment and is particularly sensitive to the BOLD effect (Haacke *et al.*, 1999).

A typical diagnostic MR image is optimized for spatial resolution and contrast to detect the particular pathology of interest. This typically means a scan time of several minutes. Although it is possible to do fMRI with a scan lasting minutes, the requirement of needing to keep a discrete set of brain regions active for such a time makes this impractical for anything other than the simplest experiment.

Speeding up the scanning process requires not only very high-performance scanner hardware, but comes at a cost to image quality. However, with the advent of fMRI, most modern scanners have the technological capability to run very fast imaging methods.

The most common fast imaging method used for fMRI is echo planar imaging (EPI). This method is able to collect data from a single "slice" through the brain in less than 100 ms, meaning that, at coarse resolution, it is possible to scan the whole brain in around 3 s (Stehling *et al.*, 1991). EPI also has the benefit of being inherently a T_2*-weighted sequence, so it is ideally suited to BOLD fMRI.

The largest drawback to using EPI is that the images often contain image distortion and signal loss. An example of this is shown in Fig. 2. The air-filled sinuses that sit below the frontal lobes of the brain cause a "hole" to appear in the EPI images, compared to the standard MRI, and the frontal lobes also appear

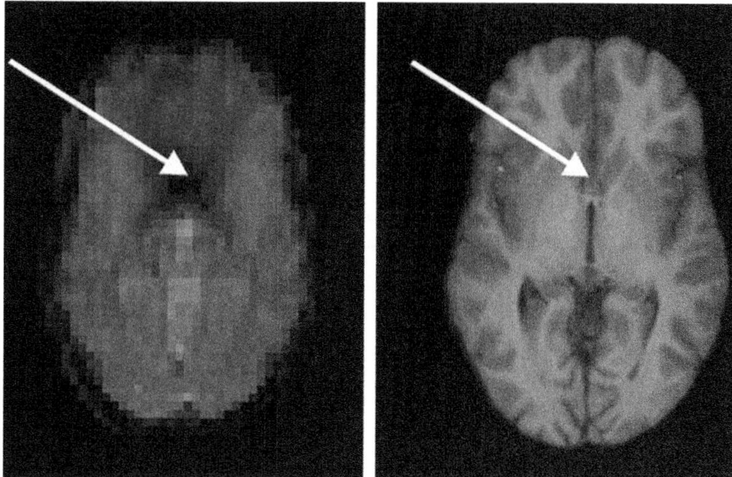

Fig. 2 An example of signal loss in the frontal lobes seen in echo planar imaging (EPI). (Left) A typical EPI scan used for fMRI and (right) the same slice as seen in a conventional MRI scan. Brain tissue that is clearly visible in the conventional MRI scan appears missing in the EPI scan, particularly in the region indicated by the arrow.

smeared out and distorted (Jezzard and Clare, 1999). Such effects mean that it is difficult to accurately detect activations in these regions of the brain. Several methods may be used to try and address this problem, such as correcting the distortions by using a "field map" (Jezzard and Balaban, 1995) by using specially designed mouthpieces graphite to compensate for the effect of air sinuses (Wilson *et al.*, 2002), or by using imaging methods similar to EPI that do not suffer from distortion (Glover and Law, 2001), although these often have their own disadvantages.

Unfortunately, the characteristics of the EPI method that make it susceptible to signal loss near sinuses are also those that make it sensitive to the BOLD effect. A typical fMRI experiment on a human subject using EPI would have image pixel sizes of 3×3 mm^2 and use a slice thickness of between 3 and 6 mm. Using thinner slices is one way of reducing signal loss near sinuses, but again this could reduce sensitivity to the BOLD effect (Merboldt *et al.*, 2000). Another parameter that affects signal loss is known as the "echo time" or TE. By reducing the echo time, signal loss is reduced, but again this comes at a cost to BOLD sensitivity. In practice, an echo time of 30–50 ms gives good results over the whole brain, but this is a parameter worth varying in initial pilot experiments to find the optimum balance in the brain regions of interest (Clare *et al.*, 2001).

One final note on rapid MRI is that these methods produce a high level of acoustic noise, often over 100 dB. This means that it is essential to provide the subject with adequate ear protection and warn them prior to the experiment.

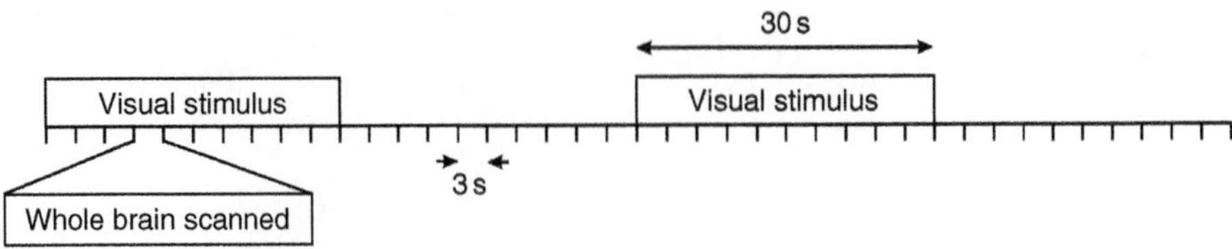

Fig. 3 A schematic diagram of a typical fMRI experiment where the whole brain is scanned every 3 s and alternating periods of visual stimulus and no stimulus are given every 30 s.

D. Experimental Design

The simplest form of fMRI experiment consists of blocks of stimulus presentation and "rest," interleaved such as illustrated in Fig. 3 for a visual stimulus. Typical timings of such a block paradigm are 30 s of stimulus and 30 s of rest, both repeated four times, with the whole brain being scanned once every 3 s. Critical to the success of the experiment is that there is a single clear difference between the task and the rest condition. It is not conceivable that the brain is completely inactive during the "rest" period, but it needs to be assumed that such activity is equally likely to be present during the task period as the rest period.

Because activations are detected by comparing serial MRI scans, any subject movement between each scan will reduce the ability to detect them. It is, therefore, important to minimize subject movement. For most short fMRI experiments, this is best done by using foam pads around the subject's head. Such pads or pillows not only provide support but also act as points of reference for the subjects as they try and keep their own head still. Many experimenters advocate the use of thermoplastic masks or bite bars to keep the subject still. While these do minimize head movement very effectively, they are often uncomfortable for the subject and usually require some time to get used to using them.

Whatever stimulus is used, it is likely that some form of visual stimulus or cue will need to be given to the subject either to stimulate the visual cortex directly, to instruct the subject in the timing and pacing of a movement task, or present cognitive stimuli such as patterns of letters to compare or remember. The most versatile way of presenting such stimuli is to use a high-quality video projector connected to a computer. This can project text or images onto a screen near the end of the scanner, at the subject's feet. Then an angled mirror above the subject's face, or a prism arrangement, enables the subject to view the screen. There are a number of more specialized systems that deliver the picture directly to glasses worn by the subject; however, the complexity and expense of these systems only make their use justified for particular applications that need higher control on what the subject sees.

Visual presentation is not the only way to present stimuli to subjects. As indicated earlier, the high acoustic noise environment of the scanner is not ideal for using auditory stimuli; however, it is possible to use MRI-compatible headphones (either pneumatic or electrostatic). Successful auditory studies have been accomplished by scanning at a slower rate, with short gaps in the scanning during which the speech or sound is played (Hall *et al.*, 1999). Other devices, such as vibrotactile stimulators to stimulate the somato-sensory cortex, thermal devices to stimulate the pain network, or olfactometers to deliver smells, have all been used in the MRI environment. As with all equipment that comes in contact with a subject, it is essential that there is no chance of it causing any harm. The scanner environment adds additional constraints, both on safety and on the ability to get high-quality MR images, so it is important to check carefully before even taking a device into the magnet room.

As well as presenting a stimulus to a subject, it is often desirable to record some response from the subject. The most simple and versatile way to do this is with an MRI compatible, four button box. The subject can rest their four fingers of one hand on each of the buttons on the box, and the response can be fed back to the control computer for recording which button was pressed and the precise timing. Interface with the computer is usually best done via a dedicated analog and digital interface card (such as from National Instruments, Austin, TX), which should be able to handle not only the signals from button boxes but also from joysticks or other analog devices, and be able to control other stimulus presentation modalities that require a digital or analog signal. Getting the subject to verbalize a response is not advisable in general because the movement of the head caused by speaking can reduce the ability to detect small activations. Additionally, it can be hard to hear any response in the noisy environment of the scanner during the experiment.

Software for cueing the experiment and presenting the stimuli is available commercially (e.g., Presentation, Neurobehavioral Systems, Albany, CA) or from research groups (e.g., DMDX, www.u.arizona.edu/~kforster/dmdx/dmdx.htm; Cogent, www.vislab.ucl.ac.uk/Cogent). Such software enables a series of stimuli to be cued up then played out sequentially and will record the nature and timing of any responses by the subject. The pacing of an experiment relative to the acquisition of the scans is critically important, as it is the final images that contain the signal of interest. While this might seem trivial, it is often the case that neither the scanner nor the stimulus presentation computer can be relied upon to keep exact time. While this timing difference may only be one-hundredths of a second, over a long scan run this can make a significant difference. It is usually possible to arrange for the scanner to output a timing (TTL) trigger at the start of acquiring each scan. This trigger can then be detected by the stimulus presentation computer and be used to start the next stimulus.

A block design paradigm, where there are relatively long blocks of stimulation and rest, is suitable for many applications, but can suffer from a number of problems. First, it may not be possible to reliably get a brain region to be active for such a long period of time. Often habituation will occur as the subject easily learns a task or loses interest in the stimulus. There are also some stimuli that need to be presented for short periods of time, such as painful ones. Second, in some cases, particularly cognitive paradigms, it is not desirable to use the same type of stimuli continually. For example, if the experiment requires the subject to discriminate between stimuli, they may quickly learn that the response stays the same for 30 s and make the cognitive part of the paradigm invalid. Third, there are some cases where it is desirable to separate out brain regions that are involved in different aspects of a task. This is particularly the case in experiments on memory, where different brain networks may be involved in the storage of information to the retrieval. To deal with the second problem, it is possible to carry out a block design experiment where the majority of stimuli are of one type in the "task" period and of the other type in the "rest" period, but there are a few of the other type added to keep the novelty component of the experiment.

An alternative to block designs are "event-related" designs. This design type is similar to that used in evoked potential EEG recordings in the brain where a single stimulus is presented at some repetition rate. In EEG, this is particularly suitable, as the electrical activity associated with the stimulus lasts less than a few hundred milliseconds. In fMRI, however, where the BOLD stimulus response takes 15–20 s to return to baseline following the stimulus, waiting such a long time between stimuli can be less suitable. This method is useful for looking for brain networks responding to different parts of a complex task (such as the memory illustration given earlier), but a more efficient use of event-related fMRI is to present the single stimuli at shorter intervals, often randomized in time. The analysis of such data is more complex, as it requires a model of how the overlapping BOLD responses to individual, closely spaced stimuli combine. However, such experiments can be highly efficient, particularly when stimuli need to be presented in some random order (Friston *et al.*, 1999).

E. Analysis of Images

In the simplest case, analysis of data consists of subtracting the average of all the images acquired during the "rest" phase of the experiment from the average of those acquired during the "task" period. While this gives a general qualitative indication of activated regions, in order to assign statistical significance to the result it is necessary to carry out a more detailed analysis. Also, this simple subtraction does not take account of the fact that the peak BOLD signal is delayed by around 6 s from the start of stimulation. In practice, typical fMRI analysis consists of three parts: preparation of fMRI data, model-based detection of the BOLD signal, and statistical inference and thresholding of the activations. If the results of a number of subjects are to be combined and compared, such as between a patient group and a control group, then an additional step of "group statistics" is required. Each of these areas is looked at in turn here. Most of these methods are available in commercial or freely available software packages (e.g., FSL, www.fmrib.ox.ac.uk/fsl; SPM, www.fil.ion.ucl.ac.uk/spm; AFNI, afni.nimh.nih.gov/afni; Brain Voyager, Brain Innovation, The Netherlands).

1. Preparation of fMRI Data

As explained in the previous section, minimizing the head motion of the subject is vital to getting good results. However, even with the best restraint methods, there is often some small residual motion that occurs in the images. This can be reduced by performing motion correction, in software, on the data. The motion correction algorithm compares each individual image with the first in the series and applies a mathematical transform to rotate or move the image until they look as similar to each other as possible (Friston *et al.*, 1996). Because the BOLD signal changes in the image are very small, they generally do not bias the motion correction. Next, the images are often spatially smoothed (blurred). The optimal detection of activations occurs when the spatial smoothness of the images is the same as the size of the region of activation. By applying spatial smoothing to the images, the ability to detect activations is often increased (Shaw *et al.*, 2003). Finally, the time course of each pixel in the image is filtered to remove long-term drifts in the signal and is sometimes filtered to smooth the time course of the signal over time.

2. Model-Based Detection of the BOLD Signal

Figure 4 shows a representation of a number of scans from an fMRI time series. If a single pixel in an activated region is selected, and its intensity is plotted over time, it displays a clear delayed response with respect to the stimulus presentation. If a mathematical model for the amount of delay and smoothing that is seen in the theoretical BOLD response with respect to the stimulus pattern is assumed (such as shown in the bottom line of Fig. 4), then a statistical measure of how likely that pixel is truly activated in response to the stimulus can be obtained by calculating the correlation coefficient between this theoretical line and the actual time course. Critical to the success of this method is the choice of mathematical model that turns the stimulus time course into a theoretical BOLD response. All of the software packages have a range of choices for this function, but a commonly used one is a gamma function convolution of the stimulus time series. The mathematical framework for this correlation-based approach, known as the general linear model (GLM), is not the only one that can be taken, and it does indeed include assumptions that may not be fully appropriate for fMRI data; however, for the majority of fMRI experiments, it is sensitive and statistically reliable (Friston *et al.*, 1995). The GLM can also be used to analyze the "event-related" fMRI experiments described earlier, again producing a model for the theoretical BOLD response given the stimulus timing pattern used. Analyzing the response through time of each pixel in the image results in a statistical "map" of the strength of correlation throughout the brain.

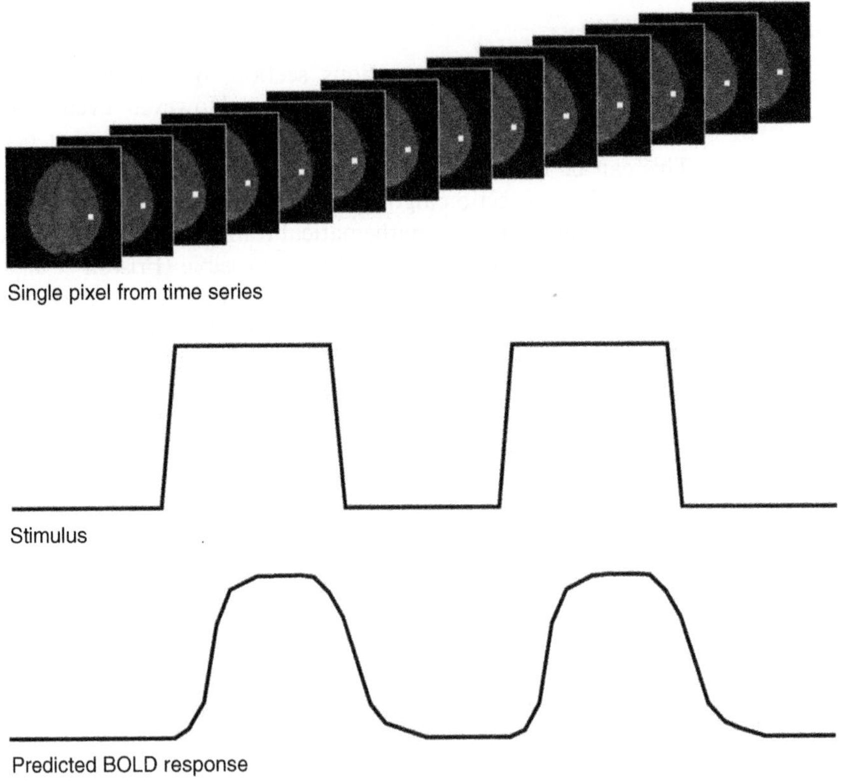

Fig. 4 Representation of the predicted BOLD response pattern (bottom line) to the stimulus (middle line) in single pixel that "activates" to that stimulus.

3. Statistical Inference and Thresholding of Activations

The output image produced by the GLM looks something like Fig. 5A. It is clear that there is a high correlation at the bottom of the image, but it is not clear yet if this is significant. It is possible to threshold the image so that only those individual pixels that have a correlation coefficient that is significant to better than $p < 0.5\%$, but in an image of approximately 10,000 pixels, we know that 50 pixels would be labeled as "activated" purely by chance. An alternative is to threshold at a much lower significant threshold (such as 0.5% divided by 10,000), but this stringent threshold risks missing genuinely activated pixels. As an alternative it is common to use information on the number of pixels near each other to increase our confidence in the result. For example, if we see 10 pixels in a block together all showing high correlation coefficients, then we can be more sure that this represents a genuine activation than if we saw one pixel on its own with a similarly high correlation coefficient. The fMRI analysis software packages all contain the

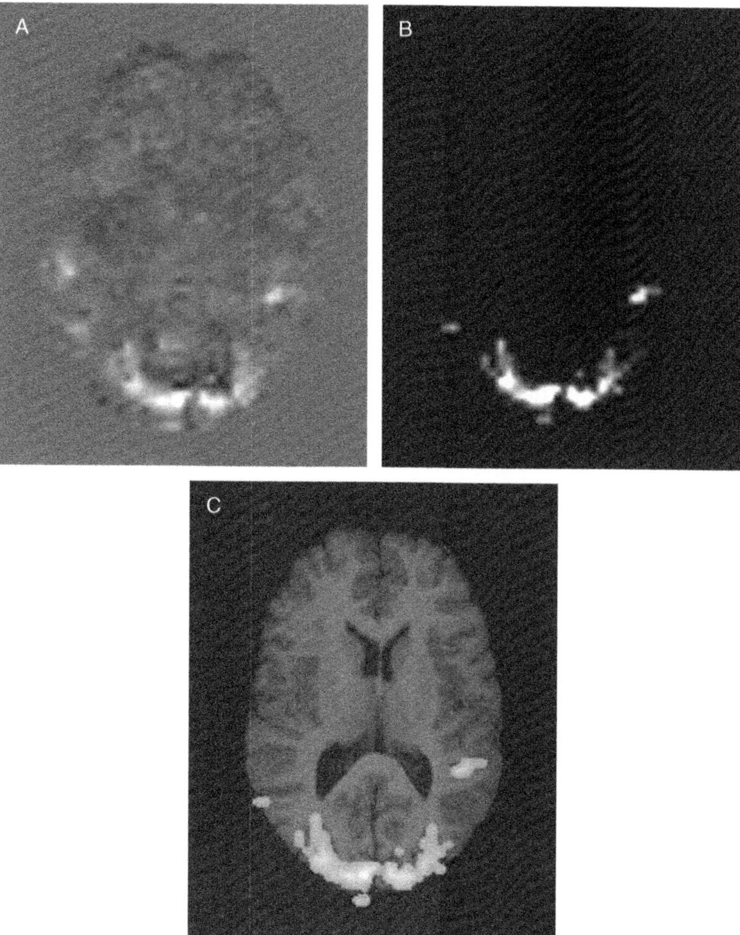

Fig. 5 (A) Statistical map obtained from the general linear output. This map is then thresholded at an appropriate p score (B) and is then overlaid on a high-quality MRI scan of the same subject's brain (C).

appropriate theory, such as that of Gaussian random field (Friston *et al.*, 1994) to threshold the activation images on the basis of both correlation coefficient (e.g., as reported as a "Z score") and pixel cluster size. What the software will output therefore is a list of pixel clusters that have a Z score of greater than say 2.3 (a good, if arbitrary, value to start with) and that have a pixel cluster size making the statistical significance (p-value) less than say 0.5%. These thresholded activation images can then be overlaid on the subject's high-quality MRI scan (to which the fMRI images have been aligned) or on a standard brain atlas, such as shown in Fig. 5C.

4. Group Comparisons

If a typical result from a group of subjects is requires or if a comparison between two groups needs to be made, then there are two additional steps that need to be performed. First, the MRI scans must be morphed to align to some standard brain template. Such brain templates have been made up of MRI scans from hundreds of individuals and are generally supplied with the software packages. Although not an ideal template, it is very common to report results with referenced to the atlas of Talairach based on a dissection of a single brain. Software for morphing to template brain and alignment to the Talairach atlas is included in most fMRI analysis packages. Once all the subjects' scans from a single study are aligned to the same template, further statistical analysis can be performed on data to show regions that are significantly activated across all subjects or ones that are differentially activated in one group relative to another.

IV. An Application of Functional MRI

The ability of the brain to reorganize functionally after injury is a fascinating but hard-to-study phenomenon. Functional MRI has been used to demonstrate the cortical changes that occur upon rehabilitation after stoke (Johansen-Berg *et al.*, 2002). Here, the experiment is described as an example of the integration of all the components described earlier to investigate brain function.

Patients with mild to moderate injury following stroke were scanned on four separate occasions, both before and after a movement therapy aimed at regaining motor control over their damaged side. In the scanner, the subjects were cued visually to tap their hand, which was resting on a wooden board, at a rate that was either 25% or 75% of their maximum tapping rate. A 6-min series of EPI scans, with an echo time of 30 ms and a repetition rate of 3 s, was recorded during tapping of first the unaffected hand and then the affected hand. A simple block design was used, similar to that illustrated in Fig. 3, with the subject resting their hand for 30 s between 30 s of hand tapping. For all scanning sessions the hand-tapping rate was kept constant, even if the subject was able on a later occasion to tap at a faster rate. This was essential for determining whether the brain activation patterns associated with performing the movements changed over time. A recovery score for each subject was also determined based on their motor performance before and after therapy.

Scans from the four sessions of each subject were analyzed together as one GLM analysis. This analysis was set up to detect not only correlations between the pixel time course and a predicted BOLD response to the stimulus but also in the same analysis, differences between the two sessions before therapy and the two sessions after therapy. This illustrates the strength of a well-designed GLM analysis; it is not necessary to individually analyze the results from each fMRI session and then look for differences in activation patterns, but it is possible to set up the analysis in such a way as to generate one statistical image with the particular result of interest, in this case the changes that have taken place after therapy.

The researchers then went on to perform a second level of analysis to obtain a summary result representing all the subjects. This was done by subtracting the pretherapy from the posttherapy activation image (unthresholded) for each subject and weighting this difference image by the recovery score for that subject. Combining these images across the group gave an image of areas where activation increases correlate with recovery across the group. The results of both the analysis of the individual subjects and the group analyses indicated that upon recovery, movement of the affected hand produced increased activity in the motor networks of the unaffected hand were being recruited to compensate for the damage on the affected side.

V. Discussion and Conclusion

The advent of fMRI has made a huge impact in the way that the brain is studied, both in the pure neuroscience setting and in a clinical context. The increasing availability of MRI scanners in hospitals throughout the world means that although the technology is expensive, it is increasingly available to researchers. This has been coupled with a solid development of tools for stimulus presentation and, importantly, for data analysis that has the sophistication and statistical rigor required for solid inference, coupled with an ease of use suitable for general laboratory use.

The next big challenge in the development of fMRI is to more fully understand, quantitatively, the relationship between the signals observed in the MRI scans and the underlying neural activity of which it is a marker. This will require not only more sophisticated imaging methodology and more complex physiological models but also way to get a closer measure of the working of the neuron *in vivo*. Here, the experiments performed on animals, as described in other chapters in this volume, will play a vital role.

References

Belliveau, J. W., Kennedy, D. N., Jr., McKinstry, R. C., Buchbinder, B. R., Weisskoff, R. M., Cohen, M. S., Vevea, J. M., Brady, T. J., and Rosen, B. R. (1991). Functional mapping of the human visual cortex by magnetic resonance imaging. *Science* **254,** 716.

Buxton, R. B. (2001). The elusive initial dip. *Neuroimage* **13,** 953.

Buxton, R. B., Wong, E. C., and Frank, L. R. (1998). Dynamics of blood flow and oxygenation changes during brain activation: the balloon model. *Magn. Reson. Med.* **39,** 855.

Chan, S. (2002). The clinical relevance and scientific potential of ultra high-field-strength MR imaging. *AJNR Am. J. Neuroradiol.* **23,** 1441.

Clare, S., Francis, S., Morris, P. G., and Bowtell, R. (2001). Single-shot T2* measurement to establish optimum echo time for fMRI: studies of the visual, motor, and auditory cortices at 3.0 T. *Magn. Reson. Med.* **45,** 930.

Frank, J. A., Anderson, S. A., Kalsih, H., Jordan, E. K., Lewis, B. K., Yocum, G. T., and Arbab, A. S. (2004). Methods for magnetically labeling stem and other cells for detection by *in vivo* magnetic resonance imaging. *Cytotherapy* **6**(6), 621–625.

Friston, K. J., Worsley, K. J., Frackowiak, R. S., Mazziotta, J. C., and Evans, A. C. (1994). Assessing the significance of focal activations using their spatial extent. *Hum. Brain Mapp.* **1,** 214.

Friston, K. J., Holmes, A. P., Poline, J. B., Grasby, P. J., Williams, S. C., Frackowiak, R. S., and Turner, R. (1995). Analysis of fMRI time-series revisited. *Neuroimage* **2,** 45.

Friston, K. J., Williams, S., Howard, R., Frackowiak, R. S., and Turner, R. (1996). Movement-related effects in fMRI time-series. *Magn. Reson. Med.* **35,** 346.

Friston, K. J., Zarahn, E., Josephs, O., Henson, R. N., and Dale, A. M. (1999). *Neuroimage* **10,** 607.

Glover, G. H., and Law, C. S. (2001). Stochastic designs in event-related fMRI. *Magn. Reson. Med.* **46,** 515.

Haacke, M. E., Brown, R. W., Thompson, M. R., and Venkatesan, R. (1999). "Magnetic Resonance Imaging." Wiley, New York.

Hall, D. A., Haggard, M. P., Akeroyd, M. A., Palmer, A. R., Summerfield, A. Q., Elliott, M. R., Gurney, E. M., and Bowtell, R. W. (1999). "Sparse" temporal sampling in auditory fMRI. *Hum. Brain Mapp.* **7,** 213.

Jezzard, P., and Balaban, R. S. (1995). Correction for geometric distortion in echo planar images from B0 field variations. *Magn. Reson. Med.* **34,** 65.

Jezzard, P., and Clare, S. (1999). Sources of distortion in functional MRI data. *Hum. Brain Mapp.* **8,** 80.

Johansen-Berg, H., Dawes, H., Guy, C., Smith, S. M., Wade, D. T., and Matthews, P. M. (2002). Correlation between motor improvements and altered fMRI activity after rehabilitative therapy. *Brain* **125,** 2731.

Kim, S. G., Hendrich, K., Hu, X., Merkle, K., and Ugurbil, K. (1994). Potential pitfalls of functional MRI using conventional gradient-recalled echo techniques. *NMR Biomed.* **7,** 69.

Leontiev, O., and Buxton, R. B. (2007). Reproducibility of BOLD, perfusion, and CMRO2 measurements with calibrated-BOLD fMRI. *Neuroimage* **35**(1), 175–184.

Liu, T. T., Wong, E. C., Frank, L. R., and Buxton, R. B. (2002). Analysis and design of perfusion-based event-related fMRI experiments. *Neuroimage* **16,** 269.

Liu, T. T., and Brown, G. G. (2007). Measurement of cerebral perfusion with arterial spin labeling: Part 1. Methods. *J. Int. Neuropsychol. Soc.* **13**(3), 517–525.

Lu, H., Golay, X., Pekar, J. J., and Van Zijl, P. C. (2003). Functional magnetic resonance imaging based on changes in vascular space occupancy. *Magn. Reson. Med.* **50**(2), 263–274.

Merboldt, K. D., Finsterbusch, J., and Frahm, J. (2000). Reducing inhomogeneity artifacts in functional MRI of human brain activation-thin sections vs gradient compensation. *J. Magn. Reson.* **145,** 184.

Miezin, F. M., Maccotta, L., Ollinger, J. M., Petersen, S. E., and Buckner, R. L. (2000). Characterizing the hemodynamic response: effects of presentation rate, sampling procedure, and the possibility of ordering brain activity based on relative timing. *Neuroimage* **11,** 735.

Ogawa, S., Lee, T. M., Kay, A. R., and Tank, D. W. (1990). Brain magnetic resonance imaging with contrast dependent on blood oxygenation. *Proc. Natl. Acad. Sci. USA* **87,** 9868.

Shaw, M. E., Strother, S. C., Gavrilescu, M., Podzebenko, K., Waites, A., Watson, J., Anderson, J., Jackson, G., and Egan, G. (2003). Evaluating subject specific preprocessing choices in multisubject fMRI data sets using data-driven performance metrics. *Neuroimage* **19,** 988.

Silva, A. C., and Koretsky, A. P. (2002). Laminar specificity of functional MRI onset times during somatosensory stimulation in rat. *Proc. Natl. Acad. Sci. USA* **99,** 15182.

Stehling, M. K., Turner, R., and Mansfield, P. (1991). Echo-planar imaging: magnetic resonance imaging in a fraction of a second. *Science* **254,** 43.

Thulborn, K. R., Waterton, J. C., Matthews, P. M., and Radda, G. K. (1982). Oxygenation dependence of the transverse relaxation time of water protons in whole blood at high field. *Biochim. Biophys. Acta* **714,** 265.

Wiggins, G. C., Triantafyllou, C., Potthast, A., Reykowski, A., Nittka, M., and Wald, L. L. (2006). 32-channel 3 Tesla receive-only phased-array head coil with soccer-ball element geometry. *Magn. Reson. Med.* **56**(1), 216–223.

Wilson, J. L., Jenkinson, M., and Jezzard, P. (2002). Optimization of static field homogeneity in human brain using diamagnetic passive shims. *Magn. Reson. Med.* **48,** 906.

PART II

Imaging of Receptors, Small Molecules, and Protein-Protein Interactions

CHAPTER 6

Positron Emission Tomography Receptor Assay with Multiple Ligand Concentrations: An Equilibrium Approach

Doris J. Doudet* and James E. Holden†

*Department of Medicine
Division of Neurology, and TRIUMF
University of British Columbia
Vancouver, British Columbia V6T 2A3, Canada

†Department of Medical Physics
University of Wisconsin
Madison, Wisconsin 53705

I. Update
 A. Pharmacological Interventions: Influence of the Acute Time Course of Pharmacological Effect
 B. Pharmacological Interventions: Acute Versus Chronic Administration
 C. Other Targets, Other Species
II. Introduction
III. Overview of *In Vivo* Receptor Assay
 A. Basic Principles
 B. Distinctions Between *In Vivo* and *In Vitro* Methods
 C. Potential Confounds in *In Vivo* Methods
 D. Mathematical Considerations
 E. Other Considerations
IV. Methods
 A. Radiochemistry and Determination of SA
 B. General Experimental Procedure
 C. Data Analysis
V. Example Applications
 A. Distinction of Density from Affinity Effects

DOI: 10.1016/B978-0-12-375043-3.00006-8

B. Sequential Versus Nonsequential Studies
C. Two-Point Studies
VI. Conclusions
References

I. Update

Our chapter on the use of multiple ligand concentrations to distinguish the effects of macromolecule density from those of affinity in PET macromolecular assays *in vivo* is presented here without change. Our work since publication has not been refinements of the method *per se*, but rather demonstrations of the nearly unlimited range of applications afforded by this single simple idea.

A. Pharmacological Interventions: Influence of the Acute Time Course of Pharmacological Effect

One of the most promising applications of the multiple ligand concentration method is the evaluation of the effects of pharmacological challenges on the response of the receptor system. A key element of the method is the comparison of results from sequential studies performed on the same day with those from multiple studies performed on separate days. In studies in rhesus monkeys with two inhibitors of the dopamine membrane uptake transporter (DAT), NS2214 and methylphenidate, the expected decrease in binding potential (BP) of raclopride, secondary to the drug-induced increase of synaptic dopamine (DA), was seen for both drugs in both sequential and nonsequential conditions (Doudet *et al.*, 2006). However, the data from the sequential studies were consistent with a corresponding decrease in receptor density, with no change in affinity, while those from the nonsequential studies were consistent with a corresponding decrease in affinity, with no change in receptor density. We hypothesized this to be the consequence of the lack of stability of the synaptic concentrations of the endogenous ligand DA in response to the pharmacological effect of the DAT inhibitors over the time frame of the sequential studies following acute administration. In contrast, the nonsequential studies were all performed at the same time following the drug interventions, which increased the likelihood that all ligand concentrations were probing the same synaptic situation. A simple model of progressively increasing synaptic DA concentrations following acute administration of a DAT inhibitor, which would cause the test ligand to have a progressively decreasing affinity with the receptor as time passed, reproduced the data from the sequential study very well, data that could only be interpreted as a decrease in receptor density if the affinity is assumed to be constant. Thus, whenever the pharmacological challenge is suspected to induce progressive changes in the synaptic environment, nonsequential studies are the better choice. In both sequential and nonsequential studies, the lowest specific activities (SA: injected radioactivity divided by coinjected ligand mass) used resulted in receptor occupancies of only 60%. The ambiguity of the results was resolved by additional studies under both conditions with SA values low enough to assure receptor occupancy near saturation (>80%). These were combined with the very high SA studies for both conditions into two-point plots. The plots from the sequential studies were nearly identical to those from the nonsequential studies, confirming that the acute drug administrations reduced binding by reducing ligand-receptor affinity. At the same time, the data exposed that this reduction in affinity is not stable over time following acute administration of these DAT inhibitors.

B. Pharmacological Interventions: Acute Versus Chronic Administration

This alternative approach, two studies with very high and very low SA values, respectively, was applied to compare the changes in receptor properties induced by acute administration with those induced by chronic administration of the DAT inhibitor NS2214. Daily administration of this inhibitor over a 4-week period gave an identical reduction in BP as that from a single acute dose. However, the low SA studies performed under the same two conditions showed that this reduction was due to affinity changes in the acute case and receptor density changes in the chronic case (Fig. 1), suggesting different adaptative responses of the receptor system to acute versus long term change in the synaptic environment.

C. Other Targets, Other Species

The wide applicability of the approach was demonstrated in a study in which the target molecule, the test ligand, and the model species were all different from those in our original report. Dihydrotetrabenazine administered at multiple

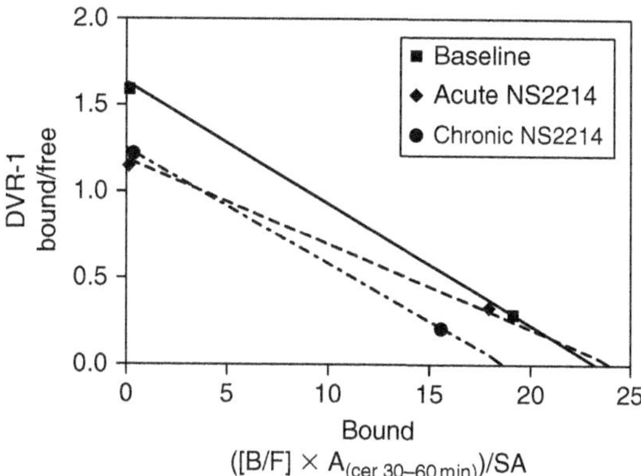

Fig. 1 Two-point Scatchard plots from studies of raclopride in rhesus monkey striatum. Both acute and chronic treatment with the DAT inhibitor NS2214 reduced the BP; however, the reduction was due to a change in affinity after an acute dose, while the reduction was due to a reduction in receptor density after the chronic treatment.

concentrations was used to perform the first reported *in vivo* assay of the density of the vesicular monoamine transporter in rat striatum (Sossi *et al.*, 2007). Large reductions of tracer binding in animals with 6-OHDA-induced lesions of the dopaminergic nigrostriatal pathway were shown to be entirely due to reductions in transporter density, with no change in ligand-transporter affinity.

II. Introduction

Among the many current modern imaging modalities, positron emission tomography (PET) presents the advantage of allowing the medical researcher to open a window into the mechanisms controlling a variety of physiological processes in health and disease. Although PET is widely used as a therapeutic and diagnostic tool in cardiology and oncology, many of these uses still rely on its more qualitative aspects. Although its diagnostic role in neurological and psychiatric disorders is limited, the true power of PET is to allow insights into the physiology and neurochemistry of the brain, where its quantitative capabilities are an asset and are being widely developed and used in human subjects, both normal controls and patients. One of the most studied aspects to date is the role of a variety of neurotransmitters and their receptors in health, aging, and disease. Although a field still in infancy, an assortment of tracers has been or is being developed for various forms of DA, serotonin, acetylcholine, opiate, glutamate, and GABA receptors. Some receptor ligands may also be used as surrogate markers of the extent of release of their presynaptic neurotransmitters, with the implied assumption that the changes in binding of the tracer to the receptor in a given subject or a given population result from a change in the competition with the endogenous ligand. Issues and questions raised by this approach have been reviewed in detail by Laruelle (2000), and although some are relevant to the subject of this chapter, they will not be reiterated here.

A challenge facing the study of living neuroreceptors is to be able to reconcile *in vivo* PET findings with those from *in vitro* postmortem studies in patients or in animal models of disorders. *In vitro* studies (or *ex vivo* studies in isolated but intact tissues) present the advantage of having direct access to the tissue, allowing not only complete control of the conditions in which the measurements are obtained but also the use of techniques leading to fully quantitative answers, such as Scatchard's (1949) methodology, which permits separate evaluation of the density and the affinity of the receptors of interest in a given condition. Knowledge of the number of receptors and of their affinity in specific brain regions, specific pathological conditions, or after acute or long-term drug therapy would greatly enhance our understanding of the pathophysiological mechanisms and the induced compensatory effects involved in idiopathic diseases or in response to injuries (such as stroke) and drug exposure. A number of attempts have been made to evaluate *in vivo* neuroreceptor characteristics. However, working with a living organism poses a number of constraints on the type of studies and the type of data that can be acquired safely and in a less invasive manner.

This chapter summarizes some of the issues associated with obtaining adequate and accurate data *in vivo* and how and why they may differ from published *in vitro* findings. We review some of the pertinent literature briefly and present the results of our own efforts in the development of an *in vivo* multiple ligand concentration receptor assay (MLCRA) method that could be applied to human patient studies with the best reproducibility, reliability, and minimal burden on the patient. All the studies reported here have been obtained using [^{11}C]raclopride, a ligand of the DA $D_{2/3}$ receptors. Raclopride is known to bind to $D_{2/3}$ with a single affinity and represents the best example currently available. Thus, studies using other ligands with different characteristics may have to be validated using similar principles as described later.

III. Overview of *In Vivo* Receptor Assay

A. Basic Principles

The routine outcome of most neuroreceptor PET studies is a BP or an equivalent. The concept of BP was introduced in the early days of the application of PET to the study of neuroreceptors by Mintun *et al.* (1984) and continues to be the most prevalent experimental endpoint, primarily because its determination from measured data is remarkably reliable and robust, regardless of the particular data acquisition and reduction methods chosen. However, it is, by definition ($BP = B_{max}/K_d$), a reflection of both the density of receptors B_{max} in the target tissue and the apparent affinity, represented inversely by the dissociation constant K_d, between those receptors and the tracer. Thus, although it is a useful and widely used indicator of altered receptor function, a change in BP does not provide information on the specific nature of the change, and a lack of change does not necessarily represent maintenance of normal function. In an effort to resolve this ambiguity, Farde *et al.* (1986) developed an elegant method to assess independently, *in vivo*, receptor density and affinity. In analogy with the *in vitro* Scatchard method, Farde's original method calls for the sequential use of multiple concentrations of test ligand (i.e., two PET scans at a very minimum, a first one at high specific activity [SA] of the tracer followed by at least one with coinjection of the specific ligand with its unlabeled form to induce a significant occupancy of the receptors). The main assumptions in the *in vivo* studies are that the tracer binds to a single receptor site and that its rates of binding and release are compatible with the length of the experiment (i.e., equilibrium in all the region of interest occurs within four to five half lives of the positron emitter with which the tracer is labeled, or a maximum of 90–100 min in the case of most ^{11}C-labeled compounds).

Variations on this theme have been reported, with the required changes in receptor occupancy in the sequential scans being induced either by prior or conjoint administration of a competitor (Delforge *et al.*, 1995, 1999; Wong *et al.*, 1986) or, in our own studies, straight administration of the tracer at low SA

(Holden *et al.*, 2002). This design was introduced in analogy with similar approaches in postmortem ligand-binding studies in preparations of dilute concentrations of membranes isolated from the tissue of interest. Despite the apparent common principle, there are many important differences between the *in vivo* MLCRA and the *in vitro* assay applied in membrane preparations. These methodological differences were addressed in detail in an earlier publication (Holden *et al.*, 2002).

B. Distinctions Between *In Vivo* and *In Vitro* Methods

Both *in vivo* and *in vitro* approaches attempt to determine the density of receptors per given unit of tissue and the apparent affinity between the receptors and the test ligand, expressed inversely as the apparent dissociation constant K_d. Although the experimental endpoints in *in vitro* MLCRA are the density of receptor molecules per mass of isolated membrane and the apparent affinity between those receptors and the labeled ligand, the determination of both of these parameters is strongly dependent on the details of the methods used to isolate and purify the membranes from the postmortem tissue, and the literature shows abundantly that both density and apparent ligand-receptor affinity values determined by *in vitro* MLCRA can vary by orders of magnitude (Riffee *et al.*, 1982; Seeman *et al.*, 1984). The main advantage of the *in vivo* MLCRA is the avoidance of the confounding effects of the membrane preparation; the bound and free concentrations of the tracer are assumed to be distinguished unambiguously on the basis of the time-course data in target and reference tissues. The upper limiting value of the kinetically determined bound component represents an accurate estimate of the true total concentration of receptors in a tissue (Delforge *et al.*, 1996, 2001). The relationship between the kinetically identified free ligand concentration (Delforge *et al.*, 1996) and the concentration of ligand actually available for binding is at the outset unknown, but its effects can be absorbed into the value of the apparent affinity between receptor and ligand. As the primary goal in both experimental contexts is to distinguish receptor density from affinity effects in measured data, this issue does not disqualify the *in vivo* compared with the *in vitro* MLCRA.

C. Potential Confounds in *In Vivo* Methods

The greatest challenge of *in vivo* MLCRA arises because the receptors are embedded in the membranes of intact, fully functioning cells in an intact, fully functioning central nervous system; the potential confounds from this lack of isolation must be accounted for to the greatest degree possible. In both *in vitro* and *in vivo* MLCRA, the measured relationship between the multiple values of the bound ligand concentrations and the free ligand concentrations with which they are equilibrated is used to evaluate single values of the total concentration of receptors and the apparent receptor-ligand affinity. The assumption is made that these values are equally valid at all ligand concentrations. The most obvious potential confound in the *in vivo* situation is that increasing antagonist concentrations may induce changes in the concentration of endogenous ligand (Gjedde and Wong, 2001), which could result in each data point being characterized by a different apparent affinity. Furthermore, circadian rhythms have been shown to alter the concentration of endogenous ligand (Smith *et al.*, 1992), which could result in compounding or opposing effects on the tracer affinity throughout the course of the day. These issues have been addressed in previous reports (Doudet *et al.*, 2003; Holden *et al.*, 2002). In particular, an approach to testing for the first of these confounds was described previously (Holden *et al.*, 2002). We believe that such a test must be performed each time a new ligand is introduced or when a previously established ligand is applied in a new experimental context.

D. Mathematical Considerations

Both *in vivo* and *in vitro* MLCRA share the controversy about the best approach for evaluating the parameters of interest from measured data. We present here two approaches, one using the linear analysis used most routinely for PET studies and another using a nonlinear approach favored by practitioners of *in vivo* MLCRA. Details of the advantages and disadvantages of each, and the considerations taken into account in our choices of analyses, were reported previously (Holden *et al.*, 2002).

E. Other Considerations

1. Radiation Dosimetry

The radiation dose has to remain within the guidelines of acceptable dosimetry, which limits the number of studies permissible within a day or even a quarter. For that reason, many PET researchers have limited their studies to two scans, one with practically null receptor occupancy from the high SA tracer and one at a significant receptor occupancy by the unlabeled analog.

2. Receptor Saturation

In living subjects it is impossible to perform total or near-total receptor saturation studies without potentially affecting the health of the subject. The degree of saturation may, however, be marginally adapted to the particular condition studied. For example, performing a study inducing 80–90% D_2 receptor occupancy by a neuroleptic such as raclopride or spiperone in a schizophrenic subject would not have the same impact as inducing the same occupancy in a parkinsonian subject. In most *in vivo* MLCRA, one usually attempts to reach about 50–60% saturation.

3. Pharmacological Interventions

In studies of acute pharmacological interventions, the performance of multiple studies requires that attention be paid to the stability of the drug effect over time, particularly the stability of the changes in endogenous ligand induced by the challenge. Changes in the synaptic concentration of endogenous ligand during the course of the two to three PET studies (acquired over 6–8 h) necessary to obtain data may interfere with the binding of the tracer by altering the apparent affinity of the tracer and thus its BP.

4. Avoidance of Blood Sampling

We developed our design and performed validation experiments in anesthetized nonhuman primates but with further studies in human subjects in mind. For this reason, we employ a data analysis method that uses the activity in a reference region devoid of the receptor of interest (cerebellum in the case of raclopride) to obtain information of the concentration of free ligand, whereas activity in the target region is assumed to provide information on the bound concentrations. Graphical methods of analysis, such as the Logan method (Logan *et al.*, 1996) or the reference tissue method (Lammertsma and Hume, 1996), provide good data without the need for a metabolite-corrected input function. In addition to avoiding arterial puncture, this approach obviates the need for metabolite analysis, which often introduces large amounts of noise and variability in the determination of the input function.

5. Equilibrium Administration

These graphical methods, however, can be sensitive to changes in blood flow brought about by disease or drug administration. Thus, we use the combination of bolus plus constant infusion administration of the PET tracer to produce a stable equilibrium between bound and free concentrations at each administered concentration (Carson *et al.*, 1997). With raclopride, we found that this equilibrium is reached within 25–30 min of the start of the tracer administration and thus remains within the time frame of the ^{11}C study.

6. Nonsequential Studies

Other concerns were the capability of the subjects, especially patients, to withstand two to three scans throughout the course of a single day and whether consecutive doses of a receptor antagonist would affect both data and the subject. We performed a simple study in normal monkeys and monkeys with drug-induced parkinsonism, comparing data obtained using a routine sequential MLCRA design (three to four consecutive scans in 1 single day) versus a nonsequential MLCRA design in which the individual scans were obtained on separate days,

days to weeks apart, in random order of SA but at the same time of day. This validation experiment also allowed us to assess both the potential effects of circadian rhythms and the effects of prior sequential administration of pharmacological doses of the unlabeled tracer. Results of this study demonstrated that baseline MLCRA studies, at least with raclopride, may be performed over several days if necessary and allow more flexibility for the patient and the physician.

7. Other Ligands

One should, however, keep in mind that each tracer has different characteristics and may present different sets of challenges. Although the methods presented here have been found sound for studies using raclopride in the striatum, further validation may be necessary when starting work with other ligands, which may have different binding and dissociation characteristics, have affinity to more than one class of receptor in a given brain region, and so forth. This chapter aims only at presenting the use of an almost ideal ligand, a blueprint of the type of studies that need to be performed before *in vivo* MLCRA can be conducted with confidence in living subjects.

IV. Methods

A. Radiochemistry and Determination of SA

One of the most important aspects of our study is that we know the SA of the ligand before we inject it into the subject. This allows improved reproducibility and less variability not only between subjects but also within subjects when repeated studies are being performed. This may represent a crucial aspect, as the concentrations of antagonist, unlabeled analog, or competitor may be a determinant in the measured K_d^{app} (Gjedde and Wong, 2001). The chemists are being told in advance of the required SA before synthesis begins.

Raclopride was synthesized as described previously (Namavari *et al.*, 1992). High SA [^{11}C]methyl iodide is produced via the gas-phase reaction of [^{11}C]methane with I_2 (Larsen *et al.*, 1997; Links *et al.*, 1997). The high SA for raclopride was greater than 1000 Ci/mmol.

1. SA Adjustment

Raclopride stock solutions are prepared by dissolving raclopride tartrate in USP water to make a 0.5-mM solution. This solution is used to prepare a 0.1-mM stock solution. Stock solution concentrations are determined precisely from standard calibration curves on analytical HPLC prior to use. The tracer production is initiated such that the final formulation will be completed 20 min (one half-life) before the anticipated time of injection. The yield in mCi is measured, and the amount of stock solution to be added is calculated using the following formula:

$$\text{ml of stock solution} = \frac{X}{2YZ}$$

where X is yield at the time of formulation (mCi), Y is desired SA in Ci/mmol at time of injection, and Z is stock solution concentration (0.1 mM). The factor of 2 in the denominator accounts for the decay occurring between the time of formulation and the time of injection.

The carrier supplied from tracer production of >1000 Ci/mmol is considered to be insignificant compared to the concentration added. The requisite volume of stock solution is added, and the time is noted. The vial is then weighed, and an aliquot for precise measurement of the SA is drawn. The remainder is sent to the PET center. An exact volume of the quality control sample is injected onto the previously prepared analytical HPLC system. The SA of the adjusted solution is confirmed, and the investigators are notified of any small adjustment of the injection time required to attain the desired exact SA.

B. General Experimental Procedure

All the examples presented in this chapter are obtained in healthy rhesus monkeys, as well as animals with MPTP-induced parkinsonism, as part of a number of studies. Detailed reports have been published (Doudet *et al.*, 2000a, 2002, 2003; Holden *et al.*, 2002). Some animals received intraperitoneal or intravenous adminstration of methamphetamine (2 mg/kg i.p.) (Doudet and Holden, 2003a) and/or a DA transporter inhibitor, methylphenidate (0.5 mg/kg i.v.) or brasofensine (0.5 mg/kg i.p.) (Doudet *et al.*, 2000b). All animal procedures are approved by the Committee on Animal Care of the University of British Columbia. Animal procedures, anesthesia regimens, and PET scan acquisition and analysis are described in detail elsewhere (Doudet *et al.*, 2000a; Holden *et al.*, 2002). Briefly, the animal is positioned prone in a stereotactic head holder. A Siemens ECAT 953–31B allows the simultaneous acquisition of 31 coronal slices through the head and brain of the monkey (in-plane resolution: 6 mm FWHM; axial resolution: 5 mm). Scan data are acquired in two-dimensional mode over 1 h. For all scans, raclopride is administered as a bolus (2.5 mCi in 1 min in 10 ml saline) followed by constant infusion (2.5 mCi in 59 min in 30 ml saline) to create a true equilibrium condition (Carson *et al.*, 1997). Scanning starts with the start of bolus injection. The scanning sequence consists of six 30-s scans, two 1-min scans, five 5-min scans, and four 7.5-min scans for a total duration of 60 min.

For the sequential acquisition method, three or four bolus/infusion injections of raclopride (specific activity: SA1 > 1000 Ci/mmol; 40 < SA2 < 20 Ci/mmol, 12 < SA3 < 9 Ci/mmol, 6 < SA4 < 3 Ci/mmol) are performed throughout the day. The scans are separated by a minimum of 2 h (SA1-SA2) and up to 3.5 h (SA3-SA4). For nonsequential studies, the SA are similar, but each raclopride scan is performed on a separate day, 1–3 weeks apart, all at the same time of day. The order of scan acquisition is random.

C. Data Analysis

1. Data Reduction

As described previously, regions of interests (ROIs) are placed over the left and right striatum (circular ROIs: 37 pixels; pixel size: 4 mm^2) in four consecutive slices and four ROIs (16 pixels each) are positioned over an area of nonspecific ^{11}C accumulation on the cerebellum in two consecutive slices (for location, see Doudet *et al.*, 2000a). Time-activity curves are obtained for each ROI and averaged for each animal into left and right striatum and cerebellum (Fig. 2).

The two MLCRA methods of parameter estimation presented in the next section, linear and nonlinear, require the equilibrium ratio *B/F* between the concentrations of bound and free ligand in the target tissue. This value was derived from the tissue-input Logan graphical method for the evaluation of equilibrium distribution volume ratios (DVRs) of reversible tracers (Logan *et al.*, 1996) using the time-activity course in the cerebellum as the input function, between 30 and 60 min postinjection, by which time equilibrium was reached at all SA used (Fig. 3). The distribution volume ratio minus one (DVR − 1) was interpreted as an estimate of the equilibrium ratio of bound and free ligand (*B/F*) in striatal regions. This graphical estimate of the bound/free ratio is represented by a variable surrounded by brackets and with a subscript g in the following equations to distinguish it from the same ratio estimated from individual measurements of *B* and *F* themselves. The other variables required by the fitting routines are these equilibrium concentrations *B* and *F* themselves. These were derived from the radioactivity concentrations in cerebellum *C*(*t*) averaged over the final 30 min of the study, the graphical *B/F* estimate, and the SA values at injection time. *B* was

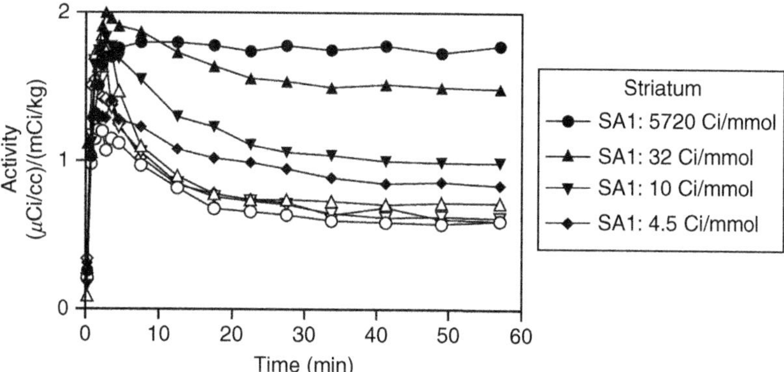

Fig. 2 Representative time courses of radioactivity concentration in the striatum (filled symbols) and cerebellum (open symbols) in a normal monkey at four decreasing SA. Constancy over time was obtained consistently in both regions during the four to five last frames, at all specific activities.

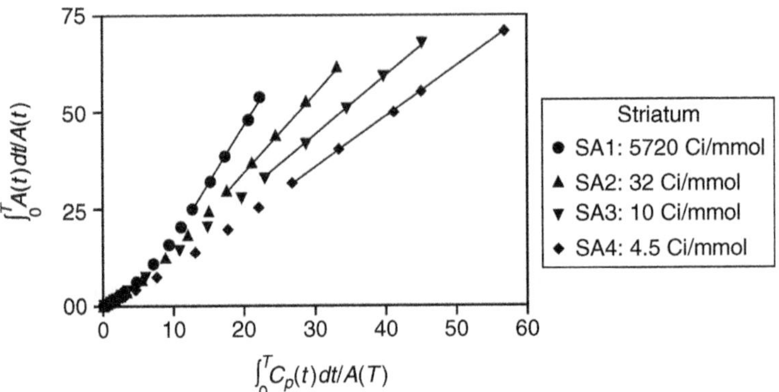

Fig. 3 Plots from the application of the tissue-input graphical estimation of DVR to data shown in Fig. 2. Linearity was observed consistently over the last four to five frames at all specific activities.

estimated as $(B/F)C/\mathrm{SA}$ and F as C/SA, where C represents the time average of $C(t)$. In summary, the measured time courses in the striatum and cerebellum are reduced to provide the estimates $(B/F)_g$ and C, which are used to compute the values provided to the parameter optimization process.

2. Parameter Optimization

We have previously reported a thorough investigation of four distinct approaches to evaluating the desired parameters BP, B_{max}, and K_d^{app} from reduced data (Holden *et al.*, 2002). We report here the two that had optimal properties. Both are based on the relationship between the bound concentration B and the free ligand concentration F with which it is equilibrated:

$$B = \frac{B_{max}F}{K_d^{app} + F} \tag{1}$$

B thus increases asymptotically to the saturated concentration B_{max} as F increases without limit, with half the receptors occupied when F reaches the value K_d^{app}. The superscript app has been added to this equilibrium dissociation constant to signify that it is the apparent value seen *in vivo* and to distinguish it from the idealized value derived from *in vitro* studies of the same ligand-receptor pair.

Both fitting equations are rearrangements of this saturation equation. The first is equivalent to the original linearization of the equation by Scatchard (1949):

$$\left(\frac{B}{F}\right)_g = \mathrm{BP} - \frac{1}{K_d^{app}}\left(\frac{B}{F}\right)_g F \tag{2}$$

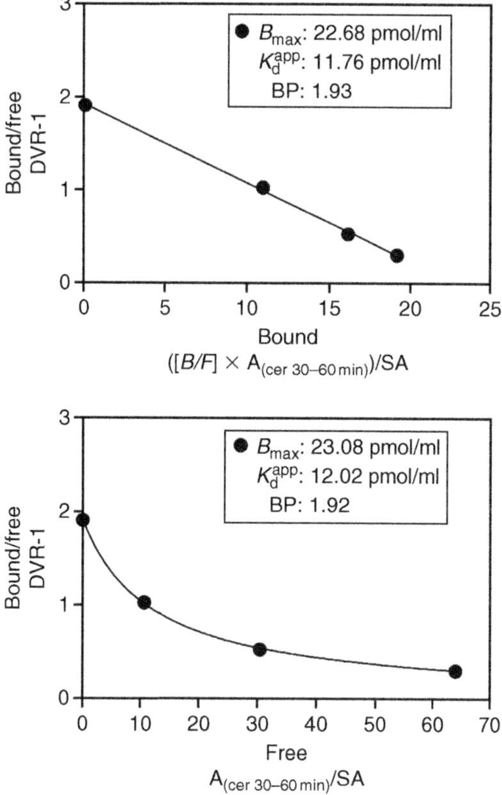

Fig. 4 Example fits from the application of two parameter-optimization approaches, linear (top) and nonlinear (bottom), to the four-point data set shown in Figs. 2 and 3. Solid curves are the model predictions of the two respective equations (see text) with the model parameters set to the optimized values shown.

Thus, $(B/F)_g$ is fitted against the bound value $(B/F)_gF$ (Fig. 4, top) with BP and K_d^{app} as optimized parameters (y-axis intercept and negative inverse of the slope, respectively). The third outcome parameter, B_{max}, is the x-axis intercept of the resulting straight line.

For the nonlinear method, the saturation equation is rearranged into

$$\left(\frac{B}{F}\right)_g = \frac{\mathrm{BP}K_d^{app}}{K_d^{app} + F} \tag{3}$$

Thus, $(B/F)_g$ is fitted against the free concentration F (Fig. 4, bottom), again with BP and K_d^{app} as optimized parameters. BP is again the y-axis intercept, and K_d^{app} is reflected in the rate of decline of the nonlinear curve. Similar to the growth of B in the saturation equation, the prediction for $(B/F)_g$ falls to half the BP value when F equals K_d^{app}. The receptor density is not represented in the graphical presentation of the curve; the value B_{max} is estimated separately as the product of the two fitted parameters.

This nonlinear parameter optimization approach was determined in our previous study to have optimal characteristics from the perspectives of the independence of the two sides of the fitting equation and the covariance observed between the two fitted parameters. However, the resulting parameters from the two approaches are nearly always statistically indistinguishable. Thus, the linear method is used in the presentation of the following example applications to illustrate changes in density or affinity, as these changes are more easily perceived from the changes in a straight line graph. Agreement between the two approaches reflects the perfect conformity of data to the saturation equation from which the fitting equations are derived. Routine comparison of the results from the two methods thus provides a simple tool for discovering systematic deviations from this conformity when the method is applied in a new experimental context.

V. Example Applications

A. Distinction of Density from Affinity Effects

Representative data sets from two experimental contexts are shown in Fig. 5. In both contexts the BP was altered significantly from the baseline value by the experimental intervention being studied, with a significant increase seen in animals that had been rendered parkinsonian by MPTP (a selective toxin of the dopaminergic nigrostriatal neurons) and a significant decrease seen in otherwise normal subjects following the acute administration of methamphetamine. Application of MLCRA showed that the increase seen in the MPTP parkinsonian model is due primarily to a change in receptor density, with no significant change in affinity (Doudet *et al.*, 2002), whereas following methamphetamine the decrease is due primarily to the change in affinity brought about by competition between raclopride and endogenous DA mobilized by the drug, with no significant change in receptor density (Doudet and Holden, 2003b).

B. Sequential Versus Nonsequential Studies

As noted earlier in Section III.E.6, our comparison of results from sequential studies performed on the same day with those from multiple studies performed nonsequentially on separate days has been motivated by several different questions. In the absence of an acute pharmacological intervention, the comparison provides assurance about the potential interference between studies and the effects of diurnal changes in the sequential case, and the effects of changes of the DA system over days or weeks in the nonsequential case. The comparison also bears on

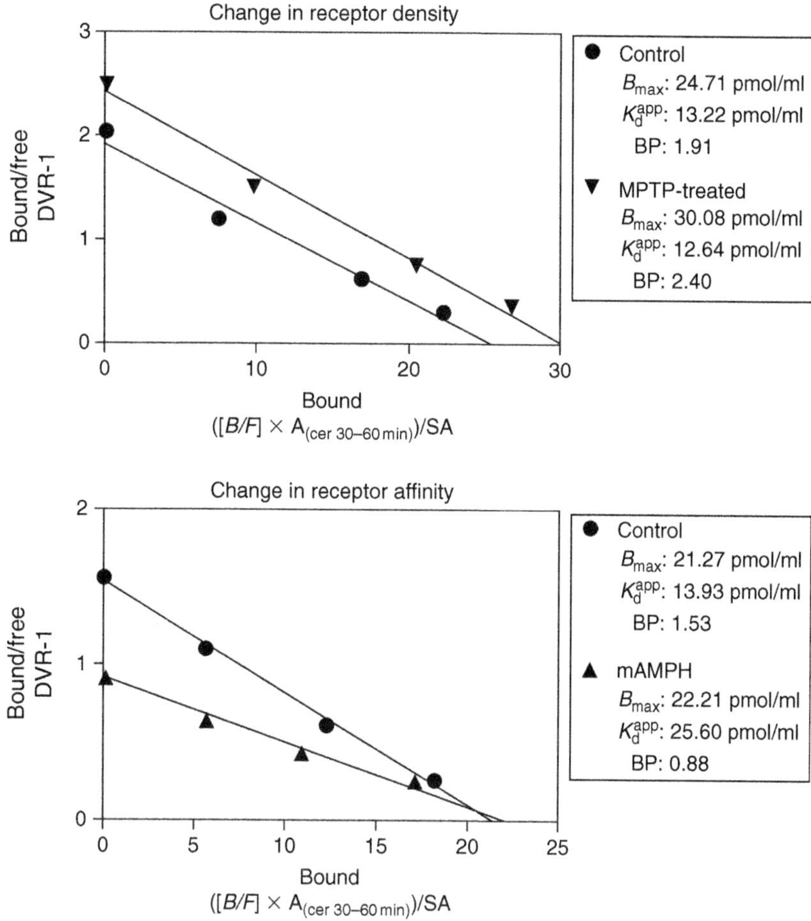

Fig. 5 Examples of the use of the MLCRA analysis. *Top*: Example of a change in receptor density. Straight-line plots were obtained using the fitted parameters in the striatum of a normal monkey (•) and in the striatum of a MPTP-treated monkey with clear clinical signs (▼). Note that in the MPTP-treated monkey, only BP and $B_{\max}$ are increased while K_d^{app} remains unchanged. *Bottom*: Example of a change in receptor affinity. Straight line plots of data in a monkey at baseline (•) and after methamphetamine (mAMPH: ▲). After methamphetamine, there is an increase in K_d^{app} and a decrease in BP in the striatum without significant changes in $B_{\max}$.

the future use of the method in a clinical setting in patients who are incapable of undergoing the rigors of sequential studies. Figure 6 shows a representative comparison under baseline conditions (Doudet *et al.*, 2003). Similar results were observed in studies in the MPTP parkinsonian model. In the absence of acute pharmacological interventions, the two approaches can be regarded as equivalent.

Following drug intervention, the comparison also provides critically important information about the evolution over time of the drug effects on the system.

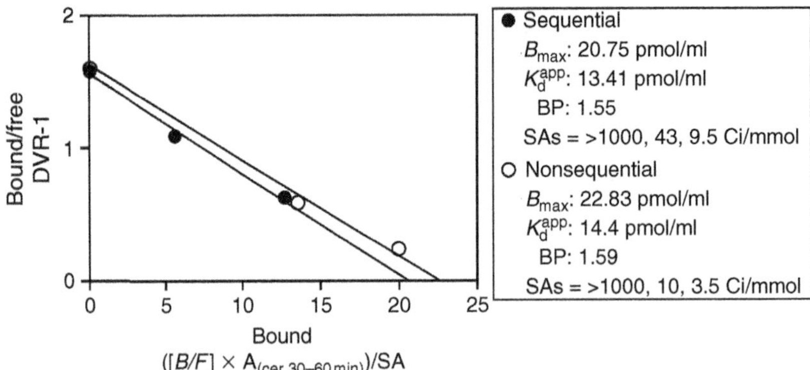

Fig. 6 Comparison of the straight-line optimization procedure used to estimate BP, B_{max}, and K_d^{app} from data measured with sequential (•) and nonsequential (○) methods in the same animal. Note the good agreement between the measures of interest, although the specific activities used were different.

Examples are not presented here, as these comparisons are a work in progress. We have observed cases such that the sequential and nonsequential results were the same, implying that the single drug administration prior to the sequential studies effected a change that was stable over time (Doudet and Holden, 2003b). However, we have also seen very significant differences between sequential and nonsequential results in other cases (Doudet *et al.*, 2000b). We interpret these to mean that the effect of those drugs on the receptor system is strongly dependent on time after drug intervention. Our validation of nonsequential studies in the absence of drug intervention supports the validity of MLCRA for the study of such drug effects if care is taken to make the multiple drug administrations in nonsequential studies as equivalent to each other as possible, particularly with regard to their timing relative to the tracer studies. However, caution must then be exercised about long-term changes in the system induced by multiple, rather than single, administrations of the drug under study.

C. Two-Point Studies

Another work in progress is our study of the use of only two SA values. We provisionally suggest that two-point studies, possibly of critical importance in clinical applications of MLCRA, may conform adequately to the assumptions of the approach to justify their ease and efficiency. Investigation of Figs. 5 and 6 reveals that the combination of the high SA point with any other data point yields a two-point plot that would not be in strong disagreement with results from a full three- or four-point analysis. However, the dependence of the measured value of $(B/F)_g$ on the desired endpoints B_{max} and K_d^{app} varies strongly with the degree of saturation, with the dependence on B_{max} increasing, and that on K_d^{app} decreasing, as saturation is increased. Our work to date strongly suggests that two-point linear analyses may require receptor saturations of 80% to be reliable, particularly in studies of acute drug interventions. In that event, the *y*- and *x*-axis intercepts would be interpreted as the true BP and B_{max} values, respectively, and the K_d^{app} value estimated from the ratio B_{max}/BP would be interpreted as the affinity measure associated with the high SA data point.

VI. Conclusions

PET studies with specific antagonists of brain neuroreceptors can distinguish between the influences of receptor density and receptor-ligand affinity by the performance of studies at multiple concentrations of the test ligand in exact analogy with the well-established methods of the postmortem receptor assay *in vitro*. This chapter attempted to convey that such *in vivo* studies have exactly the same goal as their *in vitro* counterparts, to distinguish receptor density from receptor-ligand affinity as determinants of the binding process. While considerable care and caution must be exercised in the performance and interpretation of such studies, our work to date strongly supports the claim that the approach can serve as a reliable and useful tool in both basic and clinical settings.

Acknowledgments

This work was supported by the CIHR (formerly Medical Research Council of Canada) MPO 14535. We thank Astra Research Centre for their gift of the raclopride precursor. The authors thank the staff of the UBC/TRIUMF PET program for their assistance and contribution to this work. TRIUMF is funded by a contribution by the National Research Council of Canada. The authors are grateful to Drs. T. J. Ruth (Head, PET program) and J. A. Stoessl (Director, Pacific Parkinson Research Centre). These studies would not have been possible without the assistance of S. Jivan, M. Pronk (chemists), C. English, and C. Williams (technologists). We are especially indebted to J. Grant (AHT). Special thanks are due to Dr J. Love and M. Boyd and the personnel of the UBC Animal Care Facilities for their outstanding care of the animals.

References

Carson, R. E., Breier, A., de Bartolomeis, A., Saunders, R. C., Su, T. P., Schmall, B., Der, M. G., Pickar, D., and Eckelman, W. C. (1997). Quantification of amphetamine-induced changes in [^{11}C] raclopride binding with continuous infusion. *J. Cereb. Blood Flow Metab.* **17,** 437–447.

Delforge, J., Pappata, S., Millet, P., Samson, Y., Bendriem, B., Jobert, A., Crouzel, C., and Syrota, A. (1995). Quantification of benzodiazepine receptors in human brain using PET, [^{11}C]flumazenil, and a single-experiment protocol. *J. Cereb. Blood Flow Metab.* **15,** 284–300.

Delforge, J., Syrota, A., and Bendriem, B. (1996). Concept of reaction volume in the *in vivo* ligand-receptor model. *J. Nucl. Med.* **37,** 118–125.

Delforge, J., Bottlaender, M., Loc'h, C., Guenther, I., Fuseau, C., Bendriem, B., Syrota, A., and Mazière, B. (1999). Quantitation of extrastriatal D_2 receptors using a very high-affinity ligand (FLB 457) and the multi-injection approach. *J. Cereb. Blood Flow Metab.* **19,** 533–546.

Delforge, J., Bottlaender, M., Pappata, S., Loc'h, C., and Syrota, A. (2001). Absolute quantification by positron emission tomography of the endogenous ligand. *J. Cereb. Blood Flow Metab.* **21,** 613–630.

Doudet, D. J., and Holden, J. E. (2003a). Raclopride studies of dopamine release: Dependence on presynaptic integrity. *Biol. Psychiatry* **54,** 1193–1199.

Doudet, D. J., and Holden, J. E. (2003b). Sequential versus nonsequential measurement of density and affinity of dopamine D_2 receptors with $[^{11}C]$raclopride: Effect of methamphetamine. *J. Cereb. Blood Flow Metab.* **23,** 1489–1494.

Doudet, D. J., Holden, J. E., Jivan, S., McGeer, E. G., and Wyatt, R. J. (2000a). *In vivo* PET studies of the dopamine D_2 receptors in rhesus monkeys with long-term MPTP-induced parkinsonism. *Synapse* **38,** 105–113.

Doudet, D. J., Jivan, S., English, C., and Holden, J. E. (2000b). Differential effects of amphetamine and a dopamine (DA) transporter blocker on the density and affinity of DA D_2 receptors in monkeys: PET studies with $[^{11}C]$raclopride. *Neuroimage* **11**(6), S5.

Doudet, D. J., Jivan, S., Ruth, T. J., and Holden, J. E. (2002). Density and affinity of the dopamine D_2 receptors in aged symptomatic and asymptomatic MPTP-treated monkeys: PET studies with $[^{11}C]$ raclopride. *Synapse* **44,** 198–202.

Doudet, D. J., Jivan, S., and Holden, J. E. (2003). *In vivo* measurement of receptor density and affinity: Comparison of the routine sequential method with a nonsequential method in studies of dopamine D_2 receptors with $[^{11}C]$raclopride. *J. Cereb. Blood Flow Metab.* **23,** 280–284.

Doudet, D. J., Ruth, T. J., and Holden, J. E. (2006). Sequential vs nonsequential measurement of density and affinity of dopamine D_2 receptors with $[^{11}C]$raclopride: 2: Effects of DAT inhibitors. *J. Cereb. Blood Flow Metab.* **26,** 28–37.

Farde, L., Hall, H., Ehrin, E., and Sedvall, G. (1986). Quantitative analysis of D_2 dopamine receptor binding in the living human brain by PET. *Science* **231,** 258–261.

Gjedde, A., and Wong, D. F. (2001). Quantification of neuroreceptors in living human brain. V. Endogenous neurotransmitter inhibition of haloperidol binding in psychosis. *J. Cereb. Blood Flow Metab.* **21,** 982–994.

Holden, J. E., Jivan, S., Ruth, T. J., and Doudet, D. J. (2002). *In vivo* receptor assay with multiple ligand concentrations: An equilibrium approach. *J. Cereb. Blood Flow Metab.* **22,** 1132–1141.

Lammertsma, A. A., and Hume, S. P. (1996). Simplified reference tissue model for PET receptor studies. *Neuroimage* **4,** 153–158.

Larsen, P., Ulin, J., Dahlstrom, K., and Jensen, M. (1997). Synthesis of $[^{11}C]$iodomethane by iodination of $[^{11}C]$methane. *Appl. Radiat. Isot.* **48,** 153–157.

Laruelle, M. (2000). Imaging synaptic neurotransmission with *in vivo* binding competition techniques: A critical review. *J. Cereb. Blood Flow Metab.* **20,** 423–450.

Links, J. M., Krohn, K. A., and Clark, J. C. (1997). Production of $[^{11}C]CH_3I$ by single pass reaction of $[^{11}C]CH_4$ with I_2. *Nucl. Med. Biol.* **24,** 93–97.

Logan, J., Fowler, J. S., Volkow, N. D., Wang, G. J., Ding, Y. S., and Alexoff, D. L. (1996). Distribution volume ratios without blood sampling from graphical analysis of PET data. *J. Cereb. Blood Flow Metab.* **16,** 834–840.

Mintun, M. A., Raichle, M. E., Kilbourn, M. R., Wooten, G. F., and Welch, M. J. (1984). A quantitative model for the *in vivo* assessment of drug binding sites with positron emission tomography. *Ann. Neurol.* **15,** 217–227.

Namavari, M., Bishop, A., Satyamurthy, N., Bida, G. T., and Barrio, J. R. (1992). Regioselective radiofluorodestannylation with $[^{18}F]F_2$ and $[^{18}F]CH_3COOF$: A high yield synthesis of 6-$[^{18}F]$fluoro-L-dopa. *Int. J. Rad. Appl. Instrum. A* **43,** 989–996.

Riffee, W. H., Wilcox, R. E., Vaughn, D. M., and Smith, R. V. (1982). Dopamine receptor sensitivity after chronic dopamine agonists: Striatal ^{3}H-spiroperidol binding in mice after chronic administration of high doses of apomorphine, *N-n*-propylnorapomorphine and dextroamphetamine. *Psychopharmacology (Berl.)* **77,** 146–149.

Scatchard, G. (1949). The attraction of proteins for small molecules and ions. *Ann. N. Y. Acad. Sci.* **51,** 660–672.

Seeman, P., Ulpian, C., Wreggett, K. A., and Wells, J. W. (1984). Dopamine receptor parameters detected by [^{3}H]spiperone depend on tissue concentration: Analysis and examples. *J. Neurochem.* **43,** 221–235.

Smith, A. D., Olson, R. J., and Justice, J. B., Jr. (1992). Quantitative microdialysis of dopamine in the striatum: Effect of circadian variation. *J. Neurosci. Methods* **44,** 33–41.

Sossi, V., Holden, J. E., Topping, G. J., Camborde, M. L., Kornelsen, R. A., McCormick, S. E., Greene, J., Studenov, A. R., Ruth, T. J., and Doudet, D. J. (2007). *In vivo* measurement of density and affinity of the monoamine vesicular transporter in a unilateral 6-hydroxydopamine rat model of PD. *J. Cereb. Blood Flow Metab.* **27,** 1407–1415.

Wong, D. F., Gjedde, A., and Wagner, H. N., Jr. (1986). Quantification of neuroreceptors in the living human brain. I. Irreversible binding of ligands. *J. Cereb. Blood Flow Metab.* **6,** 137–146.

CHAPTER 7

Estimation of Local Receptor Density, B'_{max}, and Other Parameters via Multiple-Injection Positron Emission Tomography Experiments

Evan D. Morris,* Bradley T. Christian,† Karmen K. Yoder,‡ and Raymond F. Muzic, Jr.§

*Departments of Diagnostic Radiology and Biomedical Engineering
Yale PET Center
Yale School of Medicine
New Haven, Connecticut 06510

†PET Physics
Waisman Laboratory for Brain imaging and Behavior
Departments of Medical Physics and Psychiatry
University of Wisconsin-Madison, Madison

‡Center for Neuroimaging
Stark Neurosciences Research Institute, and
Department of Radiology
Indiana University School of Medicine, Indianapolis, Indiana

§Departments of Radiology
Biomedical Engineering, and Oncology
Case Western Reserve University, Cleveland, Ohio

I. Update
II. Introduction
III. Theory
  A. Need for Models
  B. Compartmental Models
  C. Standard Model Equations
  D. M-I Model Equations

DOI: 10.1016/B978-0-12-375043-3.00007-X

IV. Experimental Protocol and Considerations
A. Animal Preparation
B. Measuring Blood Activity and Constructing Input Curves
C. Generation of Regional Time-Activity Curves (TACs) from PET Images
V. Models and Data Fitting
A. Implementing Model Equations
B. Parameter Estimation
C. Numerical Solution of Differential Equations
D. Parameter Estimation Considerations
VI. Results and Interpretation
A. Examination of Residuals
B. Parameter Precision
C. Model Selection/Goodness of Fit
VII. Understanding and Designing M-I Experiments
A. Sensitivity Functions
B. Using the Sensitivity Information for Design
VIII. Conclusion
References

I. Update

In the last few years, interest in "multiple-injection" (M-I) paradigms, related PET experiments, and the models required to describe them has proliferated. This development has been driven by three factors: (1) desire of PET users to study a broader range of physiological processes with imaging; (2) ongoing improvement in PET scanner sensitivity; and (3) greater availability of new tracers requiring kinetic characterization. With greater use of M-I experiments has come increased scrutiny of the details of model implementation (Salinas *et al.*, 2007). Interestingly, a number of mathematically distinct, but practically equivalent, implementations have been developed by different researchers (model implementation is discussed later in the chapter).

Recently, Vandehey *et al.* made use of the M-I approach to do a complete characterization of the kinetic parameters of two high-affinity dopamine D_2/D_3 receptor tracers ([^{18}F]fallypride and [^{11}C]FLB). Because M-I studies have the power to make precise estimates of all the individual rate constants of the model, the authors were able to identify subtle kinetic differences (specifically, the interplay between binding rate constants and blood flow parameters (Morris and Yoder, 2007)) that might make one tracer better suited to imaging competition with endogenous dopamine. Gallezot *et al.* (2008) used two different M-I protocols in baboons to estimate all of the model parameters for a popular nicotinic ligand, 2-[^{18}F]fluoro-A-85380. Because the nicotinic agonist tracer was given in nontrace amounts, it was necessary to include multiple values of the blood flow parameter, K_1, during the study. Thanks to the precise parameter estimates afforded by the

M-I approach, the authors were then able to determine the level of bias to be expected from more common methods of estimating distribution volume. Bottlaender *et al.* extended the models of Gallezot to include additional compartments for nicotine so that the effect of exogenous nicotine on tracer binding could be studied. With the assumption that nicotine was in fast equilibrium between plasma and free compartments (thereby reducing the number of model parameters), the authors used the M-I curves of A-85380 uptake (in the presence of nicotine) to derive a relationship between plasma nicotine levels and nicotinic-acetylcholine receptor (nAChR) occupancy. This method yielded less bias than if $[^{11}C]$-nicotine had been used to estimate nAChR occupancy.

The authors note that one of their early papers on $[^{11}C]$raclopride displacement by endogenous dopamine (Morris *et al.*, 1995) presaged the combined use of kinetic compartments for both multiple injections and multiple ligand species, such as was used by Bottlaender *et al.* The work of Morris *et al.* (2008) has taken a different direction of late, leading to the estimation of minute-to-minute variation in endogenous dopamine from M-I experiments with $[^{11}C]$-raclopride. Although in this work the injections of tracer did not occur within a single scan session (as is the case for the M-I experiments discussed in this chapter), the data were analyzed simultaneously by a compound model that included compartments for tracer and endogenous neurotransmitter, separately. Finally, another twist on multiple injections was recently introduced by Converse *et al.* (2004) who have pioneered PET studies that include injections of both blood flow ($[^{18}F]$fluoromethane) and receptor ligand ($[^{18}F]$fallypride) tracers in a single scan session. Unlike the other M-I studies described herein, the approach of Converse does not require a coupling of parallel compartmental models since there is no competition between $[^{18}F]$fluoromethane and $[^{18}F]$fallypride for receptor sites. Nevertheless, this new method is quite innovative in its use of a complicated dual-tracer protocol which allows for easy distinction of the contributions of each tracer to the PET data.

The M-I approach to kinetic characterization of a system is based on two concepts: (1) perturbations of the system help to reveal its inner workings and (2) parallel, coupled compartmental models are necessary to describe the system's behavior. In the following section, we outline the theory and practical application of the basic M-I protocol, which serves as the foundation for the recent advances in imaging with M-I described in Section I.

II. Introduction

Positron emission tomography (PET) is a functional imaging technique that allows an investigator to probe the biochemistry of an organism noninvasively. Because every PET study involves the injection of a radioactive molecule—a radiotracer—the practice of quantitative PET is tightly intertwined with the theory of tracer kinetics. The mission of tracer kinetics, in turn, is to estimate physiologically relevant parameters (e.g., blood flow rate, local cerebral metabolic rate, binding or dissociation rate constants) by modeling the uptake of a labeled molecule that mimics ("traces") the behavior of an endogenous or physiologically relevant exogenous chemical substance. Tracer kinetics merges experimentation and modeling. The experimental process involves both injection of a radioactive tracer and observation of local concentrations of said tracer over a period of time. (In PET, "observations" take the form of individual pixels in a time sequence of images, but this is secondary to our discussion.) Mathematically, what is needed is a model of the tracer uptake and its sequestration into various species and/or compartments. A formal comparison of model predictions with experimental observations yields estimates of model parameters; these parameters often represent the speed or magnitude of a physiological process.

Mere construction of a mathematical model, however, does not assure that each and every parameter of a model can be estimated from data. This goes to the identifiability of the parameters. Identifiability is hindered by noise in data or by ambiguity in the model structure. Identifiability is achieved through a combination of modeling parsimony and experimental design optimization. For example, no amount of optimization of an experiment could help identify the parameters n and m in the model, $Y = n \times m \times X$, where observed values of Y are related linearly to measured values of X; X is an independent and Y a dependent variable. However, as discussed later, if the model is something akin to $Y = n(m - X_1)X_2$, where both X_1 and X_2 are independent variables, then by suitably varying each of them, it may be possible to collect data that will enable an investigator to identify the parameter m as distinct from the parameter n. Roughly speaking, an appropriate experiment design would modulate the value of X_1 over a sufficient operating range, which is significant compared to m, so that the $(m - X_1)$ term did not behave effectively like the constant m.

The beauty of M-I PET experiments is that they are used to methodically perturb—and then observe—the system in question over a range of operating points so that the resultant data contain information that will differentiate the effects of parameters from one another. These complicated but elegant experiments (first conceived by Delforge *et al.*,1989, 1990) can enable the investigator to dissect out effects of otherwise highly correlated kinetic parameters such as those that describe the kinetics of a PET tracer.

What parameters do we want to distinguish? Let us focus on PET studies with receptor-ligand tracers. One can imagine that the amount of ligand bound to target receptors (specific binding) will be dependent on at least two physiological factors that have direct correlates in parameters of a kinetic model. Net receptor-mediated uptake of a tracer will be dependent on the speed of interaction of the tracer with the receptor (association and dissociation rate constants), as well as the number of the receptors in a given volume of tissue (receptor density). Not surprisingly, in the standard single-injection experimental design, the respective parameters that represent speed and number of binding sites are highly correlated. In many PET studies, it may not be necessary to distinguish the binding rate constant from the receptor density. In such cases, it would not be necessary to mount the demanding experiments or data analysis described in this chapter. However, in those specialized situations where it is important to identify the receptor density as distinct from binding rate constants for a tracer, M-I PET studies are the only way to do so.

M-I PET experiments have been carried out to closely examine the kinetics of various ligands that bind to receptors in the brain and heart (Christian *et al.*, 2004; Costes *et al.*, 2002; Delforge *et al.*, 1991, 1993, 1995, 1999; Gregoire *et al.*, 2000; Morris *et al.*, 1996; Muzic, *et al.*, 1996, 2000; Poyot *et al.*, 2001) What specialized situations might require identification of individual rate constants and receptor densities from PET data? Experiments that are intended for any of the following would be appropriate specialized applications of the techniques described herein:

- Fully evaluate the kinetics of a new tracer; determine if new tracer is different because it binds to different populations of receptors or binds to same population more avidly than established tracers.
- Accurately determine the regional variation in receptor density.
- Assess the validity of using a particular brain region as a reference region (i.e., test the assumption of no receptors but otherwise identical kinetics as a target region).
- Differentiate possible diseases of receptor (or neuronal) loss from diseases of receptor dysfunction.

This chapter is intended as a guide to graduate students, postdocs, and principal investigators who want to quickly get up to speed on key theoretical and experimental aspects of the M-I PET technique and begin to appreciate the attendant sensitivity analysis that gives the technique its power. The following discussion covers (1) the basics of the theory behind M-I PET studies, (2) practical considerations in planning and executing a successful M-I study, (3) key elements of the numerical implementation of the kinetic model and data-fitting algorithms, (4) an approach to interpretation of the parameter estimates once data are fitted, and (5) an examination of the sensitivity of PET data to the parameters and how that information can be used to improve the design of subsequent experiments.

III. Theory

A. Need for Models

PET is an imaging technique that measures radioactivity indiscriminately. No distinction can be made at measurement time between radioactivity (actually the detection of two simultaneously emitted photons) that emanates from a tracer molecule flowing with the blood, free in the extracellular space, bound to a cell protein in the intracellular space, or even from radioactivity that comes from a radionuclide attached to a metabolic product of the injected tracer. All of the aforementioned sources of radioactivity are detected and logged by the PET scanner, and all contribute to the reconstruction of a PET image. However, not all of these sources of detected signal are of equal importance to the investigator. In fact, in the case of a receptor-binding tracer molecule, the primary signal of interest is the radioactivity associated with tracer bound to a target molecule—typically a receptor or enzyme. To discern the wheat of the bound tracer signal from the chaff of the free and metabolized sources of radioactivity, the investigator must rely on a mathematical model.

B. Compartmental Models

The models used to describe PET data are usually compartmental. That is, they do not take account of spatial gradients in tracer concentration but rather assume that tissue concentrations can be properly described as well-mixed compartments. In fact, compartment models have been compared rigorously to distributed models and have been found to be satisfactory to describe PET data (Muzic and Saidel, 2003). In PET, the volume of the compartment might correspond to the volume of the voxel (if the model is being applied on a pixel-by-pixel basis) or to a larger region of interest (ROI) (if applied on the ROI level). Compartmental models are described mathematically by a series of ordinary differential equations (ODEs); one ODE is required for each compartment. Compartments typically correspond to distinct kinetic states taken on by the radiolabeled tracer. These compartments can be distinct entities physically (e.g., intra- vs. extracellular pools), distinct kinetically (e.g., bound to enzyme and bound to cell surface receptor), or distinct chemically (e.g., native vs. metabolized tracer). As long as the states represent radioactive species, they must be included in the model of the PET measurements. Sometimes, as shown later, it is necessary to model nonradioactive species as well. Usually, the tracer is introduced into the organism via bolus injection(s) and so the uptake, retention, and eventual efflux of tracer from the tissue region of interest are transient phenomena that never reach steady states. That is, the concentrations of tracer in tissue or plasma do not achieve a constant level. If the system (tracer and tissues of interest) were to reach equilibrium, the system of ODEs would reduce to a set of algebraic equations that could be solved analytically. Since this is often not the case, and certainly not true with M-I experiments, the differential equations must be solved—either analytically or numerically—to solve the model for the predicted PET activity over time in a given region (details of this procedure are given in Section V).

In most PET models of receptor-ligand interactions, we hypothesize three kinetically distinct compartments and an arterial plasma pool of tracer—all of which contribute to the measured PET radioactivity. The arterial pool is not a compartment in the mathematical sense, although it is physically distinct from tracer in tissue. Because the arterial plasma concentration in most PET studies is a measured (i.e., applied to the model as a known) quantity, its depiction does not require a differential equation. In fact, the plasma concentration (or some other input function) must exist to drive the model. If no activity is introduced into the plasma, none is ever taken up into the tissue of interest. A version of the compartmental model corresponding to free, specifically (i.e., receptor-) bound, and nonspecifically bound tracer is shown schematically in Fig. 1 (arrows between compartments connote rate constants). K_1 and k_2 are first-order constants that are related to blood flow. The term k_{on} is a second-order rate constant describing the association of tracer and receptor; k_{off} is the dissociation rate constant. B'_{max} represents the concentration of receptors available for binding. Terms k_5 and k_6 are first-order constants that measure the rates of forward and reverse nonspecific binding.

C. Standard Model Equations

In the language of mathematics, the "boxes" in Fig. 1 represent three unknown concentrations whose time-varying functions are encoded in their respective mass balances. The mass balances state that the change in concentration with time of species x (where $x = F$, B, or NS) is a function of those processes that contribute to an increase of x minus those processes that cause a loss of x

$$\frac{\mathrm{d}F}{\mathrm{d}t} = K_1 C_p - (k_2 + k_5)F - k_{on}[B'_{max} - (B + B_c)]F + k_{off}B + k_6\mathrm{NS} \quad (1)$$

$$\frac{\mathrm{d}F}{\mathrm{d}t} = k_{on}[B'_{max} - (B + B_c)]F - k_{off}B \quad (2)$$

$$\frac{\mathrm{dNS}}{\mathrm{d}t} = k_5 F - k_6 \mathrm{NS} \quad (3)$$

where C_p is the time-varying plasma radioactivity associated only with labeled native tracer. C_p is measured via blood samples. The state variables of the model, F, B, and NS, represent the time-varying concentrations of tracer (in pmol/ml) in

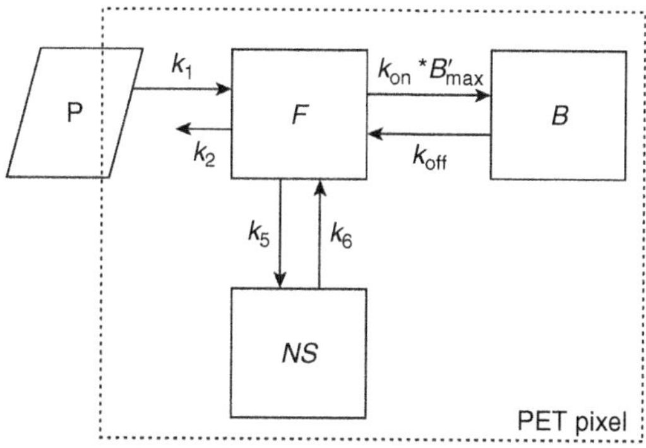

Fig. 1 Standard compartmental model used to describe dynamic PET data. The PET pixel is indicated to show that the measured quantity is a weighted sum of radioactivity in the compartments F (free), B (bound), NS (nonspecific), and some amount in the blood. P indicates that the metabolite-corrected plasma concentration is not a compartment because it is measured separately from the PET images and is assumed to be known.

free, bound, and nonspecifically bound states, respectively. B_c is the concentration of unlabeled (or "cold") tracer bound to receptors.

The part of the model of greatest interest to investigators of receptor binding is $k_{on}[B'_{max} - (B + B_c)]F$. This expression describes binding of free tracer to available receptors. It states that the concentration of available receptors is the difference between available receptors at steady state, B'_{max} (a constant), and receptors bound to either labeled, B, or unlabeled tracer, B_c (time-varying functions). *Note*: In a single-injection experiment, there is always a known relationship between labeled and unlabeled bound ligand. The ratio of the labeled to the unlabeled is the specific activity (SA is given in μCi/pmol or Bq/pmol, ratios of radioactivity to mass of ligand). Thus, the expression for available receptors is often written as $(B'_{max} - B/\text{SA})$. It will be clear why this is not adequate for modeling M-I PET data (Morris *et al.*, 1996).

Because the binding of a ligand to a receptor is a bimolecular process, it depends on available receptors, the presence of free ligand, F, and a bimolecular rate constant, k_{on}. In conventional single-injection experiments, which are predicated on injecting only a tiny ("trace") amount of radioligand, the amount of bound tracer (labeled or unlabeled) never rivals the available sites at steady state and so the term of interest, $k_{on}[B'_{max} - (B + B_c)]$, reduces to $k_{on}B'_{max}$. In this case, the model is analogous to the example described in Section II. Namely, the parameters k_{on} and B'_{max} are not uniquely identifiable and the parameter estimation problem is reduced, of necessity, to finding an effective first-order rate constant $k_3 (= k_{on}B'_{max})$.

The raison d'etre of M-I PET experiments is specifically to overcome the problem of k_{on} and B'_{max} being irretrievably correlated (i.e., unidentifiable). Why do we want to identify these parameters separately? For one, the equilibrium dissociation constant (affinity constant) K_D is the ratio of the rate constants k_{off} and k_{on}. Thus, estimation of the *in vivo* K_D for a PET ligand is effectively dependent on the estimation of k_{off} and k_{on}. Estimation of these two constants—or their ratio—is not possible from a single-injection PET study. However, if the injected mass of tracer is modulated sufficiently in the course of multiple bolus injections of tracer such that the occupancy of receptors varies over a large enough range, then the term $(B'_{max} - B - B_c)$ must be retained explicitly in the model. It then becomes possible to identify the unique roles of the association rate constant and the concentration of available receptors in the uptake and binding of a tracer. In doing so, we move toward being able to estimate the receptor number and the affinity constant separately and possibly toward using PET to distinguish a defect of receptor function from a defect of receptor number.

D. M-I Model Equations

How do we adapt the standard model equations to accommodate the description of M-I data? One approach is to treat the separate injections as separate species that compete for the same receptor sites. Figure 2 diagrams the case of three

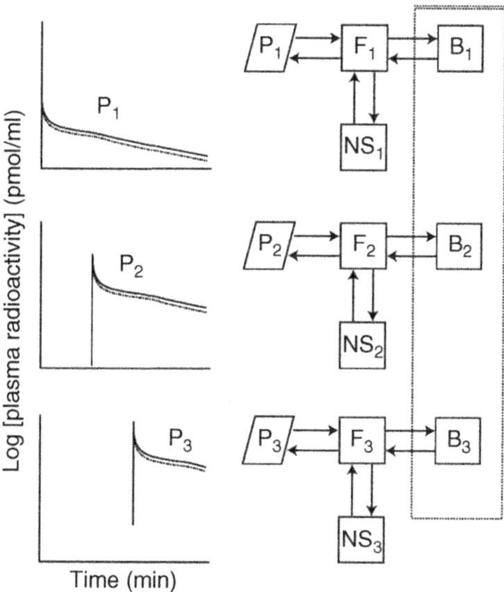

Fig. 2 Three parallel, coupled models with distinct input functions, P_1, P_2, and P_3, used to describe the dynamic time-activity curves generated from different regions of interest by a multiple-injection PET study. (*Note:* P_1 in the figure corresponds to the individual input functions $C_p^j(t - T^j)U(t - T^j)$ in the text.) All parameters are assumed to be identical across parallel models. The models are coupled because they share a common pool of receptors, B'_{max} (indicated by the dotted box surrounding all bound compartments), initially available to the tracer, regardless of injection. The injections, offset in time, that correspond to each respective subcompartmental model are illustrated to the left.

separate bolus injections of tracer. The important thing to recognize about this extension for M-I data is that the specific activity of each injection is intentionally different. Therefore, it will be necessary to somehow track the individual inputs over the entire course of the study. This is one of the subtleties of the M-I PET technique. A blood sample taken shortly after a third bolus injection will contain radioactivity that originates with each of the three injections (assuming that all three injections contain radioactivity). Figure 3 depicts the multiple injections in terms of measured radioactivity and in terms of molar quantities needed for solving the model. One approach to *a posteriori* dissection of the measured blood radioactivity is discussed at length by Morris *et al.* (1996). In brief, we might assume that all input functions have the same shape but different scales. Thus, the observed plasma radioactivity can be described as

$$C_p(t) = \sum_j S^j C_p^j(t - T^j)U(t - T^j) \tag{4}$$

where S^j is a scale factor related to injected dose, $C_p(t)$ is an analytical expression of exponentials, and $U(t - T)$ is the unit step function at time T (i.e., $U = 0$, $t < T$; $U = 1$, $t \geq T$). From Eq. (4), it is possible to recover separate C_p^j curves for each injection from the measured plasma radioactivity.

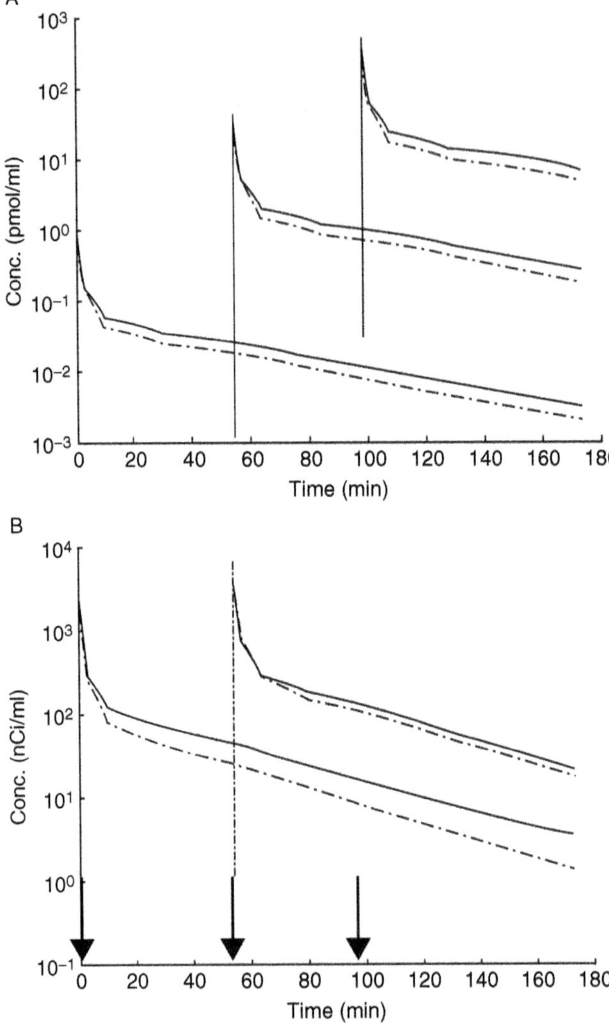

Fig. 3 (A) Input functions for each injection in terms of total ligand concentration in pmol/ml (all species (solid) and metabolite-corrected (dotted)). Metabolite-corrected molar concentrations are used to construct the input function (see text for details). (**B**) Input functions in terms of radioactivity concentration (nCi/ml). The third injection consisted of unlabeled ligand only; therefore, there is no peak of radioactivity at the time of the third injection. There is input to the system, however, that must be measured somehow or modeled based on the shape of the other input functions as described in the text. Injection times are indicated by vertical arrows.

The general model equations for multiple injections take on the following form:

$$\frac{dF^j}{dt} = K_1 C_p^j - (k_2 + k_5)F^j - k_{on}\left(B'_{max} - \sum_l B_l^j\right)F^j + k_{off}B^j + k_6 NS^j \quad (5)$$

$$\frac{dB^j}{dt} = k_{on}\left(B'_{max} - \sum_l B_l^j\right)F^j - k_{off}B^j \quad (6)$$

$$\frac{dNS^j}{dt} = k_5 F^j - k_6 NS^j \quad (7)$$

where j is the index over injection number; B_l^j is either B^j or B_c^j.

The assumption of Eqs. (5)–(7) is that the kinetic parameters (K_1, k_2, k_{on}, k_{off}, B'_{max}, k_5, k_6) are unaffected by the injection of either a high- or a low-specific activity tracer.

From the mass balance equations in Eqs. (5)–(7), we can construct the instantaneous output equation to describe the total radioactivity, $T(t)$, measured in the tissue at any moment in time as a result of one or more injections:

$$T(t) = \sum_j SA^j(t)(1 - F_v)[F^j(t) + B^j(t) + NS^j(t)] + F_v C_{wb}^j(t) \quad (8)$$

where SA^j converts the concentration associated with each injection in the tissue (F, B, and NS are in pmol/ml) into radioactivity, F_v is the blood volume fraction, and C_{wb} is the radioactivity concentration (nCi/ml) in whole blood. *Note*: The concentration of tracer in the arterial plasma (pmol/ml) is the driving force for uptake of the tracer into the tissue and, hence, the appropriate input function. However, any radioactivity in the microvasculature in the ROI contributes to the PET signal, so C_{wb} is the appropriate term for the output equation, which is in the units of the PET measurement (nCi/ml).

IV. Experimental Protocol and Considerations

M-I PET studies are sophisticated experiments, both in design and in implementation. The appropriate duration for the experiment is dependent on both the kinetics of the ligand and the half-life of the positron-emitting nuclide. In nuclear-counting experiments, the noise in the data and hence, the parameter precision are determined by the amount of radioactivity (i.e., photons) collected. From this point of view, it would be desirable to acquire PET data for as long as possible. Unfortunately, due to the expenses associated with reserving PET scanner time, veterinarian staff, and anesthetization of the animal, one of the primary considerations when designing an M-I experiment is to minimize the duration of the experiment. On the other hand, because we use these experiments to maximize precision of the parameter estimates, there is a trade-off between convenience and precision. Successful experimental optimization can help balance this and other trade-offs and achieve a desired level of parameter precision.

A. Animal Preparation

Conducting M-I studies requires a small team of personnel to ensure a successful experiment. Input from all of the team members is needed to carefully plan and design an experiment that follows the guidelines of the Institutional Animal Care and Use Committee (IACUC). A skilled veterinary staff is needed to anesthetize the animal and to insert the catheter lines for ligand injection (venous) and blood withdrawal (arterial). In general, the choice of anesthetic is determined by the investigator and the veterinary staff based on their familiarity with the anesthetic agent, ease of use, and animal safety considerations. Because M-I PET experiments measure tiny (subnanomolar) concentrations, care must be taken that any biochemical effects of the anesthetic drugs do not perturb the biochemical system under study. For example, ketamine is a widely used preanesthetic known to interact with the dopaminergic system of the brain (Smith *et al.*, 1998); therefore, a M-I study targeting the dopaminergic system should allow adequate time (>1 h) for the effects of ketamine to subside before administration of the PET ligand. Most M-I studies require a minimum of 3 h of animal anesthetization, including animal preparation (see, e.g., timeline in Table I). The entire experiment can last up to 12 h. The anesthetic must provide a stable physiological system throughout this time course, it must minimize changes in regional blood flow (which affects ligand delivery), and it must withstand possible drug-induced stimulation. For the safety of the animals, typically 1–2 weeks must be allowed between experiments for the animal to recover from the effects of the anesthesia.

The insertion of two catheters is needed for M-I studies: a venous port for the administration of ligand and an arterial port for the temporal sampling of plasma radioactivity. The ligand is generally administered into a vein as a bolus infusion (5–30 s in duration) in several milliliters of saline. A bolus infusion is needed to accurately identify the ligand delivery parameter (K_1). As nearly as possible, all injections of ligand for each experiment should be given in an identical fashion so that ligand delivery is consistent throughout each epoch of the experiment (see Section IV.B).

B. Measuring Blood Activity and Constructing Input Curves

Accurate measurement of the radioligand concentration over time in the arterial plasma is essential to precise estimation of model parameters. The input function provides the essential time-varying details of radioligand delivery to the tissue of interest. An example of three arterial plasma input functions (in terms of both molar concentration (Fig. 3A) and radioactivity (Fig. 3B)) and the plasma radioactivity curves from which they are derived are depicted in Fig. 3. The graph in

Table I
Example of a Timeline for a Multiple-Injection Pet Experiment[a]

Sample experiment measurement of D_2/D_3 receptor density in the thalamus with fallypride	
00:00:00	Preanesthesia with glycopyrolate (0.01 mg/kg)
00:30:00	Anesthesia with ketamine (10 mg/kg)/xylazine (0.5 mg/kg)
00:45:00	Intubate monkey and maintain with 1–2% isoflurane
00:60:00	Insert venous (saphenous) and arterial (femoral) catheters
01:30:00	Position monkey in PET scanner, monitor vitals
01:45:00	Acquire 10-min transmission scan for attenuation correction
02:00:00	Begin PET data acquisition
02:00:00	Injection #1, "tracer study" with high-specific activity injectate (SA_1 ~2000 mCi/μmol); withdraw blood samples periodically for analysis (~1 ml each)
02:54:00	Injection #2, "partial saturation" with low-SA injectate (SA_2 ~ 100 mCi/μmol); take blood samples
03:38:00	Injection #3, "saturation" with unlabeled fallypride only ($SA_3 = 0$ mCi/μmol); take blood samples
05:00:00	Terminate PET acquisition; remove anesthesia
05:15:00	Remove intubation when gag reflex is recovered
06:00:00	Monitor monkey during recovery from anesthesia

[a]The protocol was designed to elicit a precise estimate of B'_{max}, available receptors in the thalamus that bind [^{18}F]fallypride. In this particular design, the last injection contains only unlabeled fallypride. Note the absence of a "hot" peak at the corresponding third injection in Fig. 3B.

Fig. 3B shows measurable quantities of *radioactivity* (in nCi/ml) in the plasma. The plot displays two different measured quantities: total radioactivity in arterial plasma (solid curve) and metabolite-corrected arterial radioactivity (dash-dot line). The latter, corrected plasma concentration, is data needed for each of three input functions that drive the model, whereas whole blood radioactivity measurement (not shown) is needed for solution of the output equation (see Section III). With knowledge of the specific activity, blood data corresponding to each of the injections can be converted to input functions for the total (molar) ligand concentration, as shown in Fig. 3A. In the case of an experiment that includes a "saturation" component, the contribution of the third injection to the total ligand input function, $C_p(t)$, cannot be measured directly from the (radioactivity) blood curve, as no additional radioactivity is injected (see earlier discussion). Instead, the *shape* of the curve must be inferred from the previous injections. The scale factor, S, for the injection of unlabeled material can be determined from the ratio of the doses.

The shape of the input function is, in part, determined by the speed of the venous injection (e.g., a rapid bolus injection will result in a sharply peaked input function (blurred by dispersion as the bolus travels through the vasculature)). The blood curve is measured by withdrawing blood samples from the arterial port. The frequency of withdrawal must be matched to the anticipated shape of the input function. Blood samples are usually drawn every 5–10 s for the first several minutes following ligand injection. The samples can be drawn less frequently as the ligand begins to equilibrate between plasma and tissue(s).

As a general rule of thumb, the total volume of blood withdrawn for an experiment should not exceed 10% of the blood volume of the animal. Sampling of a 10-kg rhesus monkey would be limited to roughly 70 ml (assuming 7% of body weight is blood volume). This volume should be replaced by an iv drip of saline over the course of the experiment. The arterial blood samples are centrifuged to separate the plasma from the red blood cells. The plasma samples can be assayed further to separate the native ligand from the radiolabeled metabolic by-products. The volume of each arterial plasma sample must be large enough to yield an accurate measurement of radioactivity in the final plasma fraction (as gauged by radioactive counting statistics). In the case of primates, the volume of each arterial sample is typically 1 ml.

C. Generation of Regional Time-Activity Curves (TACs) from PET Images

As in most dynamic PET experiments, the M-I model is fitted to tissue TACs derived from PET scans yielding estimates of the kinetic parameters of interest (see Section V). Data at each time point are based on investigator-defined regions of interests (ROIs) placed on the PET images at each time. Although single-injection PET studies are sometimes analyzed in a pixel-by-pixel manner (to generate parametric maps), fitting the M-I model to data would be too demanding computationally to do so.

In most cases, ROI analysis requires that high-resolution structural image (typically a T_1-weighted MRI) is acquired and coregistered to a PET image for each PET subject. The preferred PET image (for use in registration only) is usually an image of the summed (or averaged) radioactivity over the entire duration of the PET study. The MRI allows the investigator to precisely define the exact anatomical location of ROIs, and the coregistration then gives coordinates that allow the ROIs to be applied in proper spatial orientation to each frame of PET data. Taking the average radioactivity in the ROI at each time point generates the desired TAC. Typically, PET images are not suitable as the basis for ROI templates for two reasons: (1) specific anatomy may not be resolved easily and (2) hot spots in the PET image may induce unintentional bias in the ROI placement by the investigator. Several intermodality registration algorithms (e.g., automated image registration (AIR) by Woods *et al.*, 1992, 1993) are available both in commercial medical image analysis packages (e.g., MEDx, Medical Numerics, Germantown, MD) and as stand-alone code for free download (http://bishopw.loni.ucla.edu/AIR5). The standard is now to use registration software based on a mutual information algorithm (available, e.g., in recent versions of SPM, see http://www.fil.ion.ucl.ac.uk/spm/software/).

The ROIs selected will probably depend on the characteristics of the radiotracer used. [^{18}F]Fallypride is a highly selective D_2/D_3 receptor ligand with a high-PET signal-to-noise ratio and excellent resolution in areas with low-to-moderate concentrations of D_2 receptors (e.g., cortex, thalamus) (Mukherjee *et al.*, 1995). In investigations with this ligand, several brain regions are available for analysis (in contrast, other ligands may not provide reliable data outside of brain regions with extremely high numbers of D_2/D_3 receptors (e.g., striatum) and ROIs of interest may range from very large volumes (e.g., whole striatum, whole thalamus) to smaller, more specific volumes (e.g., cortical areas, amygdala, nucleus accumbens, individual thalamic areas)). An important point to consider in selecting ROIs is their volume. Larger volumes (composed of many voxels) result in TACs with higher signal-to-noise ratios. These low-noise curves typically lead to successful data fitting and thus precise parameter estimation. Unfortunately, larger ROIs are also more prone to be heterogeneous in tissue composition and therefore lead to data that reflect an average of kinetically different regions. The investigator must also be aware that small ROIs may suffer from partial volume (PV) effect error if the structures they circumscribe are small relative to the resolution of the scanner. PV error will lead to nonlinear underestimation of the true radioactivity in the ROI and, subsequently, bias in the parameter estimates. For a review of PV error and for various approaches to correcting for it, see Kessler *et al.* (1984), Meltzer *et al.* (1996), Morris *et al.* (1999), Muller-Gartner *et al.* (1992), Muzic *et al.* (1998), Rousset *et al.* (1993, 1996, 1998), Strul and Bendriem (1999).

The resulting TACs from three brain regions generated by placing ROIs on images made in the example protocol given earlier (Table I) are shown in Fig. 4. Specific binding is highest in the striatum, moderate in the thalamus, and nearly absent in the cerebellum. We can tell this, in part, from observing (1) similarity of the decline in tracer concentration following the first and second injections and (2) the absence of deflection from the descending curve of the cerebellum at the time of the third injection. That is, injection of high- or low-specific activity does

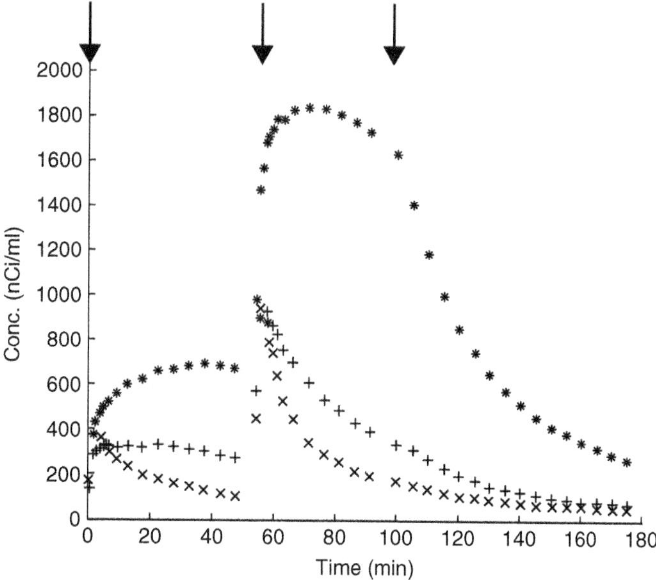

Fig. 4 Time-activity curves from the striatum (∗), thalamus (+), and cerebellum (×) from a multiple-injection study of D_2/D_3 dopamine receptors with [^{18}F]fallypride. All data are from the same animal. Injection times are indicated by vertical arrows.

not change the shape of the curve because of (1) the absence of receptors in the region and (2) the injection of cold tracer does not accentuate displacement because there is no specific binding to be displaced. The next sections address the fitting of models to data and present a resulting fit to one of the curves in Fig. 4.

V. Models and Data Fitting

A. Implementing Model Equations

This section describes the framework for relating the theoretical models (described earlier) to data that are collected (as described earlier). Since a PET scanner measures radioactivity concentration, the output equation, Eq. (8), is used to relate the radioactivity concentration (e.g., Bq/ml or μCi/ml) to the molar concentration (e.g., pmol/ml) in various compartments. However, a modification to Eq. (8) should be used in practice, as the PET scanner does not measure instantaneous radioactivity concentration. Rather, it measures concentration averaged over acquisition time intervals commonly referred to as frames. Thus, we define model$_i$ as the time-averaged concentration over frame i and compute this quantity as

$$\text{model}_i = \frac{1}{d_i}\int_{t_i}^{t_i+d_i} T(\tau)\mathrm{d}\tau \tag{9}$$

where t_i and d_i are the start time and durations of frame i and T is from Eq. (8).

To implement such an equation, it is convenient to express it in a form that can be solved with an ODE solver such as is used to solve the state equations (Eqs. (5)–(7)). Accordingly, we introduce a new expression for the integrand in Eq. (9):

$$\frac{\mathrm{d}h}{\mathrm{d}t} = T \tag{10}$$

When this differential equation, Eq. (10), is solved with initial condition $h(0) = 0$ (no radioactivity in the system at time zero), the expression for the model-predicted PET signal in time frame i is simply

$$\text{model}_i = \frac{1}{d_i}[h(t_i + d_i) - h(t_i)] \tag{11}$$

B. Parameter Estimation

In M-I studies, estimating values of model parameters as precisely as possible is often the primary goal. Parameter values provide quantitative assessments of receptor concentration, affinity, blood flow, etc. To accomplish the goal, one typically "fits a model" to data. This entails finding the values of model parameters that are most consistent with data. Mathematically, the problem is equivalent to adjusting the values of the model parameters in order to minimize the difference between the model prediction and the actual measurement of tissue radioactivity ("data"). Consider what is called the weighted least-squares objective function, which measures this difference:

$$o(\mathbf{p}) = \sum_i [w_i(\text{model}_i(\mathbf{p}) - \text{data}_i)^2] \tag{12}$$

where data_i represents data from frame "i" and $\text{model}_i(\mathbf{p})$ represents the model output, which is intended to predict data_i. Model output depends on the values of the parameter vector **p**. The task is then to adjust values of the components of **p** to make model output most closely agree with data. Mathematically, we minimize $o(\,)$ with respect to **p**. We include weights, w_i, because we do not expect to achieve perfect agreement between model and data and because we do not have uniform confidence in the measurements. The value of w_i may be specified as the reciprocal of (an estimate of) the variance of data_i, in which case the value of **p** that minimizes $o(\,)$ is a maximum likelihood estimate.[1]

While one could adjust the values of model parameters *manually* to find the ones that best explain data, such a search can often be done more efficiently and more objectively by a mathematical algorithm implemented on a computer. The Levenberg-Marquardt algorithm is popular for this application (Levenberg, 1944; Marquardt, 1963; More, 1977) Because the value of $o(\mathbf{p})$ has a complex dependence on values of the parameters, a closed form solution, which minimizes $o(\mathbf{p})$ in the general case, is not available. Consequently, an iterative approach must be used. One starts with an initial guess of the parameter values and then adjusts the components of the parameter vector **p** in order to reduce the value of $o(\mathbf{p})$. The efficiency of this process depends on having a means to predict values of $o(\mathbf{p})$ as values of **p** are altered because this provides a basis for adjusting parameter values. For this purpose, algorithms often require an estimate of the derivative of the objective function $o(\,)$ with respect to the parameter vector **p**. By differentiating Eq. (12) with respect to component j of the parameter vector, we obtain the expression

$$\frac{\mathrm{d}o}{\mathrm{d}p_j} = 2\sum_i \left[w_i(\text{model}_i - \text{data}_i)\frac{\mathrm{d}\text{model}_i}{\mathrm{d}p_j} \right] \tag{13}$$

Notably, this expression contains a term for the derivative of the model output with respect to component j of the parameter vector. These derivatives have particular significance and are given the name sensitivity functions.

One numerical approach to evaluating the sensitivity functions is to use finite differences. This approach is attractive because it is conceptually very simple: solve the model equations at one value of **p**, change the value of the jth component of **p** by a small amount denoted here as Δp_j, solve the model equations again, and then estimate the derivative as the difference in model output divided by Δp_j.

[1] Under certain assumptions about the data.

Unfortunately, in practice, this approach is not very robust. It is not at all trivial to pick a value of Δp_j small enough so that the finite differences approximate the desired derivative but not so small that the differences are dominated by "noise" or numerical imprecision.

A more robust—and recommended—approach to evaluating the sensitivity functions can be obtained by differentiating the state equations. To describe this approach, we have to take a step back and define notation for the composite set of differential equations for the state and output equations (Eqs. (5)–(7) and (10)). Recall that the equations were all of the form $dx/dt = y$ with accompanying specified initial conditions. We can group these together by defining a vector **c** and a vector-valued function $f(\,)$ that have components corresponding to the state and output equations and their variables. In the example given earlier, the vector **c** would have components

$$\mathbf{c} = [F \quad B \quad \mathrm{NS} \quad h]^{\mathrm{T}} \tag{14}$$

and the function $f(\,)$ would be defined as

$$\frac{\mathrm{d}\mathbf{c}}{\mathrm{d}t} = f(\mathbf{c}, t, \mathbf{p}) = \begin{bmatrix} \frac{\mathrm{d}F}{\mathrm{d}t} & \frac{\mathrm{d}B}{\mathrm{d}t} & \frac{\mathrm{dNS}}{\mathrm{d}t} & h \end{bmatrix}^{\mathrm{T}} \tag{15}$$

with

$$\mathbf{p} = [K_1 \quad k_2 \quad k_{\mathrm{on}} \quad k_{\mathrm{off}} \quad B'_{\mathrm{max}} \quad \ldots]^{\mathrm{T}} \tag{16}$$

The superscript T connotes the transpose; Eqs. (14)–(16) describe column vectors. The initial condition for **c**, called $\mathbf{c}_0$, is a column vector of the initial conditions of each of the state equations.

With the state and output equations expressed in this framework, we now obtain the equations needed for a robust approach to evaluating the sensitivity functions.

Specifically, by differentiating Eq. (15) and its initial condition with respect to the parameter vector **p** we obtain

$$\frac{\mathrm{d}\mathbf{S}}{\mathrm{d}t} = \frac{\partial f}{\partial \mathbf{c}}\mathbf{S} + \frac{\partial f}{\partial \mathbf{p}} \quad \text{with} \quad \mathbf{S}_0 = \frac{\partial \mathbf{c}_0}{\partial \mathbf{p}}, \tag{17}$$

which is an initial value problem like Eq. (15) except that **S** is a matrix. The rows of **S** correspond to those of **c**, whereas the columns of **S** correspond to different components of the derivatives. For example, the element in row 2, column 3 of **S** would be the derivative of B (element 2 of **c**) with respect to k_{on} (element 3 of **p**).

C. Numerical Solution of Differential Equations

Having presented a formalism of how we relate a model to experimental measurements, we next turn to the details of the numerical implementation of the solution of state, Eq. (15), and sensitivity equations, Eq. (17). These are both considered initial value problems. Numerically solving state equations entails programming Eq. (15) and selecting an appropriate ODE solver. For example, in MATLAB one could use a solver from Shampine's ODEsuite (Shampine and Reichelt, 1997), whereas in C or FORTRAN one might use a member of the LSODE family of solvers (Hindmarsh, 1983; Hindmarsh and Serban, 2002; Leis and Kramer, 1988).

Conceptually, algorithms for solving these initial value problems begin with the initial value and use the Euler formula to approximate the solution at the next time step. For example,

$$\mathbf{c}(t + \Delta t) \cong \mathbf{c}(t) + f(\mathbf{c}, t, \mathbf{p}) \cdot \Delta t. \tag{18}$$

Details of the implementation must include a strategy for selecting Δt to achieve a specified accuracy in the solution without requiring an excessive amount of computation. Fortunately, problems of this form are common and a number of algorithms are available. Generally, algorithms are classified as being designed for "stiff" or "nonstiff" equations. Details of these designations are beyond the scope of this chapter, but suffice it to say that "stiff" equations are "hard" problems to solve in that the solver is forced to take very small steps in Δt. Special algorithms have been designed for stiff equations. In comparison to nonstiff solvers, stiff solvers trade-off more complex algorithms and evaluations in each step for the ability to take larger steps.

How does one determine if equations are stiff in any given case? The pragmatic approach is to try both stiff and nonstiff solvers. Well-written solvers have built-in methods to select step size (Δt) and still keep errors in the solution within a specified range. Under such conditions, using a nonstiff solver with stiff equations (and vice versa) would lead to computationally inefficient solutions.

We alert the reader to the availability of a MATLAB-based software package that implements methods for setting up and solving models such as those used to analyze dynamic PET data. The package includes implementations of state and sensitivity equations and functions for fitting models to data in order to estimate parameters. COMKAT (Muzic and Cornelius, 2001) can be downloaded from http://comkat.case.edu. It was written by one of the authors of this chapter (R.F.M.) and is presently used by each of the authors in their research. COMKAT takes into account the details described in the preceding section so that its users do not have to be experts in numerical analysis.

D. Parameter Estimation Considerations

1. Selection of the Initial Guess

As mentioned in the previous section, algorithms estimate parameters by starting with an initial guess of the parameter values and adjusting them to minimize the value of the objective function. Care should be taken in selection of the initial guess. Algorithms often converge to the true parameter values only when the initial guess is "close enough" to the true values. How close is "close enough" is difficult to quantify in practice because it depends on the true parameter values, which are unknown, and also on the information content of data. In practice, as one is developing the fitting strategies for a particular application, one should try the estimation procedure with a range of initial guesses. Analysis of the resultant parameter estimates will provide insight into how close is "close enough."

2. Validating Parameter Estimates

When the optimization algorithm has converged to parameter values and the model output and data are in close agreement, one might assume that the parameter estimates are valid and even precise. This is not always the case. For example, there could be more than one set of parameter values that produce a model output that agrees well with data. One possibility is that there are multiple local minima in the objective function *o*( ). Another possibility is that the parameters are correlated, meaning that different combinations of parameter values will lead to essentially the same model output. Consider plotting *o*( ) as a function of values of two parameters with the height of the surface indicating the value of *o*( ). If the surface is relatively flat, then a large change in the parameter values would give rise to a small change in *o*( ). To achieve good precision in the parameter estimates, we would like to design the experiments to make the surface of *o*( ) steep. A steep objective function means that data are very sensitive to the model parameters. Moreover, we want the surface to be steep in all directions. Consider an alternative case wherein the surface is shaped like a long narrow valley aligned with the parameter axes. Changes along the valley floor make hardly any difference in the value of *o*( ). An experiment that yielded such an objective function would be insensitive to the parameter aligned with the valley, and it would not be possible to make reliable estimates for this parameter.

To investigate these possibilities, it is important to conduct simulation studies *a priori*. The basic steps of the study are as follows. (1) Create data; using representative parameter values, solve the model equations to create "perfect" data. (2) Add "noise" to perfect data to emulate the expected imprecision in the experimental data. (3) Fit simulated data with the proposed parameter estimation method. This process must be repeated numerous times with different noise realizations. Parameter estimates are then compared to the *known* values used to create data. In particular, one might calculate the error in the parameter estimates by subtracting the true values from each estimate and then summarize data in terms of the bias and precision of the estimates by calculating the mean and standard deviation of the error.

While the aforementioned techniques are important in establishing the validity of the parameter estimates, they are not necessarily complete. Simulation is but one component of validation. The next section describes another component: careful examination of the model fit to measured data.

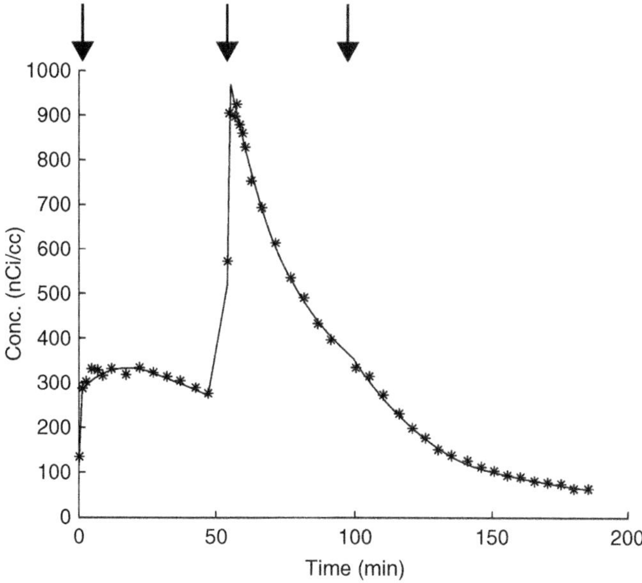

Fig. 5 Data from the time-activity curve from the thalamus (middle curve, Fig. 4). The solid curve indicates the fit of the model given in Eqs. (4)–(9) to data via with nonlinear parameter estimation described in the text. Injection times are indicated by vertical arrows.

VI. Results and Interpretation

A fit to the TAC for an ROI drawn on the thalamus (middle curve in Fig. 4) is shown in Fig. 5. This fit results in estimates of the "best" parameter values that can explain data, but how do we know if these estimates are good? There are tests that must be done. One was suggested in the previous section; namely, if fitting the model to simulated data sets reveals that multiple choices of parameters would result in equally good fits, there is little hope that fits to experimental data (which may not be strictly consistent with the model) will yield more identifiable parameters. However, assuming that the model appears to fit simulated data well and that minimizing the objective function yields unique parameters, what are the basic steps that must be followed to evaluate the quality of the results?

A. Examination of Residuals

Figure 6 shows a plot of normalized residuals derived from the fit to M-I data shown in Fig. 5. Normalized residuals, calculated as [model$_i$ – data$_i$]/S.D.(data$_i$), are a good way of determining the quality of the fit. Ideally, these residuals should be distributed normally with zero mean and unit standard deviation. Both of these conditions appear to be met in Fig. 6. The mean of the residuals will be obvious

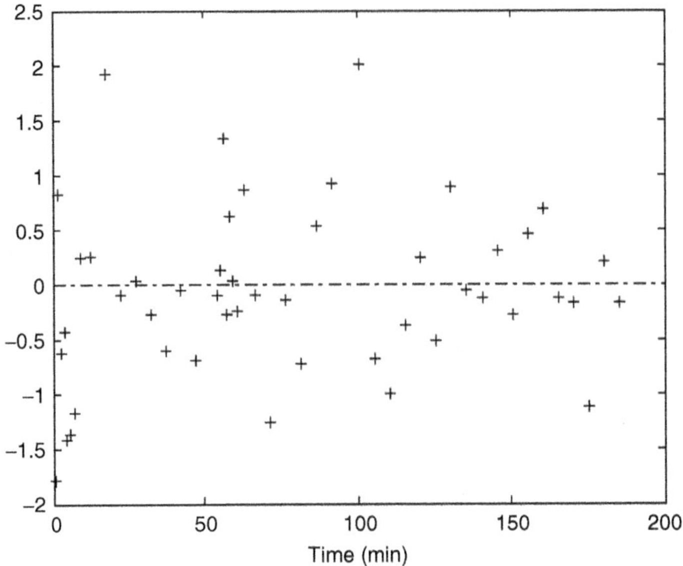

Fig. 6 Plot of the normalized residuals derived from fitted M-I thalamus data (shown in Fig. 5). Note the apparent zero-mean behavior of the residuals. See text for details.

from their plot. Any order in the pattern of the residuals, however, may indicate that the model is deficient. To determine the nonrandomness of the residuals it is useful to perform a "runs" test. A run is defined as a series of adjacent residuals that are either all positive or all negative. The fewer the number of runs, the more likely that the fit is poor and that either the model or the fitting algorithm is suspect (for examples using the runs test, see Bard, 1974).

B. Parameter Precision

If fits to data are acceptable, then the investigator will want to report his/her findings in terms of the estimated parameter values and their approximate uncertainties (variance, standard deviation, confidence intervals, correlation, etc.). To report intratrial variance, it is necessary to use an estimate of parameter variance because one fit to a data set yields only one estimate of each parameter. Many search algorithms (such as the Levenberg-Marquardt mentioned previously) will return a covariance matrix along with the optimal parameter set. The covariance matrix is usually approximated by the inverse of the weighted product of the sensitivity matrix (mentioned in the previous section) with its transpose ($\text{Cov}(\mathbf{p}) = [S^T W S]^{-1}$, where W is an $n \times n$ diagonal matrix whose elements are related inversely to the n data points in the TAC). The approximation is valid when the parameter values $\mathbf{p}$ are close to the optimal point. The diagonal elements of the resulting covariance matrix are the variances of the respective parameters. Parameters should be reported plus or minus a standard deviation (±S.D.) (square root of the variance).

Normalization of the covariance matrix by its diagonal elements yields the correlation matrix. It is prudent to examine this matrix, whose diagonal elements are unity and whose off-diagonal elements are the covariances between parameters. Highly correlated parameters (e.g., correlation >0.95) are not separable. See Table II for an example correlation matrix produced from a six-parameter fit to [^{18}F]fallypride data shown in Fig. 5. If two parameters a and b are highly correlated, then, in practical terms, only their product (or their ratio) is identified. Neither of their values individually should be trusted because an increase in one could be completely offset by a comparable decrease (or increase) in the other with no decrement to the quality of the fit and no basis for choosing one combination of parameters over another with the same product. Consider the following practical scenario. If B'_{max} is highly correlated with k_{on} (as is often the case), then there will be multiple pairs of these parameters that will be equally plausible choices to explain the acquired data. Imagine further that we are trying to compare the on rate (k_{on}) of a tracer at the serotonin transporter site in two groups of subjects, who are known to express different genetic variants of the transporter, to test the hypothesis that the binding rate will be different. If one of the groups also tends to have fewer available receptors at steady state (smaller B'_{max}) because of medication that blocks these sites (e.g., Prozac), then the medication will be a confound and the population on medication may be seen, artifactually, to have faster binding because the higher k_{on} merely balances a lower B'_{max} when data are fitted. The correlation matrix in Table II confirms that, thanks to the M-I experiment, correlations among k_{on}, B'_{max}, and k_{off} have all been minimized. In contrast, in a single-injection experiment, the correlation between k_{on} and B'_{max} would be nearly 1.

Table II
Correlation Matrix for the Data Fit Depicted in Fig. 5[a]

	K_1	k_2	k_{on}	B'_{max}	k_5	k_{off}
K_1	1	–	–	–	–	–
k_2	0.809	1	–	–	–	–
k_{on}	−0.632	−0.181	1	–	–	–
B'_{max}	0.612	0.751	*−0.197*	1	–	–
k_5	0.13	0.496	0.429	0.604	1	–
k_{off}	−0.374	−0.211	*0.416*	*0.162*	0.635	1

[a]Each element in the matrix is Corr(a, b). Diagonal elements are 1 because each parameter is completely correlated with itself. Thanks to the M-I experiment, there is very little correlation among any of the parameters B'_{max}, k_{on}, and k_{off} (see italic values). The correlation matrix is symmetric, so the top half of the matrix has not been shown; Corr(a, b) = Corr(b, a).

C. Model Selection/Goodness of Fit

Often, even well-designed experiments produce data that do not justify the use of models of the desired complexity. That is, not all parameters of the model can be identified. In these cases, it may be necessary to opt for a simpler model by fixing some parameters and not estimating them. How do we know that the simpler model is appropriate? There are a number of popular criteria that gauge "goodness of fit." One such determinant of goodness of fit is the F statistic (Landaw and DiStefano, 1984). As in all statistical testing, it is conducted with reference to the question of whether to accept or reject the null hypothesis. In the case of model selection, the null hypothesis is that the simpler model is adequate to describe data. Another popular index is the Akaike critierion (Akaike, 1976), $\text{AIC} = \ln(\text{SS}) + 2P$, where SS is the weighted sum of squares that result from the fit to data and P is the number of parameters in the model. Thus, a "good fit" will correspond to a low-AIC value, but AIC will be penalized if the fit is achieved through the use of extraneous parameters. In the case of the fit to [^{18}F]fallypride data shown for the thalamus in Fig. 5, data did not support use of both a k_5 and a k_6 parameter. It was found that setting k_6 identically to zero and estimating only k_5 was necessary and sufficient to fit data. To confirm that this was the appropriate model, the Akaike criterion was calculated for both six-parameter (k_6 set to 0) and seven-parameter fits, and the six-parameter fit was shown to be better.

VII. Understanding and Designing M-I Experiments

A. Sensitivity Functions

The sensitivity functions described earlier are key to the procedure of minimizing the least-squares objective function. They are also central to understanding how data fitting in general and the analysis of M-I data in particular work. Once we understand what the sensitivity functions tell us, we can use them to improve the design of our experiments. For an example, consider the sensitivity functions plotted in Fig. 7. These curves correspond to the derivatives of the model with respect to the six parameters, $\mathbf{p}$, that were estimated by fitting the model to data from thalamus (shown in Fig. 5). The sensitivity equations have been solved at the value of the parameters that minimized the objective function given in Eq. (12). First, we noted that the sensitivities are time-varying functions as we would expect from looking at Eq. (17). In other words, the sensitivity of the observed PET signal to any model parameter rises and falls throughout the course of the experiment. The PET signal may be most sensitive to one parameter at one moment and to another at the next. Early time data are usually the most sensitive to blood flow parameters (i.e., K_1, k_2), whereas late-time data are sensitive to receptor binding. In fact, the independent, time-varying status of each of the sensitivity functions is at the heart of parameter identifiability. In Fig. 7A and B, one can observe that the sensitivities to the K_1 and k_2 parameters are very nearly identical except that one is

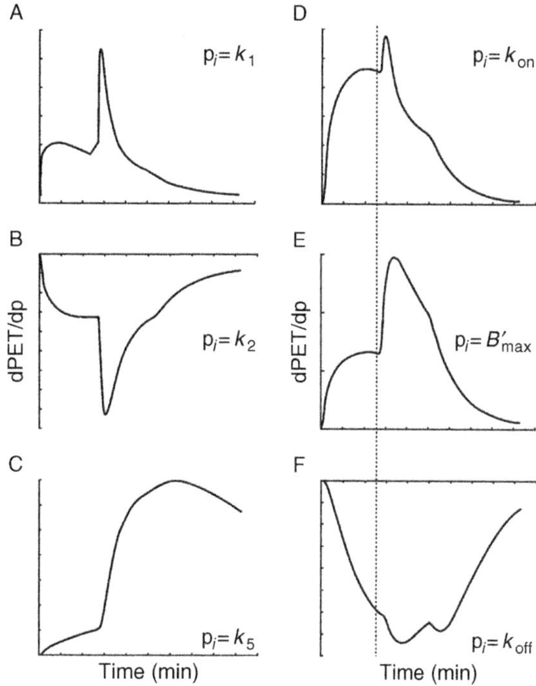

Fig. 7 Sensitivity curves for all six parameters of the model depicted in Fig. 2 evaluated over time and at the optimal parameter vector resulting from the fit to data shown in Fig. 5. Each curve is on its own scale. The vertical dotted line in D, E, and F corresponds to the time of the second injection. Everything on those plots to the left of the dotted line is the equivalent of sensitivity curves for a single injection study. See text for details.

always positive and the other always negative. We explain this behavior by noting that these two parameters are both dependent on blood flow (K_1 = extraction fraction × flow; $k_2 = K_1$/volume of distribution). As blood flow increases, more tracer is delivered to the tissue and, hence, the effect on the measurable signal is a positive one. An increase in blood flow also means that k_2, the rate at which tracer leaves the tissue, will increase and we would expect the PET signal to be diminished. The fact that these time courses mirror each other so closely means that they are not independent; in fact, they are nearly linearly dependent and so the parameters are highly correlated (Table II, Corr(K_1, k_2) = 0.809). Thus, these parameters are not identified easily from the type of experiment that was performed with [^{18}F]fallypride to estimate receptor binding in regions of moderate binding. Luckily, identification of the blood flow parameters is not the goal of the experiment. K_1 and k_2 are much better and more easily identified by an experiment involving a very sharp injection of tracer and rapid blood sampling to catch the fine detail of the input function.

More interesting from the standpoint of potential receptor-ligand characterization are the curves in Fig. 7D–F. Figure 7D–F shows the time-varying derivatives of the PET with respect to k_{on}, B'_{max}, and k_{off}, respectively. If we consider just the first epoch in each curve (to the left of the dotted line), it is very hard to distinguish the role that is played by any of these parameters. Certainly, there would be no difference in effect between raising B'_{max} or raising k_{on} during the first epoch. Recall that the first epoch is merely a single-injection experiment (with a high-SA tracer), and it is well known that k_{on} and B'_{max} are not identifiable from such a limited experiment. The effect of *lowering* k_{off} during this period would also be hard to differentiate from a concomitant rise in either of the other two parameters. As mentioned earlier in such cases, modelers must fall back to an identifiable parameter and not try to estimate both the "*m*" and the "*n*" as discussed in Section II.

If we look over the entire study duration at the sensitivity curves for k_{on}, B'_{max}, and k_{off}, we can begin to appreciate that (1) they are each distinguishable from each other and (2) it takes a sufficiently complicated experiment that manipulates occupancy to draw out differences in the processes represented by the three separate parameters. Recall that the second and third injections were termed "partial saturation" and "saturation" (see Table I). In fact, Christian *et al.* (2004) observed that there is apparently a narrow range of partial saturations that, if achieved during the second phase of the M-I experiment, yield TACs for [^{18}F]fallypride experiments, which produce estimates of k_{on} and B'_{max} that are uncoupled. If the target level of occupancy is under- or overshot in these experiments, interestingly, the parameters remain correlated in the fitting. The potential success of M-I experiments has been explained previously in terms of the sensitivity coefficients (Morris *et al.*, 1999).

B. Using the Sensitivity Information for Design

How can we use this information that appears to be contained in the sensitivity curves objectively? This is the subject of what is known as sensitivity analysis and optimal experiment design. As learned in Section VI.B, the sensitivity matrix can be used to approximate the variances of each parameter estimate. Many scalar quantities can be derived from this matrix and used to compare different experimental designs. A classical index for optimization of an experiment is the *D*-optimal criterion. "*D*" refers to the determinant of the Hessian matrix ($H \approx S^T WS$) or, equivalently, to the determinant of the inverse of the covariance matrix. In either case, to achieve a *D*-optimal design, we seek to maximize the value of the determinant of the matrix. The matrix, in turn, contains information about the collective variances of the parameters. In a physical sense, the confidence region surrounding the optimal choice of parameters in parameter space is a n_p-dimensional ellipsoid (where n_p is number of parameters) whose axes are the eigenvectors of H. Maximizing the determinant of the Hessian matrix is equivalent to minimizing the volume of this confidence region and thus reducing the possible choices of the parameter vectors that yield an equally good fit to data. That is, maximizing det(H) is equivalent to minimizing overall variance of the parameters. Many other quantities can be derived from the Hessian matrix and used as design criteria to maximize or minimize some other aspect of a parameter or parameters (for examples related to PET experiments, see Muzic *et al.*, 1994, 1996, 2000).

Because the Hessian matrix is a function of both the parameters and the experimental protocol, there are two points to consider: (1) optimal design of experiments is iterative—it must be repeated as more becomes known about parameter values upon which Hessian-based criteria depend and (2) the variances of the parameter estimates can be improved by the best choice of protocols, that is, by optimizing over a set of design variables.

1. Design Variables

What are the design variables in the typical M-I PET experiment? There are two design variables. First, the specific activities of the respective injections can be varied by mixing differing amounts of labeled and unlabeled ligand for each injection. Second, the time between injections can be varied. Because the specific activity (or equivalently the mass for a given radioactivity dose) will determine the occupancy level of receptors at a given time, we can appreciate that specific activity is the experimenter's tool for manipulating the receptor-ligand system to achieve decreased parameter correlation and increased parameter precision. In some circumstances, it may be necessary to put constraints on the design. For instance, if the total time of the experiment must be limited for reasons of convenience or safety, this will act as a constraint on the combination of times between injections. If the synthesis of the radiopharmaceutical is very difficult, it may be practically necessary to limit the design of the M-I study to a one synthesis. If so, then we constrain the choice of specific activities. In particular, the second and third injections will be limited to lower SA than the high-SA material available for the first. To investigate more about this technique, the reader is directed elsewhere for uses of optimal design in PET and tracer kinetics (Bard, 1974; Beck and Arnold, 1977; Carson *et al.*, 1983; Christian *et al.*, 2004; Delforge *et al.*, 1989, 1991; Feng *et al.*, 1999; Jacquez, 1988; Morris *et al.*, 1991; Muzic, *et al.*, 1996, 2000).

VIII. Conclusion

M-I PET studies are labor-intensive undertakings that demand not only experimental acumen but also a synthesis of mathematical and numerical expertise as well. Despite the overhead associated with such experiments, they may be the only practical means of extracting certain kinetic information about tracer uptake and behavior *in vivo* from dynamic PET images. To the extent that it may be helpful and illuminating to determine precisely the values of all the *in vivo* kinetic parameters of a tracer, it is hoped that this chapter served part as an introductory review, part as a tutorial, and part as an operating guide to a useful technique that merges functional imaging with tracer kinetics and optimal experiment design.

References

Akaike, H. (1976). In "System Identification: Advances and Case Studies." (R. K. Mehra and D. G. Lainiotis, eds.), p. **27**. Academic Press, New York.

Bard, Y. (1974). "Nonlinear Parameter Estimation." p. 213. Academic Press, New York.

Beck, J., and Arnold, K. (1977). "Parameter Estimation in Engineering and Science." p. 419. Wiley, New York.

Bottlaender, M., Valette, H., Goutal, S., Dollé, F., Hinnen, F., Bourgeois, S., Schollhorn, M. A., and Delforge, J. Brain nicotinic acetylcholine receptor occupancy by nicotine: An estimation in monkeys by using a competition multi-injection PET study with [18F]fluoro-A-85380 (submitted).

Carson, E. R., Cobelli, C., and Finkelstein, L. (1983). "The Mathematical Modeling of Metabolic and Endocrine Systems," p. 129. Wiley, New York.

Christian, B. T., Narayanan, T., Bing, S., Morris, E. D., Mantil, J., and Mukherjee, J. (2004). *J. Cereb. Blood Flow Metab.* **24,** 309.

Converse, A. K., Barnhart, T. E., Dabbs, K. A., DeJesus, O. T., Larson, J. A., Nickles, R. J., Schneider, M. L., and Roberts, A. D. (2004). PET measurement of rCBF in the presence of a neurochemical tracer. *J. Neurosci. Methods* **132**(2), 199–208.

Costes, N., Merlet, I., Zimmer, L., Lavenne, F., Cinotti, L., Delforge, J., Luxen, A., Pujol, J. F., and Le Bars, D. (2002). *J. Cereb. Blood Flow Metab.* **22,** 753.

Delforge, J., Syrota, A., and Mazoyer, B. M. (1989). *Phys. Med. Biol.* **34,** 419.

Delforge, J., Syrota, A., and Mazoyer, B. M. (1990). *IEEE Trans. Biomed. Eng.* **37,** 653.

Delforge, J., Loc'h, C., Hantraye, P., Stulzaft, O., Khalili-Varasteh, M., Maziere, M., Syrota, A., and Maziere, B. (1991). *J. Cereb. Blood Flow Metab.* **11,** 914.

Delforge, J., Syrota, A., Bottlaender, M., Varastet, M., Loc'h, C., Bendriem, B., Crouzel, C., Brouillet, E., and Maziere, M. (1993). *J. Cereb. Blood Flow Metab.* **13,** 454.

Delforge, J., Pappata, S., Millet, P., Samson, Y., Bendriem, B., Jobert, A., Crouzel, C., and Syrota, A. (1995). *J. Cereb. Blood Flow Metab.* **15,** 284.

Delforge, J., Bottlaender, M., Loc'h, C., Guenther, I., Fuseau, C., Bendriem, B., Syrota, A., and Maziere, B. (1999). *J. Cereb. Blood Flow Metab.* **19,** 533.

Feng, D., Ho, D., Lau, K. K., and Siu, W. C. (1999). *Comput. Methods Programs Biomed.* **59,** 31.

Gallezot, J. D., Bottlaender, M. A., Delforge, J., Valette, H., Saba, W., Dolle, F., Coulon, C. M., Ottaviani, M. P., Hinnen, F., Syrota, A., and Gregoire, M. C. (2008). Quantification of cerebral nicotinic acetylcholine receptors by PET using 2-[18F]fluoro-A-85380 and the multiinjection approach. *J. Cereb. Blood Flow Metab.* **28**(1), 172–189.

Gregoire, M. C., Cinotti, L., Veyre, L., Lavenne, F., Galy, G., Landais, P., Comar, D., and Delforge, J. (2000). *Eur. J. Nucl. Med.* **8,** PS–431.

Hindmarsh, A. C. (1983). In "Scientific Computing" (R. S. Stepleman, ed.), p. 55. North-Holland, Amsterdam.

Hindmarsh, A. C., and Serban, R. (2002). "User Documentation for CVODES: An ODE Solver with Sensitivity Analysis Capabilities. UCRL-MA-148813." Lawrence Livermore National Laboratory, Livermore, CA.

Jacquez, J. A. (1988). "Compartmental Analysis in Biology and Medicine," 2nd edn. The University of Michigan Press, Ann Arbor.

Kessler, R. M., Ellis, J. R., Jr., and Eden, M. (1984). *J. Comput. Assist. Tomogr.* **8,** 514.

Landaw, E. M., and DiStefano, J. J. (1984). *Am. J. Physiol.* **246,** R665.

Leis, J. R., and Kramer, M. A. (1988). *ACM Trans. Math. Softw.* **14,** 61.

Levenberg, K. (1944). *Q. Appl. Math.* **2,** 164.

Marquardt, D. (1963). *SIAM J. Appl. Math.* **11,** 431.

Meltzer, C. C., Zubieta, J. K., Links, J. M., Brakeman, P., Stumpf, M. J., and Frost, J. J. (1996). *J. Cereb. Blood Flow Metab.* **16,** 650.

More, J. J. (1977). Numerical Analysis. In "Lecture Notes in Mathematics 630" (G. A. Watson, ed.), p. 105. Springer-Verlag, New York.

Morris, E. D., and Yoder, K. K. (2007). Positron emission tomography displacement sensitivity: predicting binding potential change for positron emission tomography tracers based on their kinetic characteristics. *J. Cereb. Blood Flow Metab.* **27**(3), 606–617.

Morris, E. D., Saidel, G. M., and Chisolm, G. M., 3rd. (1991). *Am. J. Physiol.* **261,** H929.

Morris, E. D., Fisher, R. E., Alpert, N. M., Rauch, S. L., and Fischman, A. J. (1995). *In vivo* imaging of neuromodulation using positron emission tomography: Optimal ligand characteristics and task length for detection of activation. *Hum. Brain Mapp.* **3**(1), 35–55.

Morris, E. D., Alpert, N. M., and Fischman, A. J. (1996). *J. Cereb. Blood Flow Metab.* **16,** 841.

Morris, E. D., Babich, J. W., Alpert, N. M., Bonab, A. A., Livni, E., Weise, S., Hsu, H., Christian, B. T., Madras, B. K., and Fischman, A. J. (1996). *Synapse* **24,** 262.

Morris, E. D., Bonab, A. A., Alpert, N. M., Fischman, A. J., Madras, B. K., and Christian, B. T. (1999). *Synapse* **32,** 136.

Morris, E. D., Chefer, S. I., Lane, M. A., Muzic, R. F., Jr., Wong, D. F., Dannals, R. F., Matochik, J. A., Bonab, A. A., Villemagne, V. L., Grant, S. J., Ingram, D. K., Roth, G. S., *et al.* (1999). *J. Cereb. Blood Flow Metab.* **19,** 218.

Morris, E. D., Normandin, M. D., and Schiffer, W. K. (2008). Initial comparison of ntPET with microdialysis measurements of methamphetamine-induced dopamine release in rats: Support for estimation of dopamine curves from PET data. *Mol. Imaging Biol.* **10**(2), 67–73.

Mukherjee, J., Yang, Z. Y., Das, M. K., and Brown, T. (1995). *Nucl. Med. Biol.* **22,** 283.

Muller-Gartner, H. W., Links, J. M., Prince, J. L., Bryan, R. N., McVeigh, E., Leal, J. P., Davatzikos, C., and Frost, J. J. (1992). *J. Cereb. Blood Flow Metab.* **12,** 571.

Muzic, R. F., Jr., and Cornelius, S. (2001). *J. Nucl. Med.* **42,** 636.

Muzic, R. F., Jr., and Saidel, G. M. (2003). *IEEE Trans. Med. Imaging* **22,** 11.

Muzic, R. F., Jr., Nelson, A. D., Saidel, G. M., and Miraldi, F. (1994). *Ann. Biomed. Eng.* **22,** 43.

Muzic, R. F., Jr., Nelson, A. D., Saidel, G. M., and Miraldi, F. (1996). *IEEE Trans. Biomed. Eng.* **15,** 2.

Muzic, R. F., Jr., Chen, C. H., and Nelson, A. D. (1998). *IEEE Trans. Med. Imaging* **17,** 202.

Muzic, R. F., Jr., Saidel, G. M., Zhu, N., Nelson, A. D., Zheng, L., and Berridge, M. S. (2000). *Med. Biol. Eng. Comput.* **38,** 593.

Poyot, T., Conde, F., Gregoire, M. C., Frouin, V., Coulon, C., Fuseau, C., Hinnen, F., Dolle, F., Hantraye, P., and Bottlaender, M. (2001). *J. Cereb. Blood Flow Metab.* **21,** 782.

Rousset, O. G., Ma, Y., and Evans, A. C. (1998). *J. Nucl. Med.* **39,** 904.

Rousset, O., Ma, Y., Kamber, M., and Evans, A. C. (1993). *Comput. Med. Imaging Graph.* **17,** 373.

Rousset, O., Ma, Y., Marenco, S., Wong, D. F., and Evans, A. C. (1996). In "Quantification of Brain Function Using PET" (R. Myers, V. Cunningham, D. Bailey, and T. Jones, eds.), p. 158. Academic Press, San Diego.

Salinas, C., Muzic, R. F., Jr., and Saidel, G. M. (2007). Validity of model approximations for receptor-ligand kinetics in nuclear medicine. *Med. Phys.* **34**(5), 1693–1703.

Shampine, L. F., and Reichelt, M. W. (1997). *SIAM J. Sci. Comput.* **18,** 1.

Smith, G. S., Schloesser, R., Brodie, J. D., Dewey, S. L., Logan, J., Vitkun, S. A., Simkowitz, P., Hurley, A., Cooper, T., Volkow, N. D., and Cancro, R. (1998). *Neuropsychopharmacology* **18,** 18.

Strul, D., and Bendriem, B. (1999). *J. Cereb. Blood Flow Metab.* **19,** 547.

Vandehey, N. T., Moirano, J., Murali, D., Converse, A., Engle, J., Nickles, R. J., Mukherjee, J., Schneider, M., Holden, J., Davidson, R., and Christian, B. T. Considerations in choosing a tracer for measuring extrastriatal dopamine D_2/D_3 binding. *J. Cereb. Blood Flow Metab.* (in press).

Woods, R. P., Cherry, S. R., and Mazziotta, J. C. (1992). *J. Comput. Assist. Tomogr.* **16,** 620.

Woods, R. P., Mazziota, J. C., and Cherry, S. R. (1993). *J. Comput. Assist. Tomogr.* **17,** 536.

CHAPTER 8

Magnetic Resonance Imaging in Biomedical Research: Imaging of Drugs and Drug Effects

Markus Rudin, Nicolau Beckmann, and Martin Rausch

Novartis Institute for Biomedical Research
Analytical and Imaging Sciences Unit
CH-4002 Basel, Switzerland

I. Introduction
II. Drug Imaging and PK Studies
III. Noninvasive Assessment of Drug Efficacy/Pharmacodynamic Studies
   A. Qualitative Characterization of Disease Phenotype and Assessment of Drug Efficacy
   B. Quantitative Analysis: Morphometric and Physiological Imaging
IV. Disease and Efficacy Biomarkers as Bridge Between Preclinical and Clinical Drug Evaluation
V. Conclusion and Outlook
References

I. Introduction

Magnetic resonance imaging (MRI) and spectroscopy (MRS) have become established technologies in modern biomedical research, providing relevant information at various stages of the drug discovery and development process (Beckmann *et al.*, 2000, 2001; Rudin *et al.*, 1999). Strengths of MRI are (1) *high soft tissue contrast*, which is governed by a multitude of parameters; (2) *noninvasiveness*, which is of relevance when studying chronic diseases and allows for translation of study protocols from animals to humans; and (3) the high *chemical specificity* of MRS, allowing the identification of individual analytes based on compound-specific resonance frequencies, an important prerequisite for the *in vivo* study of tissue metabolism. The principal disadvantage of MRI/MRS is

ESSENTIAL BIOIMAGING METHODS
Reprinted from *Methods in Enzymology*, Volume 385 (Academic Press, 2004)

DOI: 10.1016/B978-0-12-375043-3.00008-1

the *inherently low sensitivity* due to the low quantum energy involved as compared to optical spectroscopy, leading to a low degree of spin polarization. Only nuclei with high natural abundance and high intrinsic magnetic moment, such as protons, provide sufficient signal intensity for imaging applications. In addition, exogenous contrast agents (CAs, paramagnetic or superparamagnetic compounds) with different levels of specificity are often used to modulate local signal intensities. Whereas CAs are the only source of image signal in nuclear and optical imaging methods, MRI CAs only alter the intrinsic MR signal originating from tissue water. Hence, contrast-enhanced MRI methods always suffer from a high background signal, reducing the sensitivity of the approach.

These properties of MRI/MRS have determined the applications in pharmaceutical research: the focus of applications in the last decade(s) has been the quantitative assessment of drug effects on tissue morphology, physiology, and metabolism in animal models of human disease or in patients (Beckmann *et al.*, 2000, 2001; Rudin *et al.*, 1999). It is not the scope of this chapter to provide yet another review; instead, it discusses some methodological aspects of applying MRI/MRS to biomedical research.

Preclinical *in vivo* characterization of a drug candidate comprises the study of its pharmacokinetic (PK) and pharmacodynamic properties. MRI/MRS was applied predominantly during the late phases of the discovery process, such as the optimization of a lead compound, the profiling of a potential development candidate, and during the early clinical development. More recently, molecular imaging approaches based on MRI involving target-specific contrast principles have been described that provide information relevant for target validation or the elucidation of molecular pathways (Louie *et al.*, 2000; Rudin and Weissleder, 2003; Weissleder *et al.*, 2000). These novel MRI approaches are of high potential value; nevertheless, they are severely limited by the low sensitivity of MRI, requiring high amplification of the molecular signal, and by the fact that MRI CAs are, in general, bulky and not delivered readily to the molecular target.

This chapter focuses on conventional MRI/MRS applications, discussing their role in pharmacokinetic and pharmacodynamic studies, and addresses some issues related to the development of MRI-based biomarkers.

II. Drug Imaging and PK Studies

The inherently low sensitivity of nuclear magnetic resonance has prevented any widespread attempts of using the technique for mapping the biodistribution of drug candidates *in vivo*. Let the detection limit for a given acquisition time be $p_l = 10^{12}$ spins. At a magnetic field strength of 9.4 T (proton resonance frequency $v_0 = 400$ MHz) the polarization of proton spins at room temperature is $\Delta p = \exp(-hv_0/kT) \approx 10^{-5}$ (i.e., out of 10^5 spins there is an excess of only one oriented parallel to the field and, hence, detectable). Conventional MRI maps the distribution of water protons in tissue, with the average tissue proton concentration being approximately $c_t = 80$ M. For the detection limit of 10^{12} spins, this then corresponds to a volume of

$$V = \frac{10^6(\mu l)\cdot p_l}{c_t\cdot N_A \Delta p} = 2 \times 10^{-4} \mu l \quad (1)$$

with N_A being Avogadro's number. This volume element (voxel) translates into linear pixel dimensions of 120 μm, a typical value for animal MRI studies. For endogenous metabolites studied commonly by MRS or spectroscopic imaging methods, the tissue concentration is of the order of $c_t = 1$ mM and, assuming the same data acquisition protocol, the volume would increase to 170 μl, corresponding to a voxel of $(5.5\ \text{mm})^3$.

We now apply this simple consideration to estimate drug levels that can be detected in a volume corresponding to the whole rat brain (2 ml) or rat liver (15 ml). For a compound with a molecular mass of 500 Da, doses of $c_t = 40$ and 6 mg/kg should be detectable, corresponding to tissue concentrations of 80 and 12 μM for brain and liver, respectively, assuming homogeneous distribution throughout the body and neglecting any concurrent drug clearance. However, this would be only feasible when drug signals are well separated from the signals of the endogenous metabolites at millimolar concentration, which is not the case for proton spectroscopy due to a limited chemical shift dispersion.

This is the reason why essentially all NMR drug biodistribution studies reported to date focused on magnetic nuclei such as ^{13}C, ^{19}F, and ^{31}P. Fluorine is especially promising, as its magnetic properties are comparable to those of protons, whereas the degree of polarization and hence the sensitivity is 2.5-fold and four times weaker for ^{31}P and ^{13}C for the same number of magnetic nuclei, respectively.

Given these perspectives, the attempt to image drug biodistribution using MRI/MRS approaches is not very promising. In fact, the few spectroscopic studies reported to date have sampled large detection volumes. In these cases, the spatial resolution is provided by the selectivity of the radiofrequency excitation/detection scheme using surface coils. Most of the examples relate to drugs used in oncology, and some of these PKs studies using MRS have even been translated into the clinics. A compound studied with ^{19}F MRS is 5-fluorouracyl (5-FU) (Findlay *et al.*, 1993; McSheehy *et al.*, 1998; Prior *et al.*, 1990; Schlemmer *et al.*, 1994). Such studies allowed the prediction of patient response to 5-FU based on individual PK data (Findlay *et al.*, 1993; Reese *et al.*, 2000; Schlemmer *et al.*, 1994). P MRS has been used for PK studies of ifosfamide (Payne *et al.*, 1999), whereas other cancer drugs have been investigated using ^{13}C^{12} and ^{1}H MRS (He *et al.*, 1995). In all these studies, three favorable factors apply: (1) doses of the anticancer drugs administered were relatively high (100–800 mg/kg); (2) the volume of interest sampled in the study was large (>20 ml); and (3) high specificity was achieved by studying nonendogenous nuclei (^{19}F), by exploiting unique chemical shift properties (^{31}P), or by using spectral editing techniques to distinguish drug signal from metabolite resonances (^{13}C, ^{1}H).

The percentage of drugs containing fluorine or phosphorus, however, is low (5%), and the doses commonly used are well below the values discussed. Hence, *in vivo* MRS is of limited value for PK studies and, even in the most favorable cases, the spatial and temporal resolutions achieved are rather poor. It is, therefore, not surprising that the focus of using magnetic resonance techniques has been on the pharmacodynamic readouts (i.e., on the analysis of drug effects on tissue morphology, physiology/function, and endogenous metabolism).

III. Noninvasive Assessment of Drug Efficacy/ Pharmacodynamic Studies

The vast majority of MRI/MRS applications in pharmacological research address pharmacodynamic effects of drugs in animal models of human diseases or in patients. The first step is the morphological, physiological/functional, and/or metabolic characterization of a disease phenotype on both a *qualitative* and a *quantitative* basis. The MRI signal behavior is governed by a variety of independent parameters, which are determined by the microstructural environment of the tissue water in a voxel. Those are the proton density, the various relaxation times (spin-lattice relaxation time (T_1), spin-spin relaxation or phase-memory time (T_2), free induction decay time (T_2*)) the diffusion properties of the tissue water as characterized by the apparent diffusion coefficient (ADC) or when accounting for anisotropy by the diffusion tensor, incoherent motion within a voxel due to perfusion, and coherent motion due to macroscopic blood flow. A detailed description of the various MRI contrast mechanisms is beyond the scope of this chapter and the reader is referred to the literature (Wehrli *et al.*, 1983). Pathology leads to morphological and physiological alterations and, hence, to concomitant changes of MRI contrast parameters. These changes are dynamic and will evolve as pathology evolves (Fig. 1) and may be used as a diagnostic tissue signature (Welch *et al.*, 1995). By suitable choice of the experimental parameters, the contrast-to-noise ratio (CNR) between a structure of interest and its environment can be optimized, explaining the high value of MRI as a diagnostic tool.

A. Qualitative Characterization of Disease Phenotype and Assessment of Drug Efficacy

1. Qualitative Characterization

Qualitative characterization of a disease phenotype is the basis for clinical diagnosis. The multivariate nature of the MRI signal often allows for staging of the disease, which is of relevance for the stratification of a patient/animal population to be included in drug evaluation studies. Qualitative or semiquantitative tissue characterization can also be applied to assess therapy response. As an example, the efficacy of immunosuppressive treatment in a rat kidney allograft transplantation model has been evaluated using a score accounting for

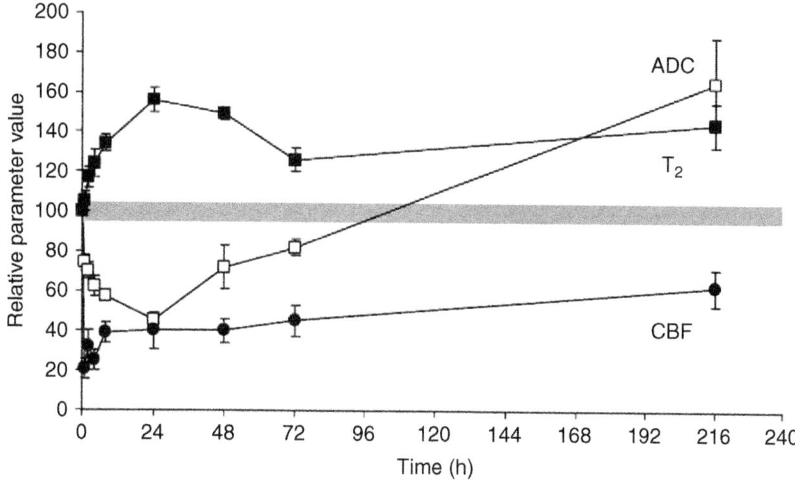

Fig. 1 Time dependence of MRI parameters in rat cerebral cortex in a model of human embolic stroke. Cerebral ischemia was induced by permanent occlusion of the left middle cerebral artery, leading to a reduction of cortical cerebral blood flow (CBF) to 20% of its contralateral value. Within minutes, the apparent water diffusion coefficient (ADC) in the affected area started to decrease, reaching a minimum of 50% of its baseline value at 24 h and pseudo-normalizing between 3 and 5 days. The most commonly used parameter for the quantitative morphometric analysis of infarct volume is the transverse relaxation time T_2, with contrast in T_2-weighted images being maximal at 24 and 48 h postinfarction. The relative profile defined by the parameters (ADC, CBF, T_2) changes as a function of time and constitutes a signature reflecting the tissue state. All values are given relative to the respective value of the contralateral, normal hemisphere (indicated by the gray line). Values represent mean ± S.E.M. (Rudin *et al.*, 2001).

morphological tissue appearance on MR images (Beckmann *et al.*, 1996). As in qualitative clinical diagnostics, the quality of such results critically depends on the skills of the interpreter. Analyses have to be carried out blindly, and even then it cannot be excluded that different operators will arrive at different conclusions.

B. Quantitative Analysis: Morphometric and Physiological Imaging

1. *In Vivo* Morphometry

Quantitative analysis of biomedical imaging data is based on morphometric or densitometric measures. Morphometric readouts are, for instance, the volume of a pathology, such as the infarct volume in stroke or the tumor volume in oncology studies, or distance measures, such as the thickness of articular cartilage in models of arthritis. Preferentially, such measures are carried out in an automated fashion, that is, with minimal operator interaction. The critical step in morphometric image analysis is image segmentation, which is relatively simple for high CNR, allowing for segmentation based on intensity thresholds (Fig. 2A). However, due to limited CNR, this approach is not generally applicable, and there is still a need to develop

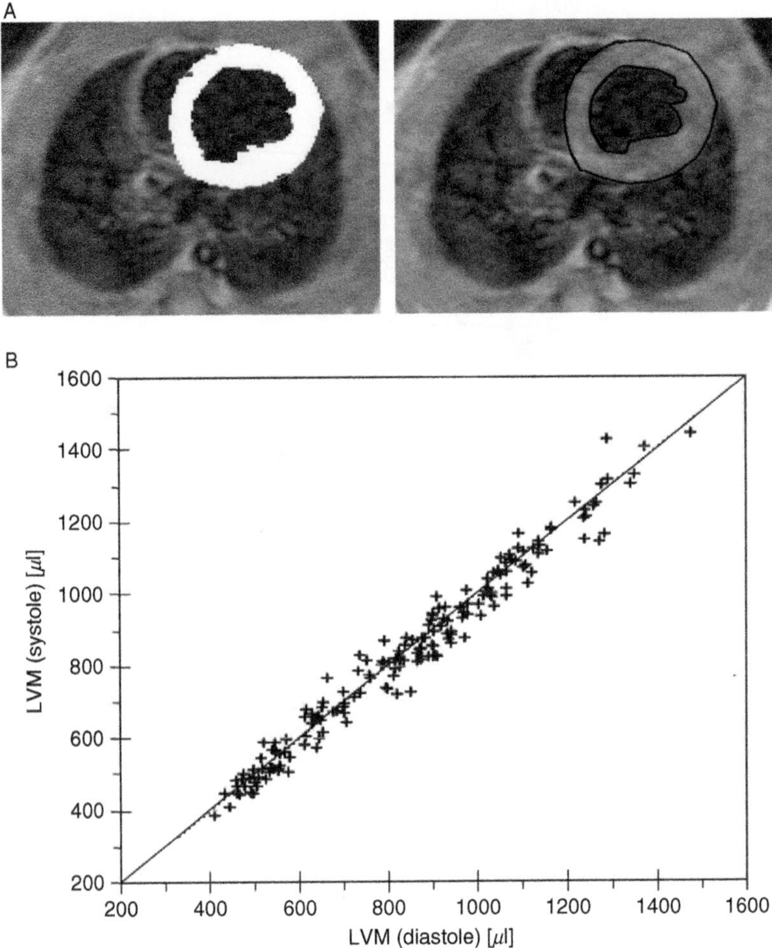

Fig. 2 *In vivo* morphometric analysis of MR images of the rat heart. One section of a transverse multislice data set covering the heart is shown. The myocardial left ventricular mass (LVM) is derived by determining the cross-sectional area in each slice either by intensity-based segmentation (A, left) or by operator-interactive tracing of the structure boundary (A, right). By adding the selected areas in all slices and multiplying with the interslice separation and the tissue density (1.05 g/cm^3), the LVM can be estimated. The reproducibility of the estimate is illustrated (B) comparing two subsequent analyses of the LVM mass, one during diastole and one during systole. The average standard deviation is 8% (Rudin *et al.*, 1991).

automated three-dimensional segmentation algorithms. For current practical applications, operator interaction is still required. Nevertheless, reproducibility is, in general, good so that the uncertainty introduced by the methodology is significantly smaller than the biological variability (Fig. 2B).

Quantitative structural information may also be derived by determining the relative or absolute values of MRI contrast parameters. Alteration of T_2 and ADC values in ischemic brain tissue following cerebral infarction indicates the severity of the ischemic insult (Rudin *et al.*, 2001); regional normalization of these values following cytoprotective therapy reflects drug efficacy (Sauter and Rudin, 1986).

2. Physiological Parameters

Quantitative densitometric analysis is applied in order to derive physiological or functional information from dynamic MRI data sets. In such experiments, the MRI signal intensity is monitored in response to a pharmacological or physiological challenge or to the passage of an exogenous CA. Derivation of physiological information from dynamic MRI data sets involves modeling within the framework of physiological models. Three examples illustrate the approach.

3. Tissue Perfusion

Assessment of tissue perfusion is based on the tracer dilution method (Meier and Zierler, 1954). Administration of an intravascular CA leads to a transient change in signal intensity in the tissue caused by a transient increase in the relaxation rate R_2 (and $R_2{}^*$), the amount of which is proportional to the local tissue concentration of the tracer $c_t(t)$:

$$\Delta R_2(t) = R_2(t) - R_{20} = \alpha_2 c_t(t) V \tag{2}$$

with R_{20} and $R_2(t)$ being the relaxation rates prior and at time t after administration of the CA, α_2 is the molar relaxivity (in $M^{-1}\ s^{-1}$) of the CA (accounting for the susceptibility difference $\Delta\chi$ between intra- and extravascular space induced by the CA), and V is the local tissue blood volume. Analysis of the tracer profile $c_t(t)$ versus t allows deriving relative hemodynamic parameters such as tissue blood flow and tissue blood volume (Rudin *et al.*, 1997). Determination of absolute hemodynamic parameters requires calibration of the perfusion maps by the arterial input function (Rausch *et al.*, 2000).

Tissue perfusion is a critical parameter for tissue survival and function, and both relative and absolute perfusion assessments are highly relevant for both diagnosis and evaluation of the therapy response. Typical applications in drug discovery are studies of focal cerebral ischemia (e.g., induced by occlusion of the middle cerebral artery in rats) (Sauter *et al.*, 1988, 2002).

4. Tissue Oxygenation

The delivery of oxygen and nutrients to tissue is critical for functional integrity or even survival; hence, the oxygenation level is a relevant parameter for the characterization of the tissue state. Ogawa *et al.* (1990) observed significant increases in proton R_2* relaxivity in rat brain during severe hypoxia, which were attributed to increased intravascular levels of deoxygenated hemoglobin. While oxygenated hemoglobin (Hb-O_2) is diamagnetic, deoxygenated hemoglobin (Hb) is paramagnetic and acts as an endogenous CA. The proton relaxation rate $\Delta R_2(=1/\Delta T_2)$ depends on the fraction of intravascular deoxyhemoglobin $(1 - Y)$ according to Scheffler *et al.* (1999)

$$\Delta R_2(f, Y) = \alpha\gamma f(1 - Y)\Delta\chi B_0 \quad (3)$$

where α is a proportionality factor, γ is the proton gyromagnetic ratio, f is the blood volume fraction, $\Delta\chi$ is the susceptibility difference between fully deoxygenated and fully oxygenated blood, and B_0 is the static magnetic field. For human hemoglobin, Y is derived from the blood oxygenation curve according to Kennan *et al.* (1994)

$$\frac{Y}{1 - Y} = \left(\frac{pO_2}{P_{50}}\right)^{2.8} \quad (4)$$

with pO_2 being the partial pressure of oxygen in blood and P_{50} the partial pressure at which 50% of the hemoglobin is oxygenated. The proton relaxation rate is highly sensitive to changes in pO_2 around normoxic levels. Determination of absolute tissue pO_2 values from measurements of MRI relaxation rates, however, is hardly feasible, as the signal intensity depends on geometrical factors describing the vascular system (vessel diameter, spacing, and orientation), the rate of water diffusion, and the static magnetic field strength (Kennan *et al.*, 1994). For the majority of practical applications, tissue oxygenation is analyzed qualitatively or semiquantitatively (relative values). This is illustrated by some examples.

Blood oxygenation level-dependent (BOLD) contrast forms the basis of brain activity studies using functional MRI (fMRI) (Kwong *et al.*, 1992; Ogawa *et al.*, 1992). Local changes in blood oxygenation are caused by neuronal activation through metabolic and hemodynamic coupling. fMRI is widely applied to study the functional architecture of the brain and for the characterization of pathologies of the central nervous system (CNS). fMRI is also used to study the CNS response to the administration of neuroactive compounds (Chen *et al.*, 1997; Reese *et al.*, 2000), providing readouts comparable to glucose utilization measurements using positron emission tomography (PET). More recently, fMRI has been applied to study functional recovery following cytoprotective treatment in a rat model of human embolic stroke (Sauter *et al.*, 2002).

Oxygenation (and perfusion) in neoplastic tissue is critical for therapy response, and knowledge of this physiological parameter would allow one to optimize treatment regimens (Gillies *et al.*, 2002). BOLD MRI has indeed been applied successfully to assess tumor blood flow and oxygenation under a variety of conditions relevant to tumor therapy (Howe and Robinson, 2001). Knowledge of the tumor oxygenation state is also relevant when studying angiogenesis. The transcription factor hypoxia-inducible factor-1 (HIF-1) is a key regulator of oxygen homeostasis, with high HIF-1 levels stimulating the formation of neovasculature (Pugh and Ratcliffe, 2003).

Gas exchange is the major function of the lungs, and ventilation can be probed by analyzing changes in the relaxation rates of lung parenchyma induced by oxygen. Molecular oxygen has a triplet ground state, that is, two unpaired electrons, is weakly paramagnetic, and thus constitutes a source of contrast in MRI. This property has been explored successfully to derive regional ventilation-related information from the human lung (Edelman *et al.*, 1996; Stock *et al.*, 1999). While qualitative and semiquantitative information is obtained readily, absolute quantification is again difficult; for example, the dissolution of O_2 in blood suggests that the tissue relaxation rates are also dependent on perfusion rates or blood volume, in addition to the degree of tissue oxygenation (Mai *et al.*, 2002).

5. Vascular Permeability

Interstitial and vascular spaces are separated by a tight barrier, which, under normal conditions, limits the free passage of molecules. Certain pathologies can be accompanied by a reduction of barrier integrity: inflammatory events, for instance, often lead to a transient increase of the vascular permeability. Angiogenesis, as often found in tumors, is characterized by the formation of new vessels with increased permeability compared to normal tissue, which can be assessed by the injection of CA into the blood circulation, followed by monitoring their accumulation in the lesions (Larsson *et al.*, 1990; Tofts and Kermode, 1991). Because the CA cannot enter the intracellular space, its distribution is restricted to two compartments: blood plasma and interstitial space. Following injection, the CA will diffuse along the concentration gradient from the circulation into the interstitial space at a rate determined by vascular permeability. Provided that the concentration of the CA remains nearly constant in the circulation over time, its concentration in tissue will reach a steady state, whose amplitude is determined by the extravascular extracellular space (i.e., the leakage space).

Quantitative assessment of vascular permeability is based on dynamic contrast-enhanced T_1 mapping (DCE-MRI), allowing one to calculate leakage rate and leakage space from the temporal profile of CA uptake. The spin-lattice relaxation rate R_1 is proportional to the concentration c_t of CA in a voxel:

$$\Delta R_1 = \alpha_1 c_t v_e \tag{5}$$

with α_1 being the molar longitudinal relaxivity of the CA and v_e its leakage space (interstitial space).

Several analytical approaches have been used for data analysis, with the two-compartment model being one of the most relevant (Tofts, 1997). In such a model, the concentration of CA in tissue c_t is determined by the leakage space v_e, the permeability surface product k, the blood volume fraction v_p, and the concentration of CA in the circulation c_p:

$$c_t(t) = k \int_0^t \exp\left(\frac{-k(t-t')}{v_e}\right) c_p dt' + v_p c_p \tag{6}$$

Because the elimination half-life time of MR CAs is usually larger than 10 min, the temporal profile of c_p can be described by a step function. Furthermore, the concentration of the tracer in circulation is often negligible in tumors compared to tissue. It is, therefore, possible to simplify Eq. (6) and model c_t by

$$c_t(t) = v_e c_{p0} \left[1 - \exp\left(-\frac{kt}{v_e}\right)\right] \tag{7}$$

where c_{p0} describes the initial concentration of the CA. The permeability of the vasculature is, hence, proportional to the initial slope of the enhancement curve (Fig. 3).

Several types of gadolinium-based CA are available for DCE-MRI. Only low-molecular-weight compounds such as GdDOTA or GdDTPA have been approved for clinical applications. Due to their small size, their diffusion rate is very high, rendering accurate determination of the initial enhancement curve often difficult. Therefore, there is a strong focus on the development of macromolecular CA providing lower diffusion rates. Macromolecular CA can be based on low molecular Gd-chelating molecules bound to larger structures such as macrocyclic arms (Turetschek *et al.*, 2001), dendrimers (Daldrup-Link *et al.*, 2000), or albumin

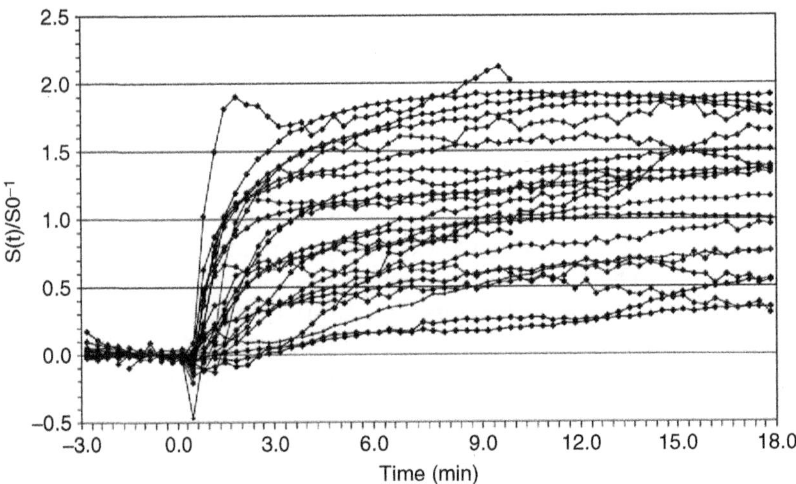

Fig. 3 Interanimal variability in a tumor xenograft model. Change in relative tumor signal intensity following administration of GdDTPA in B16 melanoma primary tumors implanted in a mouse ear. The initial uptake reflects the vascular (permeability) × (surface) product, whereas the final signal reflects the total tracer concentration in the tissue and, hence, is a measure for the extracellular leakage space. The large variability in this tightly controlled model illustrates the value of noninvasive readouts using each animal as its own control.

(Turetschek *et al.*, 2002). Because evaluation for clinical use is still ongoing, they are today used only in preclinical applications.

These three examples illustrate that while the assessment of absolute physiological parameters from MRI data is feasible, the analysis is generally not straightforward; the models used are complex and include many assumptions/approximations. Hence, the majority of physiological MRI applications use semiquantitative analysis (i.e., parameter values in the region of interest in relation to a reference tissue).

In addition to being highly desirable with regard to animal care, noninvasive imaging, provides the advantage of allowing *paired study designs*, which improve statistical power. Longitudinal studies largely eliminate effects of interindividual variation (e.g., by relating the tissue state assessed following a therapeutic intervention to baseline values prior to treatment). An example illustrates this. Pituitary hyperplasia in rats induced by chronic stimulation (4 weeks) with estradiol is considered a model for prolactinoma (Rudin *et al.*, 1988). Variability in this model is large, with the coefficient of variation (COV) for the pituitary volume following stimulation being of the order of 100%. This requires group sizes of 30–40 animals in order to detect a 50% therapy effect at a statistical level of $p \leq 0.05$. By relating the measurements following a 4-week drug treatment with the long-lasting somatostatin analog octreotide to the baseline values, this interindividual variation could be largely eliminated. The COV of the relative volume measures was found to be 5–10% only, and significant results demonstrating that octreotide treatment dose dependently reduced established hyperplasia could be demonstrated with $n = 4$ rats per group. Paired study design is attractive in case of high interindividual variability of pretreatment values as encountered frequently in cancer studies due to the inherent heterogeneity of neoplastic tissue. Even under controlled conditions (e.g., after the subcutaneous implantation of tumor xenografts) considerable data scattering is observed (Fig. 3).

The study of pharmacodynamic drug properties forms the backbone of MRI applications in drug research today. They rely on absolute or relative quantitative analysis of MRI data. While initially MRI was used predominantly to derive morphometric information *in vivo*, today physiological readouts have attracted much interest as sensitive indicators of tissue state and potentially early readouts of pharmacological efficacy.

IV. Disease and Efficacy Biomarkers as Bridge Between Preclinical and Clinical Drug Evaluation

The clinical evaluation of drug candidates that target chronic indications such as degenerative diseases involves large patient populations, is time-consuming and expensive. It is important to minimize the risk of such trials by optimizing the therapy regimen and by proper selection of the patient population. Thus, biomarkers that are indicative of the disease or provide mechanistic information on the efficacy or potential safety issues of the drug are of high value. The noninvasive character of the imaging approaches, particularly MRI and MRS, makes them attractive tools for the development of such biomarkers. A number of MRI/MRS biomarkers based on structural and functional readouts have been proposed for clinical drug evaluation in indications such as neurodegeneration, multiple sclerosis, oncology, and osteoarthritis.

For *neurodegenerative* disorders, morphological (total brain atrophy, hippocampal atrophy) and functional biomarkers (altered task-related brain activity) have been proposed. Alternatively, MRS has been applied to analyze differences in endogenous tissue metabolism in patients with mild cognitive impairment (MCI) and diagnosed Alzheimer's disease (AD) as compared to normal aging (Catani *et al.*, 2001; Kantarci *et al.*, 2002). Characteristic spectral changes were increased *myo*-inositol signals in MCI and both increased *myo*-inositol and decreased *N*-acetylaspartate signals (as marker of neuronal loss) in AD. However, in all these cases, both the sensitivity and the specificity of the proposed markers are questionable, limiting their applicability for clinical therapy evaluation. A more promising approach is based on plaque imaging using a plaque-specific PET ligand (Agdeppa *et al.*, 2003).

PET has been used extensively for characterizing pharmacokinetic and pharmacodynamic properties of drug candidates by analyzing their receptor interaction, their effects on neurotransmitter systems, or general metabolic readouts such as glucose utilization. fMRI can provide similar information on drug-induced functional responses of CNS structures. This has been demonstrated in animal studies for a number of compounds interacting with various neurotransmitter systems (Chen *et al.*, 1997; Reese *et al.*, 2000). A distinctive advantage of the fMRI method is the high spatial (100 μm) and temporal (seconds to minutes) resolution. The fMRI method does not map the drug-receptor interaction *per se*, but rather the functional consequence thereof.

Clinical end points in *oncology* trials are tumor shrinkage and ultimately patient survival. Various potential biomarkers for the early assessment of drug efficacy have been proposed comprising both markers associated with a specific mechanism (e.g., angiogenesis or apoptosis) and general disease markers (e.g., tumor metabolism or tumor proliferation). Neovascularization is essential for the growth of primary tumors and metastases; hence, the assessment of angiogenesis might predict tumor malignancy, as well as its responsiveness to therapy. A clinically established method applied to evaluate antiangiogenetic drugs is DCE-MRI using CAs such as GdDTPA, which leaks into the extracellular space (Tofts, 1997; Tofts and Kermode, 1991; Tyninnen *et al.*, 1999). Alteration in tracer uptake by the tumor reflects changes in vascular permeability (van Dijke *et al.*, 1996). Such vascular permeability measurements have indeed been used extensively to assess the effects of antiangiogenic VEGF inhibitors at both preclinical and clinical levels (Drevs *et al.*, 2002).

Efficacy biomarkers target general tumor properties such as metabolism and proliferation or microstructural changes of neoplastic tissue. MRS revealed significant alterations in tumor phospholipids and energy metabolism in response to drug treatment prior to detectable changes in tumor volume (Evelhoch *et al.*, 2000). Finally, the ADC of tissue water seems to predict successful tumor therapy. Significant increases of ADC values were observed within a few days of treatment with a cytostatic drug indicative of cell shrinkage, which was at least in part due to apoptosis (Chevenert *et al.*, 2000).

Disease progression in *degenerative joint disease* is commonly assessed by X-radiographical analysis of the joint gap. A reduction of the distance between the bone structures reflects the degeneration of articular cartilage and is a readout of advanced disease. Significant efforts have been devoted to the development of more sensitive biomarkers that could indicate subtle changes in the articular matrix that precede net structural loss. Cartilage stability is provided by a macromolecular network, with the main constituents being collagen and proteoglycans (PGs). Approaches proposed aim, therefore, at measuring the total content of macromolecules or PGs in particular. The former is based on magnetization transfer (i.e., measuring the exchange rate between bulk and macromolecular-bound water). Reduction of the macromolecular pool, particularly collagen, or loss of its structural integrity leads to a decreased exchange rate (Gray *et al.*, 1995; Laurent *et al.*, 2001). PGs are one of the major constituents of the cartilage matrix, contributing to cartilage resiliency through a negative electrostatic force. The early phase of osteoarthritis is associated with a loss of PGs, leading to an impaired biomechanical support function of cartilage, which in turn contributes to its further degradation (Grushko *et al.*, 1989). Noninvasive assessment of the PG content (e.g., using delayed gadolinium-enhanced MRI) might constitute a sensitive biomarker of osteoarthritis (Bashir *et al.*, 1999; Laurent *et al.*, 2003). This MRI technique yields an estimate of the fixed charged density (FCD) of cartilage, reflecting negatively charged side chains of PGs. The negatively charged CA Gd $(DTPA)^{2-}$ penetrates the interstitial fluid of cartilage to reach an equilibrium concentration that is governed by (1) the $Gd(DTPA)^{2-}$ concentration gradient and (2) electrostatic interactions (inversely proportional to the FCD). Quantitative analysis of the Gd-induced changes in proton relaxation rate (R_1) allows one to estimate the FCD and, hence, the PG concentration. In model systems, a good correlation between changes in relaxation rates and biochemically determined PG levels has been obtained (Laurent *et al.*, 2003), emphasizing the potential of MRI readouts as disease-relevant biomarkers.

The development of noninvasive biomarkers is highly relevant for clinical drug evaluation. They would help to stratify patient populations, optimize the therapy regimen (dosing, timing), or might even be used as surrogates for a clinical end point. Prerequisite is a careful validation of the biomarker.

V. Conclusion and Outlook

Today, *in vivo* imaging techniques, particularly MRI, have become indispensable in biomedical research. MRI is being used at various steps in drug discovery and development with focus on disease phenotyping and drug evaluation during lead optimization and compound profiling. Strengths of the MRI approach are (1) high information content (i.e., the MR signal is governed by multiple independent parameters providing high soft tissue contrast, a key characteristic for comprehensive tissue characterization) and (2) noninvasiveness, which offers advantages in study design (paired design with increased statistical power) and is a prerequisite for translational studies. The principal disadvantage of MRI is low sensitivity largely precluding PK studies. Low sensitivity is also a significant drawback in the study of target-specific (molecular imaging) applications, which have raised considerable interest recently as tools for the validation of potential drug targets, for the analysis of molecular pathways involved in drug action, and for the identification of molecular biomarkers (Rudin and Weissleder, 2003). Nevertheless, MR approaches to visualize gene expression have been described (Louie *et al.*, 2000; Weissleder *et al.*, 2000) demonstrating that target-specific information can be derived in favorable situations. MRI approaches to monitor the migration of magnetically labeled cells with high spatial resolution seem more promising as demonstrated for tracking of macrophages (Beckmann *et al.*, 2003a,b; Dousset *et al.*, 1999; Rausch *et al.*, 2001, 2002, 2003), stem cells (Hoehn *et al.*, 2002), and progenitor cells (Bulte *et al.*, 1999).

Despite the recent developments in molecular and cellular imaging, MRI in biomedical research will be used primarily for pharmacodynamic studies (i.e., for the evaluation of drug efficacy models of human disease using morphological and physiological readouts). In addition, the development of MRI-based biomarkers for translational applications such as the rapid evaluation of a therapeutic concept in the clinics will increase rapidly in importance. Molecular and cellular imaging techniques, particularly optical and nuclear methods, will complement the conventional structural and functional imaging approaches.

References

Agdeppa, E. D., Kepe, V., Petri, A., Satyamurthy, N., Liu, J., Huang, S. C., Small, G. W., Cole, G. M., and Barrio, J. R. (2003). *Neuroscience* **117,** 723.

Artemov, D., Bhujwalla, Z. M., Maxwell, R. J., Griffiths, J. R., Judson, I. R., Leach, M. O., and Glickson, J. D. (1985). *Magn. Reson. Med.* **34,** 338.

Bashir, A., Gray, M. L., Hartke, J., and Burstein, D. (1999). *Magn. Reson. Med.* **41,** 857.

Beckmann, N., Joergensen, J., Bruttel, K., Rudin, M., and Schuurman, H. J. (1996). *Transpl. Int.* **9,** 175.

Beckmann, N., Hof, R. P., and Rudin, M. (2000). *NMR Biomed.* **13,** 329.

Beckmann, N., Mueggler, T., Allegrini, P. R., Laurent, D., and Rudin, M. (2001). *Anat. Rec.* **265,** 85.

Beckmann, N., Cannet, C., Fringeli-Tanner, M., Baumann, D., Pally, C., Bruns, C., Zerwes, H. G., Andriambeloson, E., and Bigaud, M. (2003a). *Magn. Reson. Med.* **49,** 459.

Beckmann, N., Falk, R., Zurbrügg, S., Dawson, J., and Engelhardt, P. (2003b). *Magn. Reson. Med.* **49,** 1047.

Bulte, J. W., Zhang, S., van Gelderen, P., Herynek, V., Jordan, E. K., Duncan, I. D., and Frank, J. A. (1999). *Proc. Natl. Acad. Sci. USA* **96,** 15256.

Catani, M., Cherubini, A., Howard, R., Tarducci, R., Pelliccioli, G. P., Piccirilli, M., Gobbi, G., Senin, U., and Mecocci, P. (2001). *Neuroreport* **12,** 2315.

Chen, Y. C. I., Galpern, W. R., Brownell, A. L., Matthews, R. T., Bogdanov, M., Isacson, O., Keltner, J. R., Beal, M. F., Rosen, B. R., and Jenkins, B. G. (1997). *Magn. Reson. Med.* **38,** 389.

Chevenert, T. L., Stegman, L. D., Taylor, J. M. G., Robertson, P. L., Greenberg, H. S., Rehemtulla, A., and Ross, B. D. (2000). *J. Natl. Cancer Inst.* **92,** 2029.

Daldrup-Link, H. E., Shames, D. M., Wendland, M., Muhler, A., Gossmann, A., Rosenau, W., and Brasch, R. C. (2000). *Acad. Radiol.* **7,** 934.

Dousset, V., Delalande, C., Ballarino, L., Quesson, B., Seilhan, D., Coussemacq, M., Thiaudiere, E., Brochet, B., Canioni, P., and Caille, J. M. (1999). *Magn. Reson. Med.* **41,** 329.

Drevs, J., Muller-Driver, R., Wittig, C., Fuxius, S., Esser, N., Hugenschmidt, H., Konerding, M. A., Allegrini, P. R., Wood, J., Hennig, J., Unger, C., and Marme, D. (2002). *Cancer Res.* **62,** 4015.

Edelman, R. R., Hatabu, H., Tadamura, E., Li, W., and Prasad, P. V. (1996). *Nat. Med.* **2,** 1236.

Evelhoch, J. L., Gillies, R. J., Karczmar, G. S., Koutcher, J. A., Maxwell, R. J., Nalcioglu, O., Raghunand, N., Ronen, S. M., Ross, B. D., and Swartz, H. M. (2000). *Neoplasia* **2,** 152.

Findlay, M. P. N., Leach, M. O., Cunningham, D., Collins, D. J., Payne, G. S., Glaholm, J., Mansi, J. L., and McCready, V. R. (1993). *Ann. Oncol.* **4,** 497.

Gillies, R. J., Raghunand, N., Karczmar, G. S., and Bhujwalla, Z. M. (2002). *J. Magn. Reson. Imaging* **16,** 430.

Gray, M. L., Burstein, D., Lesperance, L. M., and Gehrke, L. (1995). *Magn. Reson. Med.* **34,** 319.

Grushko, G., Schneiderman, R., and Maroudas, A. (1989). *Connect. Tissue Res.* **19,** 149.

He, Q., Bhujwalla, Z. M., Maxwell, R. J., Griffiths, J. R., and Glickson, J. D. (1995). *Magn. Reson. Med.* **33,** 414.

Hoehn, M., Kustermann, E., Blunk, J., Wiedermann, D., Trapp, T., Wecker, S., Focking, M., Arnold, H., Hescheler, J., Fleischmann, B. K., Schwindt, W., and Buhrle, C. (2002). *Proc. Natl. Acad. Sci. USA* **99,** 16267.

Howe, F. A., and Robinson, S. P. (2001). *NMR Biomed.* **14,** 497.

Kantarci, K., Smith, G. E., Ivnik, J., Petersen, R. C., Boeve, B. F., Knopman, D. S., Tangalos, E. G., and Jack, C. R., Jr. (2002). *J. Int. Neuropsych. Soc.* **8,** 934.

Kennan, R. P., Zhong, J., and Gore, J. C. (1994). *Magn. Reson. Med.* **31,** 9.

Kwong, K. K., Belliveau, J. W., Chesler, D. A., Goldberg, I. E., Weisskoff, R. M., Poncelet, B. P., Kennedy, D. N., Hoppel, B. E., Cohen, M. S., and Turner, R. (1992). *Proc. Natl. Acad. Sci. USA* **89,** 5675.

Larsson, H., Stubgaard, M., Frederiksen, J. L., Jensen, M., Henriksen, O., and Paulson, O. (1990). *Magn. Reson. Med.* **16,** 117.

Laurent, D., Wasvary, J., Yin, J., Rudin, M., Pellas, T. C., and O'Byrne, E. (2001). *Magn. Reson. Imaging* **19,** 1279.

Laurent, D., Wasvary, J., Rudin, M., O'Byrne, E., and Pellas, T. (2003). *Magn. Reson. Med.* **49,** 1037.

Louie, A. Y., Huber, M. M., Ahrens, E. T., Rothbacher, U., Moats, R., Jacobs, R. E., Fraser, S. E., and Meade, T. J. (2000). *Nat. Biotechnol.* **18,** 321.

Mai, V. M., Liu, B., Polzin, J. A., Li, W., Kurucay, S., Bankier, A. A., Knight-Scott, J., Madhav, P., Edelman, R. R., and Chen, Q. (2002). *Magn. Reson. Med.* **48,** 341.

McSheehy, P. M., Robinson, S. P., Ojugo, A. S. E., Aboagye, E. O., Cannell, M. B., Leach, M. O., Judson, I. R., and Griffiths, J. R. (1998). *Cancer Res.* **58,** 1185.

Meier, P., and Zierler, K. L. (1954). *J. Appl. Physiol.* **6,** 731.

Ogawa, S., Lee, T. M., Kay, A. R., and Tank, D. W. (1990). *Proc. Natl. Acad. Sci. USA* **87,** 9868.

Ogawa, S., Tank, D. W., Menon, R., Ellermann, J. M., Kim, S. G., Merkle, H., and Ugurbil, K. (1992). *Proc. Natl. Acad. Sci. USA* **89,** 5951.

Payne, G. S., Pinkerton, C. R., and Leach, M. O. (1999). *Int. Soc. Magn. Reson. Med.* **7,** 1588.

Prior, M. J. W., Maxwell, R. J., and Griffiths, J. R. (1990). *Biochem. Pharmacol.* **39,** 857.

Pugh, C. W., and Ratcliffe, P. J. (2003). *Nat. Med.* **9,** 677.

Rausch, M., Scheffler, K., Rudin, M., and Radü, E. (2000). *Magn. Reson. Imaging* **18,** 1235.

Rausch, M., Sauter, A., Frohlich, J., Neubacher, U., Radü, E. W., and Rudin, M. (2001). *Magn. Reson. Med.* **46,** 1018.

Rausch, M., Baumann, D., Neubacher, U., and Rudin, M. (2002). *NMR Biomed.* **15,** 278.

Rausch, M., Hiestand, P., Baumann, D., Cannet, C., and Rudin, M. (2003). *Magn. Reson. Med.* **50,** 309.

Reese, T., Bjelke, B., Porszasz, R., Baumann, D., Bochelen, D., Sauter, A., and Rudin, M. (2000). *NMR Biomed.* **13,** 43.

Rudin, M., and Weissleder, R. (2003). *Nat. Rev. Drug Disc.* **2,** 123.

Rudin, M., Briner, U., and Doepfner, W. (1988). *Magn. Reson. Med.* **7,** 285.

Rudin, M., Pedersen, B., Umemura, K., and Zierhut, W. (1991). *Basic Res. Cardiol.* **86,** 615.

Rudin, M., Beckmann, N., and Sauter, A. (1997). *Magn. Reson. Imaging* **15,** 551.

Rudin, M., Beckmann, N., Porszasz, R., Reese, T., Bochelen, T., and Sauter, A. (1999). *NMR Biomed.* **12,** 69.

Rudin, M., Baumann, D., Ekatodramis, D., Stirnimann, R., McAllister, K. H., and Sauter, A. (2001). *Exp. Neurol.* **169,** 56.

Sauter, A., and Rudin, M. (1986). *Stroke* **17,** 1228.

Sauter, A., Rudin, M., and Wiederhold, K. H. (1988). *Neurochem. Pathol.* **9,** 211.

Sauter, A., Reese, T., Pórszász, R., Baumann, D., Rausch, M., and Rudin, M. (2002). *Magn. Reson. Med.* **47,** 759.

Scheffler, K., Seifritz, E., Haselhorst, R., and Bilecen, D. (1999). *Magn. Reson. Med.* **42,** 829.

Schlemmer, H. P., Bachert, P., Semmler, W., Hohenberger, P., Schlag, P., Lorenz, W. J., and vanKaick, G. (1994). *Magn. Reson. Imaging* **12,** 497.

Stock, K. W., Chen, Q., Morrin, M., Hatabu, H., and Edelman, R. R. (1999). *J. Magn. Reson. Imaging* **9,** 838.

Tofts, P. S. (1997). *J. Magn. Reson. Imaging* **7,** 91.

Tofts, P. S., and Kermode, A. G. (1991). *Magn. Reson. Med.* **17,** 357.

Turetschek, K., Floyd, E., Shames, D. M., Roberts, T. P., Preda, A., Novikov, V., Corot, C., Carter, W. O., and Brasch, R. C. (2001). *Magn. Reson. Med.* **45,** 880.

Turetschek, K., Huber, S., Helbich, T., Floyd, E., Tarlo, K. S., Roberts, T. P., Shames, D. M., Wendland, M. F., and Brasch, R. C. (2002). *Acad. Radiol.* **9,** S112.

Tyninnen, O., Aronen, H. J., Ruhala, M., Paetau, A., von Boguslawski, K., Salonen, O., Jaaskelainen, J., and Paavonen, T. (1999). *Invest. Radiol.* **34,** 427.

van Dijke, C., Brasch, R. C., Roberts, T. P., Weidner, N., Mathur, A., Shames, D. M., Desmar, F., Lang, P., and Schwickert, H. C. (1996). *Radiology* **198,** 813.

Wehrli, F. W., MacFall, J. R., and Newton, T. H. (1983). *In* "Advanced Imaging Techniques" (T. H. Newton, and D. G. Potts, eds.), p. 81, 117. Clavadel Press, San Anselmo.

Weissleder, R., Moore, A., Mahmood, U., Bhorade, R., Benveniste, H., Chiocca, E. A., and Basilion, J. P. (2000). *Nat. Med.* **6,** 351.

Welch, K. M. A., Windham, J., Knight, R. A., Nagesh, V., Hugg, J. W., Jacobs, M., Peck, D., Booker, P., Dereski, M. O., and Levine, S. R. (1995). *Stroke* **26,** 1983.

CHAPTER 9

Imaging Myocardium Enzymatic Pathways with Carbon-11 Radiotracers

Carmen S. Dence, Pilar Herrero, Sally W. Schwarz, Robert H. Mach, Robert J. Gropler, and Michael J. Welch

Department of Radiology
School of Medicine
Washington University
St. Louis, Missouri 63110

I. Introduction
II. Overview of the Production of Carbon-11
  A. Specific Activity
  B. Synthesis Modules
III. Overview of the Quality Assurance of C-11 Radiopharmaceuticals
  A. Radionuclidic Identity
  B. Radionuclidic Purity
  C. Radiochemical Purity
  D. Radioactivity Balance
  E. Chemical Purity
  F. Sterility, Apyrogenicity, Isotonicity, and Acidity
IV. Dosimetry Calculations
V. Conduct of GAP Studies
  A. Measurement of Regional Perfusion and Metabolism
  B. Metabolite Analysis
  C. Kinetic Modeling
  D. Kinetic Modeling of ^{11}C-Labeled Metabolic Radiotracers
VI. Conclusion
References

ESSENTIAL BIOIMAGING METHODS
Reprinted from *Methods in Enzymology*, Volume 385 (Academic Press, 2004)

DOI: 10.1016/B978-0-12-375043-3.00009-3

I. Introduction

Under normal conditions, the heart utilizes a variety of metabolic pathways, such as the oxidation of carbohydrates, fatty acids, lactate, and pyruvate, to meet the high-energy demands of contraction and maintenance of cellular function. The metabolic flux through each pathway is determined by the availability of substrates for each metabolic pathway in plasma, as well as hormonal status and myocardial oxygen supply. For example, the high blood levels of fatty acids during fasting result in the oxidation of fatty acids as the principal form of energy production and account for approximately 70% of the cardiac energy requirements. Consumption of a high carbohydrate meal results in an elevation of plasma glucose levels, an increase in insulin production, and an activation of glycolysis. Exercise results in the release of lactate by skeletal muscle, which is taken up rapidly by the heart, converted to acetyl-CoA, and oxidized through the tricarboxylic acid cycle (TCA). The extraordinary ability of the heart to utilize a number of different metabolic pathways and to change its metabolic preference rapidly is necessary for the maintenance of proper mechanical function under a variety of physiological conditions. Therefore, a derangement in the balance of myocardial metabolism is expected to play a key role in a number of pathological conditions leading to abnormal cardiac function.

Much of the work that resulted in the characterization of the different enzymes involved in intermediary metabolism was carried out *in vitro*. Although this seminal research provided the foundation for the fields of biochemistry and enzymology, the techniques used in the mapping of intermediary metabolism are inadequate for studying the change in metabolic processes that underlie myocardial dysfunction in human disease. While the elucidation of the different metabolic pathways was complete by the middle of the twentieth century, the study of the change in myocardial metabolism as a consequence of disease was not possible until the advent of noninvasive imaging techniques such as positron emission tomography (PET) and single photon emission computed tomography (SPECT) in the 1970s.

PET is an imaging technique developed for the *in vivo* study of metabolic functions in both healthy and diseased stages. The goal of the technique was best expressed in 1975 by Dr Michel Ter-Pogossian (Ter-Pogossian, 1977), one of the pioneers of this modality at Washington University: "Our ultimate goal is to measure *in vivo* regionally and as noninvasively as possible metabolic processes. Perhaps a term for this approach could be either *in vivo* biochemistry or functional [imaging]. The reason for seeking this goal, of course, is the application of this approach to medicine using the premise that any form of pathology either results from or is accompanied by an alteration of some metabolic pathway. Our approach to achieve the above goal consists in labeling with cyclotron-produced radionuclides, more specifically, oxygen-15, carbon-11, nitrogen-13 and fluorine-18, certain metabolic substrates, the fate of which is studied *in vivo* subsequent to their administration, by some radiation detector or imaging device, with the hope, after suitable unraveling of the metabolic model used, of measuring *in vivo* a particular pathway."

Since the early 1980s and more extensively in the mid-1990s, investigators at the Washington University School of Medicine have used PET to study the change in metabolic substrate utilization that occurs under a variety of experimental conditions, including normal aging, obesity, dilated cardiomyopathy, type 1 diabetes mellitus, and hypertension-induced left ventricular hypertrophy. This is accomplished by measuring the dynamics (i.e., uptake and washout kinetics) of radiolabeled substrates for each metabolic pathway. These studies, which utilize the radiotracers 1-[^{11}C]D-glucose, 1-[^{11}C]acetate, and 1-[^{11}C]palmitate, are collectively termed the GAP studies. This chapter provides details of the radiosynthesis, dosimetry, quality control (QC), data acquisition, and kinetic modeling that are needed to conduct this experimental paradigm successfully. These issues are discussed to help the reader new to the field gain a broad understanding of the problems faced by the PET researchers that work with short-lived isotopes and to learn some of the approaches used to solve these problems. This chapter does not include a discussion of the basic principles of PET. The reader interested in a general survey on the synthesis of ^{11}C-labeled compounds and of radiopharmaceuticals used for studying the heart is referred to Antoni *et al.* (2003) and Hwang and Bergmann (2003), respectively.

II. Overview of the Production of Carbon-11

The physical characteristics of the radionuclides used in PET are listed in Table I, along with the most common nuclear reaction to produce them in a clinical setting. Their decay mode by positron emission allows their detection outside the body after annihilation with an electron in the body. The result is the production of two photons (0.511 MeV each) at almost 180° to each other. These two photons are detected by the imaging device, which then creates images of the tissue under study. A simplified version of these events is presented in Fig. 1.

Because GAP studies require the administration of multiple radiolabeled substrates, it is necessary to use the shorter-lived positron-emitting radionuclides

Table I
Physical Characteristics of Commonly Produced Short-Lived Isotopes

Nuclide	Half-life (min)	Nuclear reaction	Max energy (MeV)	Range in H_2O (mm)	Specific activity (Ci/mmol)	Decay mode
Carbon-11	20.4	$^{14}N(p,\alpha)^{11}C$	0.96	4.1	9.22×10^6	$\beta+$ (99%)
Nitrogen-13	10.0	$^{16}O(p,\alpha)^{13}N$	1.19	5.42	18.9×10^6	$\beta+$ (100%)
Oxygen-15	2.03	$^{14}N(d,n)^{15}O$	1.70	8.0	91.7×10^6	$\beta+$ (100%)
Fluorine-18	109.7	$^{18}O(p,n)^{18}F$	0.64	2.4	1.71×10^6	$\beta+$ (97%)

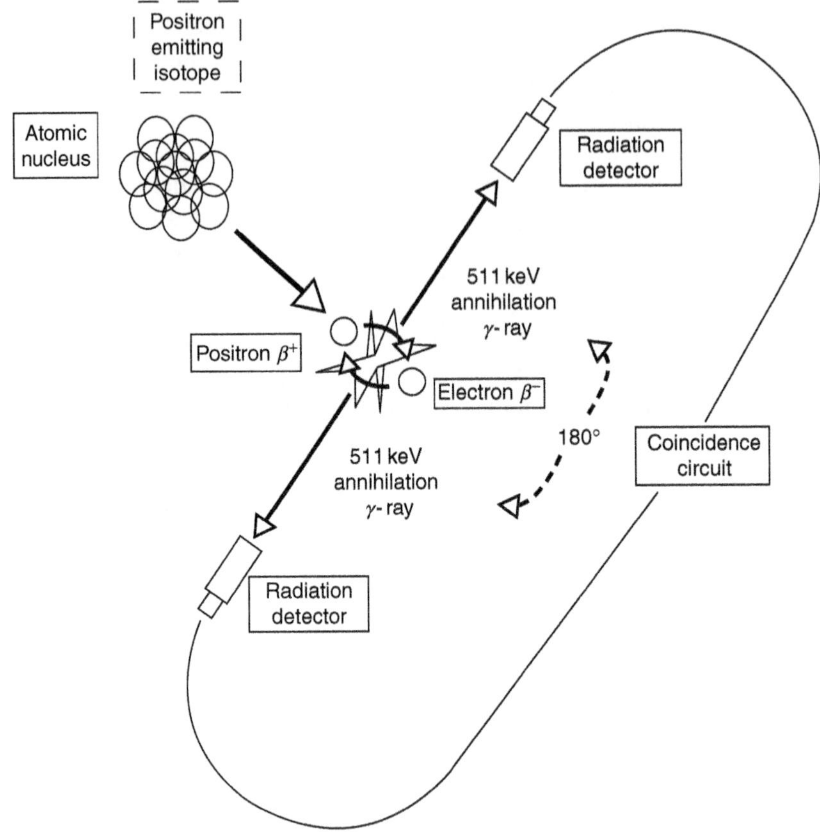

Fig. 1 Positron annihilation and coincidence detection of 0.511-MeV γ-rays.

in order to assure that sufficient radioactive decay has occurred between imaging studies. Furthermore, because it is our goal to measure the metabolic flux through each enzymatic pathway, positron-emitting versions of the metabolic substrates are best suited for this purpose. The radionuclide chosen for these studies is carbon-11, and efficient syntheses for the preparation of 1-[^{11}C]D-glucose, 1-[^{11}C] acetate, and 1-[^{11}C]palmitate have been developed in our laboratory.

Carbon-11 is produced by the $^{14}N(p,\alpha)^{11}C$ reaction using a gas target system of 0.5% oxygen in nitrogen with typical bombardments of 20–40 min at 40 μA beam power. The product obtained from the target is [^{11}C]CO_2, which is then trapped under vacuum in a specially designed stainless steel coil cooled to −196 °C with liquid nitrogen.

The transformations undergone by [^{11}C]CO_2 to produce these cardiac tracers are depicted in Fig. 2. The primary conversions shown inside the small rectangles are fast (on average, 2–5 min are needed for the conversions) and can take place on solid support systems by catalysts, as in the case of [^{11}C]CH_4 and [^{11}C]NH_4CN,

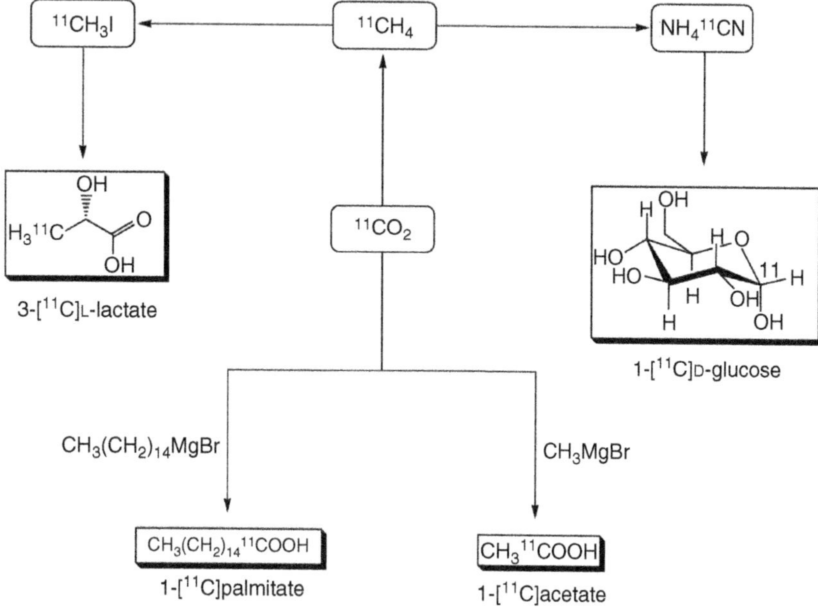

Fig. 2 Synthesis of the radiotracers used in the GAP studies.

or in the gas phase, as in the case of [^{11}C]CH_3I. It is important to remove from the [^{11}C]CO_2 gas all traces of nonradioactive oxides of nitrogen (NO_x) produced as contaminants during bombardment of the target gas. These oxides, present in about 50–150 ppm after 30 min of bombardment, may contribute to catalytic poisoning of the surface of the Pt wire inside the furnace used to produce glucose. These oxides may also lead to a lowering of radiochemical yields when using organometallic reactions (Kharasch and Reinmuth, 1954) such as the Grignard reaction used in the synthesis of 1-[^{11}C]palmitate and 1-[^{11}C]acetate. Removal of the oxides of nitrogen has a significant advantage in the reaction of carbon-11 with Grignard reagents, as it allows the use of a smaller amount of starting material and results in a significant improvement in specific activity (SA). Removal of the oxides of nitrogen is accomplished easily by placing a commercially available NO_x scrubber inline before passing the radioactive gases through to the next conversion stage. The Kitagawa gas detector solid-phase system (Matheson Gas Products tube #175SH) has been used routinely for this purpose in all of the synthesis modules described here (Dence *et al.*, 1995).

A. Specific Activity

SA is a very important parameter when working with radiopharmaceuticals. SA, defined as the amount of activity per unit mass, is expressed as the number of nuclear disintegrations per minute per mole of compound. For carbon-11, the theoretical SA of 9.2×10^6 Ci/mmol of the carrier-free radionuclide (Table I) is never achieved in practice, and dilutions to approximately 10^4 Ci/mmol are common due to the presence of traces of carbon in the gas lines, delivery systems, reagents, etc. High-SA radiotracers are very important when dealing with receptor-based compounds, gene expression experiments, and other specific uptake studies where saturation with the carrier compounds may invalidate the results.

The issue of low SA for carbon-11 compounds has been documented extensively in the literature, and a number of solutions have been offered to try to improve it. Among them are the use of ultrahigh-purity gases, a careful consideration of the target and window foil material used, and an adherence to rigid protocols for cleaning such targets and related glassware. The use of the highest quality material available is necessary for all ancillary equipment needed for isotope production, such as gas regulators, connectors, compressors, water lines, and vacuum pump oil, as all are potential sources of traces of carbon that will reduce the SA of the radiopharmaceutical. In addition, minimizing the amount of reagents used in each reaction and exploring gas- and solid-phase reactions have all been examined by chemists with some success. Because of the physiological presence of glucose, acetate, and palmitate in the human body, a very high SA for the GAP radiopharmaceuticals is of lesser concern.

B. Synthesis Modules

We have built semiautomated remote chemistry systems for the production of 1-[^{11}C]D-glucose and 1-[^{11}C]palmitate. These systems are shielded by placement within hot cells in the cyclotron area. They are relatively inexpensive and easy to construct and allow the chemist to make quick adjustments when needed during the synthesis. In contrast to the more sophisticated robotic manipulators that are also used, these remote gantries can be adapted to new, exploratory syntheses with a minimum investment of time. All the alternatives to synthesize these carbon-11 tracers (remote gantries, robotic hands, and commercially available synthesizers) share the important characteristics of reliability and very low exposure to the operator (<2 mR per synthesis). The in-house built systems are also the least expensive of the three systems.

1. 1-[^{11}C]D-Glucose

Ever since the early 1990s, the authors have been involved in the synthesis of 1-[^{11}C] D-glucose (Dence *et al.*, 1993). The result has been an improved procedure for the production of the desired compound in sufficient quantities for two simultaneous human studies and an additional animal study if needed (Dence *et al.*, 1997). This improved synthesis involves the use of a preformed sugar-borate complex of the starting substrate, D-arabinose, to effect the condensation with [^{11}C]NH_4CN. The stereochemistry of this sugar-borate complex favors the formation of glucose over mannose (ratio 1.8 ± 0.6:1). The overall chemistry illustrated in Scheme 1 is performed using a semiautomated remote system illustrated in Fig. 3.

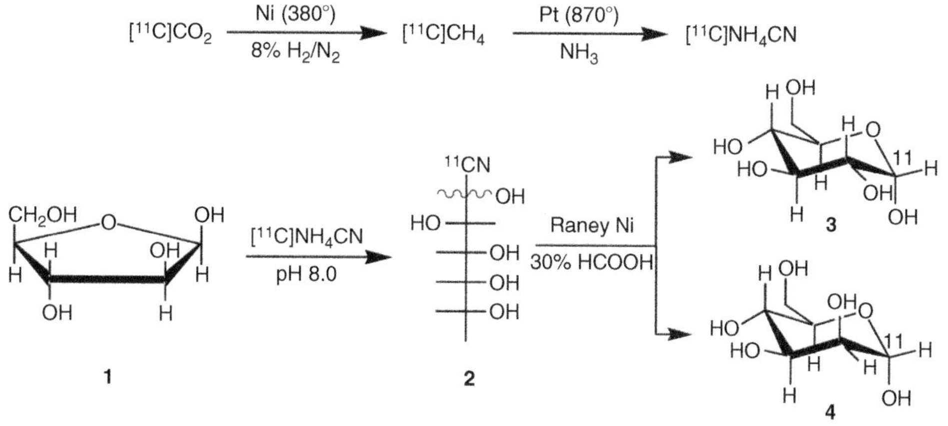

$[^{11}C]CO_2 \xrightarrow[8\%\ H_2/N_2]{Ni\ (380°)} [^{11}C]CH_4 \xrightarrow[NH_3]{Pt\ (870°)} [^{11}C]NH_4CN$

$\mathbf{1} \xrightarrow[pH\ 8.0]{[^{11}C]NH_4CN} \mathbf{2} \xrightarrow[30\%\ HCOOH]{Raney\ Ni} \mathbf{3} + \mathbf{4}$

Scheme 1 Radiosynthesis of 1-[^{11}C]D-glucose.

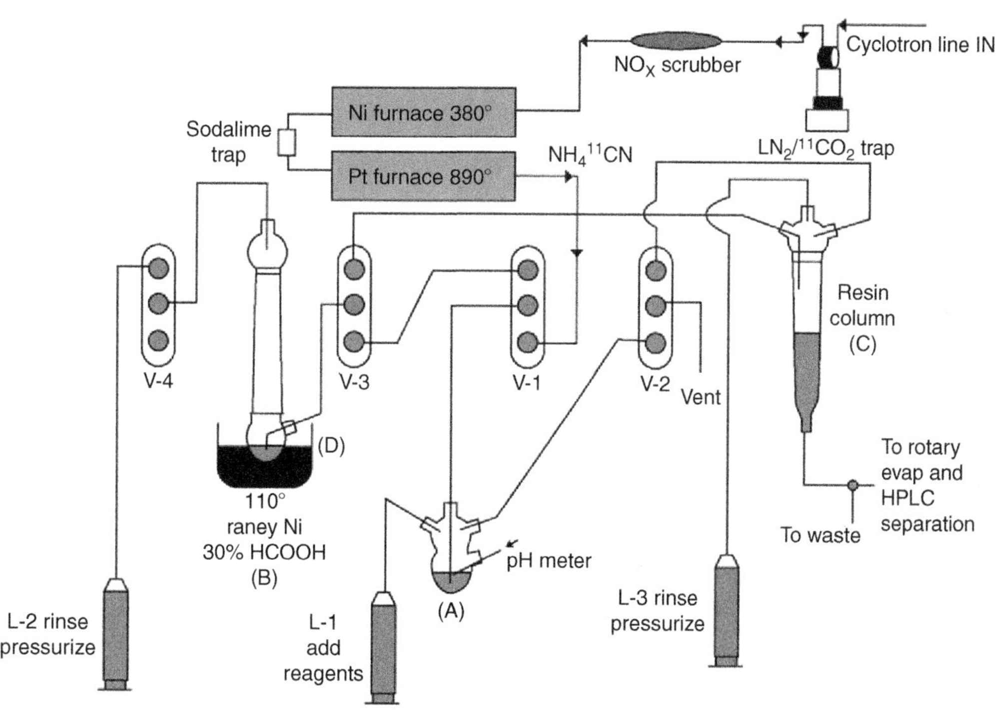

Fig. 3 Schematic of the gantry system used in the synthesis of 1-[^{11}C]D-glucose.

The reaction vessel A is a two-necked 10-ml conical flask (14/20 joints) filled with 0.5 ml of 0.01 N NaOH, and the pH probe is set in place in one of the side arms. Vessel B, a 10-ml conical vial that is modified to admit a side Teflon line, contains a freshly prepared Raney-nickel slurry (about 0.3 g) in 30% formic acid (2.0 ml). The purification column C (Bio-Rad column 26 cm long × 10 mm i.d.) contains 8.5–9.0 g of anion-exchange resin Bio-Rex 5, 100–200 mesh (OH form), and 3.5 g of cation-exchange resin AG50W-X8 100–200 mesh (H form). The purification column C is connected to the 50-ml vessel of a rotary evaporator by means of a three-way valve and a Teflon line. The rotary evaporator vessel is provided with 10–11 ml of acetonitrile to remove excess water azeotropically from the final mixture prior to high-performance liquid chromatography (HPLC) purification.

At the end of bombardment (EOB), the $[^{11}C]CO_2$ is first converted to $[^{11}C]CH_4$ in a furnace heated with a nickel-chromium resistance wire maintained at 385 °C. This furnace is provided with a borosilicate glass tube (26 cm length × 9 mm i.d.) filled in the center of the tube with small pieces of glass wool coated with 0.5 g of nickel powder on Kieselguhr (Ventron). The nickel catalyst is held in place by putting at each end of the same another small piece of glass wool and stainless steel wool. A second furnace to convert the $[^{11}C]CH_4$ to $[^{11}C]NH_4CN$ has a quartz glass column 36 cm length × 9 mm i.d., which holds 1.2 g of 0.25-mm diameter platinum wire (Aldrich 26,717–1) wound inside the quartz tube and is kept at 870–880 °C. All the connections between the two furnaces and the radiator trap for the radioactive gases are done with 1/8 o.d. Teflon tubing. The connections within valves and glassware in the gantry are made with 1/16 Teflon tubing. Two small radioactive detectors located strategically near the $[^{11}C]CO_2$ trap and vessel A help follow the flow of radioactivity during the synthesis.

The $[^{11}C]CO_2$ gas is first trapped under vacuum in a radiator trap kept at −196 °C with liquid N_2. At the end of collection, the radiator trap is brought to atmospheric pressure, and the $[^{11}C]CO_2$ is displaced from the trap with a reducing gas mixture of 8% H_2 in nitrogen. The gas is first passed through the Kitagawa purification tube to remove nonradioactive oxides of nitrogen, as described earlier. The radioactive gas then goes through the first furnace (nickel furnace) and is converted to $[^{11}C]CH_4$ by the stream of the reducing gas at 20–30 ml/min. Any unconverted $[^{11}C]CO_2$ is removed from the gas stream by a stainless steel soda-lime tube (6–8 g) placed in between the two furnaces.

Anhydrous ammonia (2 ml/min) is then added to the $^{11}CH_4/H_2/N_2$ stream, and the mixture is passed through the second furnace (platinum furnace), where it is converted to $[^{11}C]NH_4CN$. The no-carrier-added $[^{11}C]NH_4CN$ is introduced into the gantry through valve V1 and is collected in vessel A after about 5 min from EOB. After a peak reading on the radioactive detector, the ammonia flow is stopped and the pH is adjusted to approximately 9 with about 0.18 ml of 3 M glacial acetic acid. The substrate D-arabinose (10–14 mg) in 0.45 ml of 0.033 M borate buffer (pH 8.1) is added to reaction flask A and the mixture is allowed to react for 5 min at room temperature.

At the end of this incubation time, the clear reaction mixture is transferred by air pressure into flask B, where the intermediate aldonitriles are reduced with the Raney-nickel slurry. The mixture is heated under reflux for 5 min at 110 °C, is cooled for approximately 1 min, and is transferred by air pressure to resin purification column C. After the first 2–3 ml of eluate are discarded, column C is flushed dry with air to eliminate as much as possible the excess solvents used: sodium hydroxide, formic acid, acetic acid, etc. Finally, the radioactive sugars are eluted from column C by the addition of about 9 ml of water. The eluate is reduced azeotropically in the rotary evaporator under vacuum/heat to less than 0.1 ml volume, diluted with deionized (DI) water to 0.8–0.9 ml, and injected onto the preparative HPLC. 1-[^{11}C]D-Glucose is purified on a 7.8 × 300-mm Bio-Rad HPX-87P column heated to 85 °C and is then eluted with water at 1.0 ml/min. The aqueous fraction containing the 1-[^{11}C]D-glucose is collected after about 8 min in a sterile 6-ml syringe. This fraction is purified further of any remaining inorganic or metal ions by filtering through an ion-exchange chromatography Chelex cartridge (Alltech 30250). The eluate is made isotonic by the addition of 3 M NaCl, diluted to 5–7 ml with DI water, and filtered through a 0.22-μm, 25-mm vented filter to produce a sterile and pyrogen-free solution ready for injection. Current yields are from 40 to 60 mCi of final product, ready for injection, following a synthesis time of about 50 min from EOB.

2. 1-[^{11}C]Palmitate

Synthesis of 1-[^{11}C]palmitate is accomplished according to the method outlined in Fig. 2 and with the remote system detailed in Fig. 4 (Welch *et al.*, 1981, 1983). The system uses a single reaction vessel 13.5 cm long × 3.5 cm wide (B), equipped with two side arms. The lower section is in the shape of a 10-mm o.d. test tube marked at the 1-cc volume. The vessel is agitated using a standard laboratory mixer (C). A 1-mm i.d. Teflon tube (L1) is inserted through one side arm to add reagents from outside the hood. Another 1-mm i.d. Teflon tube (L2) is inserted through the second side arm to the bottom of the vessel (B). The other end of L2 enters a Teflon block (D) (4 × 5.5 cm, bored as indicated in Fig. 2). Block D is the common path for connecting the reaction vessel (B) to the waste receptacle (F) and the filtration gantry (E).

At the EOB, the [^{11}C]CO_2 produced is collected by evacuating the target gas into the cooled (−196 °C) radiator trap (A). The Grignard reagent, 0.1 M 1-pentadecylmagnesium bromide in diethyl ether (3 ml), is added to the reaction vessel (B). The Dewar (I) is lowered, the radiator trap (A) is warmed, and the [^{11}C]CO_2/N_2 is bubbled through the Grignard reagent for 1–3 min. The reaction is quenched by the addition of 3 ml of 1.0 N HCl, and 3 ml of diethyl ether is added to extract the [^{11}C]palmitate. The vessel (B) is shaken in the vortex mixer (C) and the layers are allowed to separate. The lower aqueous layer is drawn off by closing valve V2 (vent), opening valve V7 briefly to slightly pressurize the vessel (B), and then opening valve V6. The aqueous layer is pushed through the Teflon line (L2)

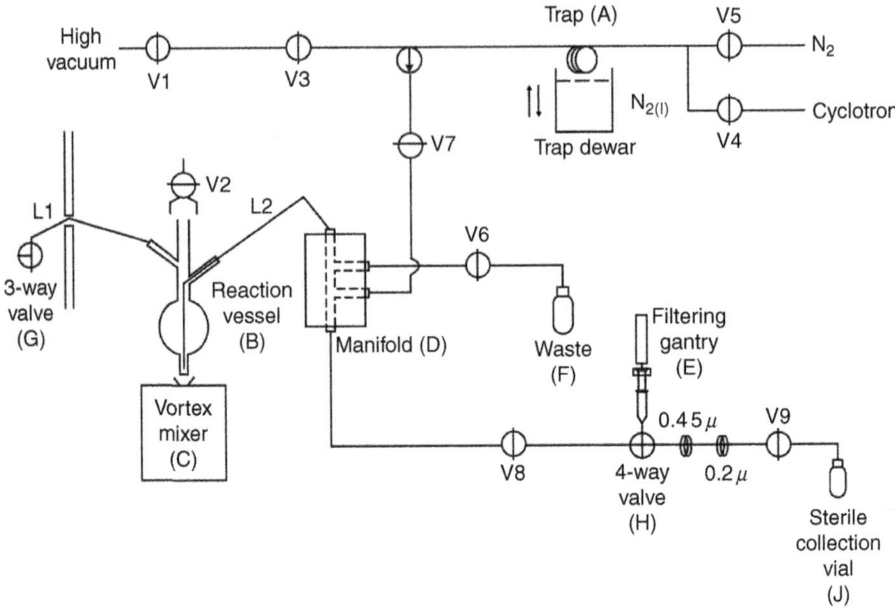

Fig. 4 Schematic of the gantry system used in the synthesis of 1-[^{11}C]palmitate.

and Teflon block (D) and into the waste receptacle (F). The remaining ether layer is washed twice with 5 ml of 0.9% sodium chloride (USP saline), and each time the lower aqueous layer is discarded into the waste receptacle (F). The ether solution is then diluted with 1 ml of 95% ethyl alcohol and the diethyl either is evaporated using a 100-ml/min flow of nitrogen through the solution, accomplished by opening valves V5, V7, and V2. Evaporation is continued until less than 1 ml of liquid (ethanol layer) is left, the nitrogen flow is reduced to 10 ml/min, and valve V5 is closed.

The ethyl alcohol solution is then diluted with 8.2 ml of a 3.5% solution of human serum albumin in USP saline (kept at ~50 °C during the synthesis) and left to stand undisturbed for 3 min to complex the fatty acid with the albumin. For the final filtration, the albumin fatty acid solution is pulled from the vessel (B) into the 12-ml syringe and is pushed through the 0.45- and 0.22-μm, 25-mm filters and into the collection vial (J). Current yields at the end of a 25–30-min bombardment are from 150 to 350 mCi of final product ready for injection in a synthesis time of 15–20 min from EOB.

3. 1-[^{11}C]Acetate

We use a *robotic system*, as well as a commercially available *synthesizer*, for the production of 1-[^{11}C]acetate. The Hudson workstation (Thermo Electron Corp., Ontario, Canada) is illustrated in Fig. 5. All platforms have been custom built and

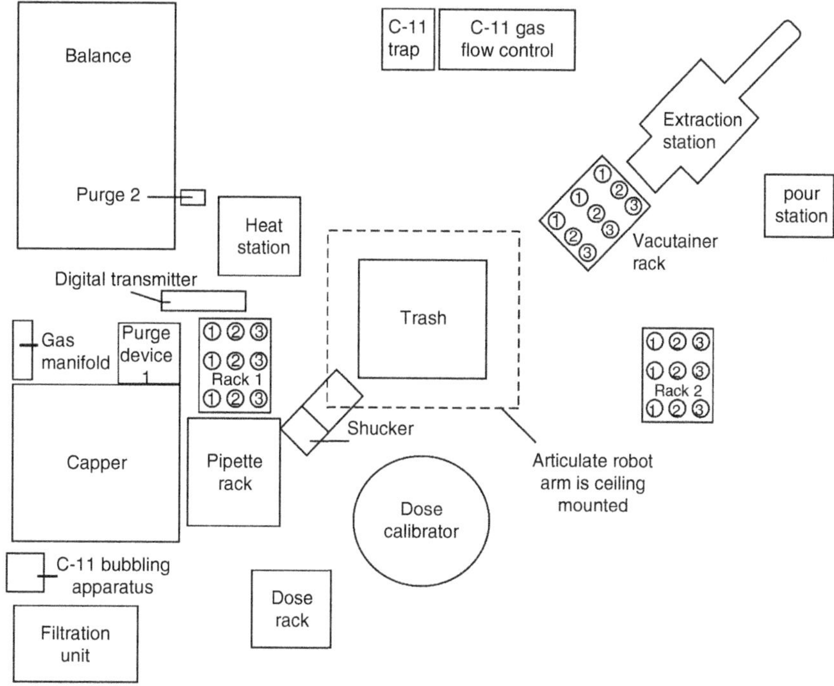

Fig. 5 Hudson robotic system for the compounding of an 1-[^{11}C]acetate injection.

include a dedicated reagent rack constructed of Plexiglas, a capping station, a nitrogen purge device, and three 3-way valves and four 2-way valves to direct the [^{11}C]CO_2 target gas and nitrogen gas flow to the trapping/reaction vessel. The capping station holds a 5-ml Reactivial (Wheaton Scientific, Millville, IL) used for trapping the [^{11}C]CO_2. A 3.5-in. × 19-gauge needle connects the inlet line for incoming target gases and nitrogen, and a 1.5-in. × 18-gauge needle connects the outlet line for venting and trapping any unreacted [^{11}C]CO_2. After the [^{11}C]CO_2 target gas addition, the system removes the cap from the Reactivial with the top-loading capping station from Hudson. The heating station is constructed from a heating block obtained from Fisher Scientific (St. Louis, MO), and an aluminum block into which a hole is drilled to accommodate the 5-ml Reactivial. A temperature controller (Model D1311 from Omega Engineering, Stanford, CT) controls the temperature of the heating block. All liquid transfers are done with disposable 1000-μl pipette tips using a pipette tip holder attached to the gripping hand of the Hudson robot that connects to a Hamilton syringe station to control pipetting and dispensing.

After cyclotron irradiation, [^{11}C]CO_2 is collected in an evacuated cold trap cooled with liquid nitrogen. The trap is removed from the liquid nitrogen, warmed, and purged using a stream of nitrogen gas (10 ml/min). The stream of nitrogen gas containing the [^{11}C]CO_2 is bubbled through 50 μl of 3 M methylmagnesium bromide diluted with 3 ml diethyl ether in a 5-ml Reactivial. USP sterile water for injection (0.25 ml) is added, and the reaction vial is placed onto a 50 °C heating block to evaporate the ether using a stream of nitrogen gas. The intermediate organometallic complex is hydrolyzed by the addition of 2 ml of 0.4 N hydrochloric acid, followed by the addition of 2 ml of USP sterile water for injection. Purification of the acidic mixture by solid phase is accomplished by the robot, which pours the solution onto the PrepSep funnel, which contains 600–700 mg of C18 resin activated previously with 5 ml of ethanol and rinsed with 10 ml of sterile water and 2–3 g of AG 11A8 ion retardation resin. The final product is filtered through a 0.22-μm, 25-mm, sterile, apyrogenic filter. Batches of 220 mCi on average at the end of 20-min syntheses are obtained routinely after a 20-min bombardment.

1-[^{11}C]Acetate is also produced routinely in our laboratory with a commercially available *chemistry synthesizer*, the CTI acetate module (Knoxville, TN) (Fig. 6). After irradiation, the target gases are passed through a needle valve into the reagent vessel; the flow of the target gas is limited to less than 100 ml/min. The stream of nitrogen gas containing the [^{11}C]CO_2 is bubbled through 50 μl of 3 M methylmagnesium bromide diluted with 1 ml diethyl ether in a 10-mm

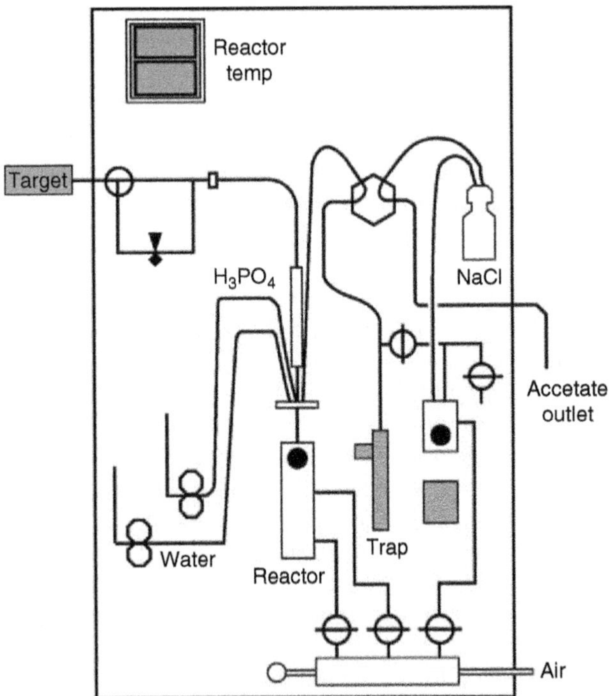

Fig. 6 CTI 1-[^{11}C]acetate synthesis module.

o.d. × 75-mm long test tube sealed with a red flange stopper top. Sterile water for injection, USP (0.25 ml) is added, and the reaction vial is heated to 145 °C. The ether is evaporated using a stream of helium gas. The intermediate is hydrolyzed by the addition of 0.5 ml of 10% phosphoric acid. The acidic mixture is then purified by heating at 145 °C for 420 s to distill 1-[^{11}C]acetate into USP saline (10 ml). The final product is passed through a 0.22-μm, 25-mm, sterile, apyrogenic filter. Average yields of 200 mCi of 1-[^{11}C]acetate are obtained routinely in a synthesis time of 20 min from EOB.

III. Overview of the Quality Assurance of C-11 Radiopharmaceuticals

Radiopharmaceuticals administered for PET procedures and which contain radionuclides of very short half-lives, such as carbon-11 (20.4 min), must be analyzed, must meet quality assurance specifications, and must be fully documented prior to administration to humans (Kilbourn *et al.*, 1985; Vera-Ruiz *et al.*, 1990). This requires various types of QC determinations, such as radionuclidic identity, radionuclidic purity, radiochemical and chemical purity, sterility, and pyrogen testing. It is important that each analytical test be validated and the limits for each test specified.

A. Radionuclidic Identity

This can be accomplished prior to release of the radiopharmaceutical by decay analysis using a dose calibrator computer program to calculate $T_{1/2}$.

B. Radionuclidic Purity

The fraction of total radioactivity that is present as the specified radionuclide should be determined from a γ-ray spectrum by means of a multichannel pulse height analyzer or a germanium detector to detect the presence of any γ photon energies other than 0.511 MeV and the sum peak at 1.02 MeV. The radionuclidic purity determination can be made three to four half-lives after the EOB with little interference from the main 0.511-MeV photopeak of the positron emitters.

C. Radiochemical Purity

The QC method for determining *radiochemical purity* (the fraction of the radiopharmaceutical that is present in the desired chemical form, with the label in the specified molecular position) is usually based on a chromatographic method with simultaneous mass and radioactivity detection. Various types of chromatographic methods such as thin-layer chromatography (TLC) or HPLC can be used. HPLC allows the in-line measurement of chemical and radiochemical purity. These chromatographic methods are performed using standards for the comparison of R_f values and retention times or for generating standard calibration curves (Kilbourn *et al.*, 1986).

D. Radioactivity Balance

For the development of new radiopharmaceuticals requiring analysis by HPLC, it is generally necessary to perform a *radioactivity balance* measurement to ensure that the total radioactivity injected onto an HPLC column is recovered at the end of the specified HPLC run time. This determination can be made by injection of an aliquot of the radiopharmaceutical (10–50 μl) onto the HPLC and collecting all the postinjection effluent solvent in a volumetric flask. The flask is then taken to the standard volume and mixed well. For example, for an HPLC run at 1.5 ml/min that lasts 10 min, a 25-ml volumetric flask is used to collect the eluate. After 10 min the flask is removed from the eluting line and a sufficient volume of water (or a solvent compatible with the HPLC solvent used) is added to bring the total volume to 25 ml. This constitutes "sample counts." The "standard counts" sample is obtained by aliquoting the original volume injected on the HPLC column (10–50 μl from the same original analyte) into another 25-ml volumetric, and adding sufficient solvent to bring the total volume to 25 ml. An aliquot from each volumetric flask is transferred into a test tube, and the samples are counted in a sodium iodide γ counter. Due to the short half-life of C-11, it is necessary to decay correct both samples to time zero and compute the percentage eluted as follows: ("counts in sample"/"counts in standard") $\times$ 100. Acceptable values should be 85% or higher. With high SA radiopharmaceuticals, some radioactivity losses are unavoidable on the HPLC tubing, column, precolumn, filters, etc. Values below 85% are usually indicative of radioactivity being retained on the chromatographic column or precolumns that need to be addressed in order to avoid inaccurate radiochemical purity determinations.

E. Chemical Purity

Analyses are required to verify the absence of any chemical impurities or solvent residues in the final preparation. Analyses also require an injection of a known standard each time a QC is performed. In this way, the accuracy of the HPLC, or of any other system that is used, is determined each time. Chemical impurities separated by HPLC are generally easy to detect if they are ultraviolet (UV) absorbing. Compounds with low UV absorption characteristics can be detected by pulsed amperometric detectors (PADs) or by HPLC mass spectrometry. The *chemical purity* requirement serves to verify the chemical identity of the product and by-products, including stereoisomeric purity, if needed (e.g., 1-[^{11}C]D-glucose vs. 1-[^{11}C]D-mannose). Ion chromatographic techniques are applied routinely to the detection of residual inorganic species in order to validate the absence of nickel, borate, and lead ions. Lead ions may potentially arise from the lead counterion of the Aminex resin of the HPLC column used in the preparative purification of the 1-[^{11}C]D-glucose preparation (Dence *et al.*, 1993).

The quantification of organic solvent residues such as ethanol, acetonitrile, and ether used in the preparation of the carbon-11 compounds is performed by gas chromatography. Separation is carried out on a Varian 3800 gas chromatograph using a capillary column DB-Wax, 30-m $\times$ 0.53-mm i.d., 1-μm film thickness (J&W Scientific). The injector and FID detector temperatures are held at 225 and 275 °C, respectively. Helium is used as a carrier at a flow rate of 7 ml/min. The column temperature is held at 40 °C for 2 min and is raised to 110 °C in 7 min. Analyses are performed on a 1.0-μl aliquot of the final injectable solution after sterile filtration.

F. Sterility, Apyrogenicity, Isotonicity, and Acidity

Tests should be performed to ensure sterility, apyrogenicity, isotonicity, and suitable acidity (pH) before administration to humans. *Sterility* should be determined postrelease on each batch of parenteral radiopharmaceutical intended for human use. The injectable drug product must be sterilized by filtration through a 0.22-μm filter as a final step in the radiosynthetic procedure. USP methods for sterility require inoculation of the radiopharmaceutical into both tryptic soy broth and fluid thioglycolate media within 24-h postend of synthesis (EOS). Because an entire lot of a PET radiopharmaceutical may be administered to one or several subjects, depending on the radioactivity remaining in the container at the time of administration, administration of the entire quantity of the lot to a single patient should be anticipated for each lot prepared. Verification of *apyrogenicity* should be made using the USP bacterial endotoxin test (BET) on each batch of every nongaseous radiopharmaceutical prepared for intravenous human administration. The USP limit for endotoxins is 175 endotoxin units (EU) per volume (V), which is the maximum volume administered in the total dose. If the $T_{1/2} \geq 20$ min, a 20-min endotoxin "limit test" must be performed prerelease (USP 46). A standard 60-min test must also be performed on each batch. The *pH* and *isotonicity* can be adjusted to physiologic values prior to the final filtration by the addition of sterile buffers or by a 0.9% sodium chloride solution.

IV. Dosimetry Calculations

All radiopharmaceuticals that are injected into humans require that absorbed dose calculations be performed. These dose calculations are needed to predict the risk involved in the use of any ionizing radiation (Stabin *et al.*, 1999). Medical internal radiation dose (MIRD) calculations require knowledge of certain parameters. These include the amount of *cumulative activity* in each of the organs of the body and the type of radiation administered.

Cumulative activity represents the time course of the radioactivity in the body that requires information on the rate of radiopharmaceutical uptake and removal (biological half-life), as well as the physical decay of the radionuclide injected (physical half-life).

Biological clearance data (percentage injected dose/organ over time) are often obtained by the performance of biodistribution studies, usually in rodents, over a time interval. If radiopharmaceuticals labeled with C-11 are used, a 2- to 3-h time interval is acceptable. Clearance can also be determined by the use of dynamic PET imaging. Mathematical models, such as the dynamic bladder model (Thomas *et al.*, 1999), can also be used to calculate the clearance. Biological clearance data are used to calculate the cumulative activity in each organ. The formula for the absorbed dose is $D = \tilde{A}S$, where $\tilde{A}$ is cumulative activity and S is absorbed dose per unit cumulative activity. The absorbed doses per unit cumulative activity can be calculated for the specific isotope used ($S = \Delta\phi/m$), where

$$\Delta\phi = 2.13\sum n_i E_i,$$

n_i is the number of particles or photons per nuclear transformation, E_i is the mean energy of the radiation, and m is the mass of the organ. These S values can also be obtained from a dosimetry computer software program MIRDOSE3 (Howell *et al.*, 1999; Stabin, 1996).

V. Conduct of GAP Studies

A. Measurement of Regional Perfusion and Metabolism

1. Data Acquisition

Figure 7 is a representation of the imaging protocol for the GAP studies. A transmission scan is initially conducted prior to administration of the radiotracer. The transmission scan consists of a data acquisition session in which a positron-emitting point source is rotated 360° around the subject to be scanned. The function of the transmission scan is to provide an accurate measurement of photon attenuation for the attenuation correction of the ensuing emission scans (i.e., a scan acquired after the administration of the radiotracer). For the measurement of myocardial blood flow (MBF), up to 0.40 mCi/kg of ^{15}O water (prepared using the method of Welch and Kilbourn, 1985) is administered as a bolus intravenously with the immediate initiation of dynamic data collection for 5 min. After allowance for decay of the ^{15}O water, up to 0.30 mCi/kg of 1-[^{11}C]acetate is injected intravenously, and a 30-min dynamic data collection is performed to measure myocardial oxygen consumption. After allowance for decay of the 1-[^{11}C]acetate, up to 0.30 mCi/kg of 1-[^{11}C]D-glucose is injected intravenously, and a 60-min dynamic data collection is performed to measure myocardial glucose metabolism. Finally, after allowance for decay of the 1-[^{11}C]D-glucose, up to 0.30 mCi/kg of

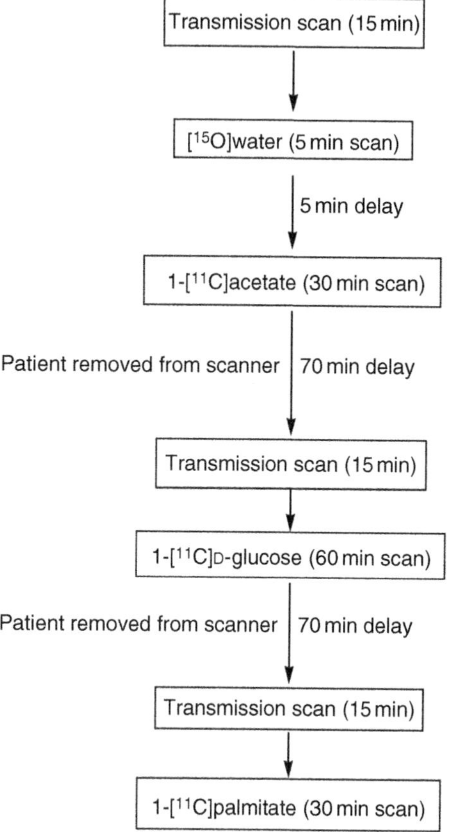

Fig. 7 Flowchart outlining the steps in conducting a GAP study.

1-[^{11}C]palmitate is injected intravenously, and a 30-min dynamic data collection is performed to measure myocardial fatty acid metabolism.

During the 1-[^{11}C]acetate, 1-[^{11}C]palmitate, and 1-[^{11}C]D-glucose scans, 8–10 venous samples are obtained to measure $^{11}CO_2$ production (in the case of 1-[^{11}C] D-glucose, 1-[^{11}C]lactate is measured as well) in order to correct the arterial input function during kinetic modeling (see Section V.C). Between each metabolic scan (i.e., between 1-[^{11}C]acetate and 1-[^{11}C]D-glucose), subjects are removed from the tomograph to increase their comfort during the study. Upon their return to the tomograph, another transmission scan is performed (a total of three transmission scans per study). Table II lists the total amount of radioactivity administered to the test subject in a typical GAP study, which is approximately 1475 mrem. This represents about 30% of the annual exposure limit for a radiation worker (e.g., personnel involved in the synthesis of PET radiotracers).

Table II
Effective Dose Equivalent (EDE) for All the Radiopharmaceuticals Administered in a Gap Study[a]

[^{15}O]Water[b]	[^{11}C]Acetate[c]	[^{11}C]Palmitate[c]	[^{11}C]d-Glucose[c]	Total
92 mrem[d]	273 mrem[d]	320 mrem[d]	790 mrem[d]	1475 mrem

[a]A measure of the biological damage caused by "ionizing" radiation, for example, γ-rays, X-rays, and β particles, is expressed by the dose equivalent, the unit of which is the rem. A special variation of the dose equivalent is the EDE, a computed uniform whole body dose that applies to nonuniform irradiation of differing organs and tissues in the body. The allowable EDE for a radiation worker in the United States is 5000 mrem. The EDE for administration of the radiopharmaceuticals listed here would be 30% of the allowable annual exposure for a radiation worker.
[b]Administered dose: 28 mCi (0.4 mCi/kg; 70 kg man).
[c]Administered dose: 21 mCi (0.3 mCi/kg; 70 kg man).
[d]EDE from unpublished dosimetry estimates.

2. Data Reconstruction and Generation of Time-Activity Curves

After data reconstruction is performed, myocardial images are reformatted from the transaxial orientation to the true short-axis views on which measurements of perfusion and metabolism will be performed. Myocardial [^{15}O]water, 1-[^{11}C]acetate, 1-[^{11}C]D-glucose, and 1-[^{11}C]palmitate images are generated and then reoriented to standard short- and long-axis views. To generate myocardial time-activity curves, regions of interest on anterior, lateral, septal, apical, and inferior myocardial walls (3–5 cm^3) are placed on three to four midventricular short- and long-axis slices of composite [^{15}O]water, 1-[^{11}C]acetate, 1-[^{11}C]D-glucose, and 1-[^{11}C]palmitate images. To generate blood time-activity curves for each tracer, a small region of interest (1 cm^3) is placed within the left atrial cavity on a midventricular slice in the horizontal long-axis orientation of each composite image. Within these regions of interest, myocardial and blood time-activity curves are generated for each of the sets of tracer data. Subsequently, blood and myocardial time-activity curves are used in conjunction with well-established kinetic models to measure MBF, oxygen consumption, glucose utilization, fatty acid utilization, and oxidation.

B. Metabolite Analysis

In order to validate the kinetic models used to study the enzymatic pathways of the heart with the carbon-11 tracers, it is necessary to account for the impact of blood acidic metabolites on the arterial input function (Herrero *et al.*, 2002a). This routinely includes the analysis of C-11 acidic metabolites present in blood, namely carbonate and lactate, following the injection of C-11 radiotracers (Dence *et al.*, 2001).

1. Determination of $[^{11}C]CO_2$

The determination is based on the loss of $[^{11}C]CO_2$ under acidic conditions. A 5-ml blood sample is withdrawn into a gray-top Vacutainer (L10330-00; Becton-Dickinson, NJ) after a specified postinjection time. Blood is spun for 5–6 min at 3500 rpm to separate the plasma. For each sample to be analyzed, a set of two test tubes are prepared, each containing 1.0 ml of 0.9 M sodium bicarbonate and 3 ml of isopropanol. To one of the test tubes, 1 ml of 0.1 N NaOH is added (labeled "basic"). To each test tube, 0.5 ml of plasma is added and the tubes are vortexed briefly and gently. The other test tube is then treated with 1 ml of 6 N HCl (labeled "acidic"). All the "acidic" test tubes are placed in a custom-made manifold and purged with a stream of nitrogen for 10 min at room temperature to eliminate $[^{11}C]CO_2$. At the end of bubbling, all the tubes are counted for radioactivity (from last-to-first collected), decay corrected to time zero, and the percentage of $[^{11}C]CO_2$ is calculated (counts "acidic"/counts "basic" × 100).

2. Total Acidic Metabolites

Following injections of 1-[^{11}C]D-glucose, blood samples are analyzed for total acidic metabolites (TAM) ([^{11}C]carbonate and [^{11}C]lactate) and residual 1-[^{11}C]D-glucose. Analysis is based on the trapping of these acidic species on an anion-exchange column while eluting the neutral species. The authors use 1.2–1.3 g of AG1-X8, in the formate form, 100–200 mesh (Bio-Rad) placed in a 6-ml disposable syringe with a glass wool plug in the bottom. The resin is rinsed with 4–6 ml of water. These columns can be prepared 24 h ahead and kept moist at room temperature. The blood samples are collected on special Vacutainer tubes (as described earlier) containing sodium fluoride and potassium oxalate to stop further glucose metabolism. About 1.0 ml of plasma is pipetted into the resin column, and DI water (in 2 + 3-ml fractions) is used to elute the nonmetabolized 1-[^{11}C]D-glucose. This eluate (5 ml total) is collected in one test tube. The acidic metabolites, [^{11}C]carbonate and [^{11}C]lactate are retained on the resin. Both eluate and resin are counted for radioactivity, and after decay correction the percentage of acidic metabolites is calculated (counts in resin/counts in eluate × 100). The percentage of [^{11}C]lactate is calculated by subtracting the percentage of CO_2 (determined as described earlier) from the percentage of TAM, and the percentage of residual glucose as 100%TAM.

C. Kinetic Modeling

After the blood time-activity curve has been corrected for its metabolites, the blood (input function) and tissue-time activity curves generated from PET cardiac images are used in conjunction with kinetic models to measure MBF and metabolism. In the kinetic modeling of PET data derived from GAP studies, the method that is typically used is the *compartmental model method*. A compartmental model is generally represented by a series of compartments linked together by arrows representing transfer between the compartments. A compartment is defined as the space in which the radiotracer is distributed uniformly (Huang and Phelps, 1986). The number of compartments that are needed to quantify the fate of the radiotracer *in vivo* is directly proportional to the number of steps in the metabolic process being investigated (Fig. 8). The arrows in Fig. 8 represent possible pathways the radiotracer can follow in a particular metabolic pathway. The symbol k above each arrow is a rate constant and denotes the fraction of the total radiotracer that would leave the compartment per unit time (turnover rate (min^{-1})).

The key assumptions of compartmental modeling are that the tracer is distributed homogeneously in each compartment and that the rate of tracer transfer from compartment 1 to compartment 2 is directly proportional to the tracer concentration in compartment 1. These assumptions make it possible to describe the system under study by n first-order, linear differential equations, where n is the number of compartments and each differential equation represents the rate of change of tracer concentration over time in a given compartment, defined as the rate of tracer *in* minus the rate of tracer *out* of the compartment. The solution to the system of differential equations gives the concentration of tracer in each compartment over time. The sum of the concentrations from all compartments (a function of the blood activity and the turnover rates of the tracer) represents the myocardial activity over the scanning period (theoretical myocardial time-activity curve). Using nonlinear least-square approaches, turnover rates (k_s values) are estimated by minimizing the differences between the PET-derived myocardial time-activity curve and the analytical curve derived from the model. A brief description of the compartmental models used in the kinetic analysis of a GAP study is outlined next.

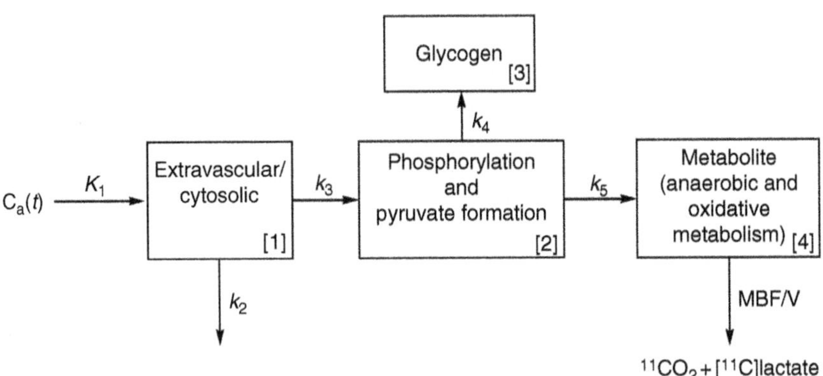

Fig. 8 Four-compartment model used for 1-[^{11}C]D-glucose. K_1 (ml/g/min), k_2, and k_3 (min^{-1}). Net 1-[^{11}C]D-glucose uptake (K, ml/g/min) = $(K_1 \times k_3)/(k_2 + k_3)$.

1. Myocardial Blood Flow

[^{15}O]Water is a freely diffusible radiotracer whose myocardial kinetics appears to be related solely to blood flow. That is, the uptake of [^{15}O]water is not altered by changes in myocardial metabolism (Bergmann *et al.*, 1989; Herrero *et al.*, 1989, 1994). The kinetics of freely diffusible tracers such as [^{15}O]water can be described by a simple one-compartment model. The approach for quantifying MBF is based on the model developed by Kety (1951, 1960a,b) for radiolabeled inert freely diffusible gases. The rate of change of myocardial tracer activity over time can be defined by a simple differential equation:

$$\frac{\mathrm{d}C_{\mathrm{T}}(t)}{\mathrm{d}(t)} = \frac{(\mathrm{MBF})C_{\mathrm{a}}(t) - (\mathrm{MBF})C_{\mathrm{T}}(t)}{\lambda} \tag{1}$$

The solution to the differential equation is shown as

$$C_{\mathrm{T}}(t) = (\mathrm{MBF})C_{\mathrm{a}}(t) * \exp\left(\frac{(\mathrm{MBF})t}{\lambda}\right) \tag{2}$$

where $C_{\mathrm{T}}(t)$ is tissue tracer concentration (counts/g); $C_{\mathrm{a}}(t)$ is arterial tracer concentration (input function) (counts/ml); MBF is myocardial blood flow per unit of tissue volume (ml/g/min); λ is the tissue/blood partition coefficient (0.92 ml/g); and * is the convolution process.

Using least-square techniques, estimates of MBF can be obtained by fitting Eq. (2) to the myocardial tissue activity $C_{\mathrm{T}}(t)$. However, because of the limited resolution of PET tomographs (8–12 mm FWHM) in relation to the thickness of the myocardium (~10 mm in humans) and effects of cardiac motion, the true tissue concentration cannot be measured directly with PET. If the object under study is less than twice the resolution of the tomograph, the true activity in the region of interest is underestimated (partial volume effect) and activity from adjacent regions is detected into the region of interest (spillover effect). The relationship between the true and the observed PET activity can be defined as

$$C_{\mathrm{TPET}}(t) = F_{\mathrm{MM}} \times C_{\mathrm{T}}(t) + F_{\mathrm{BM}} \times C_{\mathrm{a}}(t) \tag{3}$$

$$C_{\mathrm{aPET}}(t) = F_{\mathrm{BB}} \times C_{\mathrm{a}}(t) + F_{\mathrm{MB}} \times C_{\mathrm{T}}(t) \tag{4}$$

where $C_{\mathrm{T\,PET}}(t)$ is observed tissue activity (counts/g), $C_{\mathrm{T}}(t)$ is true tissue activity (counts/g), $C_{\mathrm{aPET}}(t)$ is observed blood pool activity (counts/g), $C_{\mathrm{a}}(t)$ is true blood pool activity (counts/g), F_{MM} is the tissue recovery coefficient (accounts for partial volume effects in the myocardium), F_{BM} is fraction of blood activity into tissue (accounts for spillover of blood counts into myocardium), F_{BB} is the blood recovery coefficient (accounts for partial volume effects in the blood), and F_{MB} is the fraction of tissue activity into blood (accounts for spillover of myocardium counts into blood).

If these correction factors are known *a priori*, the true blood and myocardial activity can be calculated from Eqs. (3) and (4). These correction factors can be calculated analytically if the resolution of the tomograph and the dimensions of the blood chambers and myocardial tissue are known and there is no motion present (Herrero *et al.*, 1988). However, when cardiac and respiratory motion are present and/or the measurements of cardiac chambers and tissue are not accurate, then measurement of the true blood and tissue-activity curves will be inaccurate and will result in erroneous MBF estimates. This problem is circumvented by incorporating within the blood flow model (Eq. (2)), this relationship between the true tissue activity and the PET-derived tissue activity given by

$$C_{\mathrm{TPET}}(t) = F_{\mathrm{MM}} \times \left[\mathrm{MBF}\,C_{\mathrm{a}}(t) * \exp\left(-\frac{(\mathrm{MBF})t}{\lambda}\right)\right] + F_{\mathrm{BM}} \times C_{\mathrm{a}}(t) \qquad (5)$$

where MBF is estimated along with F_{MM} and F_{BM} by fitting Eq. (5) to PET-derived tissue activity ($C_{\mathrm{T\ PET}}(t)$). This model assumes that $C_{\mathrm{a}}(t)$ can be measured directly with PET (i.e., $F_{\mathrm{BB}} = 1.0$ and $F_{\mathrm{MB}} = 0.0$ in Eq. (4)). This assumption has been validated in experimental human studies (Herrero *et al.*, 1988).

D. Kinetic Modeling of ^{11}C-Labeled Metabolic Radiotracers

For all ^{11}C-labeled metabolic radiotracers, a correction for myocardial partial volume and spillover effects was done by estimating the corresponding model turnover rates along with F_{BM} after fixing F_{MM} to values obtained from the [^{15}O] water analysis.

1. Myocardial Glucose Utilization

Myocardial glucose utilization (MGU) is obtained using a four-compartment model for 1-[^{11}C]D-glucose (Fig. 8) (Herrero *et al.*, 2002b). This model assumes that vascular 1-[^{11}C]D-glucose enters the interstitial and cytosolic component of the myocardium (compartment 1) at a rate of K_1 (ml/g/min). Once the tracer enters compartment 1, it either diffuses back into the vascular space at a rate of k_2 (min^{-1}) or it is phosphorylated and metabolized to [^{11}C]pyruvate (compartment 2) at a rate of k_3 (min^{-1}). Phosphorylated 1-[^{11}C]D-glucose can either form [^{11}C]glycogen at a rate of k_4 (min^{-1}) or be metabolized through anaerobic and oxidative pathways (compartment 4) at a rate of k_5 (min^{-1}). Radiotracer entering the metabolic pool is assumed to be unidirectional, and washout of [^{11}C]CO_2 and [^{11}C]lactate to the vasculature is assumed to be proportional to blood flow. This is an important assumption, as it enables one to "lump" all the radiolabeled intermediates in the glycolytic pathway (Fig. 9) into one compartment.

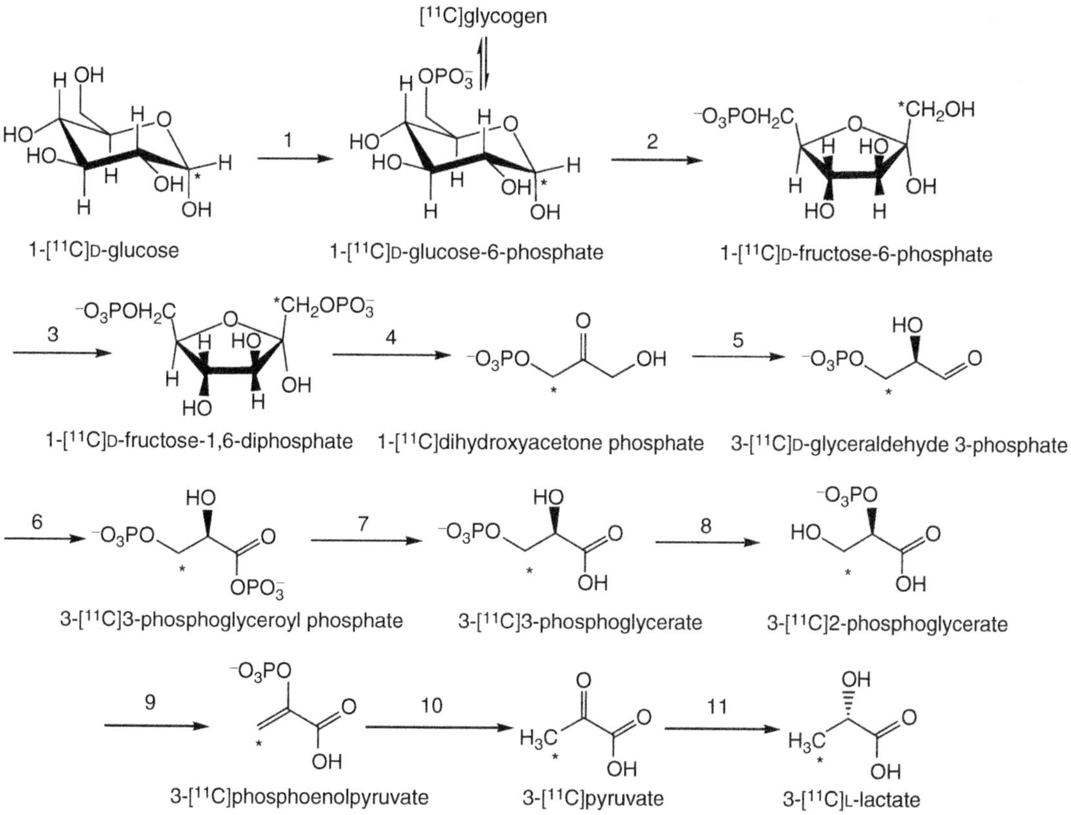

Fig. 9 Fate of the ^{11}C radiolabel in 1-[^{11}C]D-glucose in the glycolytic pathway. Enzymes: 1, hexokinase; 2, glucose phosphate isomerase; 3, 6-phosphofructokinase; 4, fructose diphosphate aldolase; 5, triosephosphate isomerase; 6, glyceraldehydephosphate dehydrogenase; 7, phosphoglycerate kinase; 8, phosphoglyceromutase; 9, enolase; 10, pyruvate kinase; 11, lactate dehydrogenase. From Nelson and Cox (2000).

Differential equations defining the model are as follows:

$$\frac{dq_1(t)}{dt} = K_1 C_a(t) - (k_2 + k_3)q_2(t) \tag{6}$$

$$\frac{dq_2(t)}{dt} = k_3 q_1(t) - (k_4 + k_5)q_2(t) \tag{7}$$

$$\frac{dq_3(t)}{dt} = k_4 q_1(t) \tag{8}$$

$$\frac{dq_4(t)}{dt} = k_5 q_2(t) - (\mathrm{MBF})q_4(t) \tag{9}$$

The solution of this set of differential equations results in the concentration of tracer in each compartment (q_1–q_4). The total radiotracer concentration in the myocardium as a function of time is then defined as the sum of the radiotracer concentrations in each compartment:

$$q_t(t) = q_1(t) + q_2(t) + q_3(t) + q_4(t) = f(C_a(t), K_1, k_2-k_5, \text{MBF}, V) \quad (10)$$

where $C_a(t)$ is arterial 1-[^{11}C]D-glucose concentration (i.e., the input function for 1-[^{11}C]D-glucose), K_1 and k_2–k_5 are turnover constants describing the transfer of radiotracer between compartments, q_n is the concentration of radiotracer in compartment n (counts/ml), V is the fractional vascular volume and is assumed to be 10% of total volume (0.1 ml/g), and f represents a function of the parameters in parentheses. The model transfer rate constants (K_1, k_2–k_5) and the spillover fraction are estimated using well-established least-square approaches by fitting the model Eq. (10) to PET myocardial time-activity curves. If one assumes steady-state conditions (i.e., differential equations are set to zero), then these estimated turnover rates (K_1, k_2–k_5) are used to calculate the net 1-[^{11}C]D-glucose uptake ($\text{GLU}_{\text{uptake}}$) and MGU as

$$\text{GLU}_{\text{uptake}}(\text{ml/g/min}) = \frac{K_1 k_3}{k_2 + k_3} \quad (11)$$

$$\text{MGU}(\text{nmol/g/ min}) = (\text{Gl}_b, \text{nmol/ml})(\text{GLU}_{\text{uptake}}, \text{ml/g/ min}) \quad (12)$$

The myocardial glucose extraction fraction (EF_{GLU}) is calculated as

$$\text{EF}_{\text{GLU}} = \frac{\text{GLU}_{\text{uptake}}}{\text{MBF}} \quad (13)$$

Hence, MGU can be calculated as the product of three key measurements—the plasma glucose level, MBF, and the myocardial glucose extraction fraction:

$$\text{MGU}(\text{nmol/g/min}) = (\text{Gl}_b)(\text{MBF})(\text{EF}_{\text{GLU}}) \quad (14)$$

where Gl_b is the plasma glucose level in nmol/ml measured from venous blood samples obtained during the PET study and EF_{GLU} is the myocardial glucose extraction fraction estimated from 1-[^{11}C]D-glucose kinetics.

2. Myocardial Oxidative Metabolism

After correction of the PET-derived blood ^{11}C activity for the $^{11}CO_2$ contribution, the blood and myocardial time-activity curves are used in conjunction with a simple one-compartment model to estimate two turnover rates: K_1 (ml/g/min) representing the net rate of 1-[^{11}C]acetate uptake into the myocardium and k_2 (min^{-1}) representing the rate at which 1-[^{11}C]acetate is converted to $^{11}CO_2$. The latter has been shown to be directly proportional to myocardial oxygen consumption (MVO_2) (Brown *et al.*, 1988; Buxton and Nienaben, 1989). MVO_2

(μmol/g/min) is then calculated from an experimentally derived linear relationship between k_2 and MVO_2 in humans (Beanlands *et al.*, 1993).

3. Myocardial Fatty Acid Metabolism

The kinetics of 1-[^{11}C]palmitate metabolism are described by a four-compartment model (Fig. 10). The model assumes that the radiotracer entering mitochondria is unidirectional and that metabolites are washed out of mitochondria into the vasculature at a rate proportional to blood flow. The differential equations describing the model are

$$\frac{dq_1(t)}{dt} = \mathrm{MBF}\left[\frac{C_a(t) - q_1}{V}\right] + k_2q_2 - K_1q_1 \tag{15}$$

$$\frac{dq_2(t)}{dt} = K_1q_1 + k_4q_3 - (k_2 + k_3 + k_5)q_2 \tag{16}$$

$$\frac{d}{dt} = k_3q_2 - k_4q_3 \tag{17}$$

$$\frac{dq_4(t)}{dt} = k_5q_2 - \left(\frac{\mathrm{MBF}}{V}\right)q_4 \tag{18}$$

The solution of this set of differential equations gives the concentration of tracer in each compartment (q_1–q_4). The total radiotracer concentration in the myocardium at any given time can be defined by the sum of the radiotracer concentrations in each compartment:

$$q_t(t) = q_1(t) + q_2(t) + q_3(t) + q_4(t) = f(C_a(t), K_1 - k_5, \mathrm{MBF}, V) \tag{19}$$

where MBF is myocardial blood flow (ml/g/min), $C_a(t)$ is concentration of 1-[^{11}C] palmitate in blood (input function of 1-[^{11}C]palmitate, counts/ml), K_1–k_5 (min^{-1}) are turnover constants describing the transfer of radiotracer between

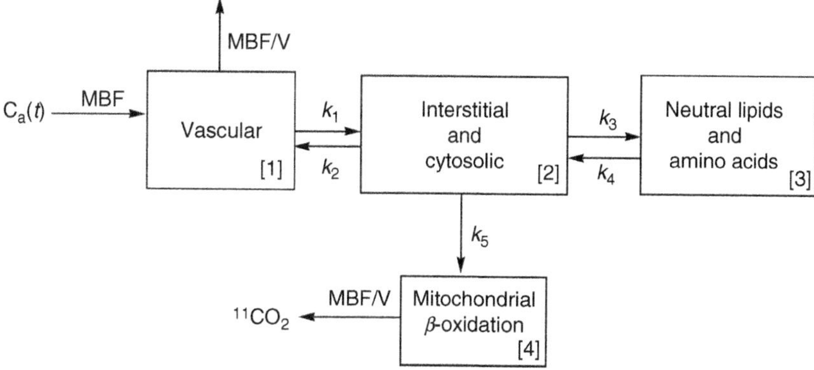

Fig. 10 The four-compartment model used in the kinetic analysis of 1-[^{11}C]palmitate.

compartments, V is the fractional vascular volume (assumed to be 10% of total volume) (0.1 ml/g), q_n is the concentration of radiotracer in compartment n (counts/ml), and q_t is the total concentration of radiotracer in the myocardium (counts/ml).

Because blood contains radiolabeled metabolites in addition to 1-[^{11}C]palmitate, the PET-derived ^{11}C blood activity must be corrected for the presence of $^{11}CO_2$ as described earlier in order to derive the true input function. MBF is fixed to values obtained with [^{15}O]water, and the fractional vascular volume is fixed at 0.1 ml/g. Similarly to the analysis of 1-[^{11}C]D-glucose, after a correction of the blood ^{11}C activity for $^{11}CO_2$, the turnover rates (K_1–k_5) and F_{BM} are estimated by fitting Eq. (19) to the PET myocardial time-activity curves after fixing F_{MM} to values obtained from [^{15}O]water analyses.

If one assumes steady-state conditions (i.e., each differential equation is set equal to zero), then key quantities such as fatty acid utilization, oxidation, and esterification (all in nmol/g/min) can be calculated from the estimated turnover rates. The model assumes that once the tracer is in the interstitial/cytosolic compartment, it can follow only three pathways: back diffusion into the vasculature (k_2), storage into neutral lipids and amino acids (esterification) (k_3), and β oxidation (k_5) (see Fig. 10). Because the proportion of arterial palmitate (a long-chain fatty acid) to the total free fatty acid concentration in blood remains constant during a wide range of free fatty acid levels, and different chains of fatty acids have comparable myocardial extraction fractions (Bergmann *et al.*, 1996), fatty acid utilization, oxidation, and esterification can be calculated from the kinetics of 1-[^{11}C]palmitate as

$$\mathrm{MFAU(nmol/g/min)} = (\mathrm{FFA_b})(\mathrm{MBF})(\mathrm{EF}_{^{11}\mathrm{C-pal}}) \tag{20}$$

where $\mathrm{FFA_b}$ is free fatty acid in blood (nmol/ml); MBF is myocardial blood flow (ml/g/min); $\mathrm{EF}_{^{11}\mathrm{C-pal}}$ is the myocardial extraction fraction of palmitate estimated from the kinetics of 1-[^{11}C]palmitate; and

$$\mathrm{MFAU(nmol/g/\,min)} = \mathrm{MFAO} + \mathrm{MFAE} \tag{21}$$

where MFAO is myocardial fatty acid oxidation, MFAE is myocardial fatty acid that is retained by the myocardium and includes esterified fatty acids, as well as intermediary metabolites, and

$$\mathrm{MFAO(nmol/g/\,min)} = k_5 q_2 \tag{22}$$

$$\mathrm{MFAE(nmol/g/\,min)} = k_3 q_2 (k_4 \text{is negligible during the study period}) \tag{23}$$

$$q_2 = \frac{K_1[\mathrm{MBFFFA_b}]}{(k_2 + k_5)(K_1 + \mathrm{MBF}/V) - (K_1 k_2)} \tag{24}$$

where q_2 is the concentration of unlabeled palmitate in compartment 2 (nmol/g), FFA_b is the fatty acid concentration in blood (nmol/ml), and V is the fractional vascular volume in myocardium (assumed to be 10% of total volume (ml/g)).

Finally, the fraction of extracted palmitate undergoing oxidation (F_{ox}) or esterification (F_{es}) can be calculated as

$$F_{ox} = \frac{\text{MFAO}}{\text{MFAU}} \tag{25}$$

$$F_{es} = \frac{\text{MFAE}}{\text{FMAU}} \tag{26}$$

VI. Conclusion

GAP studies currently represent the most thorough application of PET in the measurement of substrate utilization and oxidative metabolism in the heart. The successful completion of this research protocol requires the detailed coordination of radiochemists, cyclotron operators, cardiologists, nurses, and technicians with mathematical modelers and data analysis personnel in order to contend with the short half-lives of the radionuclides used in the imaging studies. Analysis of PET data requires sophisticated metabolite correction, image coregistration, partial volume, and spillover correction techniques in order to quantitate myocardial metabolism accurately. Nonetheless, data analyses of a typical GAP study require minimum manual data entry and, on average, are completed within 2 h from the time the myocardial PET images are reconstructed, making these types of complex studies feasible to implement in a clinical PET environment. To date, this imaging paradigm has been used to measure the changes in metabolic flux in a variety clinical research protocols, including normal aging (Kates *et al.*, 2003; Soto *et al.*, 2003), obesity (Peterson *et al.*, 2004), dilated cardiomyopathy (Davila-Roman *et al.*, 2003), type 1 diabetes mellitus, and hypertension-induced left ventricular hypertrophy (De las Fuentes *et al.*, 2003). Future studies will be directed toward the application of this paradigm in order to delineate the mechanisms responsible for the metabolic changes observed in these conditions and to assess the efficacy of novel therapies designed to reverse these metabolic abnormalities.

Acknowledgments

We thank Jeff Willits for his assistance with the illustrations and Dr Joseph B. Dence for his suggestions and reading of the manuscript. This work was conducted under NIH Grants HL13851 and RO1 AG15466.

References

Antoni, G., Kihlberg, T., and Långström, B. (2003). *In* "Handbook of Radiopharmaceuticals: Radiochemistry and Applications" (M. J. Welch and C. S. Redvanly, eds.), p. 141. Wiley, West Sussex.

Beanlands, R. S., Bach, D. S., Raylman, R., Armstrong, W. F., Wilson, V., Montieth, M., Moore, C. K., Bates, E., and Schwaiger, M. (1993). *J. Am. Coll. Cardiol.* **5,** 1389.

Bergmann, S. R., Herrero, P., Markham, J., Weinheimer, C. J., and Walsh, M. N. (1989). *J. Am. Coll. Cardiol.* **14,** 639.

Bergmann, S. R., Weinheimer, C. J., Markham, J., and Herrero, P. (1996). *J. Nucl. Med.* **37,** 1723.

Brown, M. A., Myears, D. W., and Bergmann, S. R. (1988). *J. Am. Coll. Cardiol.* **12,** 1054.

Buxton, D. B., Nienaben, C. A., Luxen, A., *et al.* (1989). *Circulation* **79,** 134.

Davila-Roman, V. G., Vedula, G., Herrero, P., de las Fuentes, L., Rogers, J. G., Kelly, D. P., and Gropler, R. J. (2003). *J. Am. Coll. Cardiol.* **40,** 271.

De las Fuentes, L., Herrero, P., Peterson, L. R., Kelly, D. P., Gropler, R. J., and Davila-Roman, V. G. (2003). *Hypertension* **41,** 83.

Dence, C. S., Powers, W. J., and Welch, M. J. (1993). *Appl. Radiat. Isot.* **44,** 971.

Dence, C. S., McCarthy, T. J., and Welch, M. J. (1995)."Proceedings 6th Workshop on Targetry and Target Chemistry"p. 216. Vancouver, Canada.

Dence, C. S., Powers, W. J., Gropler, R. J., and Welch, M. J. (1997). *J. Labeled Comp. Radiopharm.* **40,** 777.

Dence, C. S., Herrero, P., Sharp, T. L., and Welch, M. J. (2001)."12th International Symposium on Radiopharmacology."Interlaken, Switzerland, Abstract Book.

Herrero, P., Markham, J., Myears, D. W., Weinheimer, C. J., and Bergmann, S. R. (1988). *Math. Comp. Model.* **11,** 807.

Herrero, P., Markham, J., and Bergmann, S. R. (1989). *J. Comp. Assist. Tomogr.* **13,** 862.

Herrero, P., Hartman, J. J., Senneff, M. J., and Bergmann, S. R. (1994). *J. Nucl. Med.* **35,** 558.

Herrero, P., Sharp, T. L., Dence, C., Haraden, B. M., and Gropler, R. J. (2002a). *J. Nucl. Med.* **43,** 1530.

Herrero, P., Weinheimer, C. J., Dence, C. S., Oellerich, W. F., and Gropler, R. J. (2002b). *J. Nucl. Cardiol.* **9,** 5.

Howell, R. N., Wessels, B. W., and Loevinger, R. (1999). *J. Nucl. Med.* **40,** 3S.

Huang, S. C., and Phelps, M. E. (1986). *In* "Positron Emission Tomography and Autoradiography: Principles and Applications for the Brain and Heart" (M. Phelps and J. Mazziotta, eds.), p. 287. Raven Press, New York.

Hwang, D. H., and Bergmann, S. R. (2003). *In* "Handbook of Radiopharmaceuticals: Radiochemistry and Applications" (M. J. Welch and C. S. Redvanly, eds.), p. 529. Wiley, West Sussex.

Kates, A. M., Herrero, P., Dence, C. S., Soto, P., Srinivasan, M., Delano, D. G., Ehsani, A., and Gropler, R. J. (2003). *J. Am. Coll. Cardiol.* **41,** 293.

Kety, S. S. (1951). *Pharmacol. Rev.* **3,** 1.

Kety, S. S. (1960a). *Methods Med. Res.* **8,** 223.

Kety, S. S. (1960b). *Methods Med. Res.* **8,** 228.

Kharasch, M. S., and Reinmuth, O. (1954). *In* "Grignard Reactions of Non-Metallic Substances," p. 1243. Prentice Hall, New York.

Kilbourn, M. R., Dence, C. S., Lechner, K. A., and Welch, M. J. (1985). *In* "Quality Assurance of Pharmaceuticals Manufactured in the Hospital" (A. Warbick-Cerone and L. G. Johnson, eds.), p. 243. Pergamon Press, New York.

Kilbourn, M. R., Welch, M. J., Dence, C. S., and Lechner, K. A. (1986). *In* "Analytical and Chromatographic Techniques in Radiopharmaceutical Chemistry" (D. M. Wieland, M. C. Tobes and T. J. Mangner, eds.), p. 251. Springer-Verlag, New York.

Nelson, D. L., and Cox, M. M. (2000). *In* "Lehninger Principles of Biochemistry" (D. L. Nelson and M. M. Cox, eds.), p. 527. Worth Publishers, New York.

Peterson, L. R., Herrero, P., Schechtman, K. B., Racette, S. B., Waggoner, A. D., Kisreivaware, Z., Dence, C. S., Klein, S., Marsala, J., Meyer, T., and Gropler, R. J. (2004). *Circulation* (in press).

Soto, P. F., Herrero, P., Kates, A. M., Dence, C. S., Ehsani, A. A., Davila-Roman, V., Schechtman, K. B., and Gropler, R. J. (2003). *Am. J. Physiol. Heart Circ. Physiol.* **285,** H2158.

Stabin, M. G. (1996). *J. Nucl. Med.* **37,** 538.

Stabin, M. G., Tagesson, M., Thomas, S. R., Ljungberd, M., and Strand, S. E. (1999). *Appl. Radiat. Isot.* **50,** 73.

Ter-Pogossian, M. (1977). "The Developing Role of Short-Lived Radionuclides in Nuclear Medicine," p. 9. US Department of Health, Education and Welfare.

Thomas, S. R., Stabin, M. G., Chen, C. T., and Samaratunga, R. C. (1999). *J. Nucl. Med.* **40,** 102S.

Vera-Ruiz, H., Marcus, C. S., Pike, V. W., *et al.* (1990). *Nucl. Med. Biol.* **17,** 445.

Welch, M. J., and Kilbourn, M. R. (1985). *J. Labeled Comp. Radiopharm.* **22,** 1193.

Welch, M. J., Wittmer, S. L., Dence, C. S., and Tewson, T. J. (1981). *In* "Short-Lived Radionuclides in Chemistry and Biology" (J. W. Root and K. A. Krohn, eds.), ACS Advances in Chemistry Series 197p. 407. Washington, DC.

Welch, M. J., Dence, C. S., Marshall, D. R., and Kilbourn, M. R. (1983). *J. Labeled Comp. Radiopharm.* **30,** 1087.

PART III

Disease Models

CHAPTER 10

Molecular and Functional Imaging of Cancer: Advances in MRI and MRS

Arvind P. Pathak, Barjor Gimi, Kristine Glunde, Ellen Ackerstaff, Dmitri Artemov, and Zaver M. Bhujwalla

JHU ICMIC Program
Russell H. Morgan Department of Radiology and Radiological Science
The Johns Hopkins University School of Medicine
Baltimore, Maryland 21205

I. Update
II. Introduction
III. Vascular Imaging of Tumors with MRI
  A. MR Relaxation Mechanisms and the Basis of Contrast
  B. Intrinsic or Endogenous Contrast
  C. Extrinsic or Exogenous Contrast
IV. Cellular and Molecular Imaging
  A. Magnetic Resonance Detection of Cellular Targets
  B. Technical Strategies for MR Microscopy
V. Metabolic and Physiologic Spectroscopy and Spectroscopic Imaging with MRS and MRSI
  A. ^{1}H MRS
  B. ^{13}C MRS
  C. ^{31}P MRS
  D. Tumor pH
VI. Examples of Integrated Imaging and Spectroscopy Approaches to Studying Cancer
  A. MR Metabolic Boyden Chamber for Studying Cancer Cell Invasion
  B. Multinuclear MRI and MRSI of Preclinical Models of Cancer
References

ESSENTIAL BIOIMAGING METHODS

DOI: 10.1016/B978-0-12-375043-3.00010-X

I. Update

The five years since the original publication of this article have seen major advances in molecular and functional imaging using magnetic resonance imaging (MRI) and magnetic resonance spectroscopy (MRS). These advances are primarily attributable to developments in (i) stem cell biology, (ii) imaging hardware, and (iii) the synthesis of novel contrast agents.

Although biomedical research on stem cells is in its nascent stages, there has been a virtual explosion in our knowledge of their role in organogenesis. For example, neurons are produced from neural progenitor cells (NPCs), which reside in the hippocampus and the subventricular zone (Gage, 2000). These NPCs possess the ability to self-renew and generate progeny that can give rise to mature cell types such as neurons, astrocytes, and oligodendrocytes. This raises the prospect of harnessing them to repair nerve tissue damaged by neurological disease or trauma, and the ability to identify them *in vivo* would be valuable. MRS was recently used to identify NPCs in the live human brain (Manganas *et al.*, 2007). In this study, the authors used proton MRS to identify and characterize a biomarker in which NPCs were enriched and demonstrated its use as a reference for monitoring neurogenesis. To detect low concentrations of NPCs *in vivo*, they developed a signal processing algorithm that enabled the use of MRS for the analysis of the NPC biomarker in both the rodent brain and the hippocampus of humans *in vivo*, opening the possibility of investigating the role of NPCs and neurogenesis in a wide variety of human brain disorders including brain tumors.

Alterations in tissue pH underlie many pathologies and the ability to image it could offer new ways for detecting disease and tracking therapeutic efficacy in patients. For example, in tumors the extracellular pH is lower than in normal tissue and often correlates with prognosis and response to therapy. While agents for measuring pH have been developed for MRS, their low sensitivity makes it difficult to obtain a pH map at high spatial resolutions and the small pH-dependent chemical shift of such agents makes pH quantification at clinical magnetic field strengths challenging (Gallagher *et al.*, 2008). However, dynamic nuclear polarization (DNP) has recently demonstrated the potential to circumvent these problems by increasing the signal-to-noise ratio (SNR) of $>$10,000 times in liquid-state MRS (Ardenkjaer-Larsen *et al.*, 2003). A recent study demonstrated the feasibility of mapping the pH *in vivo* using hyperpolarized ^{13}C-labeled bicarobonate in a mouse tumor model (Gallagher *et al.*, 2008). Since bicarbonate is an endogenous molecule the authors propose its infusion into patients at high concentrations enabling DNP pH imaging in the clinic. Another promising advance in imaging hardware is the development of ultralow-field (ULF) or superconducting quantum interference device (SQUID)-based MRI at microtesla magnetic fields (Zotev *et al.*, 2008). Although the authors employed a prototype system to demonstrate the feasibility of human brain imaging by microtesla MRI, this technology promises to usher in a new era in molecular imaging since imaging at ULF can be performed using inexpensive and portable systems that do not subject patients to high magnetic fields. Additionally, the improved T_1-weighted contrast at low magnetic fields may allow more efficient identification of pathologies affecting T_1 (e.g., brain tumors) without the use of conventional gadolinium (Gd)-based contrast agents. An added advantage of microtesla MRI is that it can be easily integrated with complementary imaging modalities such as magnetoencephalography (MEG) (Zotev *et al.*, 2008).

Unlike optical imaging wherein one can avail of multicolored contrast agents, MRI has largely been a monochromatic method based either on signal enhancement or attenuation. However, recently Zabow *et al.* (2008) demonstrated the feasibility of multispectral MRI by developing MRI contrast agents with characteristic resonant frequencies based on their mechanical structure. Unlike conventional particulate contrast agents that produce contrast from magnetic field (i.e., resonant frequency) variations outside the particle, these engineered particles produce targeted contrast based on the direct manipulation of the signal from water within particles of a specific geometry (Zabow *et al.*, 2008).

Collectively, the above-mentioned scientific breakthroughs in conjunction with the development of "hybrid" small animal imaging systems such as PET-MRI scanners that allow us to simultaneously exploit the sensitivity of PET and the morphological resolution of MRI (Judenhofer *et al.*, 2008), herald an exciting new period in the functional and molecular imaging of cancer. Preclinical research using these innovative MRI and MRS techniques holds great potential for relieving the suffering of cancer patients by facilitating "bench-to-bedside" translation.

II. Introduction

Cancer is a disease that exhibits a degree of multiplicity and redundancy of pathways almost protean in nature. To understand and exploit molecular pathways in cancer for therapeutic strategies, it is essential not only to detect and image the expression of these pathways, but also to determine the impact of this expression on function at the cellular level, as well as within the complex system, which is a tumor. Multiparametric molecular and functional imaging techniques have several key roles to play in cancer treatment, such as revealing key targets for therapy, visualizing delivery of the therapy, and assessing the outcome of treatment. As a technique, magnetic resonance (MR) has a formidable array of capabilities to characterize function. Noninvasive multinuclear magnetic resonance imaging (MRI) and MR spectroscopic imaging (MRSI) provide a wealth of spatial and temporal information on tumor vasculature, metabolism, and physiology. MR is therefore particularly applicable to investigating a complex disease such as cancer. Several of the MRI techniques are also translatable into the clinic, and are therefore compatible with "bench to bedside" applications.

Tumor vasculature plays an important role in growth, treatment, and metastatic dissemination. The first section in this chapter therefore describes the use of MRI techniques and the underlying assumptions and mechanisms in characterizing tumor vasculature. Recent advances in the development of targeted contrast agents have significantly increased the versatility of MR for molecular imaging. Although MR techniques provide a wealth of structural and functional information, MR suffers from poor sensitivity. The second section discusses the use of targeted contrast agents and amplification strategies to increase the sensitivity of detection of molecular targets in MR molecular imaging of cancer. Technical strategies to improve the SNR for applications of MR microscopy in cancer are also included in this section. Because MR spectroscopy (MRS) and MRSI provide information on metabolism and pH, MRS applications in cancer are reviewed in Section IV. One of the most exciting aspects of MR is the ability to perform multiparametric imaging. In Section V, we present two examples of the use of multiparametric imaging in understanding cancer cell invasion and in characterizing the relationship between tumor vasculature and metabolism.

III. Vascular Imaging of Tumors with MRI

MRI techniques can be used to characterize several aspects of tumor vasculature. Tumor vasculature is typified by structural and functional anomalies that include alterations in hemodynamics, blood rheology, permeability, and drainage, and plays a critical role in cancer growth, treatment, and metastasis. Vascular MR methods are therefore useful in cancer treatment and management. An overview of the endogenous and exogenous MR contrast mechanisms utilized in characterizing tumor vasculature is presented in this section.

A. MR Relaxation Mechanisms and the Basis of Contrast

Every contrast mechanism for probing the tumor vasculature, including the use of exogenous MR contrast agents, is in some way a result of changes in the MR signal intensity brought about by changes in tissue relaxation times (T_1, T_2, or T_2*). Briefly, T_1, the spin-lattice or longitudinal relaxation time, is the time constant that characterizes the exponential process by which the magnetization returns or "relaxes" to its equilibrium position. It does so by exchanging energy with its surroundings, or lattice, at the Larmor frequency. T_1 relaxation occurs at the molecular level through several pathways, including interactions between protons in tissue water and those on macromolecules or proteins, and by interactions with paramagnetic substances (i.e., substances with unpaired electrons in their outermost shells). T_1-based MR contrast results from differences in T_1 dominating the MR signal intensity. For example, tissues with short T_1s (such as fat) appear bright in T_1-weighted MRI, since the transverse magnetization recovers to equilibrium rapidly compared with tissues with long T_1s (such as cerebrospinal fluid).

Microscopic magnetic field heterogeneities in the main field, as well as variations in local magnetic susceptibility due to the physiologic microenvironment, cause spins contributing to the transverse magnetization to lose phase coherence. The process through which this occurs is known as T_2^* relaxation. The loss in transverse coherence attributable to static magnetic field heterogeneities can be recovered using a spin-echo sequence or a refocusing pulse. However, as protons diffuse through the microscopic field inhomogeneities, they also lose phase coherence due to their Brownian random walks through the magnetic field gradients, which result in phase dispersion that cannot be reversed by the application of a refocusing pulse. This process is known as T_2 relaxation. In T_2-weighted MR images, tissues with short T_2s, such as the liver, appear dark due to the rapid decay of transverse magnetization compared with those with long T_2s, such as fat. Similarly, in T_2^*-weighted images, regions with large susceptibility gradients, such as air-tissue interfaces of the inner ear or orbits of the eye, or large veins carrying deoxygenated blood, appear hypointense.

In general, the addition of a paramagnetic solute causes an increase in the $1/T_1$ and $1/T_2$ of solvent nuclei. The diamagnetic and paramagnetic contributions to the relaxation rates of such solutions are additive and are expressed as (Lauffer, 1987):

$$\left(\frac{1}{Ti}\right)_{\text{obs}} = \left(\frac{1}{Ti}\right)_{\text{d}} + \left(\frac{1}{Ti}\right)_{\text{p}}, \quad i = 1, 2 \qquad (1)$$

where $(1/Ti)_{\text{obs}}$ is the observed solvent relaxation rate in the presence of a paramagnetic species (e.g., contrast agent), $(1/Ti)_{\text{d}}$ is the diamagnetic solvent relaxation rate in the absence of a paramagnetic species, and $(1/Ti)_{\text{p}}$ represents the additional paramagnetic contribution. In the absence of any solute-solute interactions, the solvent relaxation rates (in solution) are linearly dependent on the concentration of the paramagnetic species [M], and if $(1/Ti)$ or the relaxivity R_i, is defined as the slope of this dependence in $\text{mM}^{-1}\ \text{s}^{-1}$, we may write Eq. (1) as

$$\left(\frac{1}{Ti}\right)_{\text{obs}} = \left(\frac{1}{Ti}\right)_{\text{d}} + R_i[\text{M}], \quad i = 1, 2 \qquad (2)$$

All molecules, large and small, are in a constant state of motion, tumbling and colliding with other molecules. Intramolecular motion, as well as interaction with nearby molecules, produces fluctuations in the local magnetic field experienced by a proton. It turns out that these magnetic interactions can promote both T_1 and T_2 relaxation, but whether they do so depends on the rate at which their magnetic fields fluctuate. For example, a small molecule such as water moves quickly, so that it produces rapid magnetic fluctuations. A large molecule such as a protein moves more slowly and produces magnetic fluctuations at a correspondingly lower rate. From the relaxation theory described by Solomon (1955) and Bloembergen (1957), three primary factors that regulate the dipole-dipole interactions responsible for both T_1 and T_2 relaxation are: (1) the strength of the magnetic moment, (2) the separation between the two dipoles, and (3) the relative motion of the two dipoles.

B. Intrinsic or Endogenous Contrast

Probing tumor vasculature using intrinsic contrast produced by deoxyhemoglobin in tumor microvessels is based on the blood oxygenation level dependent (BOLD) contrast mechanism first proposed by Ogawa (1990). The concentration of endogenous paramagnetic deoxyhemoglobin is one of the primary determinants of the eventual image contrast observed. The presence of deoxyhemoglobin in a blood vessel causes a susceptibility difference between the vessel and its surrounding tissue, inducing microscopic magnetic field gradients that cause dephasing of the MR proton signal, leading to a reduction in the value of T_2* (Fig. 1). Because oxyhemoglobin is diamagnetic and does not produce the same dephasing, changes in oxygenation of the blood can be observed as signal changes in T_2*-weighted images. The functional dependence of T_2* on oxygenation in a tissue is expressed as

$$\frac{1}{T_2^*} \propto (1 - Y)b \tag{3}$$

where Y is the fraction of oxygenated blood and b the fractional blood volume. In hypoxic tumors where $0 < Y < 0.2$, the contrast produced by the method is primarily dependent on b. This method works best in poorly oxygenated tumors such as subcutaneous models, and in human xenografts with random orientation of sprouting capillaries, and it provides a fast and noninvasive measurement of tumor fractional blood volume because exogenous contrast is not required. However, the method cannot provide quantitative measurements of tumor vascular volume, vascular permeability, or blood flow. Nonetheless, this technique has been used to detect changes in tumor oxygenation and vascularization following induction of angiogenesis by external angiogenic agents (Abramovitch *et al.*, 1999), as well as to obtain maps of the "functional" vasculature in genetically modified HIF-1 (+/+ and −/−) animal models (Carmeliet *et al.*, 1998). BOLD contrast is not solely related to the oxygenation status of blood, but is also affected by factors such as oxygen saturation, the hematocrit, blood flow, blood volume, vessel orientation, and geometry (Pathak *et al.*, 2003), which should be considered when interpreting BOLD maps. In a recent study, Silva *et al.* (2000) demonstrated the feasibility of imaging blood flow in a rodent brain tumor model at a high magnetic field, using another endogenous contrast MR technique known as arterial spin labeling (ASL). In this approach, arterial blood water is used as the perfusion tracer, and it is magnetically tagged proximal to the tissue of interest, using spatially selective inversion pulses. The effect of arterial tagging on downstream images can be quantified in terms of tissue blood flow, since changes in signal intensity depend on the regional blood flow and degree of T_1 relaxation. Tissue blood flow (F) images can be computed from magnetically tagged and control images according to the expression:

$$F = \frac{\lambda}{T_1} \frac{S_{\text{control}} - S_{\text{label}}}{2\alpha S_{\text{control}}} \tag{4}$$

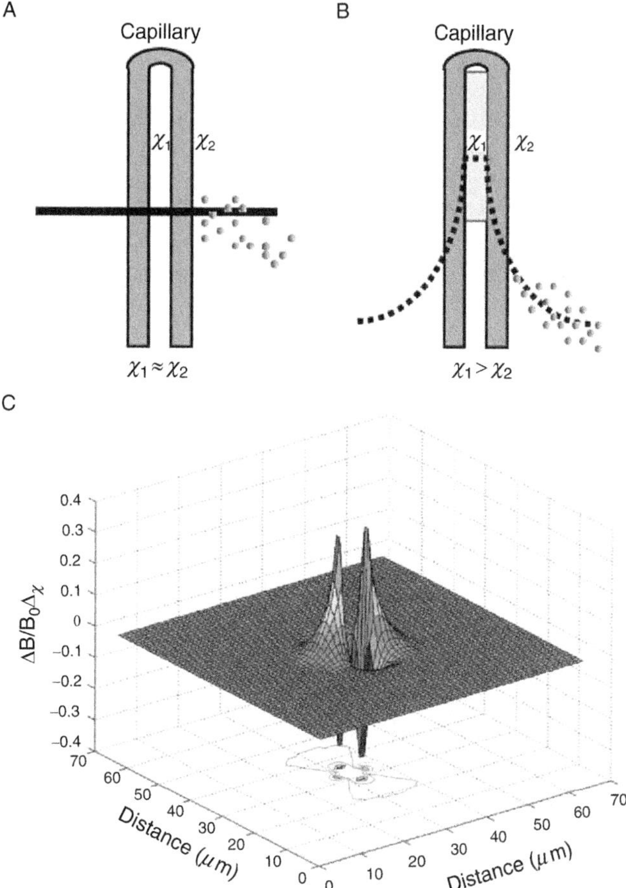

Fig. 1 Schematic illustrating the premise of the BOLD effect. (A) In the absence of a susceptibility difference between (oxygenated) blood (χ_1) and the surrounding tissue (χ_2), no microscopic field gradient is set up and diffusing water protons "see" the same local magnetic field. (B) When there is a susceptibility difference between (deoxygenated) blood (χ_1) and the surrounding tissue (χ_2), a microscopic field gradient (—) is set up and diffusing water protons "see" different local magnetic fields, leading to loss of phase coherence, reduction in T_2*, and MR signal attenuation. (C) Surface plot illustrating the three-dimensional aspects of mathematically simulated microscopic field gradients induced around a microvessel. (See plate no. 2 in the Color Plate Section.)

where $\lambda = 0.9$, is the tissue-blood partition coefficient for water, S_{control} is the control image signal intensity, S_{label} is the tagged image signal intensity, T_1 is the precalculated T_1-map, and $\alpha = 0.8$, is the tagging efficiency (Silva *et al.*, 1995). Although ASL exhibits sufficient sensitivity at high magnetic field for mapping heterogeneities in tumor blood flow, it may not do as well when the blood flow (F) is very low, since tagged arterial spins may not reach the tissue in time, relative to their T_1s (i.e., the spins will fully relax by the time they enter the imaging slice).

The advantages of vascular characterization using endogenous contrast are that the administration of an external agent is not required, making it entirely noninvasive, and repeated measurements are only limited by the constraints of anesthesia, providing dynamic data with high temporal resolution. Endogenous contrast methods, however, cannot quantify tumor vascular volume or vascular permeability, for which exogenous contrast MRI techniques are required.

C. Extrinsic or Exogenous Contrast

MR contrast agents (CA), unlike dyes or agents used with nuclear medicine or X-ray techniques, are not visualized directly in the MR image, but indirectly from the changes they induce in water proton relaxation behavior. The most commonly used MR CA are paramagnetic Gd chelates. These agents are tightly bound complexes of the rare earth element Gd and various chelating agents. The seven unpaired electrons of Gd produce a large magnetic moment that results in shortening of both T_1 and T_2 of tissue water. Because tissue T_2 values are intrinsically shorter than the corresponding T_1 values, the T_1 effect of the contrast agent predominates and tissues that take up the agent are brightened in T_1-weighted images.

Susceptibility effects of Gd-based CA resulting in the shortening of T_2 and T_2* relaxation times are also used to measure tumor vascular volume and flow. Tissues that take up the paramagnetic agent are darkened in T_2- and T_2*-weighted images. Vascular parameters can be calculated from tracer kinetics or mass balance principles, using the tissue concentration of Gd-based agents.

Several Gd complexes are either under development or in use and may be broadly classified as either low molecular weight ($\approx$0.57 kDa) agents, for example, the gadolinium diethylenetriamine pentaacetic acid (GdDTPA) compounds used clinically for contrast enhancement of various lesions, including malignant tumors, or macromolecular agents ($\approx$90 kDa) such as albumin-GdDTPA, which remain in the intravascular space for up to several hours.

Based on the physical properties of the CA used, brief descriptions of current MR methods used to characterize tumor vascularization are presented here.

1. Low Molecular Weight Contrast Agents

These are the only class of paramagnetic agents approved for routine clinical use, and there are several reports describing applications of these agents to image a variety of tumors, including breast (Furman-Haran *et al.*, 1996), brain (Aronen *et al.*, 1993), and uterine tumors (Hawighorst *et al.*, 1997). Most T_1 methods involve the analyses of relaxivity changes induced by the contrast agent to determine influx and outflux transfer constants, as well as the extracellular extravascular volume fraction based on one of several compartmental models (Tofts, 1997). Although these agents are not freely diffusible and remain in the extracellular compartment, three standard kinetic parameters that can be derived from dynamic contrast-enhanced T_1-weighted MRI of a diffusible tracer are (1) K^{trans} (min^{-1}), which is the volume transfer constant between the blood plasma and the extravascular extracellular space (EES); (2) k_{ep} (min^{-1}), which is the rate constant between the EES and blood plasmas; and (3) v_e (%), which is the volume of the EES per unit volume of tissue (i.e., the volume fraction of the EES) (Tofts *et al.*, 1999). These three parameters are related by

$$k_{ep} = \frac{K^{trans}}{v_e} \tag{5}$$

k_{ep} can be derived from the shape of the tracer concentration-time curve, but the determination of K^{trans} requires absolute values of the tracer concentration. K^{trans} has several different connotations depending on the balance between blood flow and capillary permeability in the tissue of interest. Ignoring the contribution of intravascular tracer to the total tissue concentration, as well as the possibility of further compartmentalization within the voxel, simple two-compartment (blood space and the EES) models can be broadly classified into four main types as previously described by Tofts *et al.*, 1999):

1. *Flow-limited (high permeability) or Kety Model*: This model assumes that arterial and venous blood pools have distinct CA concentrations, and because permeability (P) is high and the transendothelial flux flow (F) is limited (i.e., permeability surface area product $PS \gg F$), it assumes that the venous blood exits the tissue with a concentration that is in equilibrium with the tissue. For an extracellular tracer, the differential equation relating the tissue concentration (C_t) to the plasma concentration (C_p) is

$$\frac{dC_t}{dt} = F_\rho(1 - Hct)\left(C_p - \frac{C_t}{v_e}\right) \tag{6}$$

Here, $K^{trans} = F_\rho(1 - Hct)$, where F (ml g^{-1} min^{-1}) is the flow of whole blood per unit mass of tissue, ρ is the tissue density (g ml^{-1}), and Hct is the hematocrit, making (1 − Hct) the plasma fraction.

2. *PS-limited model*: If the flow (F) is high, the arterial and venous concentrations can be considered equal and the rate of tissue uptake is then limited by the permeability surface area product (PS) of the vessel wall and the concentration gradient between the plasma and EES compartments. Thus when $PS \ll F$, the differential equation relating the tissue concentration (C_t) to the plasma concentration (C_p) is given by

$$\frac{dC_t}{dt} = PS_\rho\left(C_p - \frac{C_t}{v_e}\right) \tag{7}$$

Here, $K^{trans} = PS_\rho(1 - Hct)$, P (cm min^{-1}) is the permeability of the vessel wall, S (cm^2 g^{-1}) is the surface area per unit mass of tissue, ρ is the tissue density (g ml^{-1}), and (1 − Hct) is the plasma fraction.

3. *Mixed flow and PS-limited model*: In the instance where tracer uptake might be limited by both flow and permeability, one can consider an additional parameter, the initial extraction ratio (E), given by

$$E = \frac{C_q - C_v}{C_a} \tag{8}$$

that describes the reduction in the blood concentration as it transits the tissue bed. The differential equation relating the tissue concentration (C_t) to the plasma concentration (C_p) is given by

$$\frac{dC_t}{dt} = EF_\rho(1 - Hct)\left(C_p - \frac{C_t}{v_e}\right) \tag{9}$$

In the flow-limited case ($PS \gg F$), ignoring tracer backflow if initial extraction is complete (i.e., $E = 1$), Eq. (9) reduces to the Kety Eq. (6). In the PS-limited case ($PS \ll F$), $E = PS/F(1 - Hct)$, and Eq. (9) reduces to Eq. (7).

4. *Clearance model*: Finally, if we define clearance (CL) as a constant relating the rate of tracer elimination from the tissue to the current tracer concentration, we can relate the tissue concentration (C_t) to the plasma concentration (C_p) as

$$\frac{dC_t}{dt} = \frac{\text{CL}}{V_t}\left(C_p - \frac{C_t}{v_e}\right) \tag{10}$$

where CL (ml min^{-1}) is the clearance and V_t (ml) is the total tissue volume. Because all of the previous differential equations have the same general form, we may formulate a generalized kinetic model as (Tofts *et al.*, 1999)

$$\frac{dC_t}{dt} = K^{\text{trans}}\left(C_p - \frac{C_t}{v_e}\right) = K^{\text{trans}}C_p - k_{ep}C_t \tag{11}$$

This model reduces to the previous forms under the appropriate boundary conditions. An excellent review of the previous models, terminology, and definitions can be found elsewhere (Tofts *et al.*, 1999). The arterial input function that these models require can be measured separately or defined in real time using voxels localized within large blood vessels. The analytic solution of the model can be derived by approximating the arterial input function [$C_a = (1 - Hct)C_p$] to a multiexponential decay as first described by Ohno *et al.* (1979). In all of the previous models, the concentration of GdDTPA is measured from changes in the T_1 relaxation rate, assuming that water is in fast exchange between the vascular and extracellular compartments. It has recently been demonstrated that the accuracy of the tissue vascular volume measurement critically depends on the validity of this assumption (Kim *et al.*, 2002).

As mentioned earlier, the low molecular weight Gd chelates employed in MRI produce both T_1 and T_2 relaxation effects. However, when high doses of these agents are employed, the induced bulk susceptibility differences between the intra- and extravascular spaces dominate the classical dipolar effects. There are two related mechanisms by which MRI contrast can be engendered from local magnetic field heterogeneities. (1) *Through diffusion*—as protons diffuse through the microscopic field inhomogeneities, they lose phase coherence due to their random Brownian motion through magnetic field gradients that are present. (2) *Through intervoxel dephasing*—even without the diffusive movement of water, there exists a heterogeneity of resonant frequencies due to the presence of microscopic field inhomogeneities within an imaging voxel, which in turn affects the MR signal intensity (in gradient-echo images) by causing intravoxel dephasing. The effect of magnetic field inhomogeneities on transverse relaxation can be characterized as (Fisel *et al.*, 1991; Kennan, 1994)

$$\frac{1}{T_2^*} = \frac{1}{T_2} + \frac{1}{T_2'} \tag{12}$$

The relaxation rate $1/T_2^*$ (R_2^*) is the rate of free induction decay or the rate at which the gradient-echo amplitude decays. The relaxation rate, $1/T_2'$ (R_2'), is the water resonance linewidth, which is a measure of the frequency distribution within a voxel. In the presence of a magnetic field perturber (such as a tumor vessel), the relative R_2 and R_2^* relaxation rates depend on the diffusion coefficient (D) of spins in the vicinity of the induced field inhomogeneities, the radius (R) of the field perturber (i.e., tumor vessel caliber), and the variation of the Larmor frequency at the surface of the perturber (Fisel *et al.*, 1991; Kennan, 1994; Weisskoff *et al.*, 1994; Yablonskiy, 1994). The two physical characteristics (R and D) can be collapsed into one term, and the proton correlation time τ_D can be described as

$$\tau_D = \frac{R^2}{D} \tag{13}$$

and the variation in the Larmor frequency ($d\omega$), at the surface of the perturber, is given by

$$d\omega = \gamma(\Delta_\chi)B_0 \tag{14}$$

where γ is the proton gyromagnetic ratio, Δ_χ is the susceptibility difference between the perturber and its background, and B_0 is the strength of the applied magnetic field. Depending on the relative magnitudes of these variables, the magnitude of the susceptibility-induced relaxation effects are commonly described by three regimes (Fisel *et al.*, 1991; Kennan, 1994; Villringer *et al.*, 1988; Weisskoff *et al.*, 1994; Yablonskiy, 1994).

1. *Fast exchange regime*: In this regime, the rate of diffusion ($1/\tau_D$) is substantially greater than the frequency variation ($d\omega$) (i.e., $\tau_D \, d\omega \ll 1$). The high diffusion rate causes all the spins to experience a similar range of field inhomogeneities within an echo time (TE), causing minimal loss of phase coherence, as well as similar loss of phase coherence between gradient-and spin-echo sequences. This is also known as the "motional-averaged" or "motional-narrowed" regime because the susceptibility-induced local magnetic field gradients are averaged out (Boxerman *et al.*, 1995; Fisel *et al.*, 1991; Kennan, 1994).

2. *Slow exchange regime*: In this regime, the rate of diffusion ($1/\tau_D$) is substantially smaller than the frequency variation ($d\omega$) (i.e., $\tau_D\ d\omega \gg 1$). Thus the phase that a proton accumulates as it passes one perturber is large (i.e., the effect is the same as it would be for the case of static field inhomogeneities). Due to the absence of motion averaging, the gradient-echo relaxation rate tends to be greater than the spin-echo relaxation rate. Also, there will be no signal attenuation on a T_2-weighted scan because the 180° pulse during the spin-echo sequence refocuses static magnetic field inhomogeneities, whereas intravoxel dephasing still occurs in a gradient-echo sequence (due to the absence of a similar refocusing RF pulse) (Fig. 2).

3. *Intermediate exchange regime*: In this regime, $\tau_D\ d\omega \sim 1$ (i.e., water diffusion is neither fast enough to be fully motionally narrowed nor slow enough to be approximated as linear gradients, making the description of the susceptibility-induced contrast more complex). In this regime, spin-echo relaxation is maximum and the gradient-echo relaxation is not very different from what it would be in the slow exchange regime (Fig. 2). In this regime, analytic solutions to estimate signal loss in the presence of diffusion become complicated due to the large spatial heterogeneity of the induced field gradients and numerical simulations are required (Boxerman *et al.*, 1995; Kennan, 1994; Weisskoff *et al.*, 1994).

From the preceding description, it is apparent that spin-echo (SE) and gradient-echo (GE) sequences have greatly differing sensitivities to the size and scale of the field inhomogeneities, resulting in a differential sensitivity to vessel caliber. The SE relaxation rate change (ΔR_2) increases, reaches a maximum for capillary-sized vessels (5–10 μm), and then decreases inversely with vessel radius. The GE relaxation rate change (ΔR_2*) increases and then plateaus to remain independent of

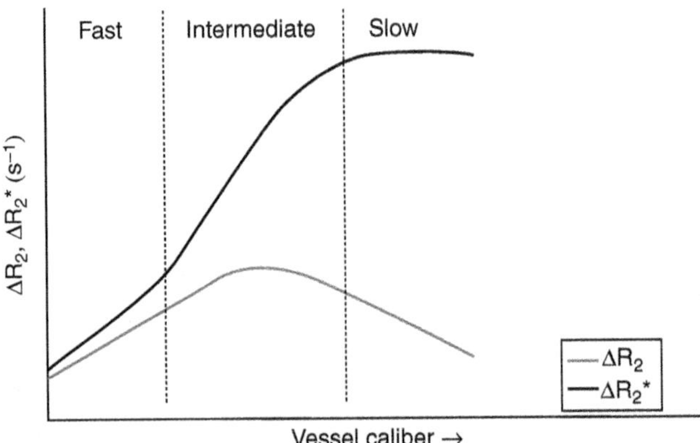

Fig. 2 Schematic to illustrate the three regimes of susceptibility-induced relaxation effects and the differential sensitivity of gradient-echo (ΔR_2*) and spin-echo (ΔR_2) relaxation rates to vessel caliber. This sensitivity to vessel size constitutes the basis for imaging macro- and microvascular blood volume, as well as imaging vessel size.

vessel radius beyond capillary-sized vessels (Fig. 2). A consequence of this result is that the SE relaxation rate changes are maximally sensitive to the microvascular blood volume, whereas the GE changes are more sensitive to the total blood volume. Based on this observation, SE sequences have been used in many tumor studies with the assumption that tumor angiogenesis is primarily characterized by an increase in the microvasculature (Aronen *et al.*, 1994). However, given the large (>20 μm) tortuous vessels usually found in tumors (Deane and Lantos, 1981; Pathak *et al.*, 2001), whether either SE or GE methods are most appropriate remains to be determined. Several investigators have acquired relative cerebral blood volume (rCBV) maps from first-pass dynamic susceptibility contrast (DSC) studies, with good spatio-temporal resolution (Maeda *et al.*, 1993; Rosen *et al.*, 1991). With this technique, preliminary results indicate that MRI-derived rCBV may better differentiate histologic tumor types than conventional MRI (Aronen *et al.*, 1994) and provide information to predict tumor grade (Maeda *et al.*, 1993). For example, to quantitatively measure relative cerebral blood volume (rCBV) or cerebral blood flow (CBF), regional changes in signal intensity versus time need to be converted into concentration versus time curves. As mentioned earlier, both empiric data and modeling indicate that for a given TE, the T_2* rate change $(\Delta R_2^* = \Delta(1/T_2^*) = (1/T^*_{2\text{postcontrast}} - 1/T^*_{2\text{precontrast}})$ is proportional to the brain tissue concentration

$$\Delta R_2^* = k[\text{conc.}] \tag{15}$$

where k is a tissue-specific MR pulse sequence and field strength-dependent calibration factor. Assuming monoexponential signal decay, signal intensity change following Gd injection is

$$S(t) = S_0 e^{-\text{TE}[\Delta R_2^*(t)]} \tag{16}$$

yielding:

$$\frac{-1}{\text{TE}} \ln\left[\frac{S(t)}{S_0}\right] = kC(t) \tag{17}$$

where S_0 is the baseline signal intensity before contrast administration, $S(t)$ is the tissue signal with contrast, TE is the echo time, and $C(t)$ is the concentration-time curve. The area under the concentration-time curve is proportional to the rCBV.

$$\frac{-1}{\text{TE}} \int_0^\infty \ln\frac{S(t)}{S_0} dt\, s \propto \text{rCBV} \tag{18}$$

These steps are summarized in Fig. 3. These curves often include contributions due to recirculation that must be eliminated before tracer-kinetic principles may be used to extract volume and flow information. This is usually accomplished by exponential extrapolation or fitting to a gamma-variate function with recirculation cut-off (Thompson *et al.*, 1964). For an instantaneous bolus injection, the central volume principle states that CBF = CBV/MTT, where MTT is the mean transit

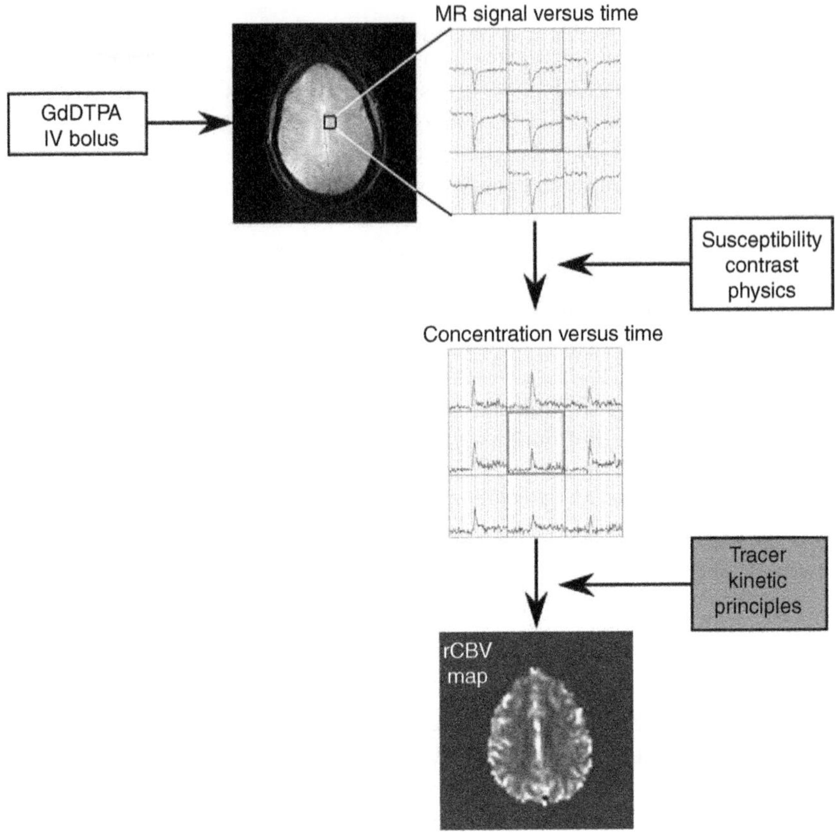

Fig. 3 Schematic of the steps involved in the generation of dynamic rCBV maps.

time of contrast agent through the vascular network (Zierler, 1962). However, most injections are of finite duration, and the observed concentration-time curve is the convolution of the ideal tissue-transit curve with the arterial input function. Thus measurement of the blood flow requires knowledge of the arterial input curve to deconvolve the observed concentration-time curve (Axel, 1980).

A potential complication with using first-pass rCBV techniques with low molecular weight Gd contrast agents is that with elevated permeability, as is often observed in tumor vasculature, or with significant blood-brain barrier (BBB) disruption, as is often the case with brain tumors, contrast agent leaks out of the vasculature into the brain or tumor tissue, resulting in enhanced T_1 relaxation effects. Signal increases due to T_1 effects may then mask signal decreases due to T_2 or T_2* effects, leading to an underestimation of rCBV. To address this issue, a method of analysis has been devised that corrects for these leakage effects when the leakage is not extreme (Donahue *et al.*, 2000). Donahue *et al.* (2000) recently showed that although GErCBV (total tumor blood volume) correlated strongly with tumor grade, when the GErCBV data were not corrected for leakage effects, the correlation with tumor grade was no longer significant. Another obstacle to the application of the central volume principle for the calculation of blood flow is the direct measurement of the mean transit time. Weisskoff (1993) has demonstrated that MTT, which relates tissue blood volume to blood flow from the central volume principle, is not the first moment of the concentration-time curve for MR of intravascular tracers, and although first-moment methods cannot be used by themselves to determine absolute flow, they do provide a useful relative measure of flow.

More recently, the differential sensitivities of GE and SE methods to vessel radius have been further exploited to provide a measure of the averaged vessel diameter by measuring the ratio of GE and SE relaxation rates ($\Delta R_2^*/\Delta R_2$). From Fig. 3 it can be seen that as the perturber (i.e., vessel) size increases, so does the ratio $\Delta R_2^*/\Delta R_2$. Dennie *et al.* (1998) have shown that using an intravascular superparamagnetic iron oxide nanoparticle (MION) contrast agent, this ratio compared favorably to a predicted ratio using histologically determined vessel sizes and the theoretical Monte Carlo modeling results. More recently, Donahue *et al.* (2000) have demonstrated that clinically, the ratio $\Delta R_2^*/\Delta R_2$ correlated strongly with tumor grade and was a promising marker for the evaluation of tumor angiogenesis in patients.

Finally, all dynamic susceptibility-based contrast measurements are made assuming that the calibration factor "k" (see Eq. (13)) is the same for all tissue types and independent of tissue condition. However, a recent study has shown that k is the same for brain gray and white matter but *not* the same for normal brain and tumor tissue (Pathak *et al.*, 2003). This difference may be attributed to the grossly different vascular morphology of tumors, due to tumor angiogenesis, compared with normal brain and/or possibly differing blood rheological factors such as hematocrit. Consequently, the sensitivity to blood volume differences between tumor and normal brain tissue may be lessened when using gradient-echo susceptibility contrast agent methods.

2. High Molecular Weight Contrast Agents

Quantitative determination of parameters of tumor vasculature with low molecular weight contrast agents is complicated by fast extravasation of the contrast agent from leaky tumor vessels. The availability of high molecular weight contrast agents such as albumin-GdDTPA (alb-GdDTPA) complexes or synthetic compounds such as polylysine-GdDTPA and Gadomer-17 provide an opportunity for quantitative determination of tumor vascular volume and vascular permeability surface area product (PS) for molecules of comparable sizes (Ogan *et al.*, 1987). The relatively slow leakage of these agents from the vasculature results in a long half-life time and complete equilibration of plasma concentrations within the tumor, independently of blood flow. Assuming fast exchange of water between all the compartments in the tumor (plasma, interstitium, cells), the concentration of the contrast agent within any given voxel is proportional to changes in relaxation rate ($1/T_1$) before and after administration of the contrast. Relaxation rates can be measured either directly using fast single-shot quantitative T_1 methods (Schwarzbauer *et al.*, 1993) or from T_1-weighted steady-state experiments (Brasch *et al.*, 1997), which provide better temporal resolution but are susceptible to experimental artifacts caused by variations in T_2 and T_2* relaxation times. Pixel-wise maps can be generated from the acquired data and processed with the appropriate model to obtain spatial maps of tumor vascular volume and vascular permeability surface area product.

A simple linear compartment model, describing uptake of the contrast agent from plasma, postulates a negligible reflux of the contrast agent from the interstitium back to the blood compartment. Blood concentrations of the contrast agent can be approximated to be constant for the duration of the MR experiment, and under these conditions, contrast uptake is a linear function of time (Fig. 4) (Patlak *et al.*, 1983; Roberts *et al.*, 2000). On a plot of contrast agent concentration versus time, the slope of the line provides the parameter PS, and the intercept of the line with the vertical axis at time zero provides the vascular volume (Fig. 4). For absolute values of these parameters, the change in relaxation rate of the blood must be quantified. Changes in blood T_1 can be obtained separately from blood samples taken before injection of the contrast agent and at the end of the experiment, or may be obtained noninvasively (Pathak *et al.*, 2004).

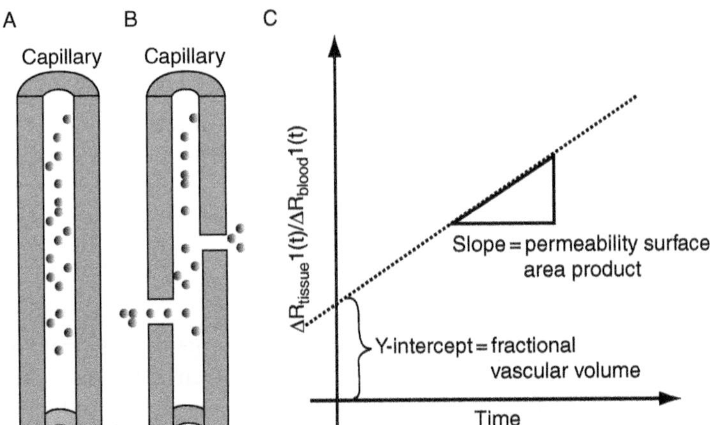

Fig. 4 Schematic illustrating (A) a blood vessel in which the macromolecular contrast agent is confined to the intravascular space. (B) In the case of a tumor vessel, due to elevated permeability, the contrast agent extravasates into the adjoining interstitial space. (C) Initially, the bulk of the T_1 relaxation effect is proportional to the intravascular space, since the contrast agent is confined to this space. The ratio of the change in relaxation rate of the tissue to that in the blood yields the fractional blood volume in that voxel. Over time, as the contrast agent extravasates into the adjoining tissue, the rate of change of the relaxation rate becomes proportional to the permeability surface area product for that vessel.

For macromolecular agents such as alb-GdDTPA (MW ≈ 90 kDa), blood concentrations equilibrate within 2–3 min and do not change for at least 40 min after an intravenous bolus injection. Tissue concentrations of the agent for a time period starting 5 min and up to 40 min after the bolus injection increase linearly with time. Therefore, the simple linear model is preferable for analysis of intrinsically noisy relaxation data because it is much more stable in comparison with nonlinear fitting algorithms required for the two compartment models discussed earlier. An example of vascular volume and permeability maps derived with this approach is shown in Fig. 5 (Bhujwalla *et al.*, 2003). This linear-model approach

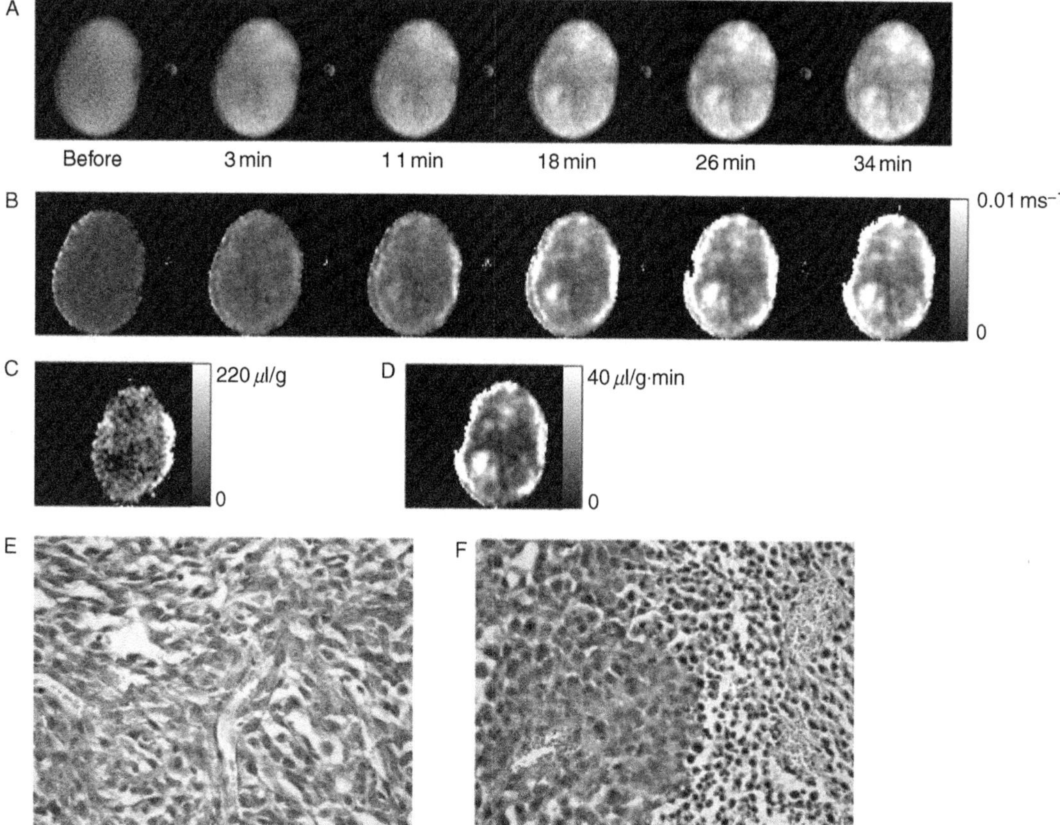

Fig. 5 (A) Raw 1 s saturation recovery images obtained from a single slice from a MatLyLu tumor, at different time points. (B) Corresponding relaxivity maps derived for this slice (using 100 ms, 500 ms, 1 s, and 7 s saturation recovery intervals) at different time points. Maps of (C) vascular volume and (D) permeability surface area product derived from the relaxivity maps for this slice. High-magnification photomicrographs from (E) viable, high-vascular volume and low-permeability regions, and (F) dying, low-vascular volume and high-permeability regions, obtained from a 5 μm-thick hematoxylin and eosin-stained section obtained from the same slice. From Bhujwalla *et al.* (2003). (See plate no. 3 in the Color Plate Section.)

was employed to detect vascular differences for metastatic versus nonmetastatic breast and prostrate cancer xenografts (Bhujwalla *et al.*, 2000). These studies not only showed that regions of high vascular volume were significantly less leaky compared with regions of low vascular volume, but that although invasion was necessary, without adequate vascularization it was not sufficient for metastasis to occur.

The accuracy of the measurement of tissue vascular volume using this approach does, however, depend on the water exchange rate between the vascular and extracellular compartments. Using a simplified model of fast exchange, where there may be intermediate to slow exchange, can lead to significant underestimation of vascular volume. Experimental approaches to minimize these errors are based on observations that the initial slope of the relaxation curve is independent of the exchange rate (Donahue *et al.*, 1996).

Large molecular weight contrast agents may also potentially be used to measure tumor blood flow by detecting the first pass of the agent through tumor vasculature, similar to the method described by Ostergaard *et al.* (1996), although this approach may not be feasible when the heartbeat is very rapid, as for rodents.

IV. Cellular and Molecular Imaging

A. Magnetic Resonance Detection of Cellular Targets

The development of targeted MR contrast agents has significantly increased the versatility of MR methods to detect receptor expression and specific cellular targets in cancer and other diseases. In the past, the intrinsically low SNR of MRI and MRS has limited the applications of MR-based methods for imaging targets at low concentrations. Here, we review strategies to improve the sensitivity of MR detection, the design and application of targeted relaxation contrast agents, and the use of signal amplification using enzymatic reactions and water exchange.

1. Sensitivity and Typical Target Concentration

The sensitivity of MR detection is a complex parameter that depends on various factors, including the resonant nucleus, the strength of the main magnetic field B_0, intrinsic relaxation times, and magnetic field inhomogeneities within the sample that are often determined by micro- and macroarchitecture of the tissue being studied. *In vivo* proton (^{1}H) MRS performed using magnetic field strengths with B_0 in the range of 4.7–11 T can detect protons in the millimolar (mM) range. This level of sensitivity can only be obtained with optimized detection schemes, radiofrequency (RF) coils, and B_0 inhomogeneity corrections (shimming) for a spatial resolution of about 10^{-2} cm^3. Proton MRS is often complicated by the background signals of water and lipids that have to be suppressed using editing sequences (Tkac *et al.*, 1999). In certain cases, MRS of different nuclei such as ^{19}F or ^{31}P is more appropriate for target-specific MRS.

As mentioned earlier, ^{1}H MRI detects signals from bulk water in the sample (proton concentration of about 90 M) and can provide spatial resolutions of about 10^{-5} cm^3. The specificity of MRI can be significantly increased by the use of MR contrast agents (CA). A single molecule of CA affects a large number of surrounding water molecules and induces substantial changes in the detected water signal. Shortening of the relaxation time by a contrast (or relaxation) agent can be detected with an appropriately weighted MRI method. CA are generally classified as "T_1 agents" or "T_2 agents." Reduction in T_1 results in increased intensities in T_1-weighted MR images (so-called positive contrast), whereas T_2 shortening produces a negative contrast or reduced brightness in T_2-weighted MR images. CA are characterized by T_1 or T_2 relaxivity, which is the reciprocal of the change in relaxation time (T_1 or T_2) per unit of concentration. Most T_1 CA are based on different chelate complexes of Gd, and T_2 CA usually incorporate a solid iron oxide core embedded in various polymer coatings. Therefore, it is convenient to express the relaxivity of the CA per unit concentration of the metal as (mM s)$^{-1}$. T_1 and T_2 relaxivities of CA are complex functions of the magnetic field B_0, temperature, and correlation times (rotational, translational, and exchange) that in turn depend on the molecular size and structure of the CA complexes. Typical T_1 relaxivity values of Gd-based CA are in the range of 5–20 mM^{-1} s^{-1} (up to 80 mM^{-1} s^{-1}) for MS-325 bound to albumin) (Caravan *et al.*, 2002). Iron oxide-based superparamagnetic CA have high T_2 relaxivities reaching 200 mM^{-1} s^{-1} (Strable *et al.*, 2001). To generate detectable contrast in MR images, the average concentration of [Gd] and [Fe] should be above 10 μM (10% shortening of the relaxation times for intrinsic T_1 of 1 s and T_2 of 100 ms, respectively).

The minimum detectable concentration of the target will depend upon the efficiency of labeling of the CA, or MR probes. To estimate the upper limit of detection, it is important to consider typical *in vivo* concentrations of molecular targets that are most abundant and are of biological and medical significance. Cell surface receptors represent such a class of molecular targets, and for highly expressed receptors (10^6 per cell), the concentration of binding sites per unit volume is about 10^{15} ml^{-1} or $\sim$1 μM, providing complete accessibility of the target to the MR probes. To enable MR detection, these targets have to be labeled with a significant number ($\gg$10) of Gd or Fe atoms; for MRS, each target should be associated with more than 10^3 of the specific chemical probes.

Different strategies are currently available to perform target-specific or molecular MRI. One strategy is to use macromolecular carriers labeled with a large number of Gd^{3+} ions, or iron oxide nanoparticles that incorporate thousands of Fe^{3+} ions, and to direct them to receptors using highly specific high-affinity probes such as monoclonal antibodies (mAb). An alternative approach is to use enzymatic signal amplification, where the activity of an endogenous or exogenous enzyme significantly amplifies the number of MR reporter molecules. Yet another approach uses the exchange between bulk water and exchangeable groups on the surface of a reporter protein or a polymer probe. This chemical exchange can be detected as a decreased intensity of the water resonance, when the specific group is irradiated with an RF field. As in the case of relaxation agents, a significant increase in sensitivity is possible because one exchangeable group affects the signal of the abundant water molecules. The following section briefly describes some of these strategies and their application to the study of cells and preclinical tumor models.

2. T_1 Contrast Agents

As discussed earlier, the unpaired electrons of paramagnetic metal ions such as Gd^{3+}(III), Mn^{2+}(II), or Fe^{3+}(III) generate strong magnetic moments that induce efficient relaxation of water molecules. The chelates of these metals can be used as efficient T_1 CA. Because of the optimum electron relaxation time and high stability of the complex, GdDTPA chelates are used most frequently. Early attempts to conjugate GdDTPA to a specific mAb for target-specific MRI were reported as early as by Unger *et al.* (1985) and subsequently by Matsumura *et al.* (1994) and Shahbazi-Gahrouei *et al.* (2001). Because only a limited number of Gd chelates can be conjugated to a single mAb without significantly reducing its binding affinity (Gohr-Rosenthal *et al.*, 1993), in these studies the contrast generated was insufficient for MR detection (Anderson-Berg *et al.*, 1986).

To increase the relaxivity per target site, multiple Gd chelates can be attached to a polymer carrier molecule such as a protein. In comparison with GdDTPA, these high molecular weight complexes have a longer circulation time and increased relaxivity. Several macromolecular CA platforms based on Gd chelates have been designed and used, including albumin-GdDTPA conjugates (Bhujwalla *et al.*, 2000; Schmiedl *et al.*, 1987), poly-L-lysine (Bogdanov *et al.*, 1993; Gohr-Rosenthal *et al.*, 1993), avidin (Artemov *et al.*, 2003a), and poly-amidoamine (PAMAM) dendrimers of different generations (Bryant *et al.*, 1999; Kobayashi *et al.*, 2001). Large molecular size CA include cross-linked liposomes and nanoparticle emulsions labeled with a large number (~50,000) of Gd^{3+} ions (Anderson *et al.*, 2000; Sipkins *et al.*, 1998; Winter *et al.*, 2003). The typical molecular size of these CA varies from about 6–8 nm for protein-based agents to ~200 nm for polymerized liposomes and nanoparticle emulsions. Interestingly, the relaxivity of a complex is a linear function of the number of Gd^{3+} ions attached to the polymer carrier (Schmiedl *et al.*, 1987) and increases with the size of the complex. It is not clear if relaxivity is saturated when standard chelate chemistry is used for sequestering Gd^{3+} ions.

Large paramagnetic Gd complexes, such as paramagnetic polymerized liposomes (Sipkins *et al.*, 1998) and Gd-perfluorocarbon nanoparticles (Anderson *et al.*, 2000; Winter *et al.*, 2003), were successfully used to image $\alpha_v\beta_3$ integrin receptors expressed on angiogenic endothelium. These nanoparticles were targeted to the receptor by mAb either covalently bound or attached via biotin-avidin linkers. Although these CA were large, the molecular target was intravascular and therefore easily accessible.

Smaller CA are necessary to image molecular targets, which require extravasation of the CA in solid tumors because of the reduced permeability and interstitial diffusion of large CA. MRI of mucin-like protein expressed in many types of gastrointestinal carcinomas was reported, using anti-mucin mAb covalently conjugated to poly-L-lysine-GdDTPA with a labeling ratio of 65 Gd^{3+} ions per molecule (Gohr-Rosenthal *et al.*, 1993). The molecular weight of the conjugate was about 200 kDa. Folate-conjugated GdDTPA magnetic dendrimers (fourth generation, up to 64 complexing sites for Gd^{3+}) were used for targeted MRI of human folate receptors in ovarian tumor xenografts (Konda *et al.*, 2000).

Recently, a two-step labeling strategy was used for *in vivo* MRI of the HER-2/*neu* receptor. The two-step labeling allows separation of the targeted CA complex into two components with relatively low molecular weight (160 kDa for mAb, and 70 kDa for avidin), which improves the delivery of the CA. Receptors were prelabeled with biotinylated anti-HER-2/*neu* mAb, and probed with an GdDTPA-avidin conjugate 12 h later. A maximum labeling efficiency of about 50 Gd per receptor was estimated, from an average of 12.5 Gd^{3+} per avidin and 4 biotins per mAb. Positive contrast in HER-2/*neu* overexpressing tumor xenografts was detected in T_1-weighted MR images using this approach (Artemov *et al.*, 2003a).

A novel concept in MR molecular imaging is enzyme-specific amplification of the T_1 relaxivity of the targeted CA. One such approach relies on the β-galactosidase-mediated catalytic removal of the protecting sugar cap from a caged Gd contrast agent (Louie *et al.*, 2000). This change in chemical structure of the compound enables a large number of water molecules to be directly coordinated by the metal, dramatically reducing water T_1 relaxation time due to inner sphere effects (Koenig and Brown, 1984).

Another approach is the enzymatic polymerization of small molecular weight Gd chelates, which results in a significant increase in T_1 relaxivity of the polymer product. Magnetic oligomers produced by polymerization of hydroxyphenol-modified GdDOTA monomers have been proposed as sensitive probes for MRI of nanomolar concentrations of oxidoreductases (peroxidase) (Bogdanov *et al.*, 2002). Low-relaxivity (3.75 $mM^{-1}\ s^{-1}$) monomeric substrates (AH) are oxidized by the peroxidase (E), thereby reducing peroxide (H_2O_2) and producing activated moeties (A^*) that self-polymerize to form high-relaxivity (11.5 $mM^{-1}\ s^{-1}$) magnetic oligomers (A_n):

$$2\mathrm{AH} + [\mathrm{E}\cdot\mathrm{H_2O_2}] \rightarrow 2\mathrm{A}^* + 2\mathrm{H_2O} + \mathrm{E} \quad n\mathrm{A}^* \rightarrow \mathrm{A}_n \tag{19}$$

This method was used for MRI of E-selectin expressed on the surface of endothelial cells using sandwich constructs of anti-E-selectin $F(ab')_2$ conjugated to peroxidase through digoxigenin (DIG)-anti-DIG Ab linkers (Bogdanov *et al.*, 2002).

3. T_2 Contrast Agents

The large combined magnetic moment (so-called Curie spin) of superparamagnetic iron oxide nanoparticles makes them effective T_2 contrast agents (Gillis *et al.*, 1999). For biocompatibility and chemical stabilization, the monocrystalline (MION) and polycrystalline (SPIO) iron oxide cores, which have diameters of ~5 and ~30 nm, respectively, are coated with a protective layer composed of biopolymers such as dextran or other polysaccharide, or a unilamellar vesicle (e.g., magnetoliposomes) (Bulte *et al.*, 1999a), resulting in diameters of 17–50 nm. Magnetodendrimers consist of a superparamagnetic iron oxide core encapsulated within a dendrimer superstructure (Bulte *et al.*, 2001; Strable *et al.*, 2001). These compounds typically demonstrate high T_2 relaxivity, often up to and above 200 $mM^{-1}\ s^{-1}$ at $B_0 = 1.5$ T. In comparison, the corresponding T_1 relaxivity of these compounds is typically below 10 $mM^{-1}\ s^{-1}$. The superparamagnetism of the iron oxide core depends upon the alignment of individual electron spins. The T_2 relaxivity of the ultra-small monocrystalline superparamagnetic iron oxide nanoparticles (MION-46L), with a magnetic core diameter of 4.6 nm, is close to 20 $mM^{-1}\ s^{-1}$ at 1.5 T magnetic field and 25 °C (Bulte *et al.*, 1999b). For larger SPIO particles, with a core diameter of 16 nm, the T_2 relaxivity at 1.5 T is 240 $mM^{-1}\ s^{-1}$. These nanoparticles produce even larger T_2* effects by inducing local disturbances in the magnetic field. These "long range" effects cause dephasing of signal from areas much larger than the size of the nanoparticle (Bulte *et al.*, 1992; Dodd *et al.*, 1999).

The high T_2 relaxation rate of these compounds makes them an attractive choice for MRI of cellular targets. Cells nonspecifically labeled with iron oxide nanoparticles by phagocytosis and pinocytosis can be detected by MRI at iron concentrations as low as 1.7×10^{-15} g per cell or 8.5×10^4 particles per cell (Weissleder *et al.*, 1997). MRI of a single T-cell, loaded with SPIO, was demonstrated by Dodd *et al.* (1999) Stem cells loaded with magnetodendrimers (9–14 pg iron per cell) were successfully imaged both *in vitro* and *in vivo* after transplantation (Bulte *et al.*, 2001). Iron oxide-based CA can be used for MRI of cellular targets with an expression level of about 10^5 $cell^{-1}$.

As with Gd-based CA, iron oxide CA can be targeted to molecular epitopes on the cell surface by chemical conjugation with mAb (or mAb fragments). Cultured lymphocytes were imaged with a mAb directed against the lymphocyte common antigen conjugated to SPIO particles (Bulte *et al.*, 1992). The conjugation was achieved using a streptavidin linker connecting the biotinylated mAb and the biotinylated dextran-coated SPIO nanoparticles. E-selectin expressing human endothelial cells were imaged using the $F(ab)_2$ fragment of anti-human E-selectin mAb conjugated to CLIO (cross-linked iron oxide) nanoparticles (Kang *et al.*, 2002). Only cells incubated with IL-1β cytokine demonstrated a negative contrast in T_2-weighted MR images. HER-2/*neu* expressing malignant breast cancer cells were detected using two-step labeling with biotinylated Herceptin mAb and streptavidin-SPIO nanoparticles (Artemov *et al.*, 2003b). An example of two-step labeling of HER-2/*neu* cell surface receptors with streptavidin-SPIO particles and biotinylated anti-HER-2/*neu* mAb (Herceptin) is shown in Fig. 6. Cell lines expressing high levels of the receptor (AU-565) generate strong negative T_2 contrast as shown in Fig. 6B. Data from these studies demonstrated a linear dependence between the concentration of the target sites and T_2 relaxivity generated by SPIO CA (Artemov *et al.*, 2003b).

The *in vivo* applications of iron oxide-targeted CA include imaging of inflammation sites with human polyclonal immunoglobulin G (IgG) attached to MION particles (Weissleder *et al.*, 1991), and imaging of apoptosis in solid tumor models exposed to a chemotherapeutic agent (Zhao *et al.*, 2001). In the latter study, SPIO particles were conjugated to the C2 domain of the protein synaptotagmin, which selectively binds to phosphatidylserine residues that relocate onto the outer leaflet of the plasma membrane in apoptotic cells (Zhao *et al.*, 2001).

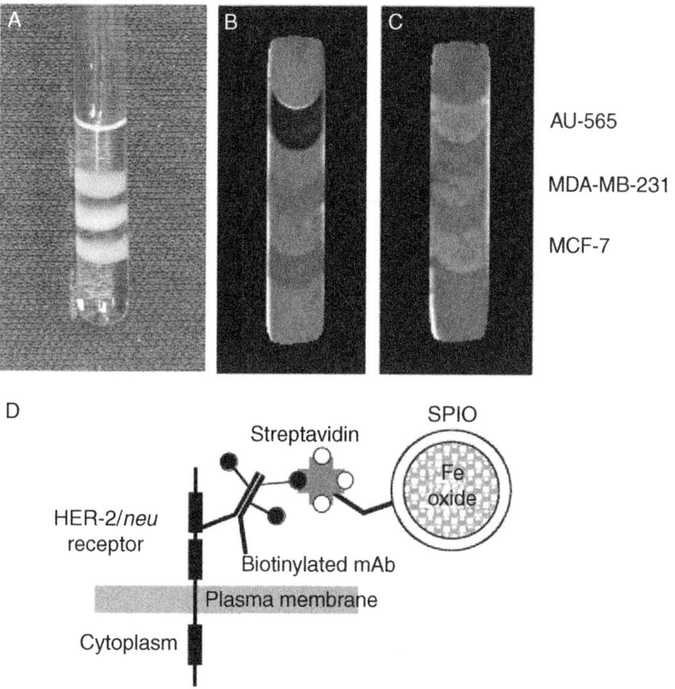

Fig. 6 MR images of AU-565, MDA-MB-231, and MCF-7 breast cancer cells embedded in agarose gel in a 5-mm NMR tube. (A) Layout of the cell sample. Cells were pretargeted with biotinylated Herceptin and a nonspecific biotinylated mAb (negative control), and probed with streptavidin SPIO microbeads as shown in (D). T_2 maps of the cell samples were reconstructed from eight T_2-weighted images acquired with a relaxation delay of 8 s and TE in the range 20–250 ms. A T_2 map of a cell sample probed with Herceptin is shown in (B), and the control cell sample treated with a nonspecific biotinylated mAb is shown in (C). Expression level of the HER-2/*neu* receptor was 2.7×10^6 for AU-565, 8.9×10^4 for MCF-7, and 4×10^4 for MDA-MB-231 cells, respectively. (See plate no. 4 in the Color Plate Section.)

Weissleder *et al.* (2000) have demonstrated a novel strategy for MR signal enhancement by the active transport of CA into cells using a transporter system. 9L glioma cells were engineered to express the modified transferrin receptor, ETR, with a knocked-down negative feedback regulation domain. These cells were loaded with MION nanoparticles conjugated to human holotransferrin (TF), which is a substrate for ETR, and imaged both *in situ* and *in vivo* using T_2*-weighted MRI. Within 1 h, up to 8×10^6 of the TF-targeted CA nanoparticles were internalized by the cells.

A significant advantage of the iron oxide nanoparticles compared with Gd-based CA is their high T_2/T_2* relaxivity, which produces strong negative MR contrast at nanomolar concentrations of the CA. However, the large molecular size (~20–30 nm) of the superparamagnetic iron oxide-based CA can be a potential problem for *in vivo* applications, since delivery may be limited. The successful applications of these CA for target-specific MRI were probably a result of highly permeable vasculature at the sites of inflammation or in treated apoptotic tumors, which permitted efficient delivery of these CA into the interstitium. The long circulation time of these agents and an efficient amplification of the label by cell internalization are other possible reasons for contrast uptake within the tumor.

4. MR Spectroscopy and Water Exchange

Of all the stable magnetic nuclei, ^{1}H MRS provides the highest sensitivity, although strong water and lipid signals pose a problem for *in vivo* detection. Another magnetic isotope that can be detected by MRS with about 80% of proton receptivity is ^{19}F. The complete absence of the natural fluorine background and a large range of chemical shifts are important advantages of the use of this isotope as a reporter for *in vivo* MR studies.

An example of the use of ^{19}F to detect a reporter enzyme is the conversion of 5-fluorocytosine (5-FC) to 5-fluorouracil (5-FU) by the bacterial or yeast enzyme, cytosine deaminase (CD). CD is not present in mammalian cells, and therefore the formation of 5-FU from 5-FC occurs only in regions where CD is expressed. The conversion of 5-FC to 5-FU was detected, *in vivo*, in solid tumors derived from cancer cells transfected with yeast CD (Stegman *et al.*, 1999). Because the chemical shift difference between 5-FC and 5-FU is approximately 1.2 ppm, and approximately 3.5 ppm between 5-FC and the fluorinated nucleotide-nucleoside products of 5-FU, all three compounds are easily resolved *in vivo*. In a similar approach, CD was covalently conjugated to mAb specific for the L6 antigen, which is expressed on the surface of the human lung adenocarcinoma cell line, H2981 (Aboagye *et al.*, 1998). *In vivo* ^{19}F MRSI of mice bearing H2981 tumors demonstrated localization of 5-FU signals within the tumor region. Although a relatively high magnetic field strength of 4.7 T was used in these studies, the available sensitivity only allowed spectroscopic images of 5-FU and 5-FC with an in-plane resolution of 6.25×6.25 mm, with a 20-mm-thick slice to be acquired within 35 min. The sensitivity and resolution of the method is also reduced by the rapid diffusion, clearance, and metabolic degradation of the compounds.

Another example of using MRS to detect an enzyme reporter is the detection of phosphocreatine produced from creatine *in vivo* in liver transfected with the murine creatine kinase enzyme (CK-B) (Auricchio *et al.*, 2001). The low sensitivity of ^{31}P MRS (~7% of photon) used in this study limits the application of this method for *in vivo* studies.

Chemical-exchange saturation transfer (CEST) permits MR detection of exchangeable protons with high sensitivity by detecting changes in the bulk water signal. Technically, changes in the water intensity are measured with and without RF irradiation at the chemical shift of the exchangeable group (Goffeney *et al.*, 2001; Guivel-Scharen *et al.*, 1998). Hydroxyl, amine, and amide protons have been used for CEST detection (Mori *et al.*, 1997). Magnetization transfer from the exchangeable proton to numerous water protons provides a sensitivity enhancement factor of over 5000 for specially optimized probes such as polyuridilic acid (imino protons) (Snoussi *et al.*, 2003). The proton transfer enhancement factor (PTE) is defined as

$$\mathrm{PTE} = \frac{2[\mathrm{H_2O}]}{[\mathrm{probe}]}\left(1 - \frac{S_{\mathrm{sat}}}{S_0}\right) \tag{20}$$

where S_{sat} and S_0 are the water signal intensities with and without RF irradiation. The number of exchangeable protons and the exchange rate constant are the key parameters that define the efficiency of the CEST probe. The proton exchange rate should be low enough to enable spectral separation of the MR signal of the exchangeable group and, on the other hand, should be sufficiently fast to allow multiple water molecules to exchange protons with the exchangeable group (Goffeney *et al.*, 2001). Increasing the chemical shift difference between the exchangeable group and water enables use of the higher exchange rates with correspondingly higher PTE. This can be achieved with paramagnetic shift reagents that introduce a large shift to the resonance frequency of the neighboring spins (Zhang *et al.*, 2001). CEST agents provide sensitivity similar or higher than paramagnetic CA (for the same number of exchangeable groups and Gd chelates). The sensitivity gain provided by CEST suggests that dedicated CEST contrast agents may be used as probes for targeted MRI.

Although the MRI probes and methods discussed here can be successfully used to image molecular targets in isolated cells, the translation of these techniques *in vivo* is not straightforward. The imaging properties of different targeted MR agents and potential areas of their application for *in vivo* MRI/MRS are summarized in Table I. The translation of these techniques into the clinic will require a substantial improvement in both CA chemistry and MRI technology.

Here, we discuss strategies based on contrast agent chemistry to achieve gain in signal. In the following paragraphs, we outline technical approaches to improve the sensitivity of MR methods.

Table I

Summary of Targeted CA Currently Available, their Applications and Potential Problems

Imaging agent	Relative sensitivity of MR detection	Potential molecular targets	MRI/MRS experimental methods	Potential problems
Iron oxide-based agents (MION, SPIO, CLIO)	High, $\sim 10^5$ target sites per cell	Cell surface receptors *in situ*, cell transporters	T_2- and T_2*-weighted and T_2 quantitative MRI	Large size of nanoparticles ($\sim$30 nm) restricts *in vivo* delivery
Gd-loaded liposomes and nanoparticle emulsions	High, $\sim 10^4$ targets per cell	Cellular markers on the endothelium in blood vessel lumen.	T_1-weighted and T_1 quantitative MRI	Very large molecular size, slow extravasation
Gd-labeled macromolecule complexes (proteins, dendrimers)	Moderately high, $\sim 10^6$ receptors per cell	Cell targets in solid tumors with leaky vasculature	T_1-weighted and T_1 quantitative MRI	Pharmacokinetics and stability of chelate complexes *in vivo*
MRS probes (5-FC)	Low, millimolar concentrations of the probe	Reporter enzymes, expressed in the cell or delivered exogenously	^1H, ^{19}F, ^{31}P MRS	Low sensitivity results in low spatial resolution
Novel probes (polymerized, CEST)	Potentially can be very high	Reporter enzymes and cell surface markers	T_1-weighted MRI, proton exchange MRI	No data

B. Technical Strategies for MR Microscopy

Traditionally, cell microscopy is performed using optical techniques. The promise of noninvasively detecting molecular events with high spatial localization and sufficient sensitivity drives the effort in MR microscopy. High-resolution MR spectroscopy has been utilized in achieving spectra of volume-limited samples (Olson *et al.*, 1995; Peck *et al.*, 1995; Subramanian *et al.*, 1998) and in performing localized spectroscopy on picoliter-scale samples (Minard and Wind, 2002; Wind *et al.*, 2000). High-resolution imaging has been implemented in the microscopic investigation of cell and tissue structures (Cho *et al.*, 1990; Glover *et al.*, 1994), of large single cells (Aguayo *et al.*, 1986), and to detect single mammalian cells (Weissleder *et al.*, 1997). Recent work in single cell tracking (Hinds *et al.*, 2003) and the study of compartmental diffusion of isolated single cells (Grant *et al.*, 2001) provides an avenue to noninvasively study disease progression and regression, response of individual cells or small cellular structures to external perturbation, immune attack, and gene therapy. Therefore, MR microscopy has promise in the noninvasive time-course study of precancerous events, early stages of tumor development, diagnosis of small tumors, and distinction of benign tumors from malignant ones.

Although MR has limited sensitivity, refinement in microfabrication and nanofabrication techniques, electronic circuitry, and pulse sequences make MR microscopy possible. The information provided from MR-derived parameters provide excellent means of obtaining high-resolution biochemical, functional, and morphologic information from cancer cells and tumors. Although the fundamental principles governing conventional MR and MR microscopy are the same, there are certain challenges distinct to microscopy. These challenges arise from molecular diffusion, low SNR resulting from small voxel size and RF coil insensitivity to the sample, and local magnetic field inhomogeneity. Several of these issues are discussed here.

1. Technical Aspects of Microscopy

a. Signal-to-Noise Ratio

One of the principal impediments in microscopy is low SNR. MR is inherently insensitive because its signal amplitude relies on a small nuclear population difference between two energy states. For example, out of 2,000,009 protons at 1.5 T, only nine protons contribute to the MR signal. Furthermore, the acquisition time varies inversely with the square of SNR. To maintain SNR, as the resolution improves from 1 mm $\times$ 1 mm $\times$ 1 mm to 100 μm $\times$ 100 μm $\times$ 100 μm, for instance, the acquisition will take 1 million times longer. Therefore, microscopy efforts focus heavily on enhancing signal amplitude and detection sensitivity.

Signal enhancement may be achieved by increasing the static magnetic field strength, although high field systems are expensive and field inhomogeneity can be a potential drawback at high field. Another approach to enhance signal is polarization of the sample. As mentioned earlier, only a handful of nuclei contribute to the MR signal. The ratio of signal-generating nuclei to the total number of nuclei can be increased by polarizing the sample. Polarization in MR is most commonly achieved through optical pumping of the noble gas isotopes ^{3}He and ^{129}Xe. Hyperpolarized gas has proven to be valuable in imaging pulmonary microstructure and function (Moller *et al.*, 2002). Hyperpolarized gases also induce cross-relaxation, thereby increasing signals from other nuclei within the environment, and they hold significant potential for MRI and MRS studies of the biologic microenvironment.

High-temperature superconducting coils also increase SNR by eliminating resistance in the RF sensor (Black *et al.*, 1993). Cryocooled probes and preamplifiers reduce thermal noise in the system, thereby increasing SNR. These noise reduction-elimination techniques are often cumbersome and expensive, and have yet to be fully optimized. The bulk of the effort in increasing sensitivity is directed toward designing and manufacturing sensitive room temperature RF coils. Improving RF sensitivity is less expensive than increasing field strength and does not require sample polarization or special cooling or superconducting circuitry. RF coils can be tailored to the sample under investigation to provide optimal SNR for that sample, providing flexibility in achieving high performance with a variety of samples.

b. RF Sensitivity

A principal challenge of MR microscopy is to increase SNR, which is proportional to RF sensitivity (Holt and Richards, 1976; Peck *et al.*, 1995):

$$\mathrm{SNR} \propto \frac{\omega_0^2 \cdot (B_1/i) \cdot v_s}{V_{\mathrm{noise}}} \tag{21}$$

where ω_0 (rad s^{-1}) is the nuclear precession frequency, $B_1/i(T/A)$ is the transverse magnetic field generated by the coil per unit current, v_s (m^3) is the sample volume, and V_{noise} (V) is the noise voltage, expressed as

$$V_{\mathrm{noise}} = \sqrt{4 \cdot k_B \cdot T \cdot R_{\mathrm{noise}} \cdot \Delta f} \tag{22}$$

where k_B (1.38×10^{-23} J K^{-1}) is Boltzman's constant, T is the temperature in K, R_{noise} (Ω) is the noise owing to the sample and coil, and Δf (Hz) is the spectral bandwidth. In the microcoil regime, sample losses are negligible and the total resistance is dominated by the coil resistance (Hoult and Lauterbur, 1979). The $(B_1/i) \cdot v_s$ term is closely correlated with the filling factor of the coil. The most effective way to increase RF sensitivity when imaging volume-limited samples is to match the coil size to the sample size. When the filling factor of the coil increases, SNR increases. Because acquisition time varies inversely with the square of SNR, increased SNR permits the investigation of biologic systems in short, physiologically relevant times. Therefore, reduction in coil size and in coil resistance, both from miniaturization and other geometric optimization, have become the foci in microcoil design.

To address the sensitivity requirements of microscopy, a new regime of RF coils called "microcoils" has been developed (Aguayo *et al.*, 1986; Lee *et al.*, 2001; Olson *et al.*, 1995; Subramanian and Webb, 1998; Subramanian *et al.*, 1998; Webb, 1997). The challenges in developing microcoils are those of fabrication and sample positioning. Volume coils must be fabricated with thin conductors and on very small capillaries that are capable of providing mechanical stability to the coil, without compromising the coil's sensing volume. With advances in microfabrication techniques, planar coils on the order of tens to hundreds of microns can be patterned to submicron resolution (Massin *et al.*, 2003) and integrated with microfluidic systems (Trumbull *et al.*, 2000) for accurate sample placement and replacement.

c. Volume Microcoils

Volume coils are conducive to investigating samples whose geometry is principally three-dimensional, and for applications requiring high field homogeneity (narrow spectral linewidth). Birdcage, saddle, solenoid, and scroll configurations are examples of volume coil geometries. We have focused on solenoid coils because they are most widely used, and on the novel "scroll" geometry because of its potential for miniaturization.

Classical analysis of on-axis sensitivity of a solenoid of numerous turns is

$$\frac{B_1}{i} = \frac{\mu_0 \cdot n}{d \cdot \sqrt{1 + (l/d)^2}} \tag{23}$$

where μ_0 ($4\pi \times 10^{-7}$ H m^{-1}) is the permeability of free space, n is the number of turns of the solenoid, d (m) is the coil diameter, and l (m) is the length of the coil. Therefore, for a fixed length to diameter ratio, as the coil diameter decreases, sensitivity increases. The previous equation was derived for the direct current (DC) approximation, where the injected current is distributed uniformly across the cross-section of the solenoid wire. Upon application of an alternating current (AC), the analysis becomes complicated owing to eddy currents generated in the coil wire governed by the Faraday induction law, which effectively push the conductive current out toward the wire perimeter. The conductive current penetration in the wire cross-section is characterized by the skin depth

$$\delta = \frac{1}{\sqrt{\mu \cdot \pi \cdot \sigma \cdot f}} \tag{24}$$

where μ (H m^{-1}) is the permeability of the wire, σ (mho m^{-1}) is its conductivity, and f (Hz) is the operating frequency. As the operating frequency increases, the skin depth decreases and current crowding at the coil perimeter increases the coil resistance. Additionally, if the coil windings are in close proximity to each other, current crowding due to the interactions of the coil windings will further increase coil resistance owing to the phenomenon of "proximity effect," also attributable to the Faraday induction law. With the wire diameter far exceeding skin depth, proximity effects and skin depth dominate resistance, whereas for wire dimensions close to skin depth, the resistance of the coil closely approximates the DC case. Therefore, fabricating microcoils with conductor thickness on the order of skin depth is advantageous to SNR, with certain provisos that are beyond the scope of this chapter but are detailed elsewhere (Peck *et al.*, 1995).

Also, solenoid microcoils have been routinely fabricated by winding thin wire on a small-diameter capillary. Although the spacing between the windings is difficult to control and reproduce (Seeber *et al.*, 2001), it is a critical factor in optimizing microcoil performance (Peck *et al.*, 1995). Solenoid microcoils have electrical leads of lengths equivalent to the length of the coil wire, and therefore losses in the leads owing to resistance and parasitic capacitance are not negligible. To minimize lead losses, a capacitor should be placed across the leads very close to the microcoil, effectively shortening the leads. However, even a nonmagnetic capacitor cannot be placed so close to the microcoil as to cause field distortion owing to magnetic susceptibility effects. The lead losses are an important part of the circuit and should be accounted for in any electrical model characterization of microcoil performance. Solenoid microcoils suffer from scalability and difficulty in fabrication. Wire thickness is a limiting factor in coil miniaturization, and multilayered solenoids are very difficult to wind. Scroll microcoils were developed to overcome these limitations (Gimi *et al.*, 2000). A scroll microcoil is a conductor ribbon wound cylindrically. To generate multiple sensing layers, the conductor is laminated with a dielectric and this ribbon is wound upon itself. Because scroll microcoils can be fabricated from sheets of very thin conductor, their dimensions are not limited by wire diameter. A thick dielectric layer makes scrolls robust and easy to wind. This microcoil geometry has the advantage of achieving very small microcoil dimensions, and with conductor thickness on the order of skin depth, which reduces resistive losses as explained earlier.

d. Surface Microcoils

Although volume coils provide a homogenous RF field and are conducive to three-dimensional geometry, there are microscopy applications where the requirements of sample geometry, loading, and positioning make surface coils more desirable. Because volume coils are wound around a capillary for mechanical stability, the capillary wall thickness can compromise valuable sensing volume for very small coils. Additionally, precise sample positioning is often not possible when using volume coils. Surface coils, on the other hand, provide a higher filling factor for certain samples, and permit greater flexibility in sample positioning and the sample's access to nutrients, drugs, and perfusates. Additionally, planar surface microcoils are well suited to investigate principally two-dimensional geometries such as cell cultures, because they provide high localized SNR in an excitation-acquisition plane close to the plane of the coil.

Current microfabrication technology is well suited for planar geometries and less amenable to geometries with high-aspect ratio (length to diameter ratio), making surface coils easier to microfabricate than volume coils. Therefore, microfabrication of surface coils offer marked flexibility in geometric parameters. A common surface configuration is that of a spiral microcoil (Eroglu *et al.*, 2003; Massin *et al.*, 2002). In contrast to a single loop coil, a spiral provides additional field sensing/focusing turns, thereby increasing the transverse magnetic field near the region of the coil. However, as the number of turns of the spiral increase, the coil resistance increases as well. After a certain number of turns, the contribution of the coil's resistance to SNR outbalances the advantage from an increased number of sensing/focusing turns. Therefore, there is an optimal number of turns of a spiral coil for maximum SNR. When the turns of the spiral are far apart, the contribution of the outer turns to the field in the central region of the coil diminishes. When the turns of the spiral are close to each other, proximity effects play a role in the coil's performance and induce losses in the coil. An optimum interturn spacing must be selected based on electrical modeling of inductive and capacitive interturn coupling. An increased number of turns of the spiral will increase the coil inductance, and the required capacitance to achieve RF resonance would be very small, making the RF circuit difficult to tune.

Surface coils provide very high localized SNR, but their SNR advantage over volume coils decreases rapidly with increasing imaging distance from the plane of the coil (Eroglu *et al.*, 2003). Surface coils generate radiant magnetic fields that create field inhomogeneities, which results in spectral broadening, and are frequently not the preferred configuration where narrow spectral linewidth is important. However, more than one surface transceiver microcoil can be used in generating the transverse magnetic field and receiving RF signal from the sample. For instance, a Helmholtz configuration would have a higher sensing region and field homogeneity than a single planar coil. To achieve high local SNR while still imaging a large field of view, several surface microcoils can be used in configurations such as a phased array (Roemer *et al.*, 1990). Parallel imaging techniques (Sodickson and McKenzie, 2001) such as SENSE, which relies on arrays of mutually coupled coils (Wright *et al.*, 1991), and SMASH (Sodickson and Manning, 1997) are now frequently used. Detailed discussion of these techniques is beyond the scope of this chapter but may be found elsewhere (Pruessmann *et al.*, 1999; Sodickson *et al.*, 2002).

Another aspect of microcoil design is that of susceptibility effects on magnetic field homogeneity. A microcoil conductor such as copper would create static field distortions owing to its diamagnetic nature. Susceptibility-compensated wire (Doty Scientific Inc., Columbia, SC) reduces this diamagnetic effect on static field distortion. For example, a composite of an aluminum core within a copper tube will reduce the wire magnetism to approximately 2% of pure copper.

Technological advances in microfabrication and electronics, development of improved contrast agents and targeted molecular probes, and the emergence of new technology such as mechanical detection of MR (Schaff and Veeman, 1997;

Sidles and Rugar, 1993) are likely to carry microscopy into the realm where subcellular detection is routine. The push toward implantable coils (Silver *et al.*, 2001), combining MR with optical imaging modalities (Wind *et al.*, 2000), and integrating microfluidics with MR systems (Trumbull *et al.*, 2000) will lead to improved cellular and subcellular detection of physiological events *in vivo*, and the detection of molecular events *in vitro*.

V. Metabolic and Physiologic Spectroscopy and Spectroscopic Imaging with MRS and MRSI

MRS and MRSI provide a wealth of information on tumor physiology and metabolism. Different metabolic information can be derived depending upon the nucleus (i.e., ^{1}H, ^{13}C, or ^{31}P) examined.

A. ^{1}H MRS

The high sensitivity of ^{1}H MRS permits proton spectra to be obtained with high spatial and temporal resolution. This is important because one of the main characteristics of tumor blood flow is its heterogeneity, which results in a heterogeneous oxygen, pH, and metabolite distribution. The ability to obtain spatially localized spectra from small voxels is necessary not only to localize the measurement to tumor tissue and minimize signal contribution from normal tissue but also to determine the spatial distribution of metabolites within the tumor to better characterize the tumor, as well as its response to therapy. Unedited proton spectra are dominated by signal from water, methyl, and methylene protons. Water suppression methods are routinely used to eliminate the signal from water during acquisition, using techniques such as VAPOR (Tkac *et al.*, 1999), CHESS (Hause *et al.*, 1985), or band selective refocusing (Shungu and Glickson, 1994; Star-Lack *et al.*, 1997). Although the intense methyl and methylene signals originating from mobile lipids can provide useful information (Al-Saffar *et al.*, 2002; Barba *et al.*, 1999; Callies *et al.*, 1993), since these signals dominate the spectrum, resonances from metabolites such as lactate and alanine, which appear near the lipid region, are obscured. The use of a long TE of 272 ms can significantly reduce signal from the mobile lipids. Localized presaturation methods are also used when the lipid signal in the tumor is localized to a peripheral region (Bhujwalla *et al.*, 1996; Shungu and Glickson, 1994). Recent methods for lipid suppression have employed gradient filtering of lactate multiple-quantum coherences (Hurd and Freeman, 1991; Sotak, 1988) and the application of adiabatic pulses for spectral editing (de Graaf *et al.*, 1995). However, coherence selection may not be optimal, and two-dimensional experiments, difference spectra, or additional phase cycling steps may be required to obtain uncontaminated spectra. He *et al.* (1995a,b) have shown that a homonuclear gradient-coherence transfer method, combined with a frequency selective pulse, is very effective in suppressing both lipid and water in a single scan.

Typically, proton spectra obtained from tumors contain resonances from taurine, total choline (choline, Cho; phosphocholine, PC; and glycerophosphocholine, GPC), total creatine (phosphocreatine and creatine), and lactate (Howe *et al.*, 1993). Figure 7 displays representative ^{1}H MR spectra obtained from an invasive and metastatic human breast cancer xenograft model, MDA-MB-231. Figure 7A is a high-resolution ^{1}H MR spectrum of a perchloric acid extract of MDA-MB-231 cells. A diffusion-weighted, water-suppressed ^{1}H MR spectrum of live perfused cells is shown in Fig. 7B, and a spectrum obtained from a representative 1 mm × 1 mm × 4 mm voxel of a ^{1}H chemical shift imaging (CSI) data set, obtained from a MDA-MB-231 tumor in a SCID mouse is shown in Fig. 7C. The CSI data set was acquired using the BASSALE sequence (Shungu and Glickson, 1994). High-resolution ^{1}H MRS resolves the $^{3}J_{\text{H-H}}$ coupling in lactate at 1.33 ppm and the N-$(CH_3)_3$ resonances of GPC, PC, and Cho (Fig. 7A insert). In perfused isolated cells, as well as in tumor xenografts, an unresolved signal of total choline-

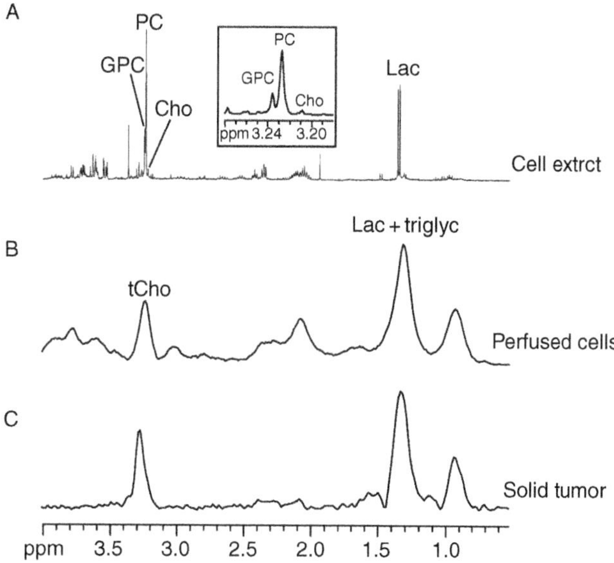

Fig. 7 ^{1}H MR spectra from (A) perchloric acid cell extracts, (B) intact cells, and (C) a 1 mm × 1 mm × 4 mm solid tumor voxel of the metastatic human breast cancer xenograft MDA-MB-231. The ^{1}H MR spectrum shown in (A) is a high-resolution spectrum of cell extracts. The insert displays a zoomed region at 3.2 ppm to demonstrate that human breast cancer cells exhibit low GPC levels, high PC levels, and high levels of total choline-containing metabolites. The diffusion-weighted, water-suppressed ^{1}H MR spectrum shown in panel (B) was acquired from intact cells perfused in our MR-compatible cell perfusion system. The ^{1}H MR spectrum shown in (C) is a representative 1 mm × 1 mm × 4 mm voxel obtained from a CSI data set acquired using the BASSALE sequence. CSI data were acquired with a TE of 272 ms and TR of 1 s within a total acquisition time of 25 min. Assignments made in the ^{1}H MR spectra are Cho, free choline; GPC, glycerophosphocholine; PC, phosphocholine; Lac, lactate; tCho, total choline-containing metabolites; Lac + Triglyc, lactate + triglycerides.

containing compounds is detected at 3.2 ppm, and a combined signal of lactate and triglycerides is detected at 1.3 ppm (Fig. 7B and C).

^{1}H MR spectra of tumors typically exhibit elevated total choline and lactate levels (Gribbestad *et al.*, 1994; Howe *et al.*, 2003; Negendank, 1992). The high levels of lactate are consistent with high glycolytic rates and poor blood flow associated with tumors (Vaupel *et al.*, 1989a). The high levels of total choline detected in breast, prostate, and different types of brain tumors primarily arise from increased PC levels in tumor cells, as confirmed by high-resolution ^{1}H MRS studies of cell extracts (Aboagye and Bhujwalla, 1999; Ackerstaff *et al.*, 2001; Bhakoo *et al.*, 1996). Molecular alterations underlying the increased PC levels observed in cancer cells include increased expression and activity of choline kinase (Ramirez de Molina *et al.*, 2002a,b), a higher rate of choline transport (Katz-Brull and Degani, 1996), and increased phospholipase D (Noh *et al.*, 2000) and phospholipase A2 (Guthridge *et al.*, 1994) activity. Thus, an increased membrane degradation or turnover combined with elevated choline kinase activity appear to cause the elevated total choline levels observed in tumor ^{1}H MR spectra, where both membrane phospholipid precursors and breakdown products contribute to the total choline signal (Aboagye and Bhujwalla, 1999). Clinically, the total choline signal has been employed for proton MRSI of cancer. MRSI is typically performed in conjunction with high-resolution anatomic MRI, and it can significantly improve the diagnosis and the assessment of cancer location and aggressiveness. Pre- and posttherapy studies have demonstrated the potential of combined MRI and MRSI to provide a direct measure of the presence and spatial extent of cancer, as well as the time course and mechanism of therapeutic response (Kurhanewicz *et al.*, 2000; Leach *et al.*, 1998). The use of elevated choline levels to detect cancer with MRS or MRSI has been demonstrated for prostate (Kurhanewicz *et al.*, 2000), brain (Li *et al.*, 2002), breast (Gribbestad *et al.*, 1999), and other cancers (Negendank, 1992).

B. ^{13}C MRS

^{13}C MRS is uniquely suited for studying glycolysis and other metabolic pathways such as choline metabolism in cancer cells and solid tumors. The flux of metabolites through various pathways can be measured through the use of labeled substrates and metabolic modeling. Two applications of ^{13}C MRS are shown in Fig. 8. [1,2-^{13}C]-choline can be utilized to follow the production of the water-soluble ^{13}C-labeled choline phospholipid metabolites PC and GPC in human MDA-MB-231 breast cancer cells as shown in Fig. 8A(i). Using a dual-phase extraction method, the lipid fraction can be recovered and measured separately to assess incorporation of [1,2-^{13}C]-choline into membrane phosphatidylcholine as shown in Fig. 8A(ii). Figure. 8B is ^{13}C MR spectra obtained *in vivo* from a RIF-1 tumor at 400 MHz using heteronuclear cross-polarization, showing the appearance of signals from ^{13}C glucose and ^{13}C lactate with time. These data can be used to determine the glycolytic rate of the tumor (Artemov *et al.*, 1998).

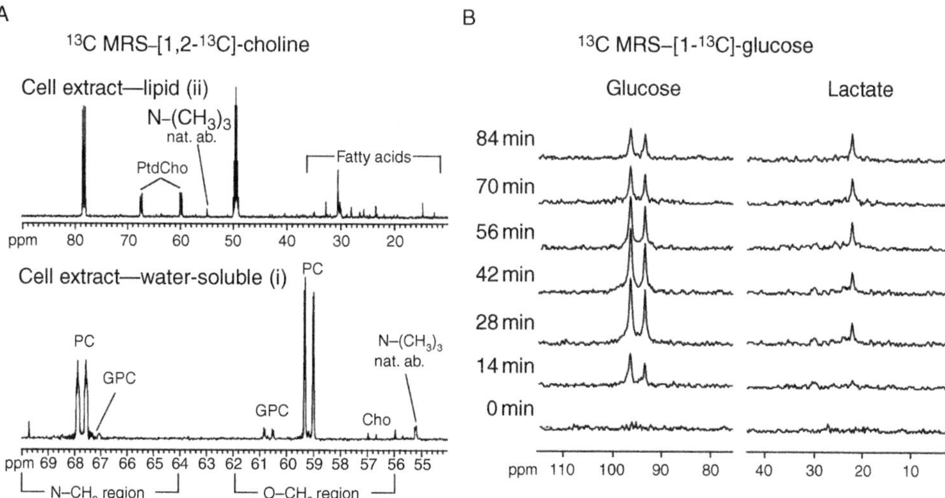

Fig. 8 (A) Representative ^{13}C MR spectra of the water-soluble (i) and the lipid fraction (ii) of MDA-MB-231 human breast cancer cells. Spectra were obtained from MDA-MB-231 cells that were labeled with 100 μM [1,2-^{13}C]-choline for 24 + 3 h and extracted using a dual phase extraction method. ^{13}C label was detected in the water-soluble metabolites glycerophosphocholine (GPC), phosphocholine (PC), and free choline (Cho), as well as in membrane phosphatidylcholine (PtdCho). (B) *In vivo* ^{13}C spectroscopy of a RIF-1 tumor obtained at 400 MHz using heteronuclear cross-polarization. The animal was injected with 900 mg kg^{-1} ^{13}C-labeled D-glucose. The specific glycolytic rate of the tumor can be determined from the kinetic analysis of ^{13}C-lactate buildup.

Although the sensitivity of ^{13}C MRS is relatively low, indirect detection methods (van Zijl *et al.*, 1993) permit the detection of the ^{13}C label with a sensitivity approaching that of the proton nucleus, and greatly increase the sensitivity of detecting ^{13}C-labeled metabolites *in vivo*. Artemov *et al.* (1995) have also demonstrated the use of heteronuclear cross-polarization transfer to increase the sensitivity of direct ^{13}C detection. One major advantage of direct ^{13}C detection is its relative insensitivity to motion compared with inverse detection methods.

^{13}C MRS studies (direct and indirect ^{13}C detection) of tumors have shown that in poorly differentiated transplanted tumors, [1-^{13}C]-labeled glucose is metabolized to lactate (Artemov *et al.*, 1998; Bhujwalla *et al.*, 1992; Constantinidis *et al.*, 1991; Schupp *et al.*, 1993). Ronen *et al.* (1994) have shown that a well-differentiated rat hepatoma (H4IIEC3) exhibited metabolic behavior similar to that of normal hepatocytes, mainly utilizing alanine as a substrate and resorting to glucose only under conditions of nutrient deprivation. When studying perchloric acid extracts of tumors or organs from animals infused with [1-^{13}C]- or [U-^{13}C]-labeled glucose, the labeling pattern of metabolites can provide insight into metabolic compartmentalization, shuttling of metabolites between cell types or organs, and metabolic fluxes in general (Bouzier *et al.*, 1999).

^{13}C-labeled lactate can be utilized as a metabolic marker for poor blood flow and oxygenation in unperturbed tumors, although this is complicated by several factors (Bhujwalla *et al.*, 1994). Glycolysis is tightly regulated by pH, ADP levels, and inorganic phosphate (Erecinska and Silver, 1989; Trivedi and Danforth, 1966). As mentioned earlier, tumors can form lactate in the absence of oxygen. Poor delivery of ^{13}C-labeled glucose to areas of low blood flow and inhibition of phosphofructokinase at low pH may confound the interpretation of ^{13}C MR spectra of tumors to obtain indices of blood flow and oxygenation from the metabolism of ^{13}C-labeled glucose (Bhujwalla *et al.*, 1994). This can be accounted for by measuring blood flow (or at least the relative heterogeneity of blood flow) to the tumor. The rate of clearance of ^{13}C-labeled lactate may also provide a measure of blood flow, provided lactate transport out of cells does not vary and lactate is not metabolized. On the other hand, an acute reduction of tumor blood flow will result in a significant increase of ^{13}C-labeled lactate. For most tumors, lactate levels seem to be equilibrated by an interplay of forces involving hemodynamics, substrate supply, hypoxia, venous clearance, glucose supply, extent of necrosis, and degree of inflammatory cell infiltrate (Terpstra *et al.*, 1996). A clear correlation between decreasing tumor oxygenation and increasing glycolytic rate was observed in a murine mammary carcinoma model, studied by volume-localized ^{13}C MRS with ^{1}H-^{13}C cross-polarization to detect the conversion of [1-^{13}C]-glucose to [3-^{13}C]-lactate (Nielsen *et al.*, 2001). Human breast cancer cells incubated with [1-^{13}C]-glucose exhibited a diminished mitochondrial energy generation, as assessed by the reduction in the flux of pyruvate utilized for mitochondrial energy generation compared with pyruvate used to replenish tricarboxylic acid cycle intermediates, which correlated with the degree of malignancy of the breast cancer cells (Singer *et al.*, 1995). ^{13}C MRS methods can also be used to detect the effect of treatment aimed at the selective inhibition of glycolysis in tumors (Floridi *et al.*, 1981). Some of these strategies have already been investigated with ^{31}P MRS (Karczmar *et al.*, 1992; Stolfi *et al.*, 1992).

[1,2-^{13}C]-choline (Fig. 8A) or other ^{13}C-labeled lipid precursors, such as [3-^{13}C]-serine, [1,2-^{13}C]-ethanolamine, or [^{13}C-methyl]-methionine, can be utilized for ^{13}C MRS studies to characterize the phospholipid metabolism of cells (Dixon, 1996; Gillies *et al.*, 1994a; Ronen and Degani, 1992). These lipid precursors can be utilized for high-resolution ^{13}C studies of cell extracts, for real-time monitoring studies of perfused isolated cells, or for infusion studies of animal tumor models. [1,2-^{13}C]-choline has been applied to further elucidate the aberrant choline phospholipid metabolism in cancer cells (Fig. 8A). ^{13}C MRS studies employing [1,2-^{13}C]-choline in a cell perfusion system demonstrated that breast cancer cells exhibit enhanced choline transport and choline kinase activity (Katz-Brull and Degani, 1996). This study also revealed that the rate of choline phosphorylation was much faster than the choline transport rate (Katz-Brull and Degani, 1996).

C. ^{31}P MRS

^{31}P MRS studies of solid tumors were among the first MR studies of solid tumors to be performed (Griffiths *et al.*, 1981) *in vivo*. Metabolites detected in ^{31}P MR spectra of solid tumors are nucleoside triphosphates (NTP), phosphocreatine (PCr), inorganic phosphate (P_i), phosphodiesters (PDE), and phosphomonesters (PME). The chemical shift of the P_i resonance yields the pH of the tumor.

Representative ^{31}P MR spectra from perchloric acid cell extracts, intact perfused cells, and solid tumors derived from an invasive and metastatic human breast cancer xenograft, MDA-MB-231, are shown in Fig. 9. High-resolution ^{31}P MRS resolves the typical coupling pattern in the NTP and nucleoside diphosphate (NDP) signals (Fig. 9A), since divalent cations were masked with ethylenediaminetetraacetic acid (EDTA) in the extract spectra. In perfused isolated cells and tumor xenografts, unresolved NTP and NDP signals are detected (Fig. 9B and C). Detection of PC and GPC, and potentially PE and GPE, in ^{31}P MR spectra renders ^{31}P MRS useful for the study of cellular phospholipid metabolism. The P_i resonance in live cells (Fig. 9B) and tumors (Fig. 9C) reflects the overall pH of the cells and the interstitium. In isolated perfused cells, two signals representing intra- and extracellular P_i can be resolved, given that the extracellular P_i concentration does not exceed physiologic values of 1 mM.

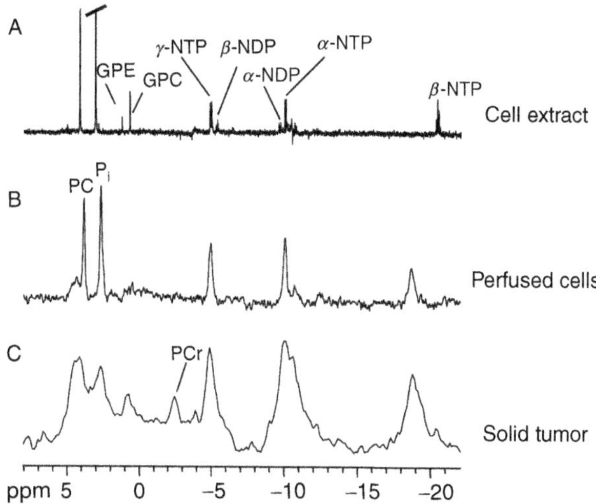

Fig. 9 ^{31}P MR spectra from (A) perchloric acid cell extracts, (B) intact cells, and (C) a solid tumor of the metastatic human breast cancer xenograft MDA-MB-231. The ^{31}P MR spectrum shown in (A) is a high-resolution spectrum of cell extracts. The ^{31}P MR spectrum shown in panel (B) was acquired from intact cells perfused in our MR-compatible cell perfusion system. The ^{31}P MR spectrum shown in (C) is from a solid MDA-MB-231 tumor inoculated in a SCID mouse. Assignments made in the ^{31}P MR spectra are: NDP, nucleoside diphosphate; NTP, nucleoside triphosphate; GPC, glycerophosphocholine; GPE, glycerophosphoethanolamine, PC, phosphocholine; PCr, phosphocreatine; P_i, inorganic phosphate.

Early results obtained from tumors suggested that levels of NTP, PCr, and P_i would reflect the efficiency of flow and oxygenation within a tumor (Evanochko *et al.*, 1984). It is likely that at a given time, a ^{31}P spectrum from a tumor will depend on glucose and oxygen consumption rates, cell density, and nutritive blood flow. However, since both glucose and oxygen delivery are dependent on blood flow, energy metabolism should be tightly coupled to blood flow. Indeed, most studies show that within a single tumor line, progressive tumor growth and the associated decline of blood flow result in a decrease of high-energy metabolites such as adenosine triphosphate (ATP) and PCr and increase of P_i (Li *et al.*, 1988; Okunieff *et al.*, 1986). Vaupel *et al.* (1989a,b) measured changes in ^{31}P MRS parameters with tumor growth and, in parallel experiments, measured tumor oxygen tensions with oxygen electrodes. A strong correlation was observed between ^{31}P MRS parameters PCr/P_i and NTP/P_i and tumor oxygenation. Rofstad *et al.* (1988) investigated the dependence of ^{31}P MRS parameters on the radiobiologic hypoxic fraction, a parameter of importance for radiation therapy, for two tumor lines with widely different hypoxic fractions. Within a given cell line the (NTP + PCr)/P_i ratio decreased with tumor volume and radiobiologic hypoxic fraction. However, when ^{31}P MRS parameters were related to hypoxic fractions across cell lines, the tumor line with the higher hypoxic fraction did not have a lower (NTP + PCr)/P_i ratio. A dissociation of the energy metabolism and the radiobiologic hypoxic fraction can exist if cells are highly glycolytic and do not require oxygen. In fact, it is possible that highly glycolytic tumors such as the 9L glioma may have a low hypoxic fraction (Moulder and Rockwell, 1984). ^{31}P MRS parameters may, however, be useful in detecting blood flow-mediated changes in tumor reoxygenation (Kallman, 1972) during a course of radiation therapy (Tozer and Griffiths, 1992).

Acute changes in tumor blood flow produce more dramatic changes in high-energy phosphates. As mentioned earlier, the action of vasoactive agents that either improve or decrease tumor blood flow has been studied over the past decade with the aim of creating hypoxia and thereby increasing response to bioreductive drugs targeted toward hypoxic cells, or improving tumor blood flow and oxygenation and sensitizing tumors to radiation (Denekamp, 1993). ^{31}P MR spectra of experimental tumors show a prompt decrease in NTP, PCr, and pH and an increase in P_i following delivery of agents known to reduce tumor blood flow (Bhujwalla *et al.*, 1990; Okunieff *et al.*, 1988). However, the direct action of some of these agents on cellular metabolism may also contribute to the metabolic changes observed (Tozer *et al.*, 1990). The dependence of NTP levels on tumor blood flow may have a threshold that may be characteristic of each tumor type, depending upon its energy requirements; blood flow rates above this threshold may not further elevate NTP levels (Bhujwalla *et al.*, 1990).

^{1}H MRS studies of choline phospholipid metabolism in cancer cells and solid tumors have been complemented by a vast array of ^{31}P MRS investigations performed *in vivo* and *in vitro* (reviewed in de Certaines *et al.*, 1993; Negendank, 1992; Podo, 1999). Phospholipid metabolites have been monitored in cancer, using

^{31}P MRS during mutant *ras*-oncogene transformation (Ronen *et al.*, 2001), drug treatment with antimicrotubule drugs (Sterin *et al.*, 2001), or the nonsteroidal anti-inflammatory agent indomethacin (Glunde *et al.*, 2002; Natarajan *et al.*, 2002). These data indicate that diverse molecular alterations and treatments arrive at common endpoints in choline phospholipid metabolism of cancer cells.

D. Tumor pH

1. ^{31}P MRS

MR measurements of pH are obtained from the chemical shift difference between P_i and an endogenous reference such as PCr or α-NTP (Moon and Richards, 1973). The P_i signal in the spectrum originates from the intra- and extracellular compartment. Tumor interstitial fluid has P_i concentrations of 1–2 mM, which is very close to the plasma P_i concentration, suggesting that pH as measured by MRS is weighted toward intracellular pH by at least 70% for tumors with extracellular volumes less than 50% (Stubbs *et al.*, 1992). Although large necrotic areas do not accumulate P_i (Tozer and Griffiths, 1992), it is likely that cells in areas with poor blood flow may have a substantially higher P_i concentration than cells in well-perfused regions of the tumor. Therefore, in such cases, the chemical shift of the P_i signal may be biased toward the pH of the cells with poor blood flow. Gillies *et al.* (1994b) have reported the use of an exogenous compound, 3-aminopropylphosphonate (3-APP), to obtain extracellular pH (pH_e) *in vivo* from a ^{31}P spectrum. Results obtained from a transplanted tumor confirm predictions, based on electrode measurements, of an acidic extracellular environment and a neutral to alkaline intracellular pH.

The more acidic (mainly extracellular) pH measured by electrodes and the neutral to alkaline (mainly intracellular) pH measured by MRS suggest that tumor cells may have increased H^+-transporting activity relative to normal tissue. Gillies *et al.* (1982) have shown that Ehrlich ascites cells can maintain intracellular pH values of 7.1 in the presence of an extracellular pH environment of 6.8. The gradient collapsed in the absence of oxygen and glucose, suggesting that the proton extrusion mechanisms were energy driven. Several *in vivo* MR studies have also demonstrated the close dependence of intracellular pH on blood flow and substrate supply. An acute reduction of blood flow usually results in a significant decrease of intracellular pH (Gillies *et al.*, 1982, 1994b; Tozer *et al.*, 1990). Similarly, the P_i signal-derived pH usually decreases with progressive growth of the tumor (Li *et al.*, 1988; Rofstad *et al.*, 1988; Vaupel *et al.*, 1989a,b). However, a human ovarian xenograft did not exhibit this decrease with growth (Rofstad and Sutherland, 1988), suggesting that different types of tumors may have different proton extrusion capabilities. Studies on the effects of hyperglycemia on tumor metabolism also suggest that significant decreases in the P_i signal-derived pH occur mainly when hyperglycemia produces a decrease of tumor blood flow or energy metabolism (Evelhoch *et al.*, 1984). In fact, an increase in glucose delivery to the tumor can increase pH and energy levels (Okunieff *et al.*, 1989).

2. ^{1}H MRS

^{1}H MRS is more sensitive than ^{31}P or ^{13}C MRS, but currently there are no ^{1}H-detectable endogenous markers to quantitatively measure tumor pH *in vivo*. ^{1}H MRS approaches to measure tumor pH have relied on compounds, such as imidazoles and aromatics, that resonate far down-field of endogenous metabolites. Ballesteros and her colleagues (Gil *et al.*, 1994) have developed an imidazole compound, (+/−)2-imidazole-1-yl-3-ethoxycarbonylpropionic acid (IEPA), which has been used to measure extracellular pH using ^{1}H MRS of breast tumor xenografts with a spatial resolution of $1 \times 1 \times 2\ \text{mm}^3$ (van Sluis *et al.*, 1999). These pH maps showed pH values ranging from 6.4 to 6.8, which were consistent with those measured with ^{31}P MRS of 3-APP. By combining MRSI of IEPA and vascular MRI using albumin-GdDTPA, Bhujwalla *et al.* (2002a) have demonstrated the feasibility of obtaining coregistered maps of vascular volume, permeability, and extracellular pH.

^{1}H MRSI techniques employing proton chemical-exchange-dependent saturation transfer (CEST) provide another strategy to measure pH *in vivo*. Magnetization transfer (MT) has been employed to evaluate proton and other nuclide chemical exchange to study chemical reactions (Alger and Shulman, 1984). Potential exogenous CEST-contrast agents have been tested, demonstrating the feasibility of a CEST-based MRI contrast agent (Ward *et al.*, 2000). Recently, the use of amide protons of endogenous mobile cellular proteins and peptides (chemical shift of 8.3 ± 0.5 ppm), which exchange with water for CEST, has been investigated by ^{1}H MRS and MRI (Zhou *et al.*, 2003). To achieve amide proton CEST contrast, amide protons were selectively irradiated with radiofrequency at 8.3 ppm, and water was imaged after several seconds of transfer, thereby calculating an MT ratio asymmetry parameter (Zhou *et al.*, 2003). However, pH maps based on the amide proton transfer (APT) contrast are difficult to quantify, since variation of several parameters, such as the concentration of amide protons and water, can affect the actual measurement. Although APT contrast images seem to provide relative pH maps, it would be desirable to achieve absolute quantification. For pH imaging of solid tumors, it would also be necessary to distinguish between intracellular and extracellular pH, which is not (yet) possible using this new ^{1}H MRS-based pH imaging technique.

VI. Examples of Integrated Imaging and Spectroscopy Approaches to Studying Cancer

MR can be used for an integrated imaging and spectroscopic imaging approach, which is extremely useful in studying a disease as complex as cancer. In this section, we have included two examples of such an approach in studying cancer cell invasion, and the vascularization and metabolism of solid tumors.

A. MR Metabolic Boyden Chamber for Studying Cancer Cell Invasion

The ability of cancer cells to invade and metastasize is one of the most lethal aspects of cancer. Cancer cells invade by secreting enzymes that degrade basement membrane. This invasive potential is commonly assayed by determining the penetration of cells into reconstituted basement membrane gel (Matrigel or extracellular matrix (ECM) gel). Invasion is then quantified by counting the number of cells that invade ECM gel-coated filters over a period of 5–72 h. However, these methods do not permit evaluation of the metabolic state of tumor cells, nor do they allow invasion to be measured dynamically in the same sample, under controlled environmental conditions, or following therapeutic interventions.

We therefore developed an invasion assay system, termed the metabolic Boyden chamber (MBC) assay (Pilatus *et al.*, 2000), to dynamically track the invasion of cancer cells into ECM gel and simultaneously characterize oxygen tensions and physiologic and metabolic parameters. In this assay, ^{1}H, ^{31}P, and ^{19}F MR experiments of cancer cells continually perfused with medium are performed on a GE Omega 400 MHz MR spectrometer with 130 G cm^{-1} shielded gradients. A schematic describing the system is shown in Fig. 10. The current design achieves a reproducible thickness of ECM gel while allowing free perfusion through the tube. By replacing Norprene tubing with less permeable Viton tubing, we obtain oxygen tensions under 1.5%, which is necessary to evaluate the impact of the hypoxic tumor environment on cancer cell invasion. We incorporate

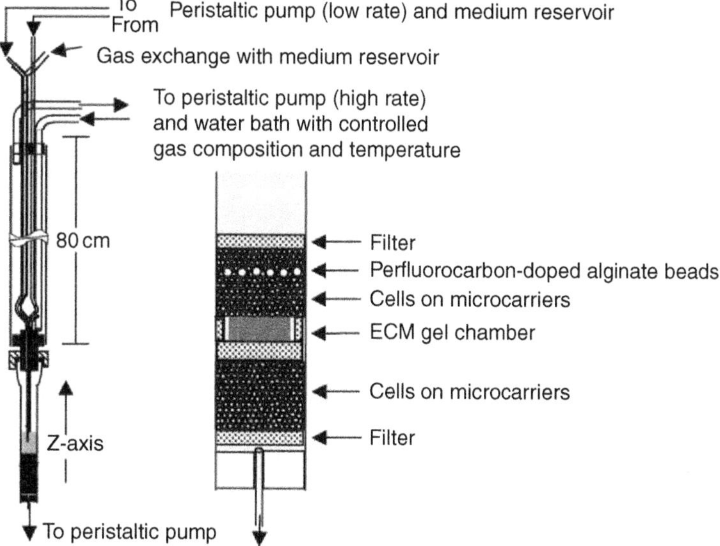

Fig. 10 Schematic of "metabolic Boyden chamber assay" demonstrating the reproducible layer of ECM gel and perfluorocarbon-doped alginate beads placed within the cell layers. Adapted from Pilatus *et al.* (2000).

perfluorotripropylamine (FTPA)-doped alginate beads in the NMR tube and embed FTPA into the ECM gel to directly measure oxygen tensions in the sample using ^{19}F MR relaxometry (McGovern *et al.*, 1993). An example of the oxygen tensions achieved in this system is shown in Fig. 11.

T_1-weighted ^{1}H MR images are used to visualize the geometry of the sample, including the ECM gel, as well as changes in the integrity of the ECM gel due to invasion and degradation. The 1D distribution of invading cells in the sample is obtained from the profile of intracellular water measured with 1D imaging along the length of the sample with a spatial resolution of 0.031 mm (zero-filled to 0.016 mm). A quantitative index of invasion is obtained from these cellular profiles. We routinely obtain localized proton spectra of intracellular water and metabolites with a slice thickness of 0.31 mm. With the current hardware, experiments with a spatial resolution of 0.312 mm (128 phase-encoding steps, 40 mm field of view (FOV)) can be performed within 9 h. The energy status of the cells, pH, and levels of choline phospholipid metabolites are obtained from ^{31}P MR spectra.

Typical invasion and metabolic data obtained with the MBC assay for the noninvasive prostate cancer cell line, DU-145, and the invasive prostate cancer cell line, MatLyLu, at comparable time points are displayed in Fig. 12. Representative T_1-weighted ^{1}H MR images demonstrating the different rates of degradation of ECM gel by three prostate cancer cell lines, MatLyLu, PC-3, and DU-145, are presented in Fig. 13. Quantitative differences in the invasion index for three

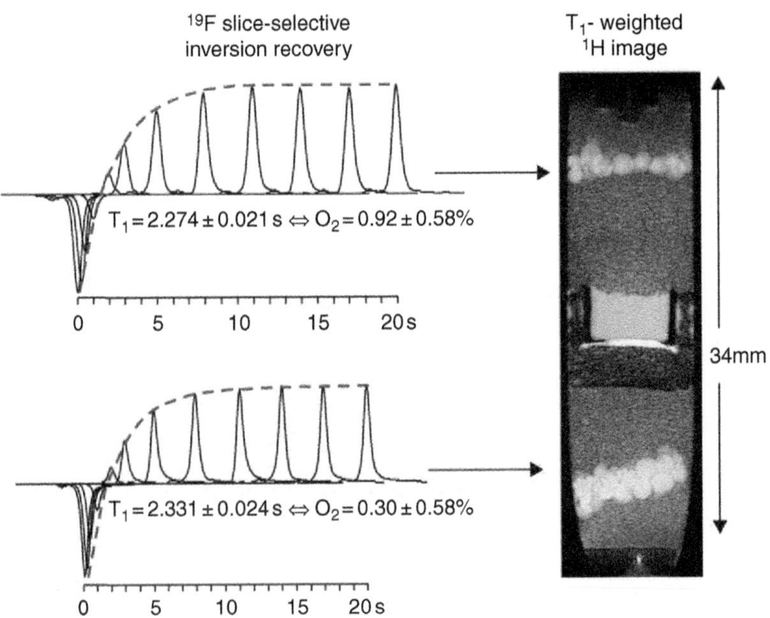

Fig. 11 Characterization of oxygen tensions in the metabolic Boyden chamber perfusion system.

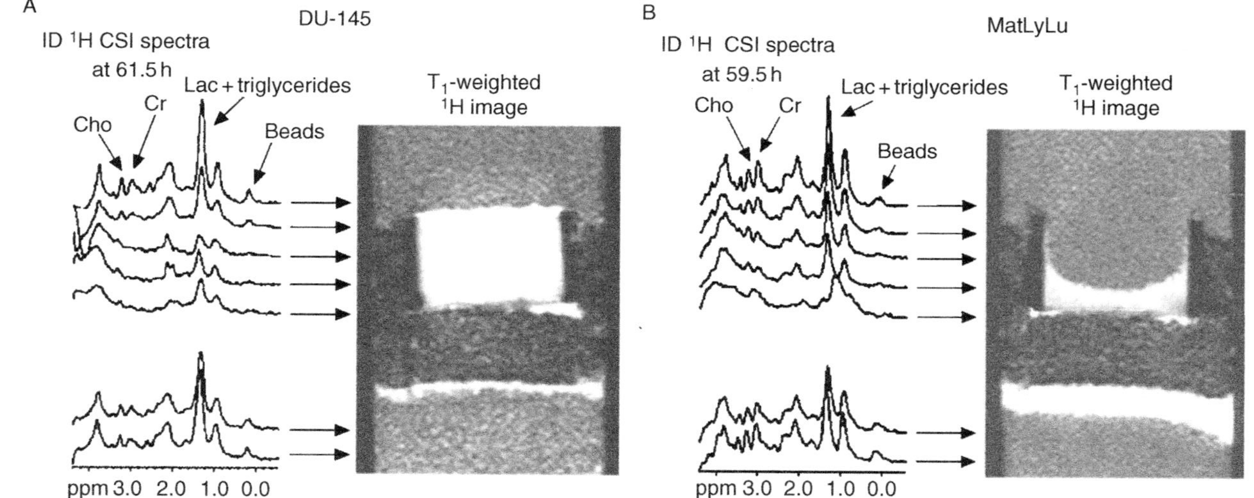

Fig. 12 Expanded ^{1}H MR image of sample showing the ECM gel region for (A) DU-145 and (B) MatLyLu cells at comparable time points. Images were obtained with TR 1 s, TE 30 ms, FOV 40 mm, slice thickness 2 mm, and an in-plane resolution of 0.078 mm. Corresponding ^{1}H MR spectra in the figure are from every third 0.31-mm-thick slice localized within the sample. Metabolites assigned are Cho (total choline), Cr (total creatine), Lac + Triglycerides (lactate and triglycerides). Signal from the beads to which the cancer cells are attached is also observed in the spectra. Adapted from Pilatus *et al.* (2000).

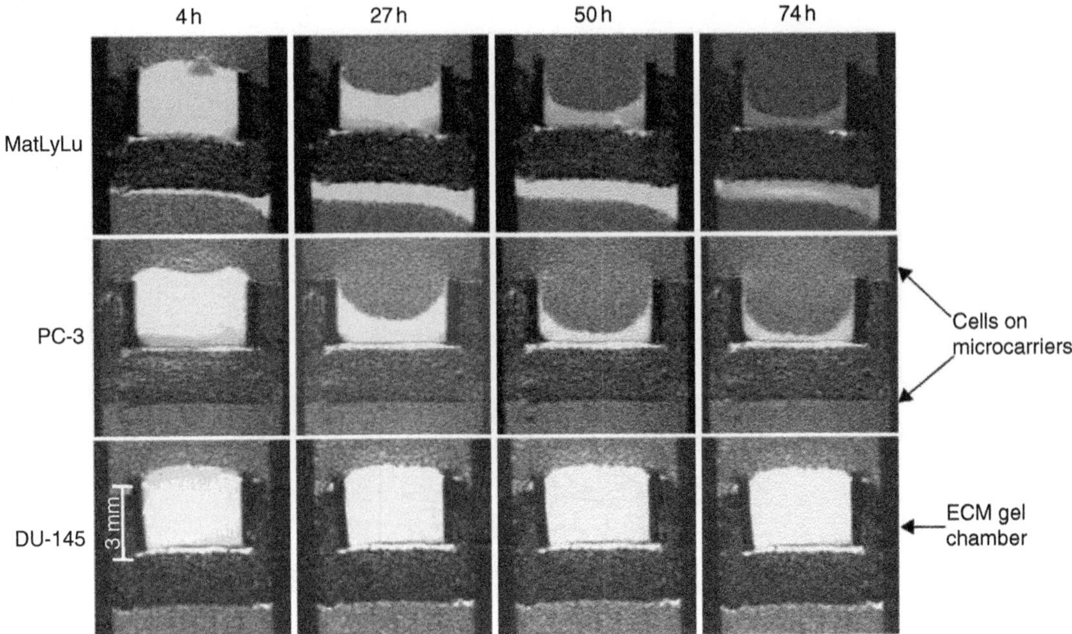

Fig. 13 "Metabolic Boyden chamber assay" demonstrating differences in invasive characteristics of three prostate cancer cell lines. The T_1-weighted ^{1}H MR images show the bright ECM gel layer, which is significantly degraded by MatLyLu and PC-3 cells, but not by DU-145 cells.

different prostate cancer cell lines are summarized in Fig. 14, and demonstrate the differences in the invasion index for the three cell lines.

B. Multinuclear MRI and MRSI of Preclinical Models of Cancer

Over the past decade, we have established several MRI and MRSI techniques to study preclinical models of cancer. From the earlier sections, it is apparent that a unique aspect of MR is its potential ability to investigate the relationships between tumor vascularization, physiology, and metabolism. Although it is useful to study these as separate characteristics, the ability to relate metabolism and vascularization within the same region of interest adds a new dimension to our understanding of how one impacts on the other for tumor models with different vascular and metastatic characteristics, or for those overexpressing a selected gene or receptor, or for tumors with different drug resistance. We have also developed combined vascular, metabolic, and extracellular pH imaging, and can perform combined vascular, metabolic, and optical imaging or positron-emission tomography (PET).

For combined metabolic and vascular imaging of tumor models, both proton spectroscopic images (SI) and vascular maps are obtained using a ^{1}H RF coil on our GE Omega 4.7-T spectrometer during a single experiment, without disturbing

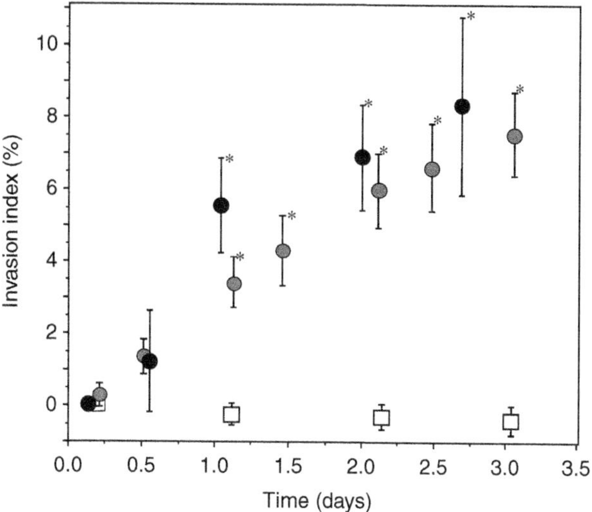

Fig. 14 Invasion index (I) for (•) MatLyLu ($n = 6$), (•) PC-3 ($n = 4$), and (□) DU-145 ($n = 4$) prostate cancer cells. Values are mean ± S.E. * Represents a statistically significant difference between MatLyLu and DU-145, and between PC-3 and DU-145 cells ($p < 0.01$).

the position of the animal or the tumor (Fig. 15). During the experiment, the body temperature of the animal is maintained at 37 °C by means of a heating blanket. Typically, we first obtain a spectroscopic imaging (SI) data set using the BASSALE pulse sequence (Bhujwalla *et al.*, 2002b; Shungu and Glickson, 1994). Images of total choline and lactate-lipid are generated from the SI acquired from a 4-mm-thick slice, with an in-plane resolution of 2 mm (zero-filled to 1 mm), FOV = 32 mm, matrix size = 16 × 16 × 512, 4 scans per phase encode step, TE = 136 ms, TR = 1 s. After SI, which is completed within 30 min, measurements of vascular volume and permeability surface area product are obtained. Vascular imaging is done as follows. Multislice relaxation rates (T_1^{-1}) of the tumor are obtained by a saturation recovery method combined with fast T_1 SNAPSHOT-FLASH imaging (flip angle = 10°, TE = 2 ms). Images of four slices matching the SI data (slice thickness of 1 mm) are acquired with an in-plane spatial resolution of 0.125 mm (matrix = 128 × 128, FOV = 16 mm, NS = 16) for three relaxation delays (100 ms, 500 ms, and 1 s) for each of the slices. An M_0 map with a recovery delay of 7 s is acquired once at the beginning of the experiment. Images are obtained before intravenous (IV) administration (via the tail vein) of 0.2 ml of 60 mg ml^{-1} albumin-GdDTPA in saline (dose of 500 mg kg^{-1}) and repeated every 5 min, starting 3 min after the injection, for up to 30 min.

Relaxation maps are computed from the data sets for three different relaxation times and the M_0 data set on a voxelwise basis (Bhujwalla *et al.*, 2000). Vascular volume and permeability product surface area (PS) maps are generated from the ratio of $\Delta(1/T_1)$ values in the images to that of blood. As described earlier

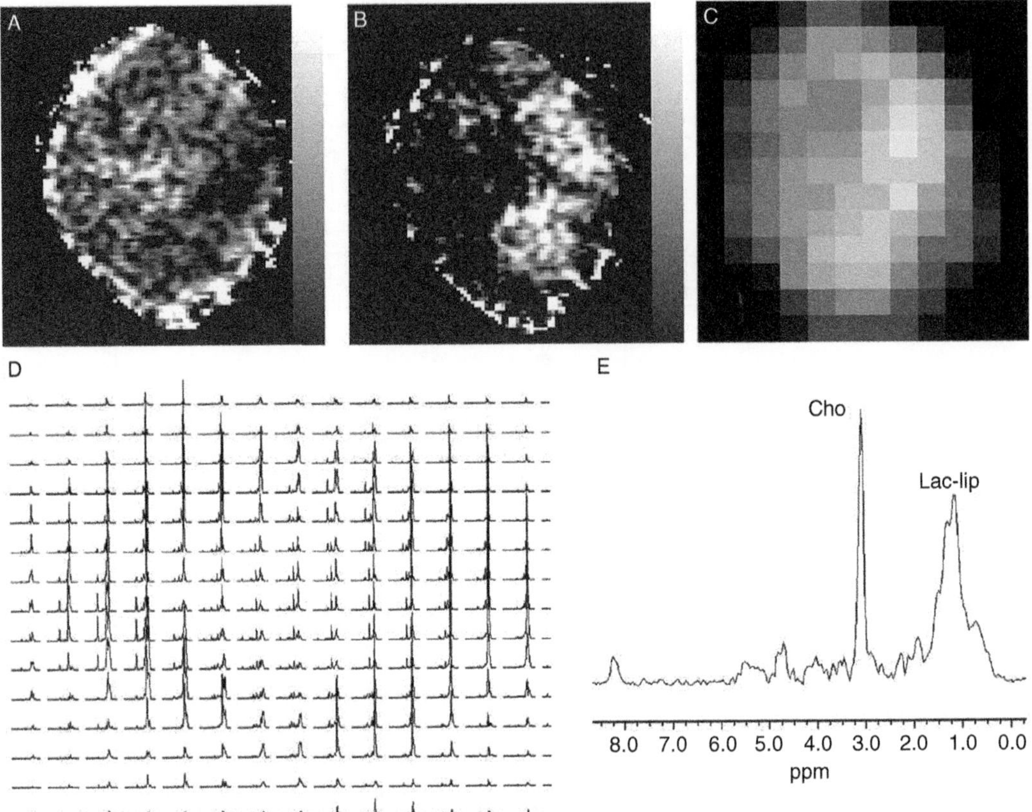

Fig. 15 Coregistered maps of (A) vascular volume, (B) permeability surface area product, and (C) total choline obtained from the central slice of a transgenic PC-3 tumor (270 mm^3). Vascular volume ranged from 0 to 126 μl g^{-1} and PSP from 0 to 3.4 μl g^{-1} min. Proton CSI spectra obtained from 1 mm × 1 mm × 4 mm voxels used to generate the total choline map are shown in (D), and the spectrum obtained from a single 1 mm × 1 mm × 4 mm voxel with large signals from total choline and lactate-lipid is shown in (E).

(see Fig. 4), the slope of $\Delta(1/T_1)$ ratios versus time in each pixel is used to compute PS (Fig. 15B), whereas the *y*-intercept is used to compute vascular volume (Fig. 15A). Thus vascular volumes are corrected for permeability of the vessels. Blood T_1 is obtained from a sample withdrawn from the inferior vena cava in terminal experiments, or the tail vein when not sacrificing the animal. A special microcoil can be used to determine T_1 of 20-μl blood samples (two drops of blood) at 4.7 T, the magnetic field used for all the *in vivo* studies presented here. Because blood T_1 can be determined from a couple of drops of blood from the tail vein without sacrificing the animal, it allows us to perform longitudinal measurements of vascular volume and permeability in the same animal. We can also use an *in vivo* tail coil that allows us to obtain blood T_1 s by using voxels localized on a tail vein blood vessel (Pathak *et al.*, 2003). T_1 maps of the tail are acquired with short TE spin-echo imaging with saturation recovery preparation and variable recovery delays. Acquisition parameters are typically TE = 5 ms, TR = 250 ms, RD = 50–200 ms, FOV = 4 mm, ST = 1 mm, matrix size = 64 × 40 for an in-plane resolution of 62.5 μm. This tail coil system has been validated with a flow phantom and provides reproducible T_1 measurements for flow rates of up to 0.5 cm s^{-1}, and its high in-plane resolution minimizes volume-averaging effects.

This approach of combined vascular and metabolic imaging can be extended to determining the relationship between any (three) colocalized parameters such as vascular volume, permeability, extracellular pH, total choline, or lactate-lipid. By displaying images for each parameter through a unique color channel (e.g., vascular volume as red, vascular permeability as green, and extracellular pH or choline or lactate as blue), it is feasible to visually inspect the interrelationship between these by fusing the color maps and determining the fractional volumes of the patterns for each tumor (Bhujwalla *et al.*, 2002a). Parametric maps of vascular volume, permeability, and pH_e can also be used to generate three-dimensional, volumetric histogram matrices (Bhujwalla *et al.*, 2002a). This display extends the conventional histogram plot to a volumetric histogram. Each voxel in the 3D display corresponds to an entry in a three-dimensional matrix of vascular volume, permeability, and pH_e. The intensity of color of the voxel represents the frequency of occurrence (histogram count) of the entry from the sampled data set. Although not presented here, these approaches of acquiring and analyzing multiparametric data can be extended to perform combined MR molecular and functional imaging to visualize molecular markers, and understand their role in tumor vascularization and metabolism.

In conclusion, with its enormous versatility, MR is certainly a method capable of effectively investigating a disease as complex as cancer. As with most methods, however, it is imperative to identify the questions most appropriate for the method. It is hoped that this chapter has succeeded in describing some of the current applications and advances of MR methods in functional and molecular imaging of cancer.

Acknowledgments

Work from the authors' program was supported through funding by NIH grants 2R01 CA73850, 1R01 CA90471, 1R01 CA82337, P20 CA86346, and P50 CA 103175.

References

Aboagye, E. O., and Bhujwalla, Z. M. (1999). Malignant transformation alters membrane choline phospholipid metabolism of human mammary epithelial cells. *Cancer Res.* **59**(1), 80–84.

Aboagye, E. O., Artemov, D., Senter, P. D., and Bhujwalla, Z. M. (1998). Intratumoral conversion of 5-fluorocytosine to 5-fluorouracil by monoclonal antibody-cytosine deaminase conjugates: Noninvasive detection of prodrug activation by magnetic resonance spectroscopy and spectroscopic imaging. *Cancer Res.* **58**(18), 4075–4078.

Abramovitch, R., Dafni, H., Smouha, E., Benjamin, L., and Neeman, M. (1999). *Cancer Res.* **59,** 5012.

Ackerstaff, E., Pflug, B. R., Nelson, J. B., and Bhujwalla, Z. M. (2001). *Cancer Res.* **61,** 3599.

Aguayo, J. B., Blackband, S. J., Schoeniger, J., Mattingly, M. A., and Hintermann, M. (1986). *Nature* **322,** 190.

Alger, J. R., and Shulman, R. G. (1984). *Q. Rev. Biophys.* **17,** 83.

Al-Saffar, N. M., Titley, J. C., Robertson, D., Clarke, P. A., Jackson, L. E., Leach, M. O., and Ronen, S. M. (2002). *Br. J. Cancer* **86,** 963.

Anderson, S. A., Rader, R. K., Westlin, W. F., Null, C., Jackson, D., Lanza, G. M., Wickline, S. A., and Kotyk, J. J. (2000). *Magn. Reson. Med.* **44,** 433.

Anderson-Berg, W. T., Strand, M., Lempert, T. E., Rosenbaum, A. E., and Joseph, P. M. (1986). *J. Nucl. Med.* **27,** 829.

Ardenkjaer-Larsen, J. H., Fridlund, B., Gram, A., Hansson, G., Hansson, L., Lerche, M. H., Servin, R., Thaning, M., and Golman, K. (2003). Increase in signal-to-noise ratio of > 10,000 times in liquid-state NMR. *Proc. Natl. Acad. Sci. USA* **100**(18), 10158–10163.

Aronen, H. J., Cohen, M. S., Belliveau, J. W., Fordham, J. A., and Rosen, B. R. (1993). *Top. Magn. Reson. Imaging* **5,** 14.

Aronen, H. J., Gazit, I. E., Louis, D. N., Buchbinder, B. R., Pardo, F. S., Weisskoff, R. M., Harsh, G. R., Cosgrove, G. R., Halpern, E. F., Hochberg, F. H., and Rosen, B. R. (1994). *Radiology* **191,** 41.

Artemov, D., Bhujwalla, Z. M., and Glickson, J. D. (1995). *Magn. Reson. Med.* **33,** 151.

Artemov, D., Bhujwalla, Z. M., Pilatus, U., and Glickson, J. D. (1998). *NMR Biomed.* **11,** 395.

Artemov, D., Mori, N., Ravi, R., and Bhujwalla, Z. M. (2003a). *Cancer Res.* **63,** 2723.

Artemov, D., Mori, N., Okollie, B., and Bhujwalla, Z. M. (2003b). *Magn. Reson. Med.* **49,** 403.

Auricchio, A., Zhou, R., Wilson, J. M., and Glickson, J. D. (2001). *Proc. Natl. Acad. Sci. USA* **98,** 5205.

Axel, L. (1980). *Radiology* **137,** 679.

Barba, I., Cabanas, M. E., and Arus, C. (1999). *Cancer Res.* **59,** 1861.

Bhakoo, K. K., Williams, S. R., Florian, C. L., Land, H., and Noble, M. D. (1996). *Cancer Res.* **56,** 4630.

Bhujwalla, Z. M., Tozer, G. M., Field, S. B., Maxwell, R. J., and Griffiths, J. R. (1990). *Radiother. Oncol.* **19,** 281.

Bhujwalla, Z. M., Constantinidis, I., Chatham, J. C., Wehrle, J. P., and Glickson, J. D. (1992). *Int. J. Radiat. Oncol. Biol. Phys.* **22,** 95.

Bhujwalla, Z. M., Shungu, D. C., Chatham, J. C., Wehrle, J. P., and Glickson, J. D. (1994). *Magn. Reson. Med.* **32,** 303.

Bhujwalla, Z. M., Shungu, D. C., and Glickson, J. D. (1996). *Magn. Reson. Med.* **36,** 204.

Bhujwalla, Z. M., Artemov, D., Natarajan, K., Ackerstaff, E., and Solaiyappan, M. (2000). *Neoplasia* **3,** 1.

Bhujwalla, Z. M., Artemov, D., Ballesteros, P., Cerdan, S., Gillies, R. J., and Solaiyappan, M. (2002a). *NMR Biomed.* **15,** 114.

Bhujwalla, Z. M., Artemov, D., and Solaiyappan, M. (2002b). Combined vascular and metabolic characterization of orthotopically implanted prostate cancer xenografts International Society for Magnetic Resonance in Medicine, Honolulu.

Bhujwalla, Z. M., Artemov, D., Natarajan, K., Solaiyappan, M., Kollars, P., and Kristjansen, P. E. (2003). *Clin. Cancer Res.* **9,** 355.

Black, R. D., Early, T. A., Roemer, P. B., Mueller, O. M., Mogro-Campero, A., Turner, L. G., and Johnson, G. A. (1993). *Science* **259,** 793.

Bloembergen, N. (1957). *J. Chem. Phys.* **27,** 572.

Bogdanov, A. A., Jr., Weissleder, R., Frank, H. W., Bogdanova, A. V., Nossif, N., Schaffer, B. K., Tsai, E., Papisov, M. I., and Brady, T. J. (1993). *Radiology* **187,** 701.

Bogdanov, A., Jr., Matuszewski, L., Bremer, C., Petrovsky, A., and Weissleder, R. (2002). *Mol. Imaging* **1,** 16.

Bouzier, A. K., Quesson, B., Valeins, H., Canioni, P., and Merle, M. (1999). *J. Neurochem.* **72,** 2445.

Boxerman, J. L., Hamberg, L. M., Rosen, B. R., and Weisskoff, R. M. (1995). *Magn. Reson. Med.* **34,** 555.

Brasch, R., Pham, C., Shames, D., *et al.* (1997). Assessing tumor angiogenesis using macromolecular MR imaging contrast media. *J. Magn. Reson. Imaging* **7,** 68–74.

Bryant, L. H., Jr., Brechbiel, M. W., Wu, C., Bulte, J. W., Herynek, V., and Frank, J. A. (1999). *J. Magn. Reson. Imaging* **9,** 348.

Bulte, J. W., Hoekstra, Y., Kamman, R. L., Magin, R. L., Webb, A. G., Briggs, R. W., Go, K. G., Hulstaert, C. E., Miltenyi, S., and The, T. H. (1992). *Magn. Reson. Med.* **25,** 148.

Bulte, J. W., Brooks, R. A., Moskowitz, B. M., Bryant, L. H., Jr., and Frank, J. A. (1999a). *Magn. Reson. Med.* **42,** 379.

Bulte, J. W., de Cuyper, M., Despres, D., and Frank, J. A. (1999b). *J. Magn. Reson. Imaging* **9,** 329.

Bulte, J. W., Douglas, T., Witwer, B., Zhang, S. C., Strable, E., Lewis, B. K., Zywicke, H. A., Miller, B., van Gelderen, P., Moskowitz, B. M., Duncan, I. D., and Frank, J. A. (2001). *Nat. Biotechnol.* **19,** 1141.

Callies, R., Sri-Pathmanathan, R. M., Ferguson, D. Y., and Brindle, K. M. (1993). *Magn. Reson. Med.* **29,** 546.

Caravan, P., Cloutier, N. J., Greenfield, M. T., McDermid, S. A., Dunham, S. U., Bulte, J. W., Amedio, J. C., Jr., Looby, R. J., Supkowski, R. M., Horrocks, W. D., Jr., McMurry, T. J., and Lauffer, R. B. (2002). *J. Am. Chem. Soc.* **124,** 3152.

Carmeliet, P., Dor, Y., Herbert, J. M., Fukumura, D., Brusselmans, K., Dewerchin, M., Neeman, M., Bono, F., Abramovitch, R., Maxwell, P., Koch, C. J., Ratcliffe, P., Moons, L., Jain, R. K., Collen, D., and Keshet, E. (1998). Role of HIF-1 in Hypoxia-mediated apoptosis, cell proliferation and tumor angiogenesis. *Nature* **394,** 485–490.

Cho, Z. H., Ahn, C. B., Juh, S. C., Ja, J. M., Friedenberg, R. M., Fraser, S. E., and Jacobs, R. E. (1990). *Philos. Trans. R. Soc. London* **333,** 469.

Constantinidis, I., Chatham, J. C., Wehrle, J. P., and Glickson, J. D. (1991). *Magn. Reson. Med.* **20,** 17.

Deane, B. R., and Lantos, P. L. (1981). *J. Neurolog. Sci.* **49,** 55.

de Certaines, J. D., Larsen, V. A., Podo, F., Carpinelli, G., Briot, O., and Henriksen, O. (1993). *NMR Biomed.* **6,** 345.

de Graaf, R. A., Luo, Y., Terpstra, M., and Garwood, M. (1995). *J. Magn. Reson. B* **109,** 184.

Denekamp, J. (1993). *J. Natl. Cancer Inst.* **85,** 935.

Dennie, J., Mandeville, J. B., Boxerman, J. L., Packard, S. D., Rosen, B. R., and Weisskoff, R. M. (1998). *Magn. Reson. Med.* **40,** 793.

Dixon, R. M. (1996). *Anticancer Res.* **16,** 1351.

Dodd, S. J., Williams, M., Suhan, J. P., Williams, D. S., Koretsky, A. P., and Ho, C. (1999). *Biophys. J.* **76,** 103.

Donahue, K. M., Weisskoff, R. M., Chesler, D. A., Kwong, K. K., Bogdanov, A. A., Mandeville, J. B., and Rosen, B. R. (1996). *Magn. Reson. Med.* **36,** 858.

Donahue, K. M., Krouwer, H. G. J., Rand, S. D., Pathak, A. P., Marzalkowski, C. S., Censky, S. C., and Prost, R. W. (2000). *Magn. Reson. Med.* **43,** 845.

Erecinska, M., and Silver, I. A. (1989). *J. Cereb. Blood Flow Metab.* **9,** 2.

Eroglu, S., Gimi, B., Roman, B., Friedman, G., and Magin, R. L. (2003). *Concepts Magn. Reson. Imaging Part. B Magn. Reson. Eng.* **17B,** 1.

Evanochko, W. T., Ng, T. C., and Glickson, J. D. (1984). *Magn. Reson. Med.* **1,** 508.

Evelhoch, J. L., Sapareto, S. A., Jick, D. E., and Ackerman, J. J. (1984). *Proc. Natl. Acad. Sci. USA* **81,** 6496.

Fisel, C. R., Ackerman, J. L., Buxton, R. B., Garrido, L., Belliveau, J. W., Rosen, R. B., and Brady, T. J. (1991). *Magn. Reson. Med.* **17,** 336.

Floridi, A., Paggi, M. G., Marcante, M. L., Silvestrini, B., Caputo, A., and De Martino, C. (1981). *J. Natl. Cancer Inst.* **66,** 497.

Furman-Haran, E., Margalit, R., Grobgeld, D., and Degani, H. (1996). *Proc. Natl. Acad. Sci. USA* **93,** 6247.

Gage, F. H. (2000). *Science* **287**(5457), 1433–1438.

Gallagher, F. A., Kettunen, M. I., Day, S. E., Hu, D. E., Ardenkjaer-Larsen, J. H., Zandt, R., Jensen, P. R., Karlsson, M., Golman, K., Lerche, M. H., and Brindle, K. M. (2008). Magnetic resonance imaging of pH *in vivo* using hyperpolarized 13C-labelled bicarbonate. *Nature* **453**(7197), 940–943.

Gillies, R. J., Ogino, T., Shulman, R. G., and Ward, D. C. (1982). *J. Cell Biol.* **95,** 24.

Gillies, R. J., Barry, J. A., and Ross, B. D. (1994a). *Magn. Reson. Med.* **32,** 310.

Gillies, R. J., Liu, Z., and Bhujwalla, Z. (1994b). *Am. J. Physiol.* **267,** C195.

Gillis, P., Roch, A., and Brooks, R. A. (1999). *J. Magn. Reson.* **137,** 402.

Gil, S., Zaderenzo, P., Cruz, F., Cerdan, S., and Ballesteros, P. (1994). *Bioorg. Med. Chem.* **2,** 305.

Gimi, B., Grant, S. C., Magin, R. L., Fienerman, A., Frolova, E., and Friedman, G. (2000). Experimental Nuclear Magnetic Resonance Conference.

Glover, P. M., Bowtell, R. W., Brown, G. D., and Mansfield, P. (1994). *Magn. Reson. Med.* **31,** 423.

Glunde, K., Ackerstaff, E., Natarajan, K., Artemov, D., and Bhujwalla, Z. M. (2002). *Magn. Reson. Med.* **48,** 819.

Goffeney, N., Bulte, J. W., Duyn, J., Bryant, L. H., Jr., and van Zijl, P. C. (2001). *J. Am. Chem. Soc.* **123,** 8628.

Gohr-Rosenthal, S., Schmitt-Willich, H., Ebert, W., and Conrad, J. (1993). *Invest. Radiol.* **28,** 789.

Grant, S. C., Buckley, D. L., Gibbs, S., Webb, A. G., and Blackband, S. J. (2001). *Magn. Reson. Med.* **46,** 1107.

Gribbestad, I. S., Petersen, S. B., Fjosne, H. E., Kvinnsland, S., and Krane, J. (1994). *NMR Biomed.* **7,** 181.

Gribbestad, I. S., Sitter, B., Lundgren, S., Krane, J., and Axelson, D. (1999). *Anticancer Res.* **19,** 1737.

Griffiths, J. R., Stevens, A. N., Iles, R. A., Gordon, R. E., and Shaw, D. (1981). *Biosci. Rep.* **1,** 319.

Guivel-Scharen, V., Sinnwell, T., Wolff, S. D., and Balaban, R. S. (1998). *J. Magn. Reson.* **133,** 36.

Guthridge, C. J., Stampfer, M. R., Clark, M. A., and Steiner, M. R. (1994). *Cancer Lett.* **86,** 11.

Hause, A., Frahm, J., Hanicke, W., and Mattaei, D. (1985). *Phys. Med. Biol.* **30,** 341.

Hawighorst, H., Knapstein, P. G., Weikel, W., Knopp, M. V., Zuna, I., Knof, A., Brix, G., Schaeffer, U., Wilkens, C., Schoenberg, S. O., Essig, M., Vaupel, P., *et al.* (1997). Angiogenesis of uterine cervical carcinoma: Characterization by pharmacokinetic magnetic resonance parameters and histological microvessel density with correlation to lymphatic involvement. *Cancer Res.* **57,** 4777–4786.

He, Q., Bhujwalla, Z. M., Maxwell, R. J., Griffiths, J. R., and Glickson, J. D. (1995a). *Magn. Reson. Med.* **33,** 414.

He, Q., Shungu, D. C., van Zijl, P. C., Bhujwalla, Z. M., and Glickson, J. D. (1995b). *J. Magn. Reson. B* **106,** 203.

Hinds, K. A., Hill, J. M., Shapiro, E. M., Laukkanen, M. O., Silva, A. C., Combs, C. A., Varney, T. R., Balaban, R. S., Koretsky, A. P., and Dunbar, C. E. (2003). *Blood* **102,** 867.

Holt, D. I., and Richards, R. E. (1976). *J. Magn. Res.* **94,** 71.

Hoult, D. I., and Lauterbur, P. C. (1979). *J. Magn. Res.* **34,** 425.

Howe, F. A., Maxwell, R. J., Saunders, D. E., Brown, M. M., and Griffiths, J. R. (1993). *Magn. Reson. Q* **9,** 31.

Howe, F. A., Barton, S. J., Cudlip, S. A., Stubbs, M., Saunders, D. E., Murphy, M., Wilkins, P., Opstad, K. S., Doyle, V. L., McLean, M. A., Bell, B. A., and Griffiths, J. R. (2003). *Magn. Reson. Med.* **49,** 223.

Hurd, R. E., and Freeman, D. (1991). *NMR Biomed.* **4,** 73.

Judenhofer, M. S., Wehrl, H. F., Newport, D. F., Catana, C., Siegel, S. B., Becker, M., Thielscher, A., Kneilling, M., Lichy, M. P., Eichner, M., Klingel, K., Reischl, G., *et al.* (2008). Simultaneous PET-MRI: a new approach for functional and morphological imaging. *Nat Med* **14**(4), 459–465.

Kallman, R. F. (1972). *Radiology* **105,** 135.

Kang, H. W., Josephson, L., Petrovsky, A., Weissleder, R., and Bogdanov, A., Jr. (2002). *Bioconjug. Chem.* **13,** 122.

Karczmar, G. S., Arbeit, J. M., Toy, B. J., Speder, A., and Weiner, M. W. (1992). *Cancer Res.* **52,** 71.

Katz-Brull, R., and Degani, H. (1996). *Anticancer Res.* **16,** 1375.

Kennan, R. P. (1994). *Magn. Reson. Med.* **31,** 9.

Kim, Y. R., Rebro, K. J., and Schmainda, K. M. (2002). *Magn. Reson. Med.* **47,** 1110.

Kobayashi, H., Kawamoto, S., Saga, T., Sato, N., Hiraga, A., Ishimori, T., Akita, Y., Mamede, M. H., Konishi, J., Togashi, K., and Brechbiel, M. W. (2001). *Magn. Reson. Med.* **46,** 795.

Koenig, S. H., and Brown, R. D., 3rd (1984). *Magn. Reson. Med.* **1,** 437.

Konda, S. D., Aref, M., Brechbiel, M., and Wiener, E. C. (2000). *Invest. Radiol.* **35,** 50.

Kurhanewicz, J., Vigneron, D. B., and Nelson, S. J. (2000). *Neoplasia* **2,** 166.

Lauffer, R. B. (1987). *Chem. Rev.* **87,** 901.

Leach, M. O., Verrill, M., Glaholm, J., Smith, T. A., Collins, D. J., Payne, G. S., Sharp, J. C., Ronen, S. M., McCready, V. R., Powles, T. J., and Smith, I. E. (1998). *NMR Biomed.* **11,** 314.

Lee, S. C., Kim, K., Kim, J., Lee, S., Han Yi, J., Kim, S. W., Ha, K. S., and Cheong, C. (2001). *J. Magn. Reson.* **150,** 207.

Li, S. J., Wehrle, J. P., Rajan, S. S., Steen, R. G., Glickson, J. D., and Hilton, J. (1988). *Cancer Res.* **48,** 4736.

Li, X., Lu, Y., Pirzkall, A., McKnight, T., and Nelson, S. J. (2002). *J. Magn. Reson. Imaging* **16,** 229.

Louie, A. Y., Huber, M. M., Ahrens, E. T., Rothbacher, U., Moats, R., Jacobs, R. E., Fraser, S. E., and Meade, T. J. (2000). *Nat. Biotechnol.* **18,** 321.

Maeda, M., Itoh, S., Kimura, H., Iwasaki, T., Hayashi, N., Yamamoto, K., Ishii, Y., and Kubota, T. (1993). *Radiology* **189,** 233.

Manganas, L. N., Zhang, X., Li, Y., Hazel, R. D., Smith, S. D., Wagshul, M. E., Henn, F., Benveniste, H., Djuric, P. M., Enikolopov, G., and Maletic-Savatic, M. (2007). Magnetic resonance spectroscopy identifies neural progenitor cells in the live human brain. *Science* **318**(5852), 980–985.

Massin, C., Boero, G., Vincent, F., Abenhaim, J., Besse, P. A., and Popovic, R. S. (2002). *Sens. Actuators A Phys.* **97,** 280.

Massin, C., Eroglu, S., Vincent, F., Gimi, B. S., Besse, P. A., Magin, R. L., and Popovic, R. S. (2003). *Transducers* 967.

Matsumura, A., Shibata, Y., Nakagawa, K., and Nose, T. (1994). MRI contrast enhancement by Gd-DTPA-monoclonal antibody in 9L glioma rats. *Acta Neurochir Suppl (Wien)* **60,** 356–358.

McGovern, K. A., Schoeniger, J. S., Wehrle, J. P., Ng, C. E., and Glickson, J. D. (1993). *Magn. Reson. Med.* **29,** 196.

Minard, K. R., and Wind, R. A. (2002). *J. Magn. Reson.* **154,** 336.

Moller, H. E., Chen, X. J., Saam, B., Hagspiel, K. D., Johnson, G. A., Altes, T. A., de Lange, E. E., and Kauczor, H. U. (2002). *Magn. Reson. Med.* **47,** 1029.

Moon, R. B., and Richards, J. H. (1973). *J. Biol. Chem.* **248,** 7276.

Mori, S., van Zijl, P. C., and Shortle, D. (1997). *Proteins* **28,** 325.

Moulder, J. E., and Rockwell, S. (1984). *Int. J. Radiat. Oncol. Biol. Phys.* **10,** 695.

Natarajan, K., Mori, N., Artemov, D., and Bhujwalla, Z. M. (2002). *Neoplasia* **4,** 409.

Negendank, W. (1992). *NMR Biomed.* **5,** 303.

Nielsen, F. U., Daugaard, P., Bentzen, L., Stodkilde-Jorgensen, H., Overgaard, J., Horsman, M. R., and Maxwell, R. J. (2001). *Cancer Res.* **61,** 5318.

Noh, D. Y., Ahn, S. J., Lee, R. A., Park, I. A., Kim, J. H., Suh, P. G., Ryu, S. H., Lee, K. H., and Han, J. S. (2000). *Cancer Lett.* **161,** 207.

Ogan, M. D., Schmiedl, U., Mosley, M. E., Grodd, W., Paajanen, H., and Brasch, R. C. (1987). *Invest. Radiol.* **22,** 665.

Ogawa, S. (1990). *Magn. Reson. Med.* **14,** 68.

Ohno, K., Pettigrew, K. D., and Rapoport, S. I. (1979). *Stroke* **10,** 62.

Okunieff, P. G., Koutcher, J. A., Gerweck, L., McFarland, E., Hitzig, B., Urano, M., Brady, T., Neuringer, L., and Suit, H. D. (1986). *Int. J. Radiat. Oncol. Biol. Phys.* **12,** 793.

Okunieff, P., Kallinowski, F., Vaupel, P., and Neuringer, L. J. (1988). *J. Natl. Cancer Inst.* **80,** 745.

Okunieff, P., Vaupel, P., Sedlacek, R., and Neuringer, L. J. (1989). *Int. J. Radiat. Oncol. Biol. Phys.* **16,** 1493.

Olson, D. L., Peck, T. L., Webb, A. G., Magin, R. L., and Sweedler, J. V. (1995). *Science* **270,** 1967.

Ostergaard, L., Weisskoff, R. M., Chesler, D. A., Gyldensted, C., and Rosen, B. R. (1996). *Magn. Reson. Med.* **36,** 715.

Pathak, A. P., Schmainda, K. M., Ward, B. D., Linderman, J. R., Rebro, K. J., and Greene, A. S. (2001). *Magn. Reson. Med.* **46,** 735.

Pathak, A. P., Rand, S. D., and Schmainda, K. M. (2003). *J. Magn. Reson. Imaging* **18,** 397.

Pathak, A. P., Artemov, D., and Brujwalla, Z. M. (2004). *Mag. Reson. Med.* **51,** 612.

Patlak, C. S., Blasberg, R. G., and Fenstermacher, J. D. (1983). *J. Cereb. Blood Flow Metab.* **3,** 1.

Peck, T. L., Magin, R. L., and Lauterbur, P. C. (1995). *J. Magn. Reson.* **108,** 114.

Pilatus, U., Ackerstaff, E., Artemov, D., Mori, N., Gillies, R. J., and Bhujwalla, Z. M. (2000). *Neoplasia* **2,** 273.

Podo, F. (1999). *NMR Biomed.* **12,** 413.

Pruessmann, K. P., Weiger, M., Scheidegger, M. B., and Boesiger, P. (1999). *Magn. Reson. Med.* **42,** 952.

Ramirez de Molina, A., Gutierrez, R., Ramos, M. A., Silva, J. M., Silva, J., Bonilla, F., Sanchez, J. J., and Lacal, J. C. (2002a). *Oncogene* **21,** 4317.

Ramirez de Molina, A., Rodriguez-Gonzalez, A., Gutierrez, R., Martinez-Pineiro, L., Sanchez, J., Bonilla, F., Rosell, R., and Lacal, J. (2002b). *Biochem. Biophys. Res. Commun.* **296,** 580.

Roberts, H. C., Roberts, T. P., Brasch, R. C., and Dillon, W. P. (2000). *AJNR* **21,** 891.

Roemer, P. B., Edelstein, W. A., Hayes, C. E., Souza, S. P., and Mueller, O. M. (1990). *Magn. Reson. Med.* **16,** 192.

Rofstad, E. K., and Sutherland, R. M. (1988). *Int. J. Radiat. Oncol. Biol. Phys.* **15,** 921.

Rofstad, E. K., DeMuth, P., Fenton, B. M., and Sutherland, R. M. (1988). *Cancer Res.* **48,** 5440.

Ronen, S. M., and Degani, H. (1992). *Magn. Reson. Med.* **25,** 384.

Ronen, S. M., Volk, A., and Mispelter, J. (1994). *NMR Biomed.* **7,** 278.

Ronen, S. M., Jackson, L. E., Beloueche, M., and Leach, M. O. (2001). *Br. J. Cancer* **84,** 691.

Rosen, B. R., Belliveau, J. W., Buchbinder, B. R., McKinstry, R. C., Porkka, L. M., Kennedy, D. N., Neuder, M. S., Fisel, C. R., Aronen, H. J., Kwong, K. K., Weisskoff, R. M., Cohen, M. S., and Brady, T. J. (1991). Contrast agents and cerebral hemodynamics. *Mag. Reson. Med.* **19,** 285–292.

Schaff, A., and Veeman, W. S. (1997). *J. Magn. Reson.* **126,** 200.

Schmiedl, U., Ogan, M., Paajanen, H., Marotti, M., Crooks, L. E., Brito, A. C., and Brasch, R. C. (1987). *Radiology* **162,** 205.

Schupp, D. G., Merkle, H., Ellermann, J. M., Ke, Y., and Garwood, M. (1993). *Magn. Reson. Med.* **30,** 18.

Schwarzbauer, C., Syha, J., and Haase, A. (1993). *Magn. Reson. Med.* **29,** 709.

Seeber, D. A., Cooper, R. L., Ciobanu, L., and Pennington, C. H. (2001). *Rev. Sci. Instrum.* **72,** 2171.

Shahbazi-Gahrouei, D., Williams, M., Rizvi, S., and Allen, B. J. (2001). *J. Magn. Reson. Imaging* **14,** 169.

Shungu, D. C., and Glickson, J. D. (1994). *Magn. Reson. Med.* **32,** 277.

Sidles, J. A., and Rugar, D. (1993). *Phys. Rev. Lett.* **70,** 3506.

Silva, A. C., Zhang, W., Williams, D. S., and Koretsky, A. P. (1995). *Magn. Reson. Med.* **33,** 209.

Silva, A. C., Kim, S. G., and Garwood, M. (2000). *Magn. Reson. Med.* **44,** 169.

Silver, X., Ni, W. X., Mercer, E. V., Beck, B. L., Bossart, E. L., Inglis, B., and Mareci, T. H. (2001). *Magn. Reson. Med.* **46,** 1216.

Singer, S., Souza, K., and Thilly, W. G. (1995). *Cancer Res.* **55,** 5140.

Sipkins, D. A., Cheresh, D. A., Kazemi, M. R., Nevin, L. M., Bednarski, M. D., and Li, K. C. (1998). *Nat. Med.* **4,** 623.

Snoussi, K., Bulte, J. W., Gueron, M., and van Zijl, P. C. (2003). *Magn. Reson. Med.* **49,** 998.

Sodickson, D. K., and Manning, W. J. (1997). *Magn. Reson. Med.* **38,** 591.

Sodickson, D. K., and McKenzie, C. A. (2001). *Med. Phys.* **28,** 1629.

Sodickson, D. K., McKenzie, C. A., Ohliger, M. A., Yeh, E. N., and Price, M. D. (2002). *Magma* **13,** 158.

Solomon, I. (1955). *Phys. Rev.* **99,** 559.

Sotak, C. H. (1988). *Magn. Reson. Med.* **7,** 364.

Star-Lack, J., Nelson, S. J., Kurhanewicz, J., Huang, L. R., and Vigneron, D. B. (1997). *Magn. Reson. Med.* **38,** 311.

Stegman, L. D., Rehemtulla, A., Beattie, B., Kievit, E., Lawrence, T. S., Blasberg, R. G., Tjuvajev, J. G., and Ross, B. D. (1999). *Proc. Natl. Acad. Sci. USA* **96,** 9821.

Sterin, M., Cohen, J. S., Mardor, Y., Berman, E., and Ringel, I. (2001). *Cancer Res.* **61,** 7536.

Stolfi, R. L., Colofiore, J. R., Nord, L. D., Koutcher, J. A., and Martin, D. S. (1992). *Cancer. Res.* **52,** 4074.

Strable, E., Bulte, J. W., Moskowitz, B. M., Vivekanandan, K., Allen, M., and Douglas, T. (2001). *Chem. Mater.* **13,** 2201.

Stubbs, M., Bhujwalla, Z. M., Tozer, G. M., Rodrigues, L. M., Maxwell, R. J., Morgan, R., Howe, F. A., and Griffiths, J. R. (1992). *NMR Biomed.* **5,** 351.

Subramanian, R., and Webb, A. G. (1998). *Anal. Chem.* **70,** 2454.

Subramanian, R., Lam, M. M., and Webb, A. G. (1998). *J. Magn. Reson.* **133,** 227.

Terpstra, M., High, W. B., Luo, Y., de Graaf, R. A., Merkle, H., and Garwood, M. (1996). *NMR Biomed.* **9,** 185.

Thompson, H. K. J., Starmer, C. F., Whalen, R. E., and McIntosh, H. D. (1964). *Circ. Res.* **14,** 502.

Tkac, I., Starcuk, Z., Choi, I. Y., and Gruetter, R. (1999). *Magn. Reson. Med.* **41,** 649.

Tofts, P. S. (1997). *J. Magn. Reson. Imaging* **7,** 91.

Tofts, P. S., Brix, G., Buckley, D. L., Evelhoch, J. L., Henderson, E., Knopp, M. V., Larsson, H. B., Lee, T. Y., Mayr, N. A., Parker, G. J., Port, R. E., Taylor, J., and Weisskoff, R. M. (1999). *J. Magn. Reson. Imaging* **10,** 223.

Tozer, G. M., and Griffiths, J. R. (1992). *NMR Biomed.* **5,** 279.

Tozer, G. M., Maxwell, R. J., Griffiths, J. R., and Pham, P. (1990). *Br. J. Cancer* **62,** 553.

Trivedi, B., and Danforth, W. H. (1966). *J. Biol. Chem.* **241,** 4110.

Trumbull, J. D., Glasgow, I. K., Beebe, D. J., and Magin, R. L. (2000). *IEEE Trans. Biomed. Eng.* **47,** 3.

Unger, E. C., Totty, W. G., Neufeld, D. M., Otsuka, F. L., Murphy, W. A., Welch, M. S., Connett, J. M., and Philpott, G. W. (1985). *Invest. Radiol.* **20,** 693.

van Sluis, R., Bhujwalla, Z. M., Raghunand, N., Ballesteros, P., Alvarez, J., Cerdan, S., Galons, J. P., and Gillies, R. J. (1999). *Magn. Reson. Med.* **41,** 743.

van Zijl, P. C., Chesnick, A. S., DesPres, D., Moonen, C. T., Ruiz-Cabello, J., and van Gelderen, P. (1993). *Magn. Reson. Med.* **30,** 544.

Vaupel, P., Kallinowski, F., and Okunieff, P. (1989a). *Cancer. Res.* **49,** 6449.

Vaupel, P., Okunieff, P., Kallinowski, F., and Neuringer, L. J. (1989b). *Radiat. Res.* **120,** 477.

Villringer, A., Rosen, B. R., Belliveau, J. W., Ackerman, J. L., Lauffer, R. B., Buxton, R. B., Chao, Y. S., Wedeen, V. J., and Brady, T. J. (1988). *Magn. Reson. Med.* **6,** 164.

Ward, K. M., Aletras, A. H., and Balaban, R. S. (2000). *J. Magn. Reson.* **143,** 79.

Webb, A. G. (1997). *Prog. Nucl. Mag. Reson. Spectrosc.* **31,** 1.

Weisskoff, R. M. (1993). *Magn. Reson. Med.* **29,** 553.

Weisskoff, R. M., Zuo, C. S., Boxerman, J. L., and Rosen, B. R. (1994). *Magn. Reson. Med.* **31,** 601.

Weissleder, R., Lee, A. S., Fischman, A. J., Reimer, P., Shen, T., Wilkinson, R., Callahan, R. J., and Brady, T. J. (1991). *Radiology* **181,** 245.

Weissleder, R., Cheng, H. C., Bogdanova, A., and Bogdanov, A. (1997). *J. Magn. Reson. Imaging* **7,** 258.

Weissleder, R., Moore, A., Mahmood, U., Bhorade, R., Benveniste, H., Chiocca, E. A., and Basilion, J. P. (2000). *Nat. Med.* **6,** 351.

Wind, R. A., Minard, K. R., Holtom, G. R., Majors, P. D., Ackerman, E. J., Colson, S. D., Cory, D. G., Daly, D. S., Ellis, P. D., Metting, N. F., Parkinson, C. I., Price, J. M., *et al.* (2000). An integrated confocal and magnetic resonance microscope for cellular research. *J. Magn. Reson.* **147**(2), 371–377.

Winter, P. M., Caruthers, S. D., Yu, X., Song, S. K., Chen, J., Miller, B., Bulte, J. W., Robertson, J. D., Gaffney, P. J., Wickline, S. A., and Lanza, G. M. (2003). *Magn. Reson. Med.* **50,** 411.

Wright, S. M., Magin, R. L., and Kelton, J. R. (1991). *Magn. Reson. Med.* **17,** 252.

Yablonskiy, D. A. (1994). *Magn. Reson. Med.* **32,** 749.

Zabow, G., Dodd, S., Moreland, J., and Koretsky, A. (2008). *Nature* **453**(7198), 1058–1063.

Zhang, S., Winter, P., Wu, K., and Sherry, A. D. (2001). *J. Am. Chem. Soc.* **123,** 1517.

Zhao, M., Beauregard, D. A., Loizou, L., Davletov, B., and Brindle, K. M. (2001). *Nat. Med.* **7,** 1241.
Zhou, J., Payen, J. F., Wilson, D. A., Traystman, R. J., and van Zijl, P. C. (2003). *Nat. Med.* **9,** 1085.
Zierler, K. L. (1962). *Circ. Res.* **10,** 393.
Zotev, V. S., Matlashov, A. N., Volegov, P. L., Savukov, I. M., Espy, M. A., Mosher, J. C., Gomez, J. J., and Kraus, R. H., Jr. (2008). Microtesla MRI of the human brain combined with MEG. *J Magn. Reson.* **194**(1), 115–120.

CHAPTER 11

A Modified Transorbital Baboon Model of Reperfused Stroke

Anthony L. D'Ambrosio,* Michael E. Sughrue,* J. Mocco,† William J. Mack,* Ryan G. King,* Shivani Agarwal,* and E. Sander Connolly, Jr.*

*Department of Neurological Surgery
Columbia University
New York, New York 10032-2699

†University of Florida
Gainesville
FL 32610-0261

I. Update
II. Introduction
 A. Animal Models of Stroke
 B. Primate Models
III. Preoperative Care
 A. Obtaining Animals and Supplies
 B. Anesthesia and Preparation
 C. Physiologic Monitoring
IV. Operative Technique
 A. Positioning
 B. Placement of ICP Monitor and Laser Doppler Probe
 C. Transorbital Approach
 D. Vessel Occlusion
V. Postoperative Care
 A. Postoperative Monitoring
 B. Criteria for Sacrifice
VI. Data Collection and Analysis
 A. Neurologic Evaluation
 B. Radiographic Imaging
 C. Infarct Volume

DOI: 10.1016/B978-0-12-375043-3.00011-1

VII. Model Application: HuEP5C7
VIII. Conclusion
References

I. Update

Stroke unfortunately remains one of the leading causes of mortality and the leading cause of morbidity in the United States. The development of an effective neuroprotective strategy depends on the successful translation of candidate interventions from animal models to humans. Rodent models of focal cerebral ischemia are the most commonly used method toward this goal; however, a number of agents with proven efficacy in these models have not produced comparable results when translated into humans. As a result, there is still significant interest in nonhuman primate models, which convey significant anatomic and physiologic homologies to the human brain and are better suited to provide clinically relevant functional outcome measurements.

We previously highlighted the application of our modified transorbital baboon model of reperfused stroke in investigated HuEP5C7, which competitively binds E-selectin and P-selectin. Since publication of this manuscript, we would like to highlight two further applications of our model. First, by combining our primate stroke model with advanced magnetic resonance spectroscopy we were able to demonstrate prominent lactate resonances and attenuated *N*-acetylaspartate peaks in the infracted hemisphere at 3 days postischemia. Furthermore, mean area under the curve from lactate spectra had a negative correlation with functional outcome, whereas *N*-acetylaspartate showed a positive correlation. These results suggest that the evaluation of these peaks may play a role in outcome prediction following cerebral infarction in higher primates (Coon *et al.*, 2006). Second, after demonstrating significant neuroprotection with sLe^{x}-glycosylated complement inhibitory protein in a murine model we evaluated this agent in our primate model of stroke (Ducruet *et al.*, 2007). The experiment was terminated prematurely following an interim analysis demonstrating greater infarct volume in the treated animals as well as a significant hypotensive response in those animals. This study highlights the importance of preclinical nonhuman primate studies, which more accurately mimic the human condition.

Although much controversy has surrounded the use of nonhuman primates in experimental laboratory work, these models remain a critical component in the preclinical evaluation of putative neuroprotectants.

II. Introduction

Stroke is the third leading cause of death in the United States, with 750,000 deaths per year, a number exceeded only by the millions of people who are left permanently debilitated or institutionalized by the disease (Bravata *et al.*, 2003).

Extensive research efforts have been undertaken in the realm of therapeutics to reduce the immense morbidity and mortality associated with this devastating disease.

Acute stroke can be subdivided into two categories: ischemic and hemorrhagic. Acute cerebral ischemia is far more common and can occur via atherosclerotic plaque rupture or vessel occlusion secondary to an embolus (Wraige *et al.*, 2003). This acute event results in an ischemic core, where tissue damage is permanent and irreversible, and a surrounding region called the penumbra (Bonaffini *et al.*, 2002; Pestalozza *et al.*, 2002). Tissues in the penumbra are believed to remain viable and could be salvaged if the appropriate measures are implemented in a timely fashion. Recent research has implicated several detrimental event cascades that are set in motion after an acute ischemic event, including leukocyte infiltration, upregulation of inflammatory mediators, platelet activation, complement upregulation, free radicals, apoptosis, and microvascular failure (Heiss, 2002). The implication of these multiple event cascades in cerebral ischemia has given researchers several promising targets for the development of novel neuroprotective strategies.

Unfortunately, although more than 49 neuroprotective agents have been tested recently in approximately 114 stroke trials, none has shown efficacy (Gladstone *et al.*, 2002). Although many of these novel agents demonstrated significant neuroprotection in preclinical rodent trials, few were tested in nonhuman primate models of cerebral ischemia. Many investigators believe that this repeated failure of promising neuroprotective agents to demonstrate efficacy in clinical trails is rooted, at least in part, in species-specific differences in anatomy, physiology, and specific responses to ischemic injury between the rodent and the human (DeGraba and Pettigrew, 2000).

A. Animal Models of Stroke

Rodent models are the most commonly used animal models of cerebral ischemia used in preclinical testing today. Across laboratories, rodent models have considerable variation in terms of technique, species, methods of anesthesia, and duration of ischemia. Earlier models of cerebral ischemia in the rat utilized permanent middle cerebral artery occlusion (MCAo) via a craniotomy (Chen *et al.*, 1986). However, as we gained a better understanding of the critical role played by reperfusion injury and progressive microvascular failure in the pathophysiology of cerebral ischemia, many investigators moved away from models of permanent ischemia and developed reperfusion models that are believed to be more physiologic.

The most commonly used model of ischemia-reperfusion (I-R) injury involves insertion of a silicon-coated suture into the internal carotid artery and advancing it intracranially to occlude MCA blood flow (Longa *et al.*, 1989). The suture is subsequently removed to allow for cerebral reperfusion. More recently, models of embolic cerebral ischemia are rapidly gaining favor. Embolic models involve the injection of an autologous clot into the MCA via an intracarotid catheter (Zhang *et al.*, 1997a,b). Other less utilized models include photothrombotic models (Wester *et al.*, 1995) and vessel occlusion using macrospheres (Gerriets *et al.*, 2003).

B. Primate Models

A variety of large animals, including dogs (Brenowitz and Yonas, 1990) and rabbits, (Yenari *et al.*, 1997) have been utilized in several models of focal cerebral ischemia. However, nonhuman primate models provide the closest representation of human pathophysiology by reducing neuroanatomic variability and physiologic responses to ischemic insult (Lake *et al.*, 1990; Meyer *et al.*, 1980). Furthermore, the primary endpoint of most clinical stroke trials is improvement of functional outcome. Primate behavior is more complex, and as a consequence, functional deficits are more similar to those seen in humans. For this reason, outcome measures are more comparable and improvements in outcome are more clinically applicable.

In an effort to address these issues, we developed a model of reperfused nonhuman primate stroke that utilized, via a transorbital approach, unilateral internal carotid artery (ICA) and bilateral anterior cerebral artery (ACA) occlusion (Huang *et al.*, 2000a). We describe specific details of our model, including several refinements made over a 5-year experience with primate reperfused stroke.

III. Preoperative Care

A. Obtaining Animals and Supplies

Test subjects are young adult male baboons, *Papio anubis*, weighing 14–23 kg (Buckshire Farms, Perkasie, PA). Animals are individually housed in stainless steel cages and uniquely identified with a body tattoo and a cage card. Upon arrival, each subject is thoroughly assessed as per our standard Institutional Review Board (IRB) protocol by the animal care team. All animals are acclimated to laboratory conditions for a minimum of 45 days prior to study initiation.

Preparing for a transorbital procedure can be an involved process. This requires advance planning to coordinate staff to provide anesthesia support, procurement of appropriate supplies (Fig. 1), use of MRI facilities, and 24-h care overnight following the procedure.

B. Anesthesia and Preparation

On the morning of surgery, the study animal is brought into a preoperative holding area and anesthetized with ketamine (Fort Dodge Animal Health, Ft. Dodge, IA) at an intramuscular (IM) dose of 5 mg/kg. The head, neck, forearm, and femoral regions are shaved with an electric clipper. Two 18- or 20-gauge peripheral intravenous (IV) catheters are placed, and 0.9% normal saline (NS) is

Materials and suppliers

Medications	Supplier
Ketamine HCl	Fort dodge animal health
Propofol	Zeneca pharmaceutical
0.5% isoflurane	Baxter
Balanced nitrous oxide	Tech air
Fentanyl	Elkins-Sinn
Cefazolin	Bristol/Meyers squibb
Vecuronium	Organon
Midazolam	Roche
Phenylephrine hydrochloride	Gensia laboratories
Lidocaine with epinephrine 1: 1,00,000	Abbott laboratories
Pentobarbital	Veterinary laboratories
Mannitol	AmVet

Anesthesia equipment	Supplier
Ohmeda 7000 ventilator	Ohmeda
Arterial blood pressure monitor	Datascope
Femoral vein catheter	Arrow international
Transurethral foley catheter	Baxter
Esophageal probe	Datascope
Parenchymal sensor	Neuromonitor, codman
Laser doppler probe (model PF2B)	Perimed, inc.

Surgical supplies	Supplier
Adjustable stereotactic frame	Stoelting
Hand-held twist drill	Neurocare
Self-retaining lid retractor	Codman
Bipolar electrocautery	Valley forge scientific
Operating microscope	Model F170, zeiss
High-speed pneumatic drill/diamond bit	Midas rex
3 micro-yasargil aneurysm clip	Aesculap
18-gauge needles	Becton-Dickinson
10, 11, and 15 scalpel blades	Henry-Schein
Gel foam	Pharmacia and Upjohn
Radiolucent methylmethacrylate	Codman cranioplastic, J&J

Pathology supplies	Supplier
2% 2,3,5-triphenyltetrazolium in 0.9% PBS	Sigma

Fig. 1 Comprehensive list of materials and manufacturers.

started. Propofol (Zeneca Pharmaceutical, Macclesfield, UK) is then given as a bolus infusion prior to oropharyngeal intubation using a size six or seven endotracheal tube. The animal is then transported to the operating room where assisted ventilation is initiated (Ohmeda 7000 ventilator) with an inhalation mixture composed of 0.5% isoflurane (Baxter, Deerfield, IL) and balanced nitrous oxide (Tech Air, West Plains, NY) and oxygen. In anticipation of the placement of additional monitoring devices, an IV bolus infusion of fentanyl (Elkins-Sinn, Cherry Hill, NJ) at 50 μg/kg is administered, followed by a continuous fentanyl infusion of 50 to 70 μg/kg/hr. The concentration of isoflurane in the inhalation anesthetic agent is maintained between 0% and 0.6%. IV cefazolin (Bristol/ Meyers Squibb, New York, NY) is administered as prophylaxis and continued for 48 h postoperatively.

Before final positioning in the head frame (Stoelting, Wooddale, IL), a continuous IV infusion of vecuronium (Organon, Roseland, NJ) is started at 0.04 mg/kg/h. Additionally, a 0.1 mg/kg IV bolus of midazolam (Roche, Indianapolis, IN) is given every 30 min. Once the transorbital approach has begun, the fentanyl infusion rate is increased to 70–100 μg/kg/h, while the isoflurane rate is decreased to $<0.5\%$.

C. Physiologic Monitoring

An intra-arterial catheter is introduced into the femoral artery for continuous systemic blood pressure monitoring to facilitate multiple specimen collections. Blood pressure is monitored (Datascope, Paramus, NJ) to maintain a mean arterial pressure (MAP) of 60–80 mm Hg. Hypotensive episodes can be treated with injections of phenylephrine hydrochloride (Gensia Laboratories, Irvine, CA). Central venous pressure (CVP) is monitored using a femoral vein catheter (Arrow International, Reading, PA) and sustained at 5 ± 2 mm Hg. An indwelling, transurethral Foley catheter (Baxter, Deerfield, IL) allows accurate urine output monitoring to guide management of fluid balance and CVP.

Arterial blood gas (ABG) analysis is performed at regular intervals (Stat profile 3, Nova Biomedical, Waltham, MA) while the respiratory rate and tidal volume are continuously adjusted to maintain a carbon dioxide pressure (P_{CO_2}) between 35 and 40 mm Hg. Continuous core body temperature is monitored using an esophageal probe (Datascope, Montvale, NJ). Continuous intracranial pressure (ICP) monitoring is accomplished with a parenchymal sensor (Neuromonitor, Codman, Piscataway, NJ). Sustained ICP of >20 mm Hg for >5 min is treated with a bolus administration of IV mannitol at 0.5 g/kg.

Before intubation and the administration of anesthesia, baseline complete peripheral blood cell counts are performed. Systemic blood pressure, CVP, cerebral perfusion pressure (CPP), and core body temperature are maintained at constant levels throughout the procedure and for the first 24 h postoperatively. During ischemia, ventilation is adjusted to maintain a P_{CO_2} similar to those at baseline (Huang *et al.*, 2000a).

IV. Operative Technique

A. Positioning

After the insertion of all indwelling catheters and before the placement of the ICP monitor and the laser Doppler probe, the animal is positioned prone, in an adjustable stereotactic frame, with two-point head fixation via the external auditory canals. The cranial base is positioned parallel to the floor, with the anterior skull base elevated approximately 15° and turned slightly to the right. Dependent pressure points are adequately padded to prevent tissue necrosis.

B. Placement of ICP Monitor and Laser Doppler Probe

A left frontal approach via a paramedian linear skin incision and two burr holes is used for the insertion of an intraparenchymal ICP monitor and a straight laser Doppler probe (Model PF2B, Perimed, Inc., Piscataway, NJ). A hand-held twist drill (Neurocare, San Diego, CA) is used to create the burr holes. The dura is cauterized and sharply incised to allow passage of the fiberoptic pressure sensor and the laser Doppler probe. The laser Doppler probe is lowered to 10 mm below the inner table of the calvarium into the cortex. The probe is immobilized with a plastic burr hole cover and secured to the cranium with contact cement. The skin incision is closed with 3–0 interrupted nylon sutures. Intraoperative measurements of ICP and local cerebral blood flow (CBF) are continually recorded throughout the procedure.

C. Transorbital Approach

Infiltration of the medial and lateral canthi of the left orbit with 0.5% lidocaine with epinephrine 1:100,000 (Abbott Laboratories, Abbott Park, IL) is performed before making an incision in the plane along the palpebral fissure. A selfretaining lid retractor is then placed. An 18-gauge needle is carefully inserted into the anterior and posterior chambers of the globe for aspiration of the vitreous and aqueous humors. Internally decompressing the globe in this manner allows it and the periorbital soft tissue to be circumferentially dissected from the walls of the orbit. The globe can be removed after transection of the optic nerve and ophthalmic artery. Care should be taken at this point to completely cauterize the ophthalmic artery to prevent unnecessary blood loss. The residual soft tissue is removed with bipolar cauterization and curettage.

The operating microscope (Model F170, Zeiss, Thornwood, NJ) is used for the remainder of the procedure. A high-speed pneumatic drill with a coarse diamond bit (Midas Rex, Fort Worth, TX) is used to remove the bone of the posteromedial orbit. The dura of the anterior cranial fossa is then incised with a No. 11 blade and the edges cauterized to reveal the anterior circle of Willis.

D. Vessel Occlusion

Microsurgical technique is used to identify the cerebral arteries and clear them from the surrounding arachnoid membrane. After reconfirmation of the stability of the physiologic variables, vessel occlusion is accomplished through the sequential placement of three micro-Yasargil (Aesculap, Center Valley, PA) aneurysm clips: (1) on the proximal segment of the left anterior cerebral artery, proximal to the anterior communicating artery (left A1), (2) on the proximal right anterior cerebral artery (right A1), and (3) across the left ICA at the level of the anterior choroidal artery so that the clip incorporates and occludes the anterior choroidal artery (left ICA). Aneurysm clip placement and operative exposure are illustrated in Fig. 2.

Previous model protocols utilized a test occlusion period to confirm ischemic cerebral blood flow using both motor evoked potential (MEP) monitoring and laser Doppler flowmetry. This test occlusion period lasted 5 min, followed by 15 min of reperfusion and then 60 min of permanent occlusion (Wintree *et al.*, 2003). After the 60-min occlusion period, the aneurysm clips were removed and the brain was allowed to reperfuse. This process is represented in Fig. 3A. In a currently submitted publication, we demonstrated excellent correlation between MEP dropout and laser Doppler flowmetry tracings during permanent occlusion (Wintree *et al.*, 2003). Because laser Doppler flowmetry (Fig. 3B) is a direct measure of CBF, we have since abandoned MEP monitoring and no longer utilize the 5-min test occlusion period. In recent trials, we have used permanent occlusion times of 60, 75, and 90 min and found the 75-min occlusion time to give the most reliable results (unpublished data).

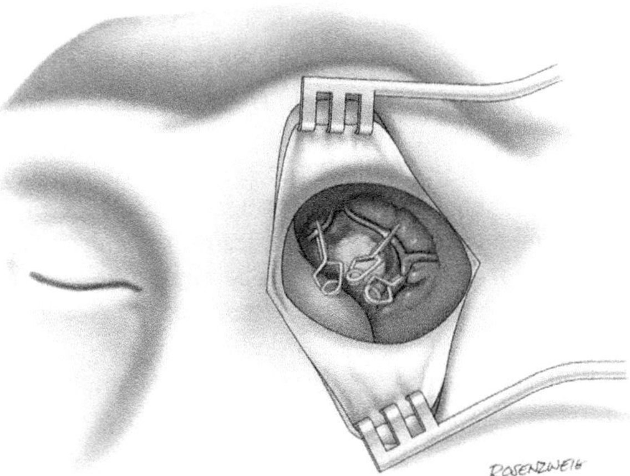

Fig. 2 Transorbital approach demonstrating placement of occlusive aneurysm clips on the internal carotid artery (ICA) and both anterior cerebral arteries (A1 segments). Reproduced with permission from Huang *et al.* (2000a,b).

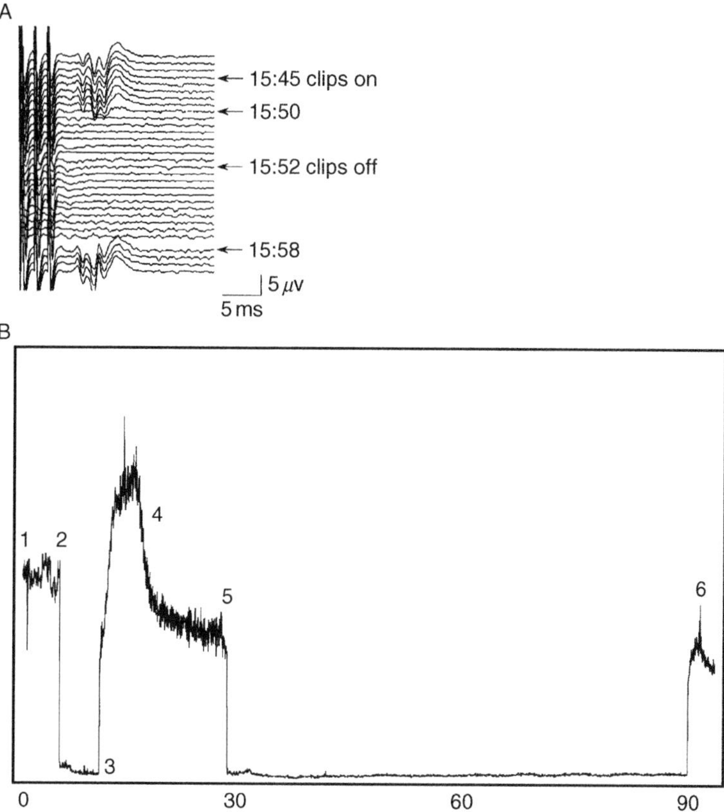

Fig. 3 (A) Representative motor evoked potential (MEP) tracing demonstrating electrophysiologic evidence of cerebral blood flow decrement and restoration with clip placement and removal, respectively. Reproduced with permission from Huang *et al.* (2000a,b). (B) Representative tracing of laser Doppler dropout following middle cerebral artery (MCA) territory occlusion. Time point 1 represents baseline cerebral blood flow (CBF). Time point 2 marks the beginning of a 5-min test occlusion period. Time point 3 represents a 15-min reperfusion period after the three temporary clips have been removed. Time point 4 demonstrates a brief period of hyperperfusion after the test occlusion period. Time point 5 represents the beginning of a 60-min permanent occlusion period. Note the immediate drop-off of CBF signal. Time point 6 represents the final removal of all three aneurysm clips and the reconstitution of CBF. Modified with permission from Wintree *et al.* (2003).

After 75 min of occlusion, the clips are removed in reverse order to permit reperfusion. A layer of gel foam (Pharmacia and Upjohn, Kalamazoo, MI) is placed over the dural defect, and the retractor is removed. Radiolucent methylmethacrylate (Codman Cranioplastic, Johnson & Johnson, Piscataway, NJ) is used to fill the orbital defect, and the eyelid is sutured closed with a running 3–0 nylon suture.

V. Postoperative Care

A. Postoperative Monitoring

At the conclusion of the surgical procedure, the animal is removed from the surgical head frame and placed supine on a padded mattress with 30° of head elevation. The fentanyl infusion is subsequently lowered to 20 μg/kg/hr, and the isoflurane is increased to 0.1–0.6%. The nitrous oxide is replaced with a balanced air and oxygen mixture. Vecuronium and midazolam are continued. The animal remains intubated and sedated with continuous physiologic monitoring and close regulation for the first 18 hours of reperfusion. Sustained ICP elevations of >20 mm Hg for >5 min are treated with IV infusions of mannitol (0.5 mg/kg/dose) as needed. Aggressive pulmonary toilet is achieved through frequent suctioning and chest physical therapy. Eighteen hours after reperfusion, the inhalation anesthetic and narcotic agents are tapered off, and the animal is permitted to regain consciousness. If the ABGs demonstrate satisfactory gas exchange, all of the indwelling catheters and monitors are removed to allow extubation and return to housing cages for observation in the animal intensive care unit. Blood samples are drawn through an arterial catheter several times throughout the postoperative period. If extubated, the animal is anesthetized prior to drawing blood with IM ketamine. Animals are continuously monitored for their ability to selfcare, eat, and drink. All wounds are examined regularly for signs of breakdown and/or infection.

B. Criteria for Sacrifice

Clinical examinations are performed several times daily. If the veterinarian determines that continued survival would be unethical secondary to devastating functional impairment prior to postoperative day 3, the animal is reintubated until day 3, at which time an MRI scan is obtained. If at any point after postoperative day 3 the animal fails neurologic examination, it is euthanized with an IV injection of pentobarbital (Veterinary Laboratories, Winnipeg, MB). Animals are survived to a maximum of 10 days, at which point they are sacrificed.

VI. Data Collection and Analysis

A. Neurologic Evaluation

Daily neurologic assessments are performed by two investigators who are blinded to all imaging data. Originally, we used the 100-point neurologic scale developed by Spetzler *et al.* (1980), with higher scores reflecting better neurologic function. With the NIH Stroke Scale (Brott *et al.*, 1989) as a template, we designed a task-oriented neurologic scoring scale that demonstrated less interobserver variability and better correlation with radiographic infarct volume (Mack *et al.*, 2003). This neurologic scoring system is shown in Fig. 4.

Task-oriented baboon neurologic scale			
Behavior (50 points)		**Motor (50 points)**	
Level of awareness (30 points)		*Tone and posture (2o points)*	
Alive	5	Sits upright with support	4
Movement/reaction to tactile stimuli	5	Sits upright without assistance	4
Aware of examiner's presence/turns head to noise	5	Stands in cage	4
Interacts with examiner/maintains attention	5	Walks around cage	4
Attempts slow movement as examiner approaches	5	Moves/jumps around cage at full speed	4
Shows teeth, growls, aggressiv/defensive movements	5		
Ability to self-care (20 points)		*Distal strength/coordination (30 points)*	
Swallows if water is placed in mouth	5	Lifts unaffected arm against gravity	3
Chews if food is placed in mouth	5	Attempts to grasp cage/bar with unaffected arm	3
Feeds from examiner's hand	5	Grasps cage/supports with unaffected arm	3
Feeds from cage	5	Shakes cage/pulls self to stand with unaffected arm	3
		Lifts affected arm against gravity	4
		Attempts to grasp cage/bar with affected arm	4
		Grasps cage/supports with affected arm	4
		Shakes cage/pulls self to stand with affected arm	4
		Preserves coordination in both arms	2

Fig. 4 Task-oriented neurologic scale. Neurologic function is assessed on a task-oriented 100-point scoring system with 50 points each given to motor and behavioral tasks. Reproduced with permission from Mack *et al.* (2003).

Animals are generally quite selfsufficient postoperatively. Most animals are able to move around their cage with a mild spastic limp. Some climb, but most do not. Additionally, most animals are capable of sitting upright without assistance. Those that cannot are assisted with a cloth sling wrapped around the upper chest and under each armpit, which is then secured to the cage. This provides adequate arm mobility in the good extremity while effectively supporting the injured arm. Animals are usually capable of using the injured arm proximally, allowing comfortable positioning during routine daily activities and sleep. Most can feed themselves adequately with the left upper extremity but generally have little useful strength on the right. Animals incapable of selffeeding are deemed unable to selfcare.

B. Radiographic Imaging

After 72 h of reperfusion, the animal is anesthetized with ketamine and sedated with an IV pentobarbital bolus and propofol infusion titrated to allow independent respiratory function for up to 6 h while the airway is maintained with an endotracheal tube. Brain MRI is then performed at this "early" time point, with the

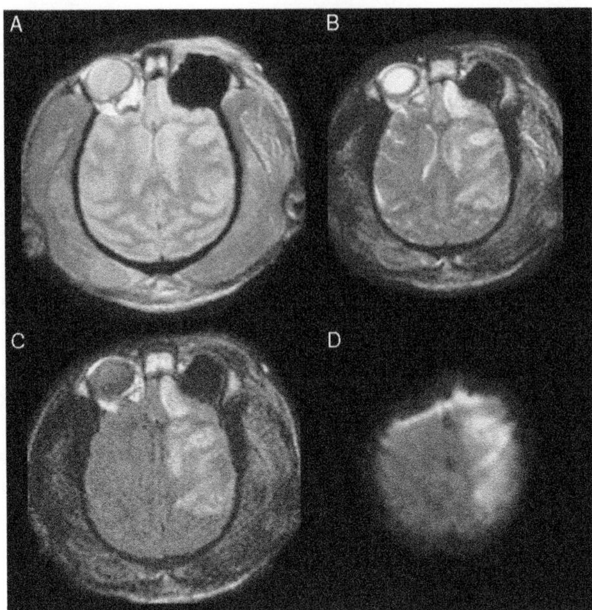

Fig. 5 Postoperative day 3 MRI demonstrating a 30% left-sided infarct. T_1-weighted (A) and T_2-weighted (B) axial images demonstrating anterior cerebral artery (ACA) and middle cerebral artery (MCA) signal changes consistent with an acute infarct. FLAIR (C) and diffusion-weighted images (D) further delineate the lesion.

acquisition of axial T_2-weighted, gradient echo, diffusion-perfusion, fluid activation inversion recovery (FLAIR), and MR angiography sequences (Fig. 5). The T_2-weighted images are acquired with a slice thickness of 3 mm and without intervening space between images. The decision for animal survival past 72 h is a clinical judgment by the veterinarian and is based on, among other things, level of alertness, respiration, and ability to selfcare. If the animal is deemed able to selfcare, it is survived out to day 10, at which time a "late" MRI is obtained before the animal is sacrificed.

C. Infarct Volume

For histologic confirmation of infarct location and correlation with MRI, the brain is removed after sacrifice with the surrounding dura intact. Three coronal sections of 5-mm thickness are collected from the ischemic ipsilateral and stereoanatomic equivalent, normal contralateral hemispheres. The first section is obtained from the medial portion of the most posterior aspect of the precentral gyrus and immersed in a solution of 2% 2,3,5-triphenyltetrazolium (TTC) (Sigma, St. Louis, MO) in 0.9% phosphate buffered saline. Additional sections are obtained immediately anterior and posterior to the first section and embedded in Tissue-Tek compound for further histologic processing. Infarcted tissue is visualized as nonstained portions of brain (Bederson *et al.*, 1986; Dettmers *et al.*, 1994).

Infarct volume is determined by two blinded observers. Areas of ischemic damage demonstrate high signal intensity in T_2-weighted MRI. Using commercially available graphics software, infarct volume can be quantified by planimetric analysis and expressed as the percentage of the total volume of the ipsilateral hemisphere.

VII. Model Application: HuEP5C7

We have used our transorbital model to test the efficacy of a variety of therapeutic interventions on infarct volume and neurologic outcome. One such study investigated a humanized monoclonal antibody, HuEP5C7, which competitively binds E-selectin and P-selectin, critical adhesion molecules implicated in both microvascular failure and inflammation following cerebral ischemia (Huang *et al.*, 2000b). Eighteen adult baboons were randomized to receive either HuEP5C7 (20 mg/kg IV, $n = 9$) or placebo ($n = 9$) immediately following a 1-h ischemic period. Serum levels of HuEP5C7, E-selectin, and P-selectin were determined at 30 min, 120 min, 24 h, 48 h, 72 h, and 9 days postoperatively. MRI scans and neurologic assessments were performed as previously outlined. Histologic examination of the infarct was analyzed to determine tissue levels of P-and E-selectin.

This study demonstrating trends toward reduced polymorphonuclear leukocyte (PMN) infiltration into the ischemic cortex, reduced infarct volumes, improved neurologic score, and improved ability to selfcare. This study suggests that HuEP5C7 is a good candidate for evaluation in clinical trials and may be a safe and effective neuroprotective agent in the future.

VIII. Conclusion

Our current model of temporary aneurysm clip occlusion of both A1 segments and the ICA at the level of the choroidal artery for 75 min, together with laser Doppler flowmetry confirmation of ischemia, allows for large and consistent hemispheric infarcts in baboons. Importantly, our animals are survivable and often recover their ability to selfcare (Huang *et al.*, 2000a,b), making postoperative neurologic assessments possible. Nonhuman primate models of cerebral I-R injury are essential in the preclinical testing of potential neuroprotective strategies for stroke. Such models provide a testing ground for novel neuroprotective agents without putting patients at risk for potential negative side effects.

References

Bederson, J. B., Pitts, L. H., Germano, S. M., Nishimura, M. C., Davis, R. L., and Bartkowski, H. M. (1986). *Stroke* **17,** 1304.

Bonaffini, N., Altieri, M., Rocco, A., and Di Piero, V.(2002). *Clin. Exp. Hypertens.* **24,** 647.

Bravata, D. M., Ho, S. Y., Brass, L. M., Concato, J., Scinto, J., and Meehan, T. P.(2003). *Stroke* **34,** 699.

Brenowitz, G., and Yonas, H.(1990). *Surg. Neurol.* **33,** 247.

Brott, T., Adams, H. P., Olinger, C. P., Jr., Marler, J. R., Barsan, W. G., Biller, J., Spilker, J., Holleran, R., Eberle, R., and Hertzberg, V.(1989). *Stroke* **20,** 864.

Chen, S. T., Hsu, C. Y., Hogan, E. L., Maricq, H., and Balentine, J. D.(1986). *Stroke* **17,** 738.

Coon, A. L., Arias-Mendoza, F., Colby, G. P., Cruz-Lobo, J., Mocco, J., Mack, W. J., Komotar, R. J., Brown, T. R., and Connolly, E. S., Jr.(2006). Correlation of cerebral metabolites with functional outcome in experimental primate stroke using *in vivo* 1H-magnetic resonance spectroscopy. *AJNR Am. J. Neuroradiol.* **27,** 1053–1058.

DeGraba, T. J., and Pettigrew, L. C.(2000). *Neurol. Clin.* **18,** 475.

Dettmers, C., Hartmann, A., Rommel, T., Kramer, S., Pappata, S., Young, A., Hartmann, S., Zierz, S., MacKenzie, E. T., and Baron, J. C.(1994). *Neurol. Res.* **16,** 205.

Ducruet, A. F., Mocco, J., Mack, W. J., Coon, A. L., Marsh, H. C., Pinsky, D. J., Hickman, Z. L., Kim, G. H., and Connolly, E. S., Jr(2007). Pre-clinical evaluation of an sLex-glycosylated complement inhibitory protein in a non-human primate model of reperfused stroke. *J. Med. Primatol.* **36,** 375–380.

Gerriets, T., Li, F., Silva, M. D., Meng, X., Brevard, M., Sotak, C. H., and Fisher, M.(2003). *J. Neurosci. Meth.* **122,** 201.

Gladstone, D. J., Black, S. E., and Hakim, A. M.(2002). Heart and Stroke Foundation of Ontario Centre of Excellence in Stroke. *Stroke* **33,** 2123.

Heiss, W. D.(2002). *J. Neural. Transm.* **63**(Suppl.), 37.

Huang, J., Mocco, J., Choudhri, T. F., Poisik, A., Popilskis, S. J., Emerson, R., DelaPaz, R. L., Khandji, A. G., Pinsky, D. J., and Connolly, E. S., Jr. (2000a). *Stroke* **31,** 3054.

Huang, J., Choudhri, T. F., Winfree, C. J., McTaggart, R. A., Kiss, S., Mocco, J., Kim, L. J., Protopsaltis, T. S., Zhang, Y., Pinsky, D. J., and Connolly, E. S., Jr. (2000b). *Stroke* **31,** 3047.

Lake, A. R., Van Niekerk, I. J., Le Roux, C. G., Trevor Hyphen Jones, T. R., and De Wet, P. D.(1990). *Am. J. Anat.* **187,** 277.

Longa, E. Z., Weinstein, P. R., Carlson, S., and Cummins, R.(1989). *Stroke* **20,** 84.

Mack, W. J., King, R. G., Hoh, D. J., Coon, A. L., Ducruet, A. F., Huang, J., Mocco, J., Winfree, C. J., Apos Ambrosio, A. L. D., Nair, M. N., Sciacca, R. R., and Connolly, E. S., Jr.(2003). *Neurol. Res.* **25,** 280.

Meyer, J. S., Yamamoto, M., Hayman, L. A., Sakai, F., Nakajima, S., and Armstrong, D.(1980). *Neurol. Res.* **2,** 101.

Pestalozza, I. F., Di Legge, S., Calabresi, M., and Lenzi, G. L.(2002). *Clin. Exp. Hypertens.* **24,** 517.

Spetzler, R. F., Selman, W. R., Weinstein, P., Townsend, J., Mehdorn, M., Telles, D., Crumrine, R. C., and Macko, R.(1980). *Neurosurgery* **7,** 257.

Wester, P., Watson, B. D., Prado, R., and Dietrich, W. D.(1995). *Stroke* **26,** 444.

Wintree, C. J., Mack, W. J., Hoh, D., King, R., Ducruet, A. F., Apos Ambrosio, A. L. D., Sughrue, M. E., McKinnell, J., and Connolly, E. S., Jr.(2003). *Acta Neurochir. (Wien)* **145,** 1105.

Wraige, E., Hajat, C., Jan, W., Pohl, K. R., Wolfe, C. D., and Ganesan, V.(2003). *Dev. Med. Child Neurol.* **45,** 229.

Yenari, M. A., de Crespigny, A., Palmer, J. T., Roberts, S., Schrier, S. L., Albers, G. W., Moseley, M. E., and Steinberg, G. K.(1997). *J. Cereb. Blood Flow Metab.* **17,** 401.

Zhang, R. L., Chopp, M., Zhang, Z. G., Jiang, Q., and Ewing, J. R. (1997a). *Brain Res.* **766,** 83.

Zhang, Z., Chopp, M., Zhang, R. L., and Goussev, A. (1997b). *J. Cereb. Blood Flow Metab.* **17,** 1081.

CHAPTER 12

Structural and Functional Optical Imaging of Angiogenesis in Animal Models

Richard L. Roberts and Pengnian Charles Lin

Department of Pathology
Vanderbilt-Ingram Cancer Center
Vanderbilt University Medical Center
Nashville, Tennessee 37232

I. Introduction
II. Intravital Microscopy and Animal Window Models
    A. The Dorsal Skin Window Chamber Model
    B. Imaging Tumor Angiogenesis and Tumor Development in the Window Chamber Model
III. Imaging of Tumor-Host Interaction and Angiogenesis Initiation Using Fluorescent Protein-Labeled Tumor Cells
    A. Imaging Tumor Vascular Response to Therapy Using the Window Model
    B. Multiphoton Laser-Scanning Microscopy in Tumor Window Model
    C. Vascular Window Model for Arthritis Angiogenesis Studies
IV. Vascular Reporter Transgenic Mouse Model
    A. Vascular-Specific Reporter Transgenic Mouse Model
V. Conclusions
References

I. Introduction

Discovery in cancer biology has moved at an accelerated pace in recent years with a considerable focus on the transition from *in vitro* to *in vivo* models. As a result, there has been a significant increase in the need to develop noninvasive, high-resolution *in vivo* imaging approaches to characterize molecular and cellular events that lead to cancer development and progression (Weissleder and Mahmood, 2001). Noninvasive molecular imaging is particularly critical for angiogenesis studies (Folkman and Beckner, 2000; McDonald and Choyke,

ESSENTIAL BIOIMAGING METHODS
Reprinted from *Methods in Enzymology*, Volume 386 (Academic Press, 2004)

DOI: 10.1016/B978-0-12-375043-3.00012-3

2003) because blood vessel formation is a multistep process, and it is strongly influenced by the microenvironment. Current *in vitro* assays cannot replicate many aspects of this dynamic process. Therefore, *in vivo* imaging in animal models is critical to elucidate mechanisms that regulate angiogenesis and to identify and validate new therapeutic targets. Traditional approaches for studying tumor development have relied on tissue biopsies and histologic analysis, which only gives a snapshot of a highly dynamic, complex process. Noninvasive molecular imaging provides an opportunity to overcome these limitations and may be critical in evaluating therapeutic responses to new antiangiogenic therapies that will be an important adjunct in translating the knowledge into clinical practice. Notably, antiangiogenic therapy is intended to target the angiogenic vessels only and will potentially cause fewer side effects because normal vessels are typically quiescent. Traditional clinical trial designs looking for the maximum toxicity dose would not apply to this new type of therapy (Cristofanilli *et al.*, 2002). Instead, identifying surrogate markers for antiangiogenic therapy is imminent. Noninvasive imaging may offer the ability to optimize therapy for each treatment and for each individual.

The ability to visualize the dynamic biologic process by *in vivo* imaging is revolutionizing many areas in biology. Recent advances in the application of fluorescent proteins have permitted microscopy to move from static images to dynamic recordings of cellular behavior in living animals (Phair and Misteli, 2001). Tissue visualization with light is probably the most common imaging in medical research, and new optical imaging approaches offer great promise for real-time monitoring of tumor development and progression in living animal models. Microscopic optical imaging methods ranging from regular microscopy, fluorescence, confocal, and multiphoton microscopy are particularly useful for elucidating structural and functional abnormalities of tumor blood vessels. They are relatively inexpensive and provide the highest resolution. Furthermore, optical imaging complements other imaging technologies such as computed tomography (CT) and magnetic resonance imaging (MRI). In this chapter, we present two animal models for microscopic optical imaging of angiogenesis.

II. Intravital Microscopy and Animal Window Models

Microscopic optical imaging methods are powerful tools for dissecting the cellular and molecular features of the microvasculature. Optical imaging offers high-resolution and real-time functional readouts in animal models. However, a major limitation of optical imaging is tissue penetration and light absorption. The most powerful current approach, multiphoton microscopy, only has the depth of imaging to hundreds of micrometers. Animal window chamber models are designed to overcome this limitation of optical imaging. A variety of window models have been developed that include the dorsal skin window model, mammary tumor window model, and cranial tumor window model (Foltz *et al.*, 1995;

Lin *et al.*, 1997; Shan *et al.*, 2003). The window chamber is a chronical model, which is installed on living animals (mice or rats). The tissues implanted in the transparent chambers in skin and other sites can be imaged over time by microscopy. The animal window models, coupled with intravital microscopy, have provided stunning insight into tumor host interaction, tumor angiogenesis initiation, and therapeutic responses of tumor blood vessels (Brown *et al.*, 2001). Rate of blood flow (BF), blood vessel diameter, vascular density, endothelium permeability, leukocyte-endothelial cell interactions, and gene expression are among the variables that can be measured by this model.

A. The Dorsal Skin Window Chamber Model

The most commonly used window chamber is the dorsal skin window chamber that is installed on the back skinfold of mice or rats (Lin *et al.*, 1997). Sterile technique is followed for this surgical procedure. The mice or rats are anesthetized, and the back of the mice or rats is shaved and has warm hair removal cream (Nair) applied for 2 min. After the cream and remaining hair have been wiped away, the back is alternately wiped with surgical sponges soaked in Hibiclens and then alcohol. The area is cleaned at least three times in this way. Then using sterile instruments, the skin is gathered from the back and sutured to a C-shaped holder, which functions to hold the skin tautly. A 10-mm diameter hole for rats or 8-mm diameter hole for mice is traced on the skin and is dissected away from the dorsal skin flap. This is done on both sides of the back for rats or one side of skin for mice, leaving a fascial plane with associated vasculature. The hole is then held vertically away from the body with a titanium superstructure (the "window chamber") that is sutured to both sides of the flap. Glass cover slips are attached to the center of the titanium saddle to cover the surgical site. A small piece of tumor or tumor cells can be placed onto the fascial plane and the chambers are sealed with glass cover slips. The C-shaped holder is then removed, and the skin surfaces adjacent to the implant are covered with Neosporin ointment. Finally, the mouse or rat is placed on a heating blanket to recover. The tissue within the chamber is approximately 200 μm thick and is semitransparent (Fig. 1).

1. Intravital Microscopy Imaging

To visualize and record tumor angiogenesis and tumor development *in vivo*, the mice or rats are anesthetized. The window chamber is placed in a special plexiglass holder to stabilize the window. The mouse or rat is then placed on a heated microscope stage for observation. One can use a regular upright microscope, fluorescent microscope, confocal microscope, or multiphoton microscope, depending on the need. Images of the vasculature of the tumor are captured by cameras and/or recorded on videotapes for further analysis. A variety of angiogenic functions and abnormalities of blood vessels in pathologic conditions can be measured in live animals.

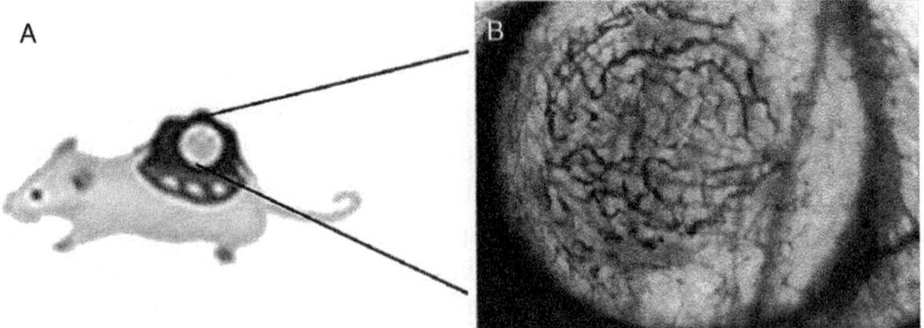

Fig. 1 Dorsal skinfold tumor window model. A small window chamber is installed on the back skinfold of mice. An 8-mm-diameter hole is dissected in the epithelium, and a fascial plane with associated vasculature remains. Tumor cells or tumor tissues can be implanted onto the fascial plane, and the chamber is sealed with glass cover slips. The chamber with tissue is approximately 1 mm thick and is semitransparent (A). Tumor growth and angiogenesis can be directly visualized and recorded in live mice by microscopy. (B) A live image of a well-vascularized tumor grown in the window chamber.

B. Imaging Tumor Angiogenesis and Tumor Development in the Window Chamber Model

Imaging studies have identified multiple cellular and molecular abnormalities that distinguish tumor vessels from their normal vessels and help explain their unusual appearance, irregular BF, and vascular leakiness. Most tumor vessels display a disorganized pattern and do not fit into the conventional hierarchy of arterioles, capillaries, and venules. We have used the tumor window model to study tumor angiogenesis and tumor development. The tumors typically grow to an observable size at 5–7 days after surgery. Tumor angiogenesis can be seen at the same time. Microscopy and recording devices are used to record the development of tumor blood vessels and tumors (Fig. 1). The following vascular and tumor indexes can be measured.

1. Tumor Vascular Length Density

The microphotographs of live tumors in the window chamber are used to obtain measurements of tumor vascular length density as an indicator of tumor vasculature. Briefly, a square grid is superimposed over the tumor images and the number of interactions between the grid and flowing vessels are counted. The vascular length density in mm/mm^3 is calculated using the formula:

$$\text{Vascular length density} = \frac{N}{4gdt}$$

where N is the average number of intersections between vessels and grid per sheet; g is the number of blocks in the grid (=54); d is the length of one grid square calibrated by a micrometer image at the same magnification; and t is the measured depth of field through which microvessels could be discerned (=0.2 mm).

2. Vessel Dilation

Vessel diameter can be measured from the images taken at each time point using the National Institutes of Health (NIH) Image 1.12 analysis program. At least 10 vessels per window and five measurements per vessel are taken. The mean of the vessel size (vessel dilation, VD) will be used for comparison. VD index is calculated using VD at each time point divided by VD at time 0.

3. Vessel Tortuosity

Tumor vessels and angiogenic vessels in pathologic conditions commonly display tortuous morphology compared with straight and uniform normal blood vessels. The vascular length (L) between two points (4 mm apart) of the same vessel is measured from the images. At least 10 vessels per window are measured, and the mean of the vessel length is used for analysis. Tortuosity index is calculated as $L/4$ mm. Vessel tortuosity (VT) is equal to 1 in normal blood vessels (straight vessels) and is larger than 1 in tortured vessels.

4. Vascular Permeability

Leaky blood vessels are common in tumors due to defective endothelial barrier function. The vascular leakiness is important because it contributes to the high-interstitial pressure in tumors and may facilitate angiogenesis by releasing plasma into tissues and forming a scaffold for endothelial cell function. To measure the vascular permeability (VP), we have used fluorescence-labeled tracers. Extravasated dye increases the fluorescent intensity in the vicinity of any chosen blood vessel over time. The leakiness of individual tumor vessels can be measured with direct microscopic visualization. Local VP is calculated as Fn/F0 at the vicinity area of a chosen blood vessel at each time point. Fn is the fluorescent intensity at n time point after the injection of dye. F0 is the measurement prior to the injection of dye. One should keep in mind that VP correlates with molecular mass, which reflects the pore size of tumor blood vessels. Depending on tumor type and location, the cutoff size varies.

5. Blood Flow

BF velocity in each vessel can be measured by the following methods. (1) One can perform a single line scanning using confocal microscopy or multiphoton microscopy and then count the number of red blood cells (RBCs) that go by. (2) One can record BF velocity using a VCR recorder. Because vessel size and BF velocity can be easily measured, a relative index of BF can be calculated as $\mathrm{BF} = V \times S$, where V is the velocity and S is the size of the vessel.

6. Hypoxia

Hypoxia is a common feature of tumors, an important stimulus for angiogenesis, and a potential target for imaging. Hypoxia regulates angiogenesis through induction and stabilization of a transcription factor, hypoxia-inducible factor (HIF). HIF binds to an 8-base pair (bp) hypoxia-response element (HRE) in the promoter region of angiogenic genes and induces angiogenic factor production. A hypoxia reporter construct has been developed (5HREhCMVmpd2EGFP), of which enhanced green fluorescent protein (EGFP) is under the control of HRE (Vordermark *et al.*, 2001). Hypoxia can be directly visualized by the expression of EGFP in tumor cells harboring this construct.

7. Tumor Size

To obtain the tumor size, hematoxylin and eosin (H&E) stained sections representing the largest cross-sectional area of each tumor are photographed and the thickness (t) and the diameter (d) of tumors are measured from the microphotographs. Tumor volumes, which are assumed to approximate a flat cylinder in shape, can be calculated using the formula:

$$\text{Tumor volume (mm}^3) = 3.14t\left(\frac{d}{2}\right)^2$$

Alternatively, one can implant fluorescent protein-labeled tumor cells in the window chamber model (Fig. 2). The fluorescence intensity of the tumor can be used as a relative index of the tumor size.

III. Imaging of Tumor-Host Interaction and Angiogenesis Initiation Using Fluorescent Protein-Labeled Tumor Cells

Tumor cells labeled with green fluorescent protein (GFP), or another fluorescent or bioluminescent reporter can be noninvasively localized and measured in preclinical models by optical imaging. Optical imaging has the ability to study cellular and molecular events in living animals. We have used the tumor cells labeled with GFP in a tumor vascular window model to examine the initiation of tumor angiogenesis and tumor-host interaction. A murine mammary tumor line transfected with GFP (4T1-GFP) was implanted into the window chamber (Li *et al.*, 2000). Using this approach, we examined tumor development in the same living mouse over time using fluorescent microscopy coupled with a digital camera. We were able to visualize tumor formation from a single tumor cell (Fig. 2). Several intriguing observations were obtained from this study.

1. *Tumor cells alter the host "normal vasculature" morphology*. Implantation of only 50 tumor cells in the window chamber caused dramatic vascular morphologic changes in just a few days (Fig. 2A and B). The surrounding host "normal" vessels became dilated and torturous.

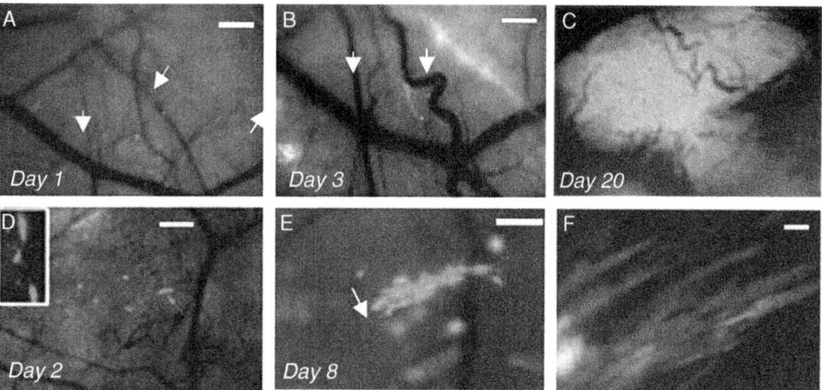

Fig. 2 Optical imaging of tumor-host interaction and tumor angiogenesis using the window chamber model. A small window chamber is installed on the back skinfold of a Balb/c mouse. Approximately 20 cells of a murine mammary tumor line transfected with EGFP (4T1-GFP) are implanted onto the fascial plane in the window chamber, and their growth is followed serially after the initial implantation. A vascularized "green tumor" forms from a single cell (green dot in Panel A) over the period of 20 days after tumor cell implantation (A-C). Interactions of tumor cells and host vasculature can be seen directly. Tumor cells change the local environment, and the surrounding normal blood vessels become dilated and tortuous, as indicated by arrows, in a few days after tumor cell implantation (A-B). Reciprocally, host environment affects tumor cell behavior. 4T1 is an epithelium tumor line and displays cobblestone-like morphology *in vitro*. However, the cells become spindle-shaped, with a fibroblast-like morphology after implantation *in vivo* (D-F). The cells migrate toward surrounding blood vessels. Size bars represent 20 μm. (See Plate no. 5 in the Color Plate Section.)

2. *Host environment alters tumor cell behavior.* 4T1 is an epithelial tumor line, which has a typical cobblestone-like morphology when cultured *in vitro*. However, a few days after implantation *in vivo* the cells became enlongated or polarized. The tumor cells underwent epithelial-to-mesenchymal transformation (EMT) indicative of cell motility, and they migrated toward nearby blood vessels (Fig. 2D and F). When the cells reached to the blood vessels, they grew around the vessel and formed a cuff, and then grew along the vessels. This suggests that tumor cells not only actively recruit blood vessels, but they also actively search for blood vessels for nutrients and oxygen. It is a mutual recruitment involving tumor-host interaction.

3. *Tumor angiogenesis starts at a much earlier time than textbooks suggest.* The traditional view is that tumor angiogenesis does not start until a tumor reaches 1–2 mm^3 in size. However, we observed that the earliest tumor angiogenesis started when there were only 300–400 cells in the tumor model (Fig. 2).

A. Imaging Tumor Vascular Response to Therapy Using the Window Model

Development of imaging parameters that reflect the efficacy of angiogenesis inhibitors has great potential. Notably, antiangiogenic therapy is intended to target the angiogenic vessels. It causes fewer side effects because normal vessels are typically quiescent. Traditional clinical trial design looking for the maximum toxicity dose would not apply to this new type of therapy. Identifying surrogate markers for antiangiogenic therapy is imminent. Optical imaging in tumor window models can be used to study the tumor vascular responses to therapy, as well as evaluate the efficacy of antiangiogenic reagents. Using the window model, we observed the heterogeneous response of tumor blood vessels to irradiation that exists among different types of tumors grown in the same host (C57-BL6). Two different types of tumors were implanted into the tumor windows. Vascularized tumors developed in 1 week, at which time they were treated with local irradiation. Irradiation treatment induced a dose- and time-dependent destruction to tumor blood vessels within the window. Radiation-sensitive tumor vessels in melanoma B16F0 showed a rapid and marked regression following 3 Gy of irradiation. Radiation-resistant tumor vessels in glioma GL261 did not respond to 3 Gy treatment and showed little response even at 6 Gy (Fig. 3). This finding indicates that tumors change the local environment and affect vascular response to therapy.

In addition, we evaluated the combination therapy of antivascular endothelial growth model (VEGF) with irradiation on tumor vasculature using the tumor window model. First, we established a vascularized tumor in the window model, then we treated the tumors with local irradiation in combination with two different VEGF inhibitors. We observed that blocking VEGF activation by using either a soluble VEGF receptor or a small VEGF receptor kinase inhibitor enhanced irradiation-induced tumor vascular destruction (Geng *et al.*, 2001).

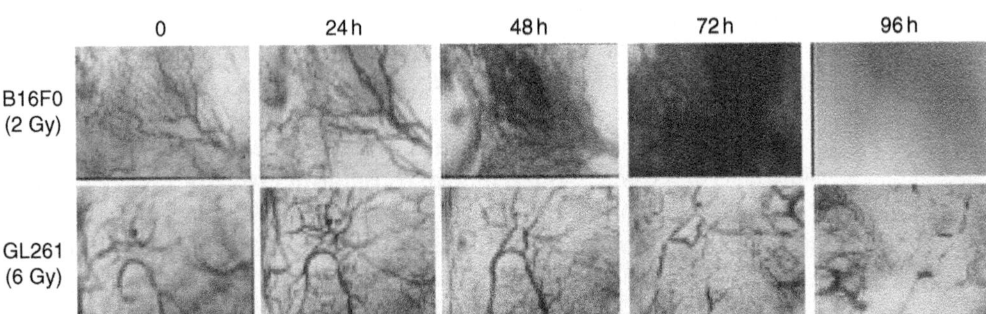

Fig. 3 Optical imaging of tumor vascular response to therapy using the window model. The dorsal window frame is applied to the back skinfold of C57-BL6 mice after removal of the epidermis. Tumor cell lines GL261 and B16F0 are implanted into the window skinfold. Angiogenesis in the implanted tumor occurs over the course of 7 days. At that time, the tumor is treated with local irradiation with 3 Gy for B16F0 melanoma and 6 Gy for GL261 glioma. The tumor vascular responses are photographed daily by microscopy. Magnification is 40×.

B. Multiphoton Laser-Scanning Microscopy in Tumor Window Model

The multiphoton laser-scanning microscope (MPLSM) offers significant advancements in depth of tissue penetration into intact samples, improved signal-to-noise ratio, and longer sample lifetimes over other optical sectioning techniques. Rakesh Jain's group has used MPLSM combined with EGFP and chronic animal window models to generate high-resolution, three-dimensional imaging in deeper regions of tumors, which provide powerful insight into gene expression, angiogenesis, physiologic function, and drug delivery in tumors (Brown *et al.*, 2001). They used transgenic mice that express EGFP under the control of the VEGF promoter. A tumor window model was installed on the back skinfold of the mice, and VEGF expression during tumor development was evaluated.

A few intriguing observations were obtained. (1) Tumor cells induce VEGF promoter activity in host cells (Fig. 4). Implantation of tumor cells in the window chamber activates VEGF expression in host stromal cells, and these cells exhibit fibroblast-like morphology. (2) Optical cross-sectioning by MPLSM shows that tumors induce VEGF promoter activity in a 35–50-μm-thick layer of host stromal cells interfacing the tumor (Fig. 4A). Below that layer, EGFP-positive stromal cells are seen at least 200 μm into the tumor (Fig. 4B). (3) EGFP-positive host cells inside the tumor frequently are parallel with angiogenic vessels (Fig. 4C). A thin (1 μm) nonfluorescent sheath often lies between the blood vessels and fluorescent cells (Fig. 4D), which presumably represents endothelial cells, pericytes, or

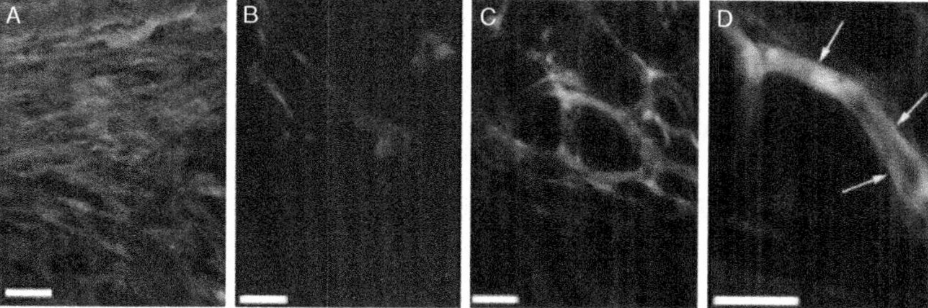

Fig. 4 Multiphoton laser-scanning microscopy imaging of tumor angiogenesis. This figure is adapted from Rekesh Jain's publication, with permission (Brown *et al.*, 2001). A MCaIV tumor is grown in transgenic mice that express EGFP under the control of the VEGF promoter (green). The tumor vasculature is highlighted by TMR-BSA injected systemically (red) (A-B). Two optical sections of the same region within the tumor, at different depths, showing the three-dimensional resolution and depth of penetration of MPLSM. (A) A highly fluorescent (GFP-expressing) layer is seen within the first 35–50 m of the tumor-host interface. (B) 200 m deeper inside the tumor, EGFP-expressing host cells have successfully migrated into the tumor and tend to colocalize with angiogenic blood vessels. (C) A maximum intensity projection of 27 optical sections, spaced 5 m apart and beginning 45 m from the tumor surface. Colocalization of VEGF-expressing host cells with angiogenic vessels is readily apparent. (D) A single optical section of a vessel from (C) taken at twice the magnification. A thin, nonfluorescent layer is apparent at many locations (arrows). Scale bars are 50 μm. (See Plate no. 6 in the Color Plate Section.)

basement membrane. Clearly, this type of study can generate novel information about the mechanisms of tumor angiogenesis, which probably cannot be achieved with other imaging technologies.

C. Vascular Window Model for Arthritis Angiogenesis Studies

Inflammation and angiogenesis are two fundamental processes that underlie pathologic disorders. Tissue injury induces inflammation, and inflammation triggers angiogenesis, which in turn initiates tissue repair and tissue growth. Rheumatoid arthritis is an inflammatory disease as well as an angiogenic disease. We established an *in vivo* synovium vascular window model to study angiogenesis in arthritis. This model is adopted from the tumor window model. We installed a window frame on the back skinfold on syngeneic DBA/1 J mice. A 0.1-mm^3 piece of rheumatoid arthritis synovium isolated from a mouse paw joint with collagen-induced arthritis (in DBA/J background) was then placed onto the fascial plane, saline solution was added, and the chamber was then sealed with a glass cover slip to form a semitransparent chamber. Rheumatoid arthritis synovium in window chambers were photographed using a microscope for vascular length density measurement. As expected, arthritis synovium is highly angiogenic because it produced high levels of angiogenic factors. Implantation of synovium isolated from an arthritic mouse paw into the window chamber induced dramatic angiogenesis within 8 days, and the synovium survived. In contrast, implanted normal joint tissue failed to induce angiogenesis, and the tissue died within days (Fig. 5). This model can be used to study angiogenesis in arthritis synovium, as well as evaluate angiogenic inhibitors for arthritis treatment.

IV. Vascular Reporter Transgenic Mouse Model

A. Vascular-Specific Reporter Transgenic Mouse Model

Two families of receptor tyrosine kinase, the vascular endothelial growth factor receptor family (VEGF-R) and the Tie family (including Tie1 and Tie2), are expressed mainly or predominantly on vascular endothelial cells. Therefore, transgenic mice harboring the promoters of the vascular-specific genes to drive a reporter gene can be valuable tools for imaging vasculature in living animals. Indeed, several lines of transgenic mice have been developed to display vascular-specific reporter gene expression. Here, we will use Tie2-GFP mice as an example (Motoike *et al.*, 2000; Phillips *et al.*, 2001). Because Tie2 is an endothelium-specific receptor, transgenic mice containing the Tie2 promoter to drive GFP expression exhibit vascular-specific GFP expression and display "green blood vessels" (Fig. 6). This model allows direct visualization of blood vessels *in vivo* without any treatment. Here, we present a few examples of using the mice for imaging angiogenesis.

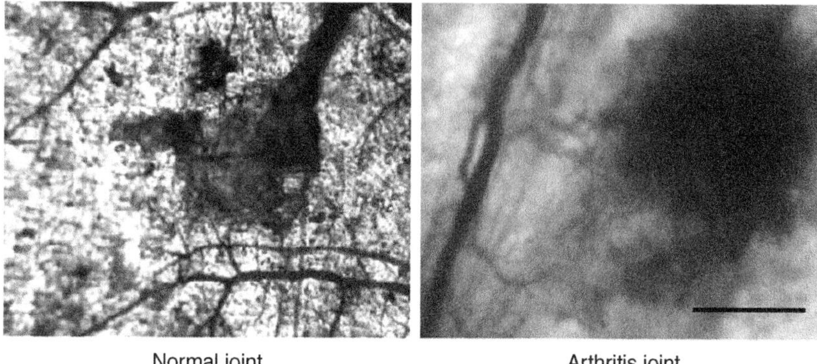

Fig. 5 Arthritis synovium window chamber model. A novel vascular window model is established on the back skinfold of a DBA mouse to study arthritis-induced angiogenesis. Synovium samples were isolated from a donor mouse paw with collagen-induced arthritis (CIA). A small piece of CIA synovium (right panel) or a normal joint tissue (left panel) was implanted in the vascular window. The photos were live pictures taken from mouse synovium windows. Magnification is 40×. Bar represents 1 mm. (See Plate no. 7 in the Color Plate Section.)

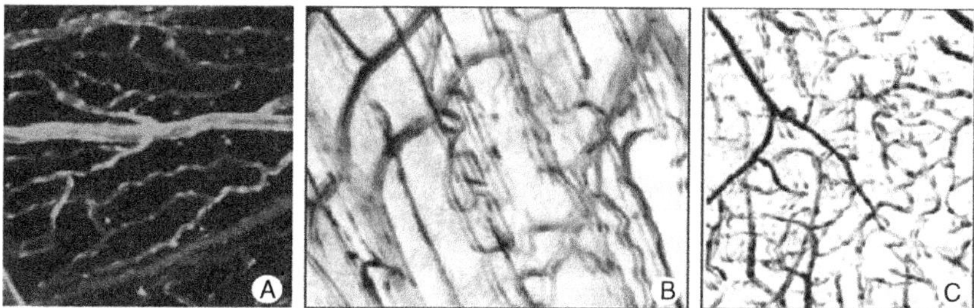

Fig. 6 (A) Conjunctiva capillaries in a Tie2-GFP mouse. Often all elements of the microcirculatory system show uniformly strong fluorescence. This image was obtained noninvasively in a lightly anesthetized Tie2-GFP mouse using a Zeiss 510 confocal microscope. (B) Anaglyph showing 3D structure of microcirculatory network in skeletal muscle of Tie2-GFP mouse. The Z-series stack of images was obtained from the medial quadriceps muscle of an anesthetized mouse through the incised skin. Arterioles (A) and venules (V) can be distinguished from capillaries. (C) Anaglyph showing 3D structure of subpial microvessel network in fixed mouse brain. (See Plate no. 8 in the Color Plate Section.)

1. Laser-Scanning Confocal Imaging of the Vascular System in Tie2-GFP Mice

We have established a noninvasive, high-resolution imaging system to examine the microcirculation in the ear dermis and conjunctiva in living Tie2-GFP mice. Using laser-scanning confocal microscopy (LSCM) to image tissues from 8- to 10-week-old Tie2-GFP mice, we have observed that in the capillary endothelial cells the most intense fluorescence is localized around the nucleus (Fig. 6A and B), and this is consistent with the stereotypical structure of the capillary endothelial cell and its highly attenuated nature. The cytoplasm of endothelial cells is highly attenuated, often measuring 50–100 nm in thickness, thus providing a short distance required for the diffusion of nutrients from the blood to the tissues. Electron micrographs of capillary endothelial cells have shown that the major fraction of the cytoplasm is located in the perinuclear region of the cell, where the cytoplasm is expanded to accommodate the nucleus. Furthermore, in the Tie2-GFP mouse, GFP is expressed as a cytosolic protein that is not restricted from the nucleus. Noninvasive fluorescence imaging of the conjunctival microvasculature and the ear dermal microcirculation in living Tie2-GFP mice showed some variation in fluorescence intensity in different segments of the vascular tree, with relatively stronger staining in small arterioles and venules compared with the fluorescence intensity of the capillary endothelial cells.

a. Imaging Procedures

Live Tie2-GFP mice were imaged directly by LSCM. The mice were lightly anesthetized with ketamine and then placed on the stage of a microscope. The tissue was examined in a Zeiss 510 LSCM with either a 10 × 0.5 NA air lens, a 20 × 0.75 NA air lens, or a 40 × 1.3 NA oil immersion lens. Working distance is a limiting factor when using high-NA oil immersion lenses, and the use of tissue sections is useful to circumvent these potential problems. Z-sectioning and 3D reconstruction was all done with Zeiss 510 hardware and software (Carl Zeiss, Inc., Oberkochen, Germany).

2. Corneal Angiogenesis Assay

The corneal micropocket assay is a simple, clean, and reliable assay to evaluate angiogenesis (Lin *et al.*, 1997). Capillary vessels sprout from the limbus into the avascular cornea upon stimulation with an angiogenic pellet implanted in a mouse cornea. Typically, when a corneal assay is established in a normal mouse, we cannot see any early events until BF has been established at approximately 4–6 days after pellet implantation. However, Tie2-GFP mice present a unique opportunity. Because vascular endothelium is labeled with GFP, one can visualize and record this dynamic process from the very beginning without relying on the establishment of circulation in matured vessels (Fig. 7). The corneas obtained from these animals showed a complex proliferation of capillaries that uniformly expressed high levels of GFP. This result confirms that Tie2 promoter activity remains activated at high levels in growth factor-induced corneal neovascularization and that Tie2-GFP is a suitable probe for noninvasive LSCM imaging in living mice.

a. Establishment of Mice Corneal Assay

The corneal micropocket assay is relatively simple and easy to perform. Briefly, angiogenic factors such as basic fibroblast growth factor (bFGF) or VEGF are combined with sterile Hydron casting solution (Interferon Sciences, New Brunswick, NJ), and the solution is pipetted onto the surface of 1.5 mm diameter Teflon rods (Dupont Co., Wilmington, DE). The pellets, containing approximately

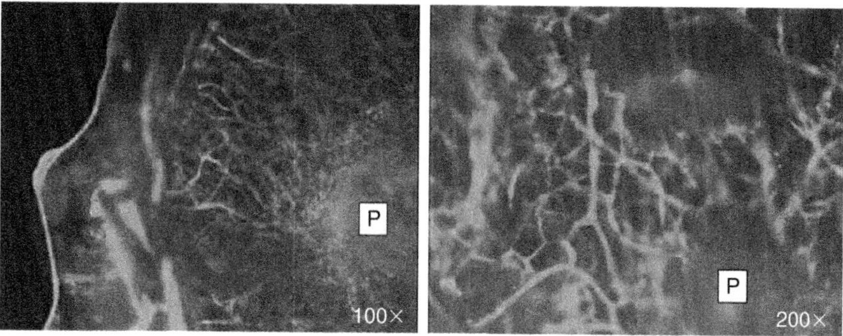

Fig. 7 Corneal micropocket assay in Tie2-GFP mice. A small surgical micropocket is created in the Tie2-GFP mouse cornea 1 mm from the limbus, and a small pellet containing bFGF (25 ng/pellet) is implanted in the pocket afterwards. Mouse cornea is harvested 5 days after pellet implantation and flatly mounted on a glass cover slip. Images are taken from fluorescent microscopy. P, Pellet.

25 ng/pellet of angiogenic factors, are air-dried in a laminar hood for 1 h and refrigerated overnight. The following day, pellets are rehydrated with a drop of phosphate buffered saline (PBS) buffer and then placed in a surgically created pocket within the cornea stromal, 1 mm from the limbus laterally of Tie2-GFP mice. At day 5 postimplantation, mice are anesthetized and corneas are removed and imaged by confocal microscopy. Measurements of the neovascular area, microvessel diameter, and assessment of length and branching complexity are made using Metamorph software (distributed by Universal Imaging Corp., a subsidiary of Molecular Devices, Downingtown, PA). Alternatively, one can directly image corneal angiogenesis in living animals.

3. Intravascular Fluorescent Probes as Markers of Capillary Perfusion and Permeability

We have used fluorescent tracer to image capillary perfusion and permeability. Intravenous injection of 0.1 mg rhodamine B dextran in 50 μl PBS in Tie2-GFP mice showed that in both mouse ear skin microvascular elements and mouse conjunctival capillary beds, rhodamine B dextran fills all fluorescent capillaries and only rarely flows through capillary segments that are negative for the GFP signal. This result reflects, in part, the extreme sensitivity of the confocal microscope and indicates the feasibility of this technique to monitor the patents of the endothelial cell lumen. It is generally possible to visualize blood cells within capillary lumen based on their negative staining characteristics against the background of fluorescence in the capillary. Also, it is normally possible to discern the movement of blood cells through the capillaries, and this provides information concerning rate of BF through specific capillary segments in a microcirculatory bed. We have found that in both conjunctival and dermal capillaries, flow rates are not uniform across all parts of a microvascular bed, although how the rate of flow is regulated remains unclear.

Dual fluorescence microangiography can measure capillary permeability using two fluorescent probes, and this method appears to be more sensitive to subtle changes in capillary permeability than single probe methods (Russ *et al.*, 2001). This system has been used in studies of the retinal vasculature and utilizes simultaneous imaging of two fluorescent tracers with distinct excitation and emission properties, and the two probes differ in molecular size. The relative molecular size of the two probes is important for determining capillary permeability. One of the tracers must be large (>70 kDa) in order for the probe to remain confined within the vasculature, whereas the other is small and is free to cross the vascular barrier. The fluorescence intensity of the two tracers in the interstitial tissues is monitored following injection and directly reflects permeability, whereas comparison of the fluorescence intensity between the large feeding arteries and the large veins in the field is used to calculate the extraction of diffusing tracer by the microcirculation.

a. Methods

For capillary perfusion measurement, fluorescein dextran (70 kDa) or rhodamine B dextran (70 kDa) are injected into the tail veins of anesthetized mice and the mice are mounted for imaging by confocal microscopy. In the seconds immediately following injection, the entire vascular system is defined by the intravascular contrast. However, transcapillary transport of tracer from the blood to the tissues occurs at different rates in different tissues, presumably due to permeability characteristics of the endothelial barrier in the different tissues. Because of this, over time, the microvascular anatomy becomes less distinct. For a detailed protocol of dual fluorescence permeability imaging (Russ *et al.*, 2001). Briefly, a mixture of sodium fluorescein (376 kDa) to indicate vessel leak and Texas red-dextran (70 kDa) to indicate vessel filling are injected intravenously into a mouse prepped for imaging by either wide-field epifluorescence as described (Russ *et al.*, 2001) or by confocal imaging. For confocal imaging, immediately following the dye injection, the gain and offset functions of the red and green channels are adjusted to maximize the dynamic range in the microvascular bed of interest. Another mouse is then prepped and mounted on the microscope and injected with dye as before, and a time series of data points are then collected and analyzed as described (Russ *et al.*, 2001).

4. BF Velocity Measurement in Living Animals

For these studies, isolated mouse RBCs are labeled with fluorescein isothiocyanate (FITC) or Texas red-dextran by standard techniques (Seylaz *et al.*, 1999) and the fluorescent cells are injected intravenously into the mouse. LSCM has confirmed uniform labeling of all RBCs by this technique. We have found that when time-lapse recordings are made using rapid laser scan speeds (scan time 20–100 μs), we can easily track the particle in capillaries, venules, and arterioles in multiple successive frames (Fig. 8A). Because the field size is constant for a given objective

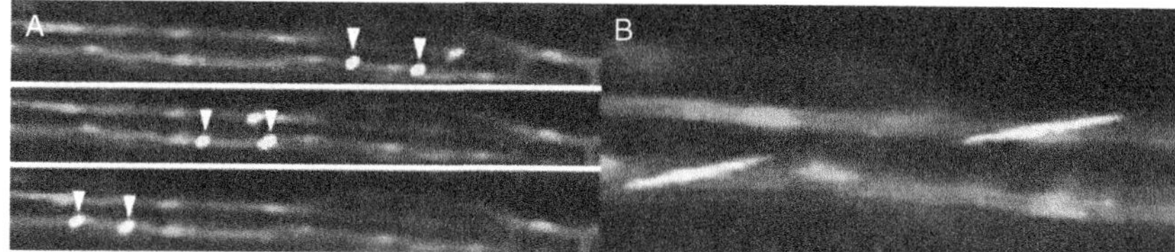

Fig. 8 Blood velocity measurements by LSCM. (A) Skeletal muscle capillaries from Tie2-GFP mice are depicted and show three successive frames from a time-lapse sequence, and it is possible to track a pair of fluorescent RBCs in each of the three frames. (B) The same capillaries imaged with slow scan speed show streaked RBCs. In *A*, the direct calculation of $\Delta d/\Delta t$ (comparing top to bottom) measurement of the distance traveled reveals the particle velocity at 0.26 pixel/ms. Velocity calculated from $\Delta d/\Delta t$ in streaks in *B* is 0.27 pixel/ms. (See Plate no. 9 in the Color Plate Section.)

lens and the frame acquisition rate is constant and known, the velocity of fluorescent particles in individual microvessels up to 200 μm beneath the muscle surface can easily be determined using the formula:

$$\text{Velocity} = \frac{\Delta d}{\Delta t}$$

where Δd is the distance the cell traveled and Δt is the time interval.

Alternatively, we have found that by using slower scan rates, LSCM is ideal for automatically determining the instantaneous flow velocity of labeled RBCs in the microvasculature in a single scan (Kleinfeld *et al.*, 1998; Seylaz *et al.*, 1999). In laser-scanning images, moving objects are often diagonally streaked (Fig. 8B) and the slope of the streak is related to the velocity of the moving particle. This method of determining particle velocity takes advantage of the precise control of the laser-scanning mechanism that scans the field in horizontal lines, pixel by pixel, over time. The streak results because time is required for the laser-scanning mechanism to scan a horizontal line of pixels. The labeled cell moves during this time interval and occupies a different position in the subsequent horizontal line of pixels. Thus, the position of moving objects is different in each successive horizontal line scan. Because the pixel dimensions are constant and the time per pixel is constant and known, the slope of the streak gives the change in position over the change in time, from which the instantaneous particle velocity can be calculated by using velocity $= \Delta d/\Delta t$, where Δd is the distance the cell traveled and Δt is the time interval.

In addition, Z-series stacks of images of the microvasculature, including capillaries, arterioles, and venules, have been obtained. These stacks are rendered off-line into 3D images and/or are digitized to measure microvessel diameter. In addition, recordings obtained in living, anesthetized mice have demonstrated that at rest there is tremendous variability in the flow rates between adjacent capillaries, and even in the same capillary over time. However, in studies in which we analyzed BF velocity in the same capillary bed over time intervals up to 20 min, we have found very consistent flow over the 20-min period in individual capillaries. Tie2-GFP mice show relatively uniform fluorescence in all the elements of the skeletal muscle microvascular system, including arterioles, venules, and capillaries (see Fig. 6B). Use of these animals will confirm that unperfused capillaries are included in the analysis, which cannot be done by other methods.

a. Methods

RBCs are fluorescently labeled by two different protocols, including reaction of the cells with FITC and hypotonic loading of the cells with sulforhodamine 101. Mouse RBCs are obtained by drawing cells from the inferior vena cava in a heparinized syringe. The cells are separated from serum by low-speed centrifugation in a table-top centrifuge and rinsed two times in heparinized saline and one time in 100 mM sodium bicarbonate (pH 8.0). The cells are resuspended in 1 ml of 100 mM sodium bicarbonate and incubated with 250 μg of FITC dissolved in 50 μl dimethylsulfoxide (DMSO) at room temperature for 30 min. Then the cells are washed three times and resuspended in 200 μl of heparinized saline. RBCs have also been loaded with sulforhodamine 101 by hypotonic shock treatment. Sulforhodamine 101 (0.2 mg) is added to 0.9 ml of distilled water, followed by the addition of 0.5 ml whole mouse blood for 20 min at room temperature. One hundred microliters of 10 $\times$ PBS are then added, and the cells are centrifuged at low speed and rinsed three times in heparinized saline. For *in vivo* imaging, labeled RBCs are intravenously injected into the tail veins of anesthetized Tie2-GFP mice that are mounted on the confocal microscope and imaged by standard methods. For experiments where tracking of individual particles is desired, rapid scan rates are used. Alternatively, in experiments in which instantaneous velocity of populations of RBCs is desired, slow scanning speeds are used.

V. Conclusions

Advances in the biomedical sciences have been accelerated by the development and utilization of new imaging technologies. With animal models widely used in the biologic sciences, finding ways to conduct *in vivo* experiments more accurately and efficiently becomes a key factor in the success of medical research. Optical imaging is inexpensive and high resolution (up to a single cell level or even subcellular level), and it allows real-time imaging. Optical imaging not only provides powerful tools with which to study the molecular mechanisms of tumor angiogenesis, identifies therapeutic targets, and validates the targets in animal models, but it will also be a valuable measurement for monitoring drug response in patients. In addition, optical imaging can easily combine with other imaging technologies. The combination of different imaging modalities will provide a detailed story about the molecular and cellular abnormalities of tumor blood vessels and will generate valuable information about the action of angiogenesis inhibitors in cancer patients.

Acknowledgments

We thank Laura DeBusk at Vanderbilt University Medical Center for her critical reading of the manuscript. This work was supported in part by a grant (CA87756) from the National Cancer Institute (P. C. L.), by the Vanderbilt-Ingram Cancer Center (CA68485), the Vanderbilt In Vivo Imaging Center (CA 86283), and the Vanderbilt Diabetes Center (DK20593).

References

Brown, E. B., Campbell, R. B., Tsuzuki, Y., Xu, L., Carmeliet, P., Fukumura, D., and Jain, R. K. (2001). *Nat. Med.* **7,** 864.
Cristofanilli, M., Charnsangavej, C., and Hortobagyi, G. N. (2002). *Nat. Rev. Drug Discov.* **1,** 415.
Folkman, J., and Beckner, K. (2000). *Acad. Radiol.* **7,** 783.
Foltz, R. M., McLendon, R. E., Friedman, H. S., Dodge, R. K., Bigner, D. D., and Dewhirst, M. W. (1995). *Neurosurgery* **36,** 976; discussion 984.
Geng, L., Donnelly, E., McMahon, G., Lin, P. C., Sierra-Rivera, E., Oshinka, H., and Hallahan, D. E. (2001). *Cancer Res.* **61,** 2413.
Kleinfeld, D., Mitra, P. P., Helmchen, F., and Denk, W. (1998). *Proc. Natl. Acad. Sci. USA* **95,** 15741.
Li, C. Y., Shan, S., Huang, Q., Braun, R. D., Lanzen, J., Hu, K., Lin, P., and Dewhirst, M. W. (2000). *J. Natl. Cancer Inst.* **92,** 143.
Lin, P., Polverini, P., Dewhirst, M., Shan, S., Rao, P. S., and Peters, K. (1997). *J. Clin. Invest.* **100,** 2072.
McDonald, D. M., and Choyke, P. L. (2003). *Nat. Med.* **9,** 713.
Motoike, T., Loughna, S., Perens, E., Roman, B. L., Liao, W., Chau, T. C., Richardson, C. D., Kawate, T., Kuno, J., Weinstein, B. M., Stainier, D. Y., and Sato, T. N. (2000). *Genesis* **28,** 75.
Phair, R. D., and Misteli, T. (2001). *Nat. Rev. Mol. Cell Biol.* **2,** 898.
Phillips, C. L., Arend, L. J., Filson, A. J., Kojetin, D. J., Clendenon, J. L., Fang, S., and Dunn, K. W. (2001). *Am. J. Pathol.* **158,** 49.
Russ, P. K., Gaylord, G. M., and Haselton, F. R. (2001). *Ann. Biomed. Eng.* **29,** 638.
Seylaz, J., Charbonne, R., Nanri, K., Von Euw, D., Borredon, J., Kacem, K., Meric, P., and Pinard, E. (1999). *Cereb. Blood Flow Metab.* **19,** 863.
Shan, S., Sorg, B., and Dewhirst, M. W. (2003). *Microvasc. Res.* **65,** 109.
Vordermark, D., Shibata, T., and Brown, J. M. (2001). *Neoplasia* **3,** 527.
Weissleder, R., and Mahmood, U. (2001). *Radiology* **219,** 316.

CHAPTER 13

MRI of Animal Models of Brain Disease

Rob Nabuurs,* David L. Thomas,† John S. Thornton,‡ Mark F. Lythgoe,§ and Louise van der Weerd*,¶

*Department of Radiology
Molecular Imaging Laboratories Leiden
Leiden University Medical Center
Leiden, The Netherlands

†Department of Medical Physics and Bioengineering
University College London
London, United Kingdom

‡Lysholm Department of Neuroradiology
National Hospital for Neurology and Neurosurgery
London, United Kingdom

§Department of Medicine and Institute of Child Health
Centre for Advanced Biomedical Imaging
University College London
London, United Kingdom

¶Department of Anatomy and Embryology
Molecular Imaging Laboratories Leiden
Leiden University Medical Center
Leiden, The Netherlands

I. Introduction
II. Biophysical Background and Methods
   A. Relaxation
   B. Diffusion
   C. Perfusion
   D. MTC
III. Applications of MRI to Experimental Neuropathology
   A. Cerebral Ischemia
   B. Epilepsy
   C. Neurodegenerative Disorders
   D. CNS Inflammation
IV. Conclusion
   References

ESSENTIAL BIOIMAGING METHODS

DOI: 10.1016/B978-0-12-375043-3.00013-5

How to Avoid Pittfalls: Tips and Tricks

- Be careful with prolonged periods of anesthesia; this changes the physiology of the animal, like tissue oxygenation, blood flow and hydratation, leading to changes in relaxation times, tissue shrinkage, etc. Likely to occur >2 h. For the above reason always keep the same order of sequences to allow better comparison.
- Maintain body temperature by an MRI-compatible heating pad or warm air. When using warm air, be aware that the animal dehydrates quickly. For longer experiments, you may have to infuse physiological salt solution intraperitonally to compensate for fluid loss.
- Rodent's eyes stay open under anesthesia, so use eye ointment prior to the experiment to prevent dehydration.
- Choose your anesthesia carefully according to your purpose. Laboratory animal manuals give a detailed overview of the side effects of anesthesia on animal physiology. This is particularly important for metabolic or functional MRI studies.
- When studying metabolites or brain function, take the circadian rhythm of the animals into account, that is, schedule all experiments at the same time of the day.
- Movement artifacts can be reduced by carefully securing the head in the MRI coil. Often ear bars are used, however, be very careful not to pierce the eardrums. As an alternative, cheek pads may be used. If you are using a breathing mask that covers most of the head, the head can be secured inside the mask with pieces of memory foam (ear plugs).
- Always use a closely fitting RF coil to optimize coil loading and thereby signal-to-noise ratios (SNR). A small surface coil gives better SNR, at the expense of inhomogeneous signal.
- Whenever possible, MRI should be followed by histological confirmation. If you use *ex vivo* MRI for high-resolution data, always image the perfusion-fixed brain inside the skull to avoid tissue distortion. One-to-one correlation remains tricky, but adding spatial markers for both MRI and histology is often helpful to find the same location.
- Always place reference tubes next to the animal head to assess image quality. The tubes should be filled with distilled water containing a relaxing agent (e.g., 1 mM $CuSO_4$). The tube can be used to check the accuracy of quantitative sequences, SNR, or to calculate contrast-to-noise ratios in weighted sequences.

I. Introduction

The present review will be restricted to the most common application of magnetic resonance imaging (MRI) in the brain, namely the depiction of hydrogen nuclei (protons) of mobile water molecules. The utility of MRI with respect to animal models of disease lies in the sensitivity of the technique to both micro- and macroscopic molecular motions. Nervous tissue consists of 70–80% water by weight, these water molecules being distributed through a variety of microscopic environments and physiological compartments. It is possible to generate MR images whose contrast reflects, amongst other factors, random molecular rotational motions (T_1 and T_2), random translational motion (diffusion), exchange with macromolecular protons (MTC) and blood flow (perfusion). The concentration and mobility of water molecules is modified in many pathologies and this is the basis of the high sensitivity of MRI to cerebral disease processes.

Furthermore, MRI contrast agents can also change these parameters allowing detection. In recent years this led to the emerging field of molecular and cellular imaging, where contrast agents targeted against disease-specific hallmarks or cells labeled with such agents are explored for early diagnostics and therapy follow-up. Also within the field of experimental neuroimaging this has taken a leap. Some examples will be briefly discussed here, a much more extensive review is given by Hoehn *et al.* (2008).

II. Biophysical Background and Methods

Some important principles are discussed here to provide a background for the rest of this article. For a more detailed introduction to MRI we refer to various excellent textbooks (Gadian, 1995; Smith and Lange, 1999). Protons possess a nuclear magnetic moment (or "spin"). In the absence of an external magnetic field these magnetic moments are randomly distributed in every direction. In the presence of a magnetic field however, a thermal equilibrium is achieved between spins oriented parallel and antiparallel to the magnetic field. The result is a net macroscopic magnetic moment, the bulk magnetization (M_0), orientated in the direction of the external field (conventionally taken to be the z-axis). The individual spins precess around the z-axis at the Larmor frequency (ω, rad s^{-1}), which is proportional to the external magnetic field (B_0, T):

$$\omega = \gamma B_0 \tag{1}$$

where γ is a constant called the gyromagnetic ratio (26.751×10^7 rad T^{-1}s^{-1} for protons).

A. Relaxation

M_0 is proportional to the total number of protons present in the sample, and hence is also called the proton density. To be able to distinguish the magnetization M_0 from the external magnetic field, M_0 is rotated by 90° into the transverse (xy) plane using a radiofrequency (RF) pulse at the Larmor frequency. Immediately following this 90° pulse, the initial magnetization level can be detected. In time, the thermal equilibrium is restored, and the magnetization vector returns to the z-axis.

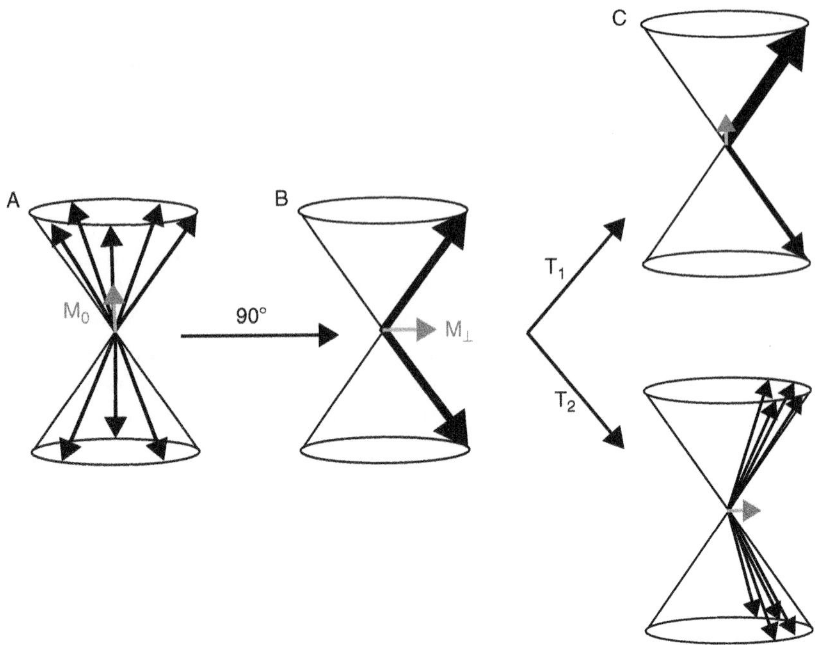

Fig. 1 Schematic representation of the nuclear magnetic resonance principle. (A) The sample magnetization M_0 arises from the uneven distribution of the spins (black arrows) between two different states, either parallel or anti-parallel to the main magnetic field B_0. The spins precess around the main magnetic field direction with the Larmor frequency ω. (B) After the application of a 90° pulse, the original distribution is shifted into the horizontal plane and phase coherence is established (the spins are all aligned along the same axis). The result is a sample magnetization $M_\perp$. (C) The spins return to the original distribution through T_1 relaxation. The loss of phase coherence is called T_2 relaxation. Both processes occur simultaneously but are depicted separately in the picture.

The characteristic times involved in this process are the spin relaxation times: longitudinal relaxation time (T_1) for the restoration of the magnetization along the z-axis, and the transverse relaxation time (T_2) for the decay in the xy-plane (Fig. 1).

1. T_2 and T_2*

The transverse relaxation time T_2 is also called the spin-spin relaxation time, referring to the molecular interactions behind the transverse relaxation process. The protons experience intramolecular dipolar interactions between two protons within the same molecule, as well as intermolecular interactions with protons of neighboring molecules. This interaction becomes more efficient when the contact time between protons is relatively long, for example, in viscous media. When the rotational correlation time of the molecules is short, as is the case for free water molecules, T_2 is relatively long (~3 s). Water molecules interacting with macromolecules or solid surfaces generally have slower tumbling rates, which leads to a reduction in the relaxation time. Because water mobility often varies substantially between tissue types, and changes in situations of cellular stress, T_2-dependent contrast is very commonly used in MRI studies.

In addition to these spin-spin interactions, the transverse magnetization is also perturbed by small local magnetic field differences. This results in different (local) Larmor precession frequencies of the spins under observation and thus in a loss of phase coherence causing a faster decay of the magnetization in the xy-plane. The corresponding apparent relaxation time is called T_2^* to distinguish it from the intrinsic transverse relaxation time T_2.

This field-disturbing effect can be exploited as a source of contrast in tissue, since such magnetic field inhomogeneities typically occur at interfaces of structures with differing magnetic susceptibilities, like soft tissue and bone, or tissue and blood. T_2^* contrast is of specific importance in blood oxygenation level dependent (BOLD) imaging, which is widely used in functional MRI investigations (Ogawa *et al.*, 1998). The paramagnetic nature of deoxygenated blood generates magnetic field gradients in blood vessels and surrounding tissues, leading to signal loss in T_2^*-weighted images. Fast T_2^*-weighted imaging is performed continuously to track transient changes in the magnetic field disturbances associated with the balance between oxyhemoglobin and deoxyhemoglobin in the blood, thus providing information on local neuronal activity. The second important application of T_2^* contrast is its use in contrast enhanced MRI (Modo and Williams, 2002). Specific exogenous (super)paramagnetic contrast agents, analogous to the tracers used in nuclear medicine, are being developed continuously in order to target specific areas or molecules, thus providing a means to map molecular events *in vivo*. Most commonly used T_2/T_2^* contrast agents are iron oxide particles, causing hypointensities on the corresponding images by lowering T_2/T_2^*, hence the name "negative" contrast agents.

a. T_2 and T_2^* measurements

Measuring relaxation times rather then making weighted images allows the quantification of observed changes. As already described, for detection the bulk magnetization M_0 is rotated by 90° into the xy-plane. The ensuing loss of phase coherence due to T_2^* effects can be reversed by the application of a series of 180° RF pulses following the initial 90° RFpulse, forming the so-called spin-echo (SE) sequence. The restoration of coherent magnetization between the 180° pulses is called an echo. The amplitude of this echo is only attenuated by T_2 relaxation (Fig. 2).

T_2^* can be measured by means of gradient echoes. In the SE sequence the 180° pulse reverses the effects of local field inhomogeneities, whereas in a gradient echo sequence the echo is generated by reversing a magnetic field gradient. The main difference between a spin echo and a gradient is that the gradient echo does not refocus the dephasing due to field inhomogeneities, and therefore the echo is weighted according to T_2^* rather than T_2. In addition to its use in T_2^* imaging,

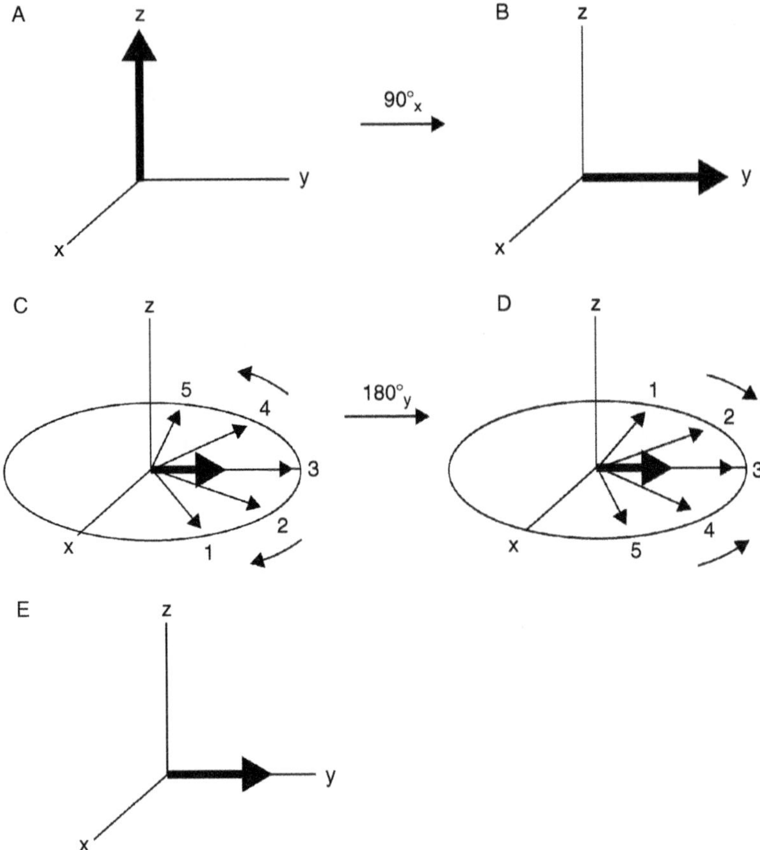

Fig. 2 (A) Diagram showing the fanning out and refocussing of magnetization in the course of a spin-echo sequence. (B) After the application of a 90° pulse, the original distribution is shifted into the horizontal plane. (C) The loss of phase coherence is primarily due to T_2* effects. (D) The 180° pulse flips the spins in the xy-plane, and the magnetization refocusses along the y-axis. The attenuation of the net magnetization vector is due to T_2 relaxation.

gradient echoes are commonly used in rapid imaging sequences, as the echo time can be made much shorter than in spin echo sequences.

2. T_1

The other relaxation time must be considered is the longitudinal relaxation time T_1, also referred to as the spin-lattice relaxation time. The mechanisms behind this relaxation are complex, but it is facilitated by the presence of microstructures (macromolecules, membranes etc.), also called the lattice, that via dipolar interactions can absorb the energy of the excited protons. This energy transfer is most efficient when the rotational correlation rate of the molecules is in the same range as the Larmor frequency. In practice, this means that T_1 becomes shorter as the molecular mobility decreases, but increases again for very slow molecular motion, as in solids. Both T_1 and T_2 reflect the properties of the physical microenvironment of water in tissue, albeit not in exactly the same way. Commonly used paramagnetic contrast agents (e.g., gadolinium or manganese-containing particles) decrease the longitudinal relaxation time T_1 leading to positive contrast.

a. T_1 measurements

The most well-known sequence to measure T_1 is the inversion recovery (IR) sequence. This sequence starts with a 180° RF pulse causing inversion of M_0, which then gradually recovers to its equilibrium. To detect the amount of magnetization left, a 90° pulse is applied after a range of delay times. This rotates the magnetization into the *xy*-plane, where it can be detected (Fig. 3). From the different delay times and the corresponding residual magnetization levels, T_1 can be calculated.

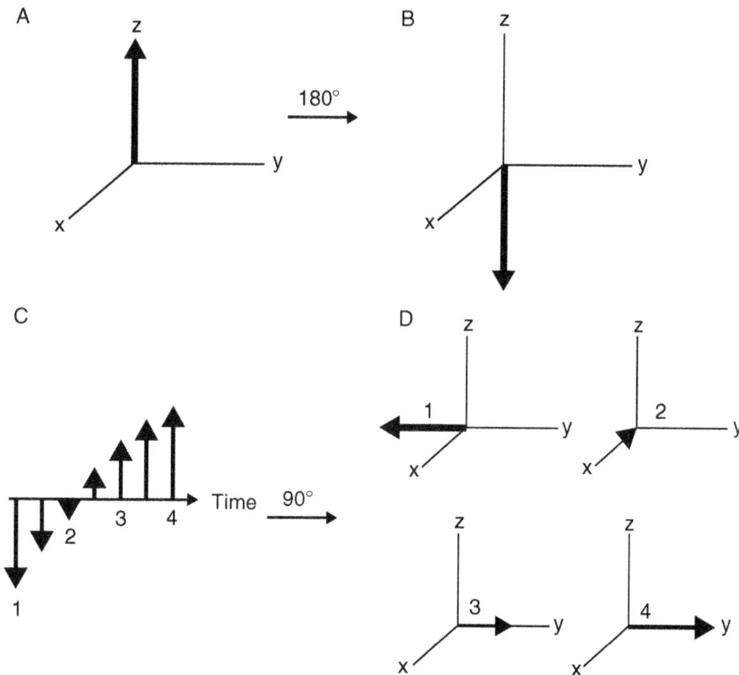

Fig. 3 (A) Diagram showing the magnetization changes during an IR sequence. (B) The 180° pulse inverts the magnetization M_0. (C) In time, the magnetization returns to equilibrium due to T_1 relaxation. (D) 90° pulses are applied to detect the residual magnetization at a number of time points. After each 90° pulse, a waiting time is introduced to let the magnetization return to equilibrium, after which the next cycle of 180°-90° pulses is performed.

B. Diffusion

Up to now, the translational motion of individual water molecules has not been considered. However, all molecules in a fluid are subject to Brownian movements, the extent of this motion depending on the temperature and the viscosity of the fluid. When an ensemble of molecules is followed in time, the root mean square displacement (x, m) shows a $\sqrt{t}$ dependence:

$$x = \sqrt{2dDt} \tag{2}$$

where D is the bulk diffusion coefficient of the fluid ($m^2 s^{-1}$), t is the displacement time (s), and d (=1, 2, or 3) is the dimensionality of the diffusion displacement. Normally, the displacement distribution of all molecules is Gaussian, where the mean displacement distance increases with increasing displacement times. However, if the molecules encounter barriers to diffusion, for example, cell membranes, these determine the maximum displacement. These boundary restrictions imply that the displacement distribution is no longer Gaussian and is going to depend on the diffusion time. As a result, the measured apparent diffusion coefficient (ADC) is smaller than the intrinsic D. This ADC value is sensitive to the number of barriers, their geometry and their permeability: in other words to the tissue microstructure.

The above is true if isotropic diffusion can be assumed, that is, diffusion that exhibits no directionality. Many biological tissues have a microstructure that favors molecular motion in a certain direction. In the brain, diffusional anisotropy occurs primarily in white matter tracts, caused by the myelin sheaths and other structures surrounding the nerve fibers, which restrict diffusion perpendicular to the axonal length. The anisotropic diffusion that arises when displacement along one direction occurs more readily than along another is defined by a diffusion tensor, and diffusion tensor imaging (DTI) is the term used for measurements of the full diffusional properties of the sample in all three dimensions (Moseley *et al.*, 1991).

1. Diffusion measurements

The ADC can be measured using a pulsed field gradient (PFG) experiment. In this experiment a sequence of two pulsed magnetic field gradients of equal magnitude but opposite sign and separated by an interval Δ temporarily change the resonance frequency of the observed spins [Eq. (1)] as a function of their position. If the spins remain at exactly the same position, the effects of the opposing gradient pulses compensate each other. However, as soon as translational motion occurs, the gradients induced frequency shifts do not exactly compensate each other anymore and a phase shift occurs. Because diffusion is random in all directions, no net phase shift results, but phase coherence is partially lost, resulting in attenuation of the echo amplitude (Fig. 4). The amount of this attenuation is

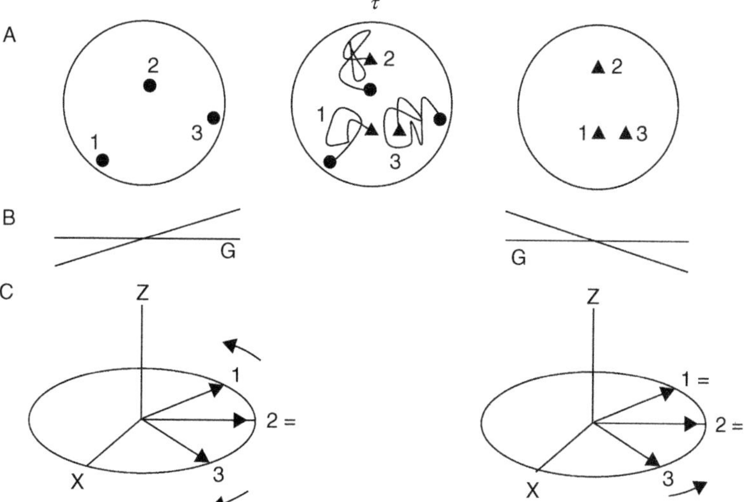

Fig. 4 (A) Water diffusion for three different spins within a sample. (B) Two diffusion gradients are applied with opposite sign and a delay time τ between them. (C) Diffusing spins experience different phase shifts (dependent on their position in the direction of the applied diffusion gradient) and are incompletely refocused, leading to a net loss in signal intensity.

determined by the length, amplitude and separation of the gradient pulses, summarized in the so-called *b* factor, and by the mean translational distance traveled during the interval Δ, which depends on the ADC. The signal intensity in a diffusion-weighted image (DWI) can therefore be described as

$$S_b = S_0 e^{-b \cdot \mathrm{ADC}} \tag{3}$$

where S_b is the DWI signal intensity and S_0 is the signal without any diffusion gradients applied.

C. Perfusion

Perfusion (or cerebral blood flow, CBF) is the amount of blood delivered to the capillary bed of a block of tissue in a certain period of time (units ml blood/100 g/min), and is closely related to the delivery of oxygen and other nutrients to the tissue. It is this quantity which determines the energy status of the tissue, and for this reason much effort has been put into its measurement. Two main MRI approaches have been developed for CBF measurement: bolus tracking and arterial spin labeling (ASL).

1. Bolus Tracking

A bolus of paramagnetic contrast agent is injected intravenously into the subject. Soon after, the contrast agent passes through the vasculature of the brain, and causes the signal of a T_2 or T_2*-weighted image to change due to a difference in magnetic susceptibility between the intra- and extravascular compartments. This reduction is transient as the bolus of contrast agent washes through the vasculature of the tissue. The passage of the bolus is relatively fast (of the order of seconds), particularly in small animals. It is therefore important to acquire images as quickly as possible, in order to characterize the signal time course accurately, which is crucial for the quantification of CBF. The rate at which successive bolus tracking experiments can be performed is limited by the clearance rate of the contrast agent from the vasculature. Residual levels of contrast agent will reduce the signal change induced by subsequent boluses and therefore reduce the precision of the CBF measurement, and repeated injections of contrast agents such as gadolinium are eventually limited by their toxicity (Shellock and Kanal, 1999).

To calculate CBF values from the bolus passage time course, the arterial input function (AIF), that is, the concentration of contrast agent entering the voxel of interest at a certain time point, needs to be known. The AIF is usually estimated from the signal time course within a major artery, such as the middle cerebral artery. Although not impossible in small animals (Perman *et al.*, 1992; Porkka *et al.*, 1991), reliable characterization is not straightforward due to the small size of arteries. Additionally, the AIF should strictly define the entry of contrast agent into the voxel of interest, and this may be different to the passage of the bolus through a major artery, due to delay and dispersion effects between the two locations (Calamante *et al.*, 2000; Ostergaard *et al.*, 1996). As a result, reliable quantification of CBF can be problematic, and so summary parameters have been widely used as an alternative. Their advantage is that they are quick and easy to calculate, with minimal assumptions required; their disadvantage is that they do not give values for the real physiological variables CBF and cerebral blood volume (CBV), and depend on experimental conditions, for example, injection rate, vascular geometry and cardiac output. Figure 5 illustrates the most commonly used summary parameters: bolus arrival time (BAT), time to peak (TTP), maximum peak concentration (MPC), mean transit time index (MTT_i), relative CBV (rel. CBV) and relative CBF index (rel. CBF_i). These parameters are related to different aspects of the cerebral hemodynamics, for example, BAT, the time after injection at which contrast agent begins to arrive in the voxel of interest, can provide information about the role of collateral blood supply when CBF is compromised. MTT_i is an approximation of the average time for any given particle of tracer to pass through the tissue, and gives an indication of different vascular territories. The CBF value obtained from the rel. CBV ("relative" because it does not take the AIF into account) and MTT_i is dubbed relative CBF_i. Although the use of summary parameters does not provide absolute values for CBF and CBV, it provides a useful tool for the investigation of perfusion during normal and ischemic conditions.

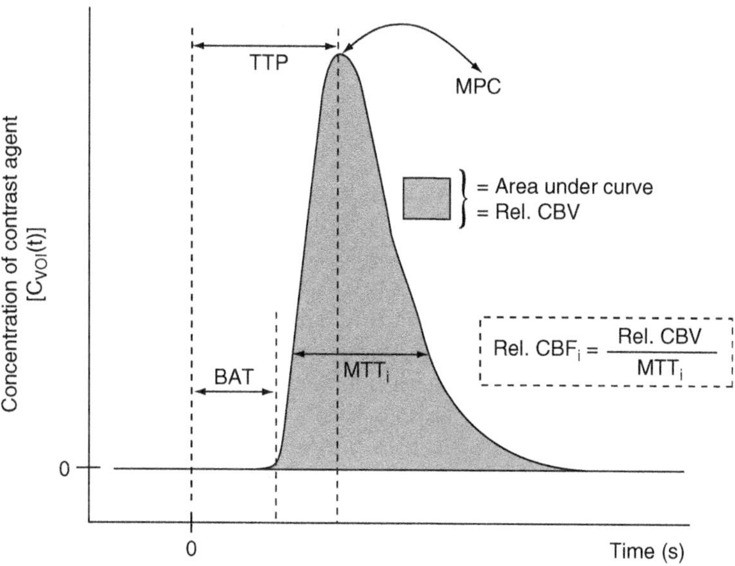

Fig. 5 Schematic representation of the concentration time curve observed in brain tissue following intravenous injection of a paramagnetic contrast agent. The summary parameters illustrated are: BAT, bolus arrival time; TTP, time to peak; MPC, mean peak concentration; MTT_i, mean transit time index; rel. CBV, relative cerebral blood volume; and rel. CBF_i, relative cerebral blood flow index.

2. Arterial Spin Labeling

ASL is a CBF measurement method that uses magnetically labeled blood water as an endogenous tracer. It is appealing for imaging animal models of brain disease because it does not require injection of exogenous tracers and places no restriction of the number of repeat measurements that can be made in a single study. This makes ASL well suited to the monitoring of CBF during experimental time courses in animal models. The images obtained with ASL can be converted into CBF maps (with units of ml/100 g/min) as long as certain other MR parameters (such as T_1 and labeling efficiency) are also measured.

In ASL, perfusion-weighted images are generated by labeling inflowing blood water by inversion of its longitudinal magnetization. Two images must be acquired: one in which spin labeling is performed (the labeled image) and one in which spin labeling is not performed (the control image). The difference between the two images is proportional to the amount of labeled blood that enters the imaging slice during the time between labeling and image acquisition, and therefore is also proportional to CBF. Spin labeling can be achieved using several alternative approaches, which has given rise to a family of ASL techniques that will now be discussed in turn.

a. CASL Measurements

The original ASL approach (Detre *et al.*, 1992) is now generally known as *continuous* ASL (or CASL), because inflowing blood magnetization is inverted continuously over a period of several seconds prior to image acquisition. This allows an accumulation of spin labeled water as it is deposited in the perfused cerebral tissue. The measurement approach is illustrated in Fig. 6. A magnetic field gradient is applied to give the proton magnetization a position-dependent frequency spread. An RF pulse of 1–3 s is applied with a frequency offset corresponding to water protons flowing through the carotid and vertebral arteries in the neck. This causes inversion of flowing spins via a process known as flow-induced adiabatic inversion (Dixon *et al.*, 1986). Following the labeling RF pulse, an image is acquired using a rapid imaging technique (e.g., EPI). A problem associated with the labeling RF pulse is chemical exchange of protons between water and macromolecules which causes the water magnetization to decrease (the MT effect; see also magnetization transfer contrast (MTC) imaging below). For this reason, an RF pulse with the reverse frequency offset is applied for the control image, which results in the same MT effect in the labeled and control image, and the only difference between the images is due to the perfusion-weighting.

b. PASL Measurements

Soon after the introduction of CASL, alternative approaches using shorter adiabatic inversion pulses were proposed, known as *pulsed* ASL (PASL). They have the advantage of a lower RF energy deposition than CASL due to the short (~10 ms) inversion pulses, but also have a lower intrinsic SNR for the perfusion signal. One of the PASL approaches is known as flow-sensitive alternating inversion recovery, or *FAIR* (Fig. 6). This technique uses a pair of IR images, one following a slice-selective inversion pulse and the other following a nonselective (global) inversion pulse. The slice-selective IR image is flow-sensitive because the inflowing blood water magnetization is fully relaxed, and so accelerates the apparent T_1 relaxation of the tissue that it flows into. In the nonselective IR case, both tissue and inflowing blood magnetization are inverted, greatly reducing the flow sensitivity. Since the same inversion time is used in both the slice-selective and nonselective acquisitions, the signal from the static tissue is the same in both, but a difference between the images is observed in the presence of flow.

Perfusion can be quantified using ASL images and some additional information such as T_1 (for a description of the principles, see Calamante *et al.*, 1999a,b; Thomas *et al.*, 2000). An important factor that affects the accuracy of CBF quantification is a parameter known as the transit time. Following spin inversion, blood water travels through the vascular tree until it reaches the capillary bed and exchanges into the cerebral tissue. During this time (the transit time), the spin label decays at a rate determined by the T_1 of arterial blood (T_{1a}). This must be accounted for in order to achieve accurate CBF quantification. Transit time effects are particularly problematic in CASL, where the labeling plane must be a minimum distance from the imaging slice to ensure that it coincides with a major artery.

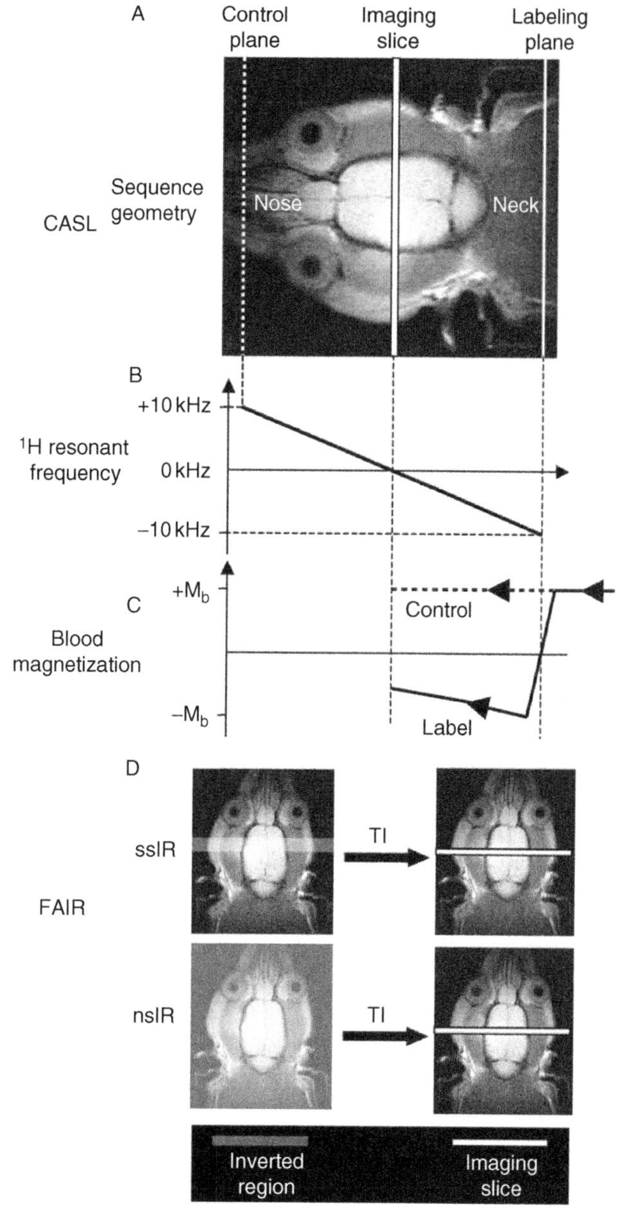

Fig. 6 (A) Continuous arterial spin labeling (CASL). Axial MR image of the rat brain showing the relative positions of the imaging slice (coronal) and the labeling and control planes. (B) A magnetic field gradient causes water protons to resonate over a range of frequencies dependent on their position, so that the labeling plane corresponds to −10 kHz and the control plane to +10 kHz. (C) By simultaneously applying a −10 kHz off-resonance RF pulse, blood water ^{1}H spins are inverted as they flow through the inversion plane (spin labeled). The control plane does not intersect any major arteries and so application of a +10-kHz RF pulse causes MT effects but not spin labeling. (D) Pulsed arterial spin labeling (PASL). In FAIR, a pair of images is also acquired, one following a slice-selective inversion (upper) and the other following a nonselective inversion (lower). The difference between the images is caused by the difference in the magnetization state of the inflowing blood water.

With PASL, transit times tend to be less because the labeling region can be placed immediately adjacent to the imaging slice. To decrease the sensitivity to transit time effects, the sequences can be modified by inserting a post labeling delay, which allows time for all the blood to travel from where it was labeled into the imaging region (Alsop, 1996; Luh *et al.*, 1999; Wong *et al.*, 1998).

D. Magnetization Transfer Contrast

A certain fraction of protons in tissue exist in a so-called "bound" state, that is, their motion is restricted because they are part either of macromolecules, or of water molecules within the hydration layers around macromolecules. These protons posses very short T_2 relaxation times (<100 μs) and hence are not accessible by standard SE MRI methods. (With currently available small-bore technology, minimum echo times are of the order of several ms, and hence the signal from these protons has already decayed before signal acquisition.) While simple models for proton relaxation behavior predict that such a proton population will have some influence upon T_1 and T_2, Wolff and Balaban (1989) proposed the method of MTC imaging (Henkelman *et al.*, 2001), as a more direct means of probing these "bound" protons.

MTC imaging is based on an inverse Fourier relationship between T_2 and the range of frequencies over which protons respond to RF excitation: protons in the "bound" fraction possess a very short T_2 and hence exhibit a broad resonance width ($\sim$20 kHz) in the frequency domain. Conversely, bulk water protons have a long T_2 with a correspondingly narrow ($\sim$10 Hz) frequency domain resonance (Fig. 7A). This difference can be used to excite the "bound" fraction independently from the bulk protons. If RF energy is supplied at a frequency offset from the central Larmor frequency (typically 1–5 kHz) the magnetization in the "bound" fraction will be reduced by saturation, while, in the absence of exchange, the bulk water pool would remain unaffected (Fig. 7B). However, on the time-scale of a typical MRI experiment there is a significant exchange of magnetization between the two proton fractions, either by chemical exchange or by magnetic interactions. Since the "bound" proton magnetization has been reduced by the off-resonance irradiation, such exchange also leads to a reduction in both the magnitude of the observable bulk water magnetization and its associated T_1 (Fig. 7C). The degree of reduction depends upon both the relative sizes of the two fractions and upon the rate of magnetization exchange between them: both of these factors may be influenced by tissue pathology.

1. MTC Measurements

In its most simple form (e.g., Ordidge *et al.*, 1991), the MTC imaging experiment involves collecting an image (S_s) which is preceded by a long ($\sim$3 s) saturating off-resonance RF pulse, followed by a second image (S_0) without a presaturation pulse. The magnetization transfer ratio (MTR) is then quantified as

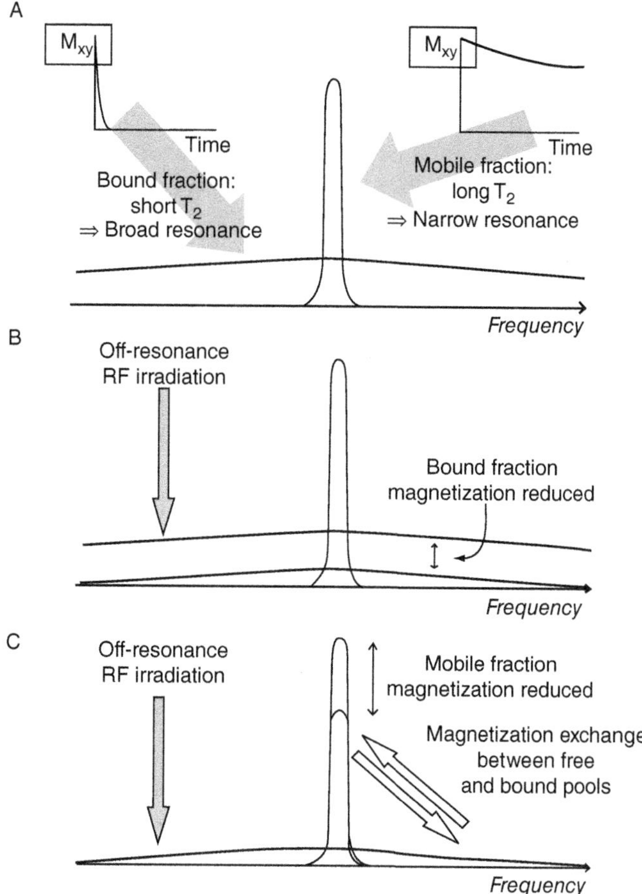

Fig. 7 Schematic diagrams showing the origins of magnetization transfer contrast. (A) Macromolecular-bound protons possess a very short T_2 and hence a broad resonance response in the frequency domain. Mobile water protons conversely exhibit a narrow frequency domain line-width. (B) In the absence of exchange, the application of RF energy at a frequency away from resonance perturbs only the bound proton fraction, causing the magnetization of this pool to reduce towards zero. (C) Exchange of magnetization between free and bound protons causes a reduction in the magnetization of the mobile pool, and hence an observable reduction in MR image intensity.

$$\mathrm{MTR} = \frac{S_0 - S_s}{S_0} \tag{4}$$

A high MTR signifies the presence of a significant proton pool associated with macromolecules or cellular microstructure *and* a significant exchange of magnetization between these protons and those of the bulk water. Reduction of the MTR suggests a disruption of tissue microstructure, the most successful application of

MTC in experimental neuroscience being the investigation of pathological disruption of white matter due to demyelination.

In order to reduce imaging time, selective saturation of the "bound" fraction may also be achieved by pulsed methods whereby gradient-echo images with short TR are obtained with a low angle excitation pulse preceded by a short (~10 ms) off-resonance pulse (Dousset *et al.*, 1992). If the repetition time is sufficiently short (~100 ms) compared to the T_1 relaxation time of the "bound" pool, an equilibrium is established after a number of cycles, resulting in substantial saturation of the "bound" fraction.

It should be noted that unless total selective saturation of the bound pool is achieved, a situation impossible to achieve in practice, the magnitude of the MTC effect is dependent upon the duration, intensity and frequency offset of the off-resonance pulses. Caution is therefore required in the quantitative comparison of MTC imaging results obtained using differing experimental schemes.

III. Applications of MRI to Experimental Neuropathology

The following section contains an overview of some the possibilities for MRI investigations of cerebral pathology in experimental animal models (for an extensive review of applications, see Van Bruggen and Roberts, 2002).

A. Cerebral Ischemia

The use of MRI in experimental neuroimaging stroke research has focused on a number of areas which include the use of MRI both as a diagnostic and as a predictive tool (Thomas *et al.*, 2000). Some of the most important topics are the investigation of the underlying processes that lead to cell death (Hoehn-Berlage, 1995); defining and understanding the concept of the penumbra (Hossmann, 1994) as a possible salvageable region, and related to that possible therapies for the treatment of stroke (Fischer and Brott, 2003; Rudin *et al.*, 1999; Wu *et al.*, 2007).

1. ADC Changes Following a Stroke

It is now well established that following a stroke the ADC of water decreases minutes after the reduction in blood supply (Moseley *et al.*, 1990) (e.g., Fig. 8; Lythgoe *et al.*, 1999). Yet it was first demonstrated, by the use of DWI, that following occlusion of the middle cerebral artery (MCAO), the ADC decreases and the corresponding ischemic lesion in both rat and cat are visible within minutes and expands primarily during the first 2 h (Roussel *et al.*, 1994). Although the lesion size has nearly fully evolved at 2 h, the ADC value continues to decrease for a period of up to 4–6 h following MCAO (40% of control) (Knight *et al.*, 1994), with some studies reporting the lowest ADC values at 24–48 h (40–50% of control) (Hoehn-Berlage, 1995). In the chronic stages of cerebral ischemia, the ADC of

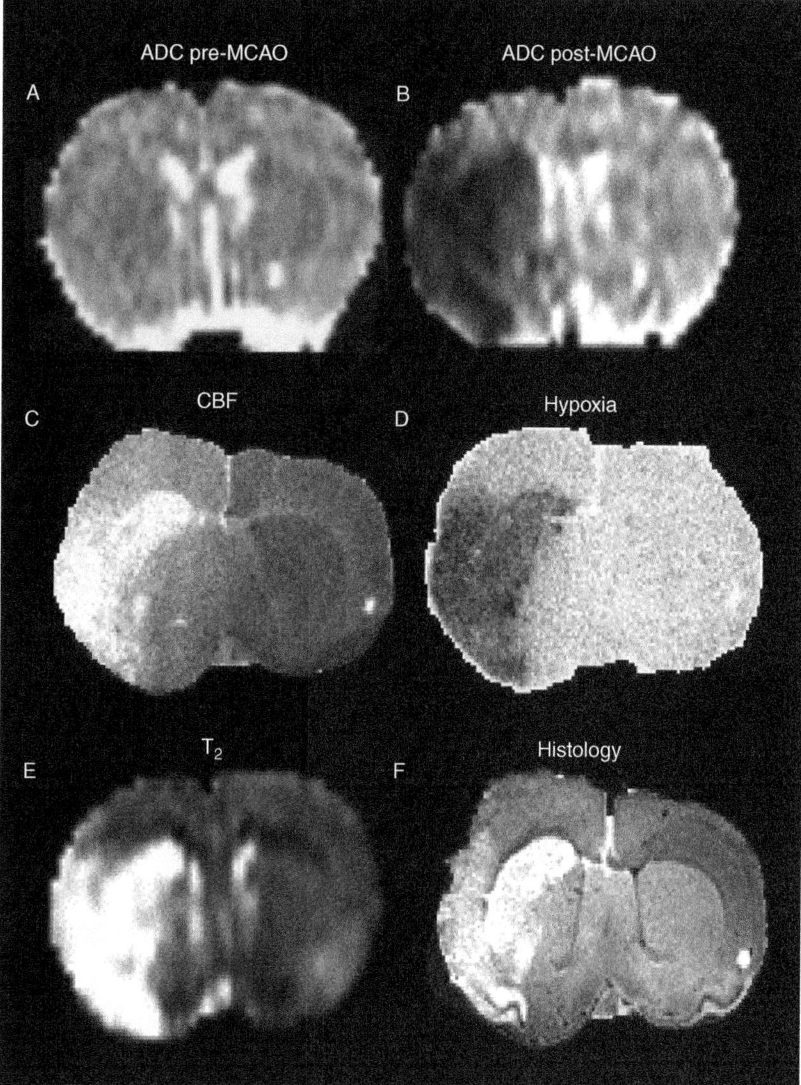

Fig. 8 MR and autoradiographic images from a rat brain before and after intraluminal suture occlusion of the middle cerebral artery: (A) ADC image pre MCA occlusion; images of (B) ADC, (C) CBF, and (D) hypoxia 2 h post-MCA occlusion; and (E) MR T_2 image and (F) histology 7 h post MCA occlusion. Following permanent middle cerebral artery occlusion in the rat, the ADC decreases and the lesions area at 2 h is comparable with the area of hypoxia. The area of blood flow decrease is larger than the area of hypoxia or ADC decrease, indicating the so called "diffusion/perfusion mismatch" region. The area of infarction, as indicated by the H and E stain, was similar to the area of T_2 increase at 7 h, which matched the area of ADC change at 2 h (Lythgoe *et al.*, 1999).

water exhibits a different pattern. Approximately 24–48 h after a vessel occlusion, the ADC starts to rise again and slowly returns to a normal value at 3 days (Knight *et al.*, 1991). Following this, a subsequent increase in the diffusion of water above that of the ischemic control can be observed after 1 week (Knight *et al.*, 1994). The elevated ADC of tissue water (or pseudo-normalization) above control values, is associated with cellular lysis or the loss of cellular barriers, combined with an excessive accumulation of edematous water (Pierpaoli *et al.*, 1993).

2. CBF Following a Stroke

While DWI may provide unique information about the effect of an ischemic insult as early as a few minutes postocclusion, it is clearly desirable to obtain information regarding the integrity of the vascular bed. MRI experiments in rat and cat models of focal cerebral ischemia demonstrate an absence of contrast agent in the ischemic core of the lesion (Quast *et al.*, 1993). Interestingly, in the periphery of the lesion, a diffusion-perfusion mismatch can be observed, that is perfusion deficits not great enough to cause energy failure may go unnoticed on DWI. A cat model of hypoperfusion shows the same pattern, that is, the DWIs show no evidence of abnormality in the territory of the occluded MCA, whereas the dynamic susceptibility contrast (DSC-MRI) blood flow measurements show decreased CBF throughout the MCA region (Derugin and Roberts, 1994). This early work using MRI has been followed by studies using noninvasive ASL techniques for the quantitation of CBF in animal models (Lythgoe *et al.*, 2002). By combining DWI and CBF data, three different tissue areas can be assigned following an ischemic insult: areas with normal perfusion and diffusion, denoting normal tissue; tissue that has a CBF decrease without diffusion changes corresponding to a region of hypoperfusion; and a region in which there is a concomitant diffusion and perfusion decrease, corresponding to a severely compromised region (Calamante *et al.*, 1999a,b).

3. The Penumbra

The term *penumbra* was introduced to designate a zone of brain tissue with moderate ischemia and impaired neuronal function, with the neuronal paralysis being fully reversed upon reperfusion (Astrup *et al.*, 1981). Currently, the term has a wider definition and is used to describe a region of ischemic tissue peripheral to the core where viable neurons may be found, and thus may be potentially salvageable with suitable intervention or therapy (Hossmann, 1994; Kinouchi *et al.*, 1993). Penumbral zones can be delineated using several different imaging modalities, each of which have definitions that rely on the underlying mechanisms of that technique (Hossmann, 1994). Moseley *et al.* (1990) observed an ADC decrease in an animal model of cerebral ischemia; this reduction of tissue water diffusion is attributed to an osmotically obliged shift of extracellular water to intracellular compartments, as a result of a disruption of ion homeostasis and formation of cytotoxic edema.

The region of signal intensity change in DWI corresponds closely to the region of periinfarct acidosis, but also encompasses the area of ATP depletion (infarct core). Therefore, it was postulated that the outer margin of the DWI visible lesion corresponds with that of the penumbra (Kohno *et al.*, 1995). However, this is only part of the picture, as it is now acknowledged that regions of DWI change that normalize on reperfusion may proceed on to infarction at a later time point (van Lookeren Campagne *et al.*, 1999) and that the areas of so-called diffusion-perfusion mismatch need to be considered as well (Baird and Warach, 1998; Meng *et al.*, 2004).

4. Spreading Depression

The occurrence of transient waves of membrane depolarization known as *spreading depression* (*SD*) emanating from an infarct core, has been suggested as one mechanism for the expansion of tissue injury into the penumbral zone (Nedergaard and Astrup, 1986). During SD the metabolic rate of the tissue increases in response to the greatly enhanced energy demands of the activated ion exchange pumps (Kocher, 1990). In the penumbra, flows are suppressed and as a result, the increased metabolic demand is not compensated by an increase in oxygen and glucose (Back *et al.*, 1994). Eventually ATP stores will be depleted, followed by the cascade of pathophysiological events leading to tissue infarction. Using DWI and ADC maps to monitor cell volume change (Latour *et al.*, 1994), and gradient-echo MRI to following apparent changes in blood flow, both of these consequences can be imaged (Gardner Medwin *et al.*, 1994; Gyngell *et al.*, 1994). The change in ADC associated with SD has been used to study the pathological basis by which SD leads to infarct growth and the mechanism whereby neuroprotective drugs may have their therapeutic effect (Rother *et al.*, 1996; Takano *et al.*, 1996).

5. Brain Reorganization Following Stroke

Stroke patients show some functional recovery over time, which is commonly thought to be associated with brain plasticity. BOLD MRI studies have demonstrated changes in activation patterns following a stroke (Dijkhuizen *et al.*, 2001; Hoehn *et al.*, 2001). With the use of behavioral tests and MRI in a rat stroke model, Dijkhuizen *et al.* (2001) assessed the correlation between temporal changes in sensorimotor function, brain activation patterns and cerebral ischemic damage. Unilateral stroke induced acute dysfunction of the contralateral forelimb, which significantly recovered at later stages. Forelimb impairment was accompanied by loss of fMRI activation in the lesioned cortex. At 3 days after stroke, extensive fMRI responses were detected in the contralesional hemisphere. After 14 days, they found reduced involvement of the contralesional hemisphere, and significant responses in the lesion periphery. A further study suggests that the degree of shift of activation balance toward the contralesional hemisphere early after stroke increases with the extent of tissue injury and that functional recovery is associated mainly with preservation or restoration of activation in the ipsilesional hemisphere (Dijkhuizen *et al.*, 2003).

6. Other MRI Contrast Mechanisms for Imaging Stroke

During the last few years animal studies have demonstrated that several MRI parameters provide additional information to the now clinically implemented T_2, diffusion and perfusion measurements.

Since BOLD MRI is sensitive to changes in regional tissue oxygenation status (Ogawa *et al.*, 1998), it can be used to monitor acute deoxygenation following induction of ischemia as well as reoxygenation after reperfusion (Roussel *et al.*, 1995). BOLD MR signal intensity, measured by T_2*-weighted MRI, drops immediately upon the onset of ischemia, and rises when reflow occurs. A transient overshoot in signal intensity during reperfusion has been described and may reflect postreperfusion hyperemia (de Crespigny *et al.*, 1992). These hemodynamic responses indirectly report on local changes in CBF, CBV and oxygen extraction fraction and their individual contributions cannot easily be distinguished. Early changes in T_2 values have been reported in conditions of ischemia (Calamante *et al.*, 1999a,b; Grohn *et al.*, 1998) and oligemia (Lythgoe *et al.*, 2000). In the latter studies of cerebral ischemia, two patterns were observed following an initial T_2 decrease: (i) T_2 values remained depressed throughout the study without an ADC change indicating a mild hypoperfusion condition (Calamante *et al.*, 1999a,b; Grohn *et al.*, 1998); (ii) T_2 and ADC values are decreased throughout the study, indicating a severe hypoperfusion condition (Calamante *et al.*, 1999a,b; Roussel *et al.*, 1995). Further, early detection (within 15 min) of ischemia (Calamante *et al.*, 1999a,b) and oligemia (Lythgoe *et al.*, 2000) are possible using the MRI parameter T_1. The underlying mechanism for this change is still unclear, but may depend of tissue oxygenation status. These data highlight that changes in T_2 and T_1 and are not always related to vasogenic edema and early changes in these parameters may provide information as to the pathophysiological nature of ischemia or oligemia. Recently, this potential has been further underlined by studying the changes within the temporal T_2 profile to differentiate between areas prone to selective neuronal necrosis and the development of cerebral infarction within subcortical regions (Wegener, 2006).

In deciding whether tissue is suitable for treatment, it is necessary to distinguish compromised yet recoverable from permanently damaged tissue. To this end, Grohn *et al.* (2000) have demonstrated early detection of irreversible cerebral ischemia in the rat using a parameter known as $T_{1\rho}$ (T_1 in the rotating frame), which probes specific spin populations taking place in the macromolecules or in the macromolecular-water interface.

Recently, manganese-enhanced MRI was used to study brain plasticity after stroke (Van der Zijden, 2007). Manganese enhancement is based on the uptake of Mn^{2+} through voltage-gated calcium channels, and as such is a tool to track neuronal connectivity and activity *in vivo*.

B. Epilepsy

Although the majority of experimental epilepsy research has been performed outside the neuroimaging field, there has been increasing interest following some early nuclear magnetic resonance spectroscopy investigations, and more recently imaging studies using MRI. The present goal of imaging is to characterize both the metabolic derangement and brain injury associated with seizures, using functional (diffusion and perfusion imaging) and structural (T_1 and T_2) neuroimaging.

1. Short-Term Changes

Following kinate injection in the rat brain, tissue damage is detectable by MRI, in which the T_1-weighted images provide better lesion contrast than the T_2 approach, and DWI shows improved contrast for edematous tissue (King *et al.*, 1991). BOLD MRI shows increases in blood flow that were associated with minor behavioral seizure signs in a similar model, but as seizure activity progresses the signal intensity remains near control values possibly due to the increased oxygen extraction of the tissue (Ogawa and Lee, 1992). Zhong *et al.* (1993) used diffusion-weighted MR imaging to investigate changes associated with epilepsy. Following intraperitoneal injection of bicuculline in the rat, the ADC in the brain decreases 14–18% during seizures. No changes occur in T_1 or T_2. This result demonstrates that during a seizure the ADC changes in a similar fashion to that reported in ischemia (Thomas *et al.*, 2000), but under different circumstances as the blood flow is increased and the ATP stores are only modestly reduced. This ADC decrease during seizure activity leads to the provisional hypothesis that the ADC change may be due to perturbations in intracellular cytosolic streaming (Duong *et al.*, 1998; Zhong *et al.*, 1993). Furthermore, ADC normalization is different between brain areas ranging from 1 to 7 days. More importantly, it has also been shown that delayed processes caused by status epilepticus can also lead delayed diffusion increase resulting from an ongoing epileptic process (Nairismagi, 2004; Tokumitsu *et al.*, 1997). There is still no complete explanation for the ADC change in stroke or epilepsy (Thomas *et al.*, 2000).

2. Long-Term Changes

The long-term temporal evolution of lesion development, investigation of epileptic activity and tissue damage are well suited to the noninvasive nature of MRI. Several studies have now monitored T_2, ADC and blood brain barrier (BBB) breakdown following epilepsy (Roch *et al.*, 2002; Tokumitsu *et al.*, 1997). In parts of the cortex, and in the amygdala, the T_2 was increased by 24 h, then progressively normalized by 5–9 days and finally increased again in the chronic phase (9 weeks). The chronic T_2 increase corresponds to gliosis, and characterizes the initial step leading to development of epilepsy that could result from spontaneous seizures (Roch *et al.*, 2002). The earlier hypothesis that increased T_2 could be directly correlated with cell death has to be revised while its relation with histological staining for neurodegeneration should not obvious correlation (Dube, 2004; Nairismagi, 2004). This highlights the importance of careful interpretation of MRI data before taking conclusion about what is going on at the cellular level, for example, correlation with histology remains a necessity.

Several studies have assessed whether volumetric changes of several brain structures occurred in period following seizures with some studies going up to 6 months, as can be found summarized by Grohn *et al.* (2007). In general, decreased hippocampal volume together with increased ventricles indicates progressive atrophy, possibly caused by neuronal death.

C. Neurodegenerative Disorders

Neurodegenerative disorders such as Alzheimer's disease (AD) or Parkinson's disease (PD) are devastating progressive illnesses. A combination of MRI approaches such as pharmacological MRI, DTI, and anatomical studies of brain atrophy is particularly useful to understand the etiology and progression of these diseases (Choi *et al.*, 2003; Van Bruggen and Roberts, 2002).

1. Parkinson's Disease

The disease is characterized by striatal dopamine depletion resulting in progressive loss of motor control and the characteristic symptoms of the disease. Experimental models of PD fall into two major categories: pharmacological, for example reserpine or amphetamine administration to deplete dopamine, a largely reversible treatment, and lesioning using neurotoxins which is permanent. Imaging experimental models has largely been in the domain of PET imaging with the availability of radioligands to monitor both pre- and postsynaptic function (Brownell *et al.*, 1998). This methodology has now been largely supplanted by functional MRI (Pelled *et al.*, 2002) or pharmacological MRI (a term used to describe drug induced functional MRI changes) techniques with activity induction by levodopa (Jenkins *et al.*, 2002), D1 and D2 receptor agonists (Zhang *et al.*, 2001), amphetamine (Chen *et al.*, 1999) or dopamine transporter agonists (Chen *et al.*, 1997). Using more classical anatomical MRI sequences, temporal signal changes in T_1 and T_2 have been used to map regions of degeneration after lesioning in nonhuman primates (Miletich *et al.*, 1994) and attempts have been made to correlate T_1 relaxation times with the abnormal accumulation of iron in degenerating dopaminergic neurons in a neurotoxin rat model (Hall *et al.*, 1992).

2. Alzheimer's Disease

AD is the most common dementia in Western societies. Pathohistological findings include widespread neuronal degeneration resulting in brain atrophy, neurofibrillary tangles and neuritic plaques containing β-amyloid ($A\beta$). Especially the latter, typically ranging in size from 16 to 250 μm, form a specific hallmark of the disease, and are known to be present even before clinical onset of the disease. Therefore, in recent years much effort has been put into the development of noninvasive methods, like MRI, to detect these Aβ plaques for diagnostics and possible therapies. Nowadays with several transgenic AD mouse models at hand developing Aβ plaques multiple groups have been able image these Aβ deposition in living animal using either T_2 or T_2*-weighted imaging methods (Anderson, 2007; Braakman *et al.*, 2006; Jack, 2005; Vanhoutte, 2005). Due to partial voluming it was not possible to image plaques of all sized. It has been postulated that contrast originated by the colocalization of iron within the plaques. However, this lead to overestimation of the plaque size, which was clearly depicted on T_2* imaging. Furthermore, in comparison to conventional spin echo imaging less plaques could be detected, suggesting other effects play a role in generating contrast to. Correlating MRI plaque load with histopathological findings to investigate its sensitivity has shown only plaques over 35 μm could be detected. Therefore, regional changes in T_2 over time have been studied by creating quantitative T_2 maps. The decreased T_2 values correlated nicely with increase plaque load (Braakman, 2006; Falangola, 2007).

Other groups have tried to develop Aβ targeting contrast agents to overcome these detection limits. For example, using magnetically labeled Aβ1–40 peptide in an Alzheimer's transgenic mouse, which has a high affinity to Aβ, enabled the detection of Aβ plaques after opening the blood-brain barrier using manitol (Fig. 9) (Wadghiri *et al.*, 2003).

3. Huntington's Disease

This inherited disease is characterized by degeneration of GABAergic neurons localized mainly within the deep gray matter of the basal ganglia. Experimental models are based on acute lesioning using GABAergic antagonists or chronic lesioning using systemic administration of 3-nitroproprionic acid (Borlongan *et al.*, 1997; Hantraye, 1998). Since the discovery of the gene mutation for the disease, new transgenic mouse models are being developed (Menalled and Chesselet, 2002). Imaging data are largely PET-based, mapping regions of reduced metabolism indicative of cell loss (Araujo *et al.*, 2000). Striatal lesions are visible with T_2-weighted and DWI protocols (Hantraye *et al.*, 1992), although at acute time-points only diffusion-weighted imaging provides sufficient sensitivity (Verheul *et al.*, 1993).

D. CNS Inflammation

The inflammatory response is part of the hosts' defence to injury and infection, but can exacerbate tissue injury when excessive or inappropriate. It has become clear that inflammation contributes not only to the archetypal CNS inflammatory disease, multiple sclerosis (MS), but also to a wide variety of acute neurological

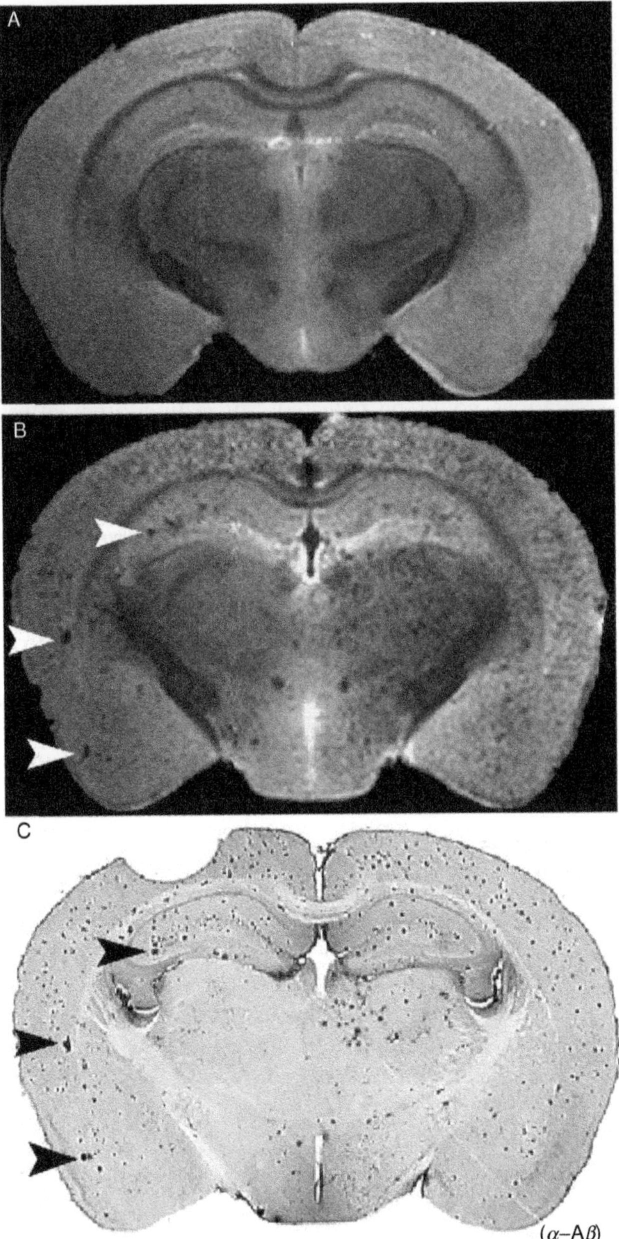

Fig. 9 Aβ plaques were detected with *ex vivo* μMRI after injection of Gd-DTPA-Aβ1–40 with mannitol. *Ex vivo* T_2-weighted SE coronal μMR images show (A) 6-month-old control and (B) APP/PS1-transgenic mouse brains. Both brains were extracted and prepared for imaging 6 h after carotid injection of Gd-DTPA-Aβ1–40 with 15% mannitol. Note the obvious matching of many larger plaques (arrowheads) between μMRI (B) and immunohistochemistry (C). (courtesy of Y. Z. Wadghiri and coworkers) Moet dus nog veranderd worden afhankelijk van het te kiezen nieuwe figuur.

and chronic neurodegenerative diseases, such as stroke, head trauma, AD, prion disease and HIV-related dementia. Despite this, little is known of the effects of inflammatory processes within the CNS, or their contribution to MR images of human neuropathologies.

1. Multiple Sclerosis

Despite a wealth of studies, the pathogenesis of MS is still not fully understood. A primary goal of animal studies is to determine the relationship between the histopathology of a disease and the MRI signal changes. Experimental allergic encephalopathy (EAE) is an autoimmune CNS disorder that can be induced in susceptible species, such as mice, rats, guinea pigs and nonhuman primates (Brok *et al.*, 2001; Gold *et al.*, 2000). However, few of these models adequately represent all of the features of human MS, and the lesions evolve spontaneously at any site within the brain and often exhibit varying temporal progressions. An alternative model is the delayed-type hypersensitivity (DTH) model in the rat (Matyszak and Perry, 1995) which involves sensitization of the immune system to a non-CNS antigen previously deposited in the brain. This model exhibits all the primary features of MS lesions: T-cell and macrophage infiltratration, BBB breakdown, edema and tissue damage, and primary demyelination. A major advantage of this model for longitudinal MRI studies is that the site of the lesion is precisely dictated by the location of the intracerebral antigen injection.

MRI findings in the EAE models include increased T_1, increased T_2 and contrast enhancement (Richards *et al.*, 1995a,b; Verhoye *et al.*, 1996), thus corresponding broadly to those found most commonly in MS patients. However, only a relatively small number of studies have investigated correlations between MRI and histopathology obtained at the same time point. An increase in T_2 has been found to correspond to regions of macrophage recruitment and edema in both guinea pig (Grossman *et al.*, 1987) and rat EAE models (Duckers *et al.*, 1997). However, T_2 changes were also associated with demyelination in the rat (Duckers *et al.*, 1997), but not in the guinea pig (Grossman *et al.*, 1987). In the *Callithrix jacchus* marmoset model of EAE increased proton density and T_2 appear to be associated with regions of either perivascular cuffing, demyelination or perivascular gliosis (Jordan *et al.*, 1999). The variability of these findings suggest that T_2-weighted MRI alone is not a reliable method of distinguishing purely inflammatory lesions from either demyelinating or remyelinating lesions (Hart *et al.*, 1998; Jordan *et al.*, 1999). In MS patients, areas which are enhanced following an injection of an MRI contrast agent, are generally considered to be a sensitive indicator for disease activity. In both guinea pig (Hawkins *et al.*, 1990) and rat (Morrissey *et al.*, 1996) models of EAE, BBB breakdown has been found to correlate with macrophage recruitment. In contrast, in the *C. jacchus* marmoset EAE model, which arguably provides the most accurate representation of the relapsing-remitting form of MS, contrast-enhancing areas correlated solely with acute, actively demyelinating lesions (Hart *et al.*, 1998). However, recent work in the rat DTH model

(Newman *et al.*, 2001) has demonstrated that axonal injury and inflammatory events occurring within a lesion are not restricted to the period of BBB breakdown and contrast enhancement. These findings suggest that MS disease progression may persist despite an intact BBB, and, consequently, contrast-enhancement may not be an accurate marker of disease activity. It has been suggested that a more appropriate method may be to monitor monocyte infiltration ("the major source of demyelination in EAE") via cells labeled with iron oxide particles which may be detected by MRI, thereby allowing assessment of the inflammatory activity induced by EAE (Rausch *et al.*, 2003).

Other imaging modalities have been used less frequently, but have yielded some interesting findings. It has been suggested that DTI may distinguish between acute and chronic EAE lesions (Richards *et al.*, 1995a,b), such that in acute lesions diffusion increases in all directions, probably as a consequence of edema, whilst in chronic lesions diffusion only increases perpendicular to the main axon axis, possibly reflecting demyelination. Measurements of magnetization transfer ratio (MTR) in EAE (Gareau *et al.*, 2000) have suggested that decreases in MTR, which are frequently assumed to reflect demyelination in human MS, may in fact result from inflammatory related changes to white matter structure rather than myelin loss *per se*. In contrast, the short component of tissue water T_2 may more accurately reflect myelin content (Gareau *et al.*, 2000). New contrast agents have recently provided an alternative approach to imaging EAE. It has been shown that the use of a superparamagnetic iron oxide contrast agent enables macrophage recruitment to the CNS to be followed *in vivo* (Dousset *et al.*, 1999).

IV. Conclusion

The combination of appropriate imaging techniques and suitable animal models of disease can greatly elucidate our understanding of human brain pathologies. This experimental imaging partnership has contributed to the development of novel imaging techniques, to the promotion of better diagnostic and prognostic measures, and to elucidation of the basic mechanisms of cellular injury leading to improved therapies.

Acknowledgments

The authors thank Dr N. R. Sibson and Dr N. G. Harris for their contribution to the manuscript. We also acknowledge the Wellcome Trust and the BBSRC for their support of the work carried out at Radiology and Physics Unit of the Institute of Child Health, Great Ormond Street Hospital and the Wellcome Trust High Field MR Research Laboratory.

References

Alsop, D. C., and Detre, J. A. (1996). Reduced transit-time sensitivity in noninvasive magnetic resonance imaging of human cerebral blood flow. *J. Cereb. Blood Flow Metab.* **16,** 1236–1249.

Anderson, S. A., and Frank, J. A. (2007). MRI of mouse models of neurological disorders. *NMR Biomed.* **20,** 200–215.

Araujo, D. M., Cherry, S. R., Tatsukawa, K. J., Toyokuni, T., and Kornblum, H. I. (2000). Deficits in striatal dopamine D(2) receptors and energy metabolism detected by *in vivo* micropet imaging in a rat model of Huntington's disease. *Exp. Neurol.* **166,** 287–297.

Astrup, J., Siesjo, B. K., and Symon, L. (1981). Thresholds in cerebral ischemia: The ischaemic penumbra. *Stroke* **12,** 723–725.

Back, T., Kohno, K., and Hossmann, K. A. (1994). Cortical negative DC deflections following middle cerebral artery occlusion and KCl-induced spreading depression: Effect on blood flow, tissue oxygenation, and electroencephalogram. *J. Cereb. Blood Flow Metab.* **14,** 12–19.

Baird, A. E., and Warach, S. (1998). Magnetic resonance imaging of acute stroke. *J. Cereb. Blood Flow Metab.* **18,** 583–609.

Borlongan, C. V., Koutouzis, T. K., and Sanberg, P. R. (1997). 3-Nitropropionic acid animal model and Huntington's disease. *Neurosci. Biobehav. Rev.* **21,** 289–293.

Braakman, N., Matysik, J., van Duinen, S. G., *et al.* (2006). Longitudinal assessment of Alzheimer's beta-amyloid plaque development in transgenic mice monitored by *in vivo* magnetic resonance microimaging. *J. Magn. Reson. Imaging* **24,** 530–536.

Brok, H., Bauer, J., Jonker, M., *et al.* (2001). Non-human primate models of multiple sclerosis. *Immunol. Rev.* **183,** 173–185.

Brownell, A. L., Livni, E., Galpern, W., and Isacson, O. (1998). *In vivo* PET imaging in rat of dopamine terminals reveals functional neural transplants. *Ann. Neurol.* **43,** 387–390.

Calamante, F., Gadian, D. G., and Connelly, A. (2000). Delay and dispersion effects in dynamic susceptibility contrast MRI: Simulations using singular value decomposition. *Magn. Reson. Med.* **44,** 466–473.

Calamante, F., Lythgoe, M. F., Pell, G. S., *et al.* (1999). Early changes in water diffusion, perfusion, T1 and T2 during focal cerebral ischaemia in the rat studied at 8.5T. *Magn. Reson. Med.* **41,** 479–485.

Calamante, F., Thomas, D. L., Pell, G. S., Wiersma, J., and Turner, R. (1999). Measuring cerebral blood flow using magnetic resonance imaging techniques. *J. Cereb. Blood Flow Metab.* **19,** 701–735.

Chen, Y. C., Galpern, W. R., Brownell, A. L., *et al.* (1997). Detection of dopaminergic neurotransmitter activity using pharmacologic MRI: Correlation with PET, microdialysis, and behavioral data. *Magn. Reson. Med.* **38,** 389–398.

Chen, Y. I., Brownell, A. L., Galpern, W., *et al.* (1999). Detection of dopaminergic cell loss and neural transplantation using pharmacological MRI, PET and behavioral assessment. *Neuroreport* **29**(10), 2881–2886.

Choi, I. Y., Lee, S. P., Guilfoyle, D. N., and Helpern, J. A. (2003). *In vivo* NMR studies of neurodegenerative diseases in transgenic and rodent models. *Neurochem. Res.* **28,** 987–1001.

de Crespigny, A. J., Wendland, M. F., Derugin, N., Kozniewska, E., and Moseley, M. E. (1992). Real-time observation of transient focal ischemia and hyperemia in cat brain. *Magn. Reson. Med.* **27,** 391–397.

Derugin, N., and Roberts, T. P. L. (1994). New and reproducible technique for experimentally induced middle cerebral artery stenosis. *Microsurgery* **15,** 70–72.

Detre, J. A., Leigh, J. S., Williams, D. S., and Koretsky, A. P. (1992). Perfusion imaging. *Magn. Reson. Med.* **23,** 37–45.

Dijkhuizen, R. M., Ren, J., Mandeville, J. B., *et al.* (2001). Functional magnetic resonance imaging of reorganization in rat brain after stroke. *Proc. Natl. Acad. Sci. USA* **98,** 12766–12771.

Dijkhuizen, R. M., Singhal, A. B., Mandeville, J. B., *et al.* (2003). Correlation between brain reorganization, ischemic damage, and neurologic status after transient focal cerebral ischemia in rats: A functional magnetic resonance imaging study. *J. Neurosci.* **15**(23), 510–517.

Dixon, W. T., Du, L. N., Faul, D. D., Gado, M., and Rossnick, S. (1986). Projection angiograms of blood labeled by adiabatic fast passage. *Magn. Reson. Med.* **3,** 454–462.

Dousset, V., Grossman, R. I., and Ramer, K. N. (1992). Lesion characterization in experimental allergic encephalomyelitis and multiple sclerosis by magnetization transfer imaging. *Radiology* **182,** 483–491.

Dousset, V., Ballarino, L., Delalande, C., *et al.* (1999). Comparison of ultrasmall particles of iron oxide (USPIO)-enhanced T2-weighted, conventional T2-weighted, and gadolinium-enhanced T1-weighted MR images in rats with experimental autoimmune encephalomyelitis. *Am. J. Neuroradiol.* **20,** 223–227.

Dube, C., Yu, H., Nalcioglu, O., and Baram, T. Z. (2004). Serial MRI after experimental febrile seizures: Altered T2 signal without neuronal death. *Ann. Neurol.* **56,** 709–714.

Duckers, H. J., Muller, H. J., Verhaagen, J., Nicolay, K., and Gispen, W. H. (1997). Longitudinal *in vivo* magnetic resonance imaging studies in experimental allergic encephalomyelitis: Effect of a neurotrophic treatment on cortical lesion development. *Neuroscience* **77,** 1163–1173.

Duong, T. Q., Ackerman, J. J. H., Ying, H. S., and Neil, J. J. (1998). Evaluation of extra- and intracellular apparent diffusion in normal and globally ischemic rat brain via ^{19}F NMR. *Magn. Reson. Med.* **40,** 1–13.

Falangola, M. F., Dyakin, V. V., Lee, S. P., *et al.* (2007). Quantitative MRI reveals aging-associated T2 changes in mouse models of Alzheimer's disease. *NMR Biomed.* **20,** 343–351.

Fischer, M., and Brott, T. G. (2003). Emerging therapies for actute ischemic stroke. *Stroke* **34,** 359–361.

Gadian, D. G. (1995). NMR and Its Applications to Living Systems Oxford University Press, Oxford.

Gardner Medwin, A. R., Van Bruggen, N., Williams, S. R., and Ahier, R. G. (1994). Magnetic resonance imaging of propagating waves of spreading depression in the anaesthetised rat. *J. Cereb. Blood Flow Metab.* **14,** 7–11.

Gareau, P. J., Rutt, B. K., Karlik, S. J., and Mitchell, J. R. (2000). Magnetization transfer and multicomponent T2 relaxation measurements with histopathologic correlation in an experimental model of MS. *J. Magn. Reson. Imaging.* **11,** 586–595.

Gold, R., Hartung, H. P., and Toyka, K. V. (2000). Animal models for autoimmune demyelinating disorders of the nervous system. *Mol. Med. Today* **6,** 88–91.

Grohn, O., and Pitkanen, A. (2007). Magnetic resonance imaging in animal models of epilepsy-noninvasive detection of structural alterations. *Epilepsia* **48**(Suppl. 4), 3–10.

Grohn, O. H. J., Lukkarinen, J. A., Oja, J. M. E., *et al.* (1998). Noninvasive detection of cerebral hypoperfusion and reversible ischemia from reductions in the magnetic resonance imaging relaxation time,T2. *J. Cereb. Blood Flow Metab.* **18,** 911–920.

Grohn, O. J., Kettunen, M. I., Makela, H. I., *et al.* (2000). Early detection of irreversible cerebral ischemia in the rat using dispersion of the magnetic resonance imaging relaxation time, T1rho. *J. Cereb. Blood Flow Metab.* **20,** 1457–1466.

Grossman, R. I., Lisak, R. P., Macchi, P. J., and Joseph, P. M. (1987). MR of acute experimental allergic encephalomyelitis. *Am. J. Neuroradiol.* **8,** 1045–1048.

Gyngell, M. L., Back, T., Hoehn-Berlage, M., Kohno, K., and Hossmann, K. A. (1994). Transient cell depolarization after permanent middle cerebral artery occlusion: An observation by diffusion-weighted MRI and localised 1H-MRS. *Magn. Reson. Med.* **31,** 337–341.

Hall, S., Rutledge, J. N., and Schallert, T. (1992). MRI, brain iron and experimental Parkinson's disease. *J. Neurol. Sci.* **113,** 198–208.

Hantraye, P. (1998). Modeling dopamine system dysfunction in experimental animals. *Nucl. Med. Biol.* **25,** 721–728.

Hantraye, P., Leroy-Willig, A., Denys, A., *et al.* (1992). Magnetic resonance imaging to monitor pathology of caudate-putamen after excitotoxin-induced neuronal loss in the nonhuman primate brain. *Exp. Neurol.* **118,** 18–23.

Hart, B. A., Bauer, J., Muller, H. J., *et al.* (1998). Histopathological characterization of magnetic resonance imaging-detectable brain white matter lesions in a primate model of multiple sclerosis: A correlative study in the experimental autoimmune encephalomyelitis model in common marmosets (*Callithrix jacchus*). *Am. J. Pathol.* **153,** 649–663.

Hawkins, C. P., Munro, P. M., MacKenzie, F., *et al.* (1990). Duration and selectivity of blood-brain barrier breakdown in chronic relapsing experimental allergic encephalomyelitis studied by gadolinium-DTPA and protein markers. *Brain* **113,** 365–378.

Henkelman, R. M., Stanisz, G. J., and Graham, S. J. (2001). Magnetization transfer in MRI: A review. *NMR Biomed.* **14,** 57–64.

Hoehn, M., Himmelreich, U., Kruttwig, K., and Wiedermann, D. (2008). Molecular and cellular MR imaging: Potentials and challenges for neurological applications. *J. Magn. Reson. Imaging* **27,** 941–954.

Hoehn, M., Nicolay, K., Franke, C., and van-der-Sanden, B. (2001). Application of magnetic resonance to animal models of cerebral ischemia. *J. Magn. Reson. Imaging* **14,** 491–509.

Hoehn-Berlage, M. (1995). Diffusion-weighted NMR imaging: Application to experimental focal cerebral ischemia. *NMR Biomed.* **8,** 345–358.

Hoehn-Berlage, M., Eis, M., Back, T., Kohno, K., and Yamashita, K. (1995). Changes of relaxation times (T1, T2) and apparent diffusion coefficient after permanent middle cerebral artery occlusion in the rat: Temporal evolution, regional extent, and comparison with histology. *Magn. Reson. Med.* **34,** 824–834.

Hossmann, K. A. (1994). Viability thresholds and the penumbra of focal ischemia. *Ann. Neurol.* **36,** 557–565.

Jack, C. R., Jr., Wengenack, T. M., Reyes, D. A., *et al.* (2005). *In vivo* magnetic resonance microimaging of individual amyloid plaques in Alzheimer's transgenic mice. *J. Neurosci.* **25,** 10041–10048.

Jenkins, B. G., Chen, Y. I., and Mandeville, J. B. (2002). Pharmacological magnetic resonance imaging. *In* "Biomedical Imaging in Experimental Neuroscience" (N. van-Bruggen, and T. P. Roberts, eds.). CRC Press, Boca Raton, FL.

Jordan, E. K., McFarland, H. I., Lewis, B. K., *et al.* (1999). Serial MR imaging of experimental autoimmune encephalomyelitis induced by human white matter or by chimeric myelin-basic and proteolipid protein in the common marmoset. *Am. J. Neuroradiol.* **20,** 965–976.

King, M. D., van-Bruggen, N., Ahier, R. G., *et al.* (1991). Diffusion-weighted imaging of kainic acid lesions in the rat brain. *Magn. Reson. Med.* **20,** 158–164.

Kinouchi, H., Sharp, F. R., Koistinaho, J., Hicks, K., Kamii, H., and Chan, P. H. (1993). Induction of heat shock hsp70 mRNA and HSP70 kDa protein in neurons in the 'penumbra' following focal cerebral ischemia in the rat. *Brain Res.* **619,** 334–338.

Knight, R. A., Dereski, M. O., Helpern, J. A., Ordidge, R. J., and Chopp, M. (1994). Magnetic resonance imaging assessment of evolving focal cerebral ischemia. Comparison with histopathology in rats. *Stroke* **25,** 1252–1261.

Knight, R. A., Ordidge, R. J., Helpern, J. A., Chopp, M., Rodolosi, L. C., and Peck, D. (1991). Temporal evolution of ischemic damage in rat brain measured by proton nuclear magnetic resonance imaging. *Stroke* **22,** 802–808.

Kocher, M. (1990). Metabolic and hemodynamic activation of postischaemic rat brain by cortical spreading depression. *J. Cereb. Blood Flow Metab.* **10,** 564–571.

Kohno, K., Hoehn-Berlage, M., Mies, G., Back, T., and Hossmann, K. A. (1995). Relationship between diffusion-weighted MR images, cerebral blood flow, and energy state in experimental brain infarction. *Magn. Reson. Imaging* **13,** 73–80.

Latour, L. L., Hasegawa, Y., Formato, J. E., Fisher, M., and Sotak, C. H. (1994). Spreading waves of decreased diffusion coefficient after cortical stimulation in the rat brain. *Magn. Reson. Med.* **32,** 189–198.

Luh, W. M., Wong, E. C., Bandettini, P. A., and Hyde, J. S. (1999). QUIPSS II with thin-slice TI_1 periodic saturation: A method for improving accuracy of quantitative perfusion imaging using pulsed arterial spin labeling. *Magn. Reson. Med.* **41,** 1246–1254.

Lythgoe, M. F., Williams, S. R., Busza, A. L., *et al.* (1999). The relationship between magnetic resonance imaging and autoradiographic markers of cerebral blood flow and hypoxia in an animal stroke model. *Magn. Reson. Med.* **41,** 706–714.

Lythgoe, M. F., Thomas, D. L., Calamante, F., *et al.* (2000). Acute changes in MRI diffusion, perfusion, T1 and T2 in a rat model of oligemia produced by partial occlusion of the middle cerebral artery. *Magn. Reson. Med.* **44,** 706–712.

Lythgoe, M. F., Thomas, D. L., and Calamante, F. (2002). MRI measurement of cerebral perfusion and the application to experimental neuroscience.*In* "Biomedical Imaging in Experimental Neuroscience" (N. van-Bruggen, and T. P. Roberts, eds.). CRC Press, Boca Raton, Florida.

Matyszak, M. K., and Perry, V. H. (1995). Demyelination in the central nervous system following a delayed-type hypersensitivity response to bacillus Calmette-Guerin. *Neuroscience* **64,** 967–977.

Menalled, L. B., and Chesselet, M. F. (2002). Mouse models of Huntington's disease. *Trends Pharmacol. Sci.* **23,** 32–39.

Meng, X., Fisher, M., Shen, Q., Sotak, C. H., and Duong, T. Q. (2004). Characterizing the diffusion/perfusion mismatch in experimental focal cerebral ischemia. *Ann. Neurol.* **55**(2), 207–212.

Miletich, R. S., Bankiewicz, K. S., Quarantelli, M., *et al.* (1994). MRI detects acute degeneration of the nigrostriatal dopamine system after MPTP exposure in hemiparkinsonian monkeys. *Ann. Neurol.* **35,** 689–697.

Modo, M., and Williams, S. C. R. (2002). MRI and novel contrast agents for molecular imaging. *In* "Biomedical Imaging in Experimental Neuroscience" (N. van-Bruggen, and T. P. Roberts, eds.). pp. 293–322. CRC Press, Boca Raton, Florida.

Morrissey, S. P., Stodal, H., Zettl, U., *et al.* (1996). *In vivo* MRI and its histological correlates in acute adoptive transfer experimental allergic encephalomyelitis. Quantification of inflammation and oedema. *Brain* **119,** 239–248.

Moseley, M. E., Cohen, Y., Mintorovitch, J., *et al.* (1990). Early detection of regional cerebral ischemia in cats: Comparison of diffusion- and T2-weighted MRI and spectroscopy. *Magn. Reson. Med.* **14,** 330–346.

Moseley, M., Kucharczyk, J., and Asgari, H. (1991). Anisotropy in diffusion-weighted MRI. *Magn. Reson. Med.* **19,** 321–326.

Nairismagi, J., Grohn, O. H., Kettunen, M. I., Nissinen, J., Kauppinen, R. A., and Pitkanen, A. (2004). Progression of brain damage after status epilepticus and its association with epileptogenesis: A quantitative MRI study in a rat model of temporal lobe epilepsy. *Epilepsia* **45,** 1024–1034.

Nedergaard, M., and Astrup, J. (1986). Infarct rim: Effect of hyperglycemia on direct current potential and (14C)-deoxyglucose phosphorylation. *J. Cereb. Blood Flow Metab.* **6,** 607–615.

Newman, T. A., Woolley, S. T., Hughes, P. M., Sibson, N. R., Anthony, D. C., and Perry, V. H. (2001). T-cell- and macrophage-mediated axon damage in the absence of a CNS-specific immune response: Involvement of metalloproteinases. *Brain* **124,** 2203–2214.

Ogawa, S., and Lee, T. (1992). Blood oxygenation level dependence MRI of the rat brain: Effects of seizure induced by kainic acid in the rat. *Proc. Soc. Magn. Reson. Med.* **1,** 501.

Ogawa, S., Menon, R. S., Kim, S. G., and Ugurbil, K. (1998). On the characteristics of functional magnetic resonance imaging of the brain. *Annu. Rev. Biophys. Biomol. Struct.* **27,** 447–474.

Ordidge, R. J., Helpern, J. A., Knight, R. A., Qing, Z. X., and Welch, K. M. A. (1991). Investigation of cerebral ischemia using magnetization transfer contrast (MTC) MR imaging. *Magn. Reson. Imaging* **9,** 895–902.

Ostergaard, L., Weisskoff, R. M., Chesler, D. A., Glydensted, C., and Rosen, B. R. (1996). High resolution measurement of cerebral blood flow using intravascular tracer bolus passages. Part I: Mathematical approach and statistical analysis. *Magn. Reson. Med.* **36,** 715–725.

Pelled, G., Bergman, H., and Goelman, G. (2002). Bilateral overactivation of the sensorimotor cortex in the unilateral rodent model of Parkinson's disease—A functional magnetic resonance imaging study. *Eur. J. Neurosci.* **15,** 389–394.

Perman, W. H., Gado, M. H., Larson, K. B., and Perlmutter, J. S. (1992). Simultaneous MR acquisition of arterial and brain signal time curves. *Magn. Reson. Med.* **28,** 74–83.

Pierpaoli, C., Righini, A., Linfante, I., Tao-Cheng, J. H., Alger, J. R., and Di Chiro, G. (1993). Histopathological correlates of abnormal water diffusion in cerebral ischaemia: Diffusion-weighted MR imaging and light and electron miscrosopy study. *Radiology* **189,** 439–448.

Porkka, L., Neuder, M., Hunter, G., Weisskoff, R. M., Belliveau, J. W., and Rosen, B. R. (1991). Arterial input function measurement with MRI.Proceedings of SMRM 10th Annual Meeting, p. 120 (Abstract).

Quast, M. J., Huang, N. C., Hillman, G. R., and Kent, T. A. (1993). The evolution of acute stroke recording by multimodal magnetic resonance imaging. *Magn. Reson. Imaging* **11,** 465–471.

Rausch, M., Hiestand, P., Baumann, D., Cannet, C., and Rudin, M. (2003). MRI-based monitoring of inflammation and tissue damage in acute and chronic relapsing EAE. *Magn. Reson. Med.* **50,** 309.

Richards, T. L., Alvord, E. C. J., He, Y., *et al.* (1995a). Experimental allergic encephalomyelitis in non-human primates: Diffusion imaging of acute and chronic brain lesions. *Mult. Scler.* **1,** 109–117.

Richards, T. L., Alvord, E. C. J., Peterson, J., *et al.* (1995b). Experimental allergic encephalomyelitis in non-human primates: MRI and MRS may predict the type of brain damage. *NMR Biomed.* **8,** 49–58.

Roch, C., Leroy, C., Nehlig, A., and Namer, I. J. (2002). Magnetic resonance imaging in the study of lithium-pilocarpine model of temporal lobe epilepsy in adult rats. *Epilespia* **43,** 325–335.

Rother, J., de Crespigny, A. J., D'Arceuil, H. E., Iwai, K., and Moseley, M. E. (1996). Recovery of the apparent diffusion coefficient after ischemia-induced spreading depression relates to cerebral perfusion gradient. *Stroke* **27,** 980–987.

Roussel, S. A., Van Bruggen, N., King, M. D., Houseman, J., Williams, S. R., and Gadian, D. G. (1994). Monitoring the initial expansion of focal ischaemic changes by diffusion-weighted MRI using a remote controlled method of occlusion. *NMR Biomed.* **7,** 21–28.

Roussel, S. A., Van Bruggen, N., King, M. D., and Gadian, D. G. (1995). Identification of collaterally perfused areas following focal cerebral ischemia in the rat by comparison of gradient echo and diffusion-weighted MRI. *J. Cereb. Blood Flow Metab.* **15,** 578–586.

Rudin, M., Beckmann, N., Porszasz, R., Reese, T., Bochelen, D., and Sauter, A. (1999). *In vivo* magnetic resonance methods in pharmaceutical research: Current status and perspectives *NMR Biomed.* **12,** 69–97.

Shellock, F. G., and Kanal, E. (1999). Safety of magnetic resonance imaging contrast agents. *J. Magn. Reson. Imaging* **10,** 477–484.

Smith, R., and Lange, R. (1999). Understanding Magnetic Resonance Imaging. CRC Press, Boca Raton, Florida.

Takano, K., Latour, L. L., Formato, J. E., *et al.* (1996). The role of spreading depression in focal ischemia evaluated by diffusion mapping. *Ann. Neurol.* **39,** 308–318.

Thomas, D. L., Lythgoe, M. F., Pell, G. S., Calamante, F., and Ordidge, R. J. (2000). The measurement of diffusion and perfusion in biological systems using magnetic resonance imaging. *Phys. Med. Biol.* **45,** R97–R138.

Tokumitsu, T., Mancuso, A., Weinstein, P. R., Weiner, M. W., Naruse, S., and Maudsley, A. A. (1997). Metabolic and pathological effects of temporal lobe epilepsy in rat brain detected by proton spectroscopy and imaging. *Brain Res.* **2**(744), 57–67.

Van Bruggen, N., and Roberts, T. P. L. (2002). Biomedical Imaging in Experimental Neuroscience. CRC Press, Boca Raton, Florida.

van der Zijden, J. P., Bouts, M. J., Wu, O., *et al.* (2008). Manganese-enhanced MRI of brain plasticity in relation to functional recovery after experimental stroke. *J. Cereb. Blood Flow Metab.* **28,** 832–840.

Vanhoutte, G., Dewachter, I., Borghgraef, P., Van, L. F., and Van der, L. A. (2005). Noninvasive *in vivo* MRI detection of neuritic plaques associated with iron in APP[V717I] transgenic mice, a model for Alzheimer's disease. *Magn. Reson. Med.* **53,** 607–613.

van Lookeren Campagne, M., Thomas, G. R., Thibodeaux, H., *et al.* (1999). Secondary reduction in the apparent diffusion coefficient, increase in cerebral blood volume and delayed neuronal death following middle cerebral artery occlusion and early reperfusion in the rat. *J. Cereb. Blood Flow Metab.* **19,** 1354–1364.

Verheul, H. B., Balazs, R., Berkelbach van der Sprenkel, J. W., Tulleken, C. A., Nicolay, K., and Van Lookeren, C. M. (1993). Temporal evolution of NMDA-induced excitoxicity in the neonatal rat brain measured with 1H nuclear magnetic resonance imaging. *Brain Res.* **6**(618), 203–212.

Verhoye, M. R., Gravenmade, E. J., Raman, E. R., Van-Reempts, J., and Van-der-Linden, A. (1996). *In vivo* noninvasive determination of abnormal water diffusion in the rat brain studied in an animal model for multiple sclerosis by diffusion-weighted NMR imaging. *Magn. Reson. Imaging* **14,** 521–532.

Wadghiri, Y. Z., Sigurdsson, E. M., Sadowski, M., *et al.* (2003). Detection of Alzheimer's amyloid in transgenic mice using magnetic resonance microimaging. *Magn. Reson. Med.* **50,** 293–302.

Wegener, S., Weber, R., Ramos-Cabrer, P., *et al.* (2006). Temporal profile of T2-weighted MRI distinguishes between pannecrosis and selective neuronal death after transient focal cerebral ischemia in the rat. *J. Cereb. Blood Flow. Metab.* **26,** 38–47.

Wolff, S. D., and Balaban, R. S. (1989). Magnetization transfer contrast (MTC) and tissue water proton relaxation *in vivo*. *Magn. Reson. Med.* **10,** 135–144.

Wong, E. C., Buxton, R. B., and Frank, L. R. (1998). Quantitative imaging of perfusion using a single subtraction (QUIPSS and QUIPSS II). *Magn. Reson. Med.* **39,** 702–708.

Wu, O., Sumii, T., Asahi, M., Sasamata, M., Ostergaard, L., Rosen, B. R., Lo, E. H., and Dijkhuizen, R. M. (2007). Infarct prediction and treatment assessment with MRI-based algorithms in experimental stroke models. *J. Cereb. Blood Flow Metab.* **27**(1), 196–204.

Zhang, Z., Andersen, A., Grondin, R., *et al.* (2001). Pharmacological MRI mapping of age-associated changes in basal ganglia circuitry of awake rhesus monkeys. *Neuroimage* **14,** 1159–1167.

Zhong, J., Petroff, O. A. C., Pritchard, J. W., and Gore, J. C. (1993). Changes in water diffusion and relaxation properties of rat cerebellum during status epilepticus. *Magn. Reson. Med.* **30,** 241–246.

CHAPTER 14

Magnetic Resonance Imaging in Animal Models of Pathologies

Pasquina Marzola, Stefano Tambalo, and Andrea Sbarbati

Department of Morphological and Biomedical Sciences
Section of Anatomy
University of Verona
Verona, Italy

I. Update
II. Introduction
III. Bacterial Infections
  A. Bacterial Thigh Infection
  B. Pneumonia
IV. Ischemic Pathologies
  A. Permanent MCAO
V. Neoplastic Pathologies
  A. Colon Carcinoma
VI. Lipid Accumulation in Metabolic-Degenerative Disorders
  A. Ob-ob Mice
VII. Conclusions
References

I. Update

Whole animal imaging methods are receiving increasing attention in both fundamental and applied research. This chapter, originally written in 2004, describes experimental approaches based on magnetic resonance imaging (MRI) used to investigate several experimental models of human pathologies. Methods described 5 years ago are still largely valid, although important hardware and software improvements have greatly advanced MRI techniques. For example, new contrast agents able to reversibly bind to plasma proteins have been applied in the study of tumor angiogenesis by dynamic-contrast-enhanced MRI. These contrast agents

ESSENTIAL BIOIMAGING METHODS

DOI: 10.1016/B978-0-12-375043-3.00014-7

have low molecular weight (500 Da), but, thanks to their binding properties, show increased sensitivity to alterations induced by antiangiogenic drugs when compared to standard macromolecular or low molecular weight contrast agents (see Marzola *et al.*, Preda *et al.*, 2005). Imaging of cerebral ischemia is still based on the assessment of alterations in ADC/T2 and tissutal perfusion, although innovative approaches, for example functional MRI (fMRI), have been proposed (Weber *et al.*, 2006). New acquisition sequences and methods have been also proposed for imaging of pulmonary pathologies. The above methodological advancements have been mentioned in the updated version of the manuscript.

Nonetheless, in our opinion the real novelty in small animal imaging is represented by the so-called multimodality imaging, that is, the integration of two or more imaging modalities to fully capture the specific strength of each technique in a single study. For example, MRI, which offers high space resolution and soft tissue contrast, can be combined with positron emission tomography (PET) which can provide high sensitivity and metabolic information (Judenhofer *et al.*, 2008).

A representative example of multimodality approach has been recently reported by our group (Galiè *et al.*, 2007). We have investigated the relationship between tumor perfusion (assessed by MRI) and tumor metabolism (assessed by PET) in experimental models of carcinoma and mesenchymal tumors. Surprisingly, we have observed that, within a given tumor, regions with high vascular perfusion exhibit low uptake of fluorodeoxyglucose (FDG), therefore reduced metabolism, and that mesenchymal tumors exhibit higher vascular perfusion and lower FDG uptake than carcinomas. By using the above approach, we have provided *in vivo* evidence of vascular/metabolic reciprocity that has important implications both in experimental models and in clinical diagnosis.

II. Introduction

Animal models of human pathologies are useful at a fundamental level to understand the dynamics of a disease and its underlying mechanisms. They also play a fundamental role in pharmaceutical research. Animal models of diseases are used in several phases of pharmaceutical research, from the drug target identification to the efficacy tests of the experimental drug. MRI is a well recognized tool for *in vivo* characterization of animal models of human pathologies in preclinical research. Because of its noninvasiveness, high soft tissue contrast, and high space resolution, which can reach 50–100 μm in small laboratory animals, MRI constitutes a powerful morphologic technique. MR signal is sensitive to a number of parameters, including proton density, water proton relaxation times (T_1, T_2, and T_2*), microscopic water self-diffusion, and macroscopic flow (i.e., blood flow in arteries). Thanks to its multiparameter dependence, MRI is not a pure morphologic technique, but it also provides physiologic, functional, and metabolic information. Examples range from neuronal activation in brain (fMRI) induced by stimuli or drugs (Marota *et al.*, 1999, 2000), assessment of organ viability after transplantation (Beckmann *et al.*, 2000), assessment of blood volume and flow in brain (Calamante *et al.*, 1999), and characterization of neovasculature in tumors (Bhujwalla *et al.*, 1999; Gossmann *et al.*, 2002). The availability of contrast agents with different physical, chemical, and biologic properties further enhances the usefulness of the technique. Standard low molecular weight ($\approx$500 Da) contrast agents that are widely used in clinics are characterized by a rapid equilibrium between vascular and extracellular space. At the equilibrium distribution, such agents are markers of tissue integrity (e.g., blood-brain barrier defects), whereas their dynamic penetration in tissues can be used as a marker of tissue microcirculation (Yuh, 1999). However, a number of applications require the use of contrast agents with different properties. For example, high molecular weight contrast agents have been used in preclinical research for characterization of tumor blood volume and microvessel permeability (Brasch *et al.*, 2000).

Iron-based nanoparticles that are characterized by a long blood halftime have been used as markers of cerebral blood volume alteration induced by somatosensory stimulation or drug administration. Several pathologies are now recognized to have a genetic origin, and consequently, genetically modified animals play an important role in this field (Beckmann *et al.*, 2001). Compared with the traditional invasive techniques, MRI allows repeated observations of the same subject during the time evolution of the pathology or therapy follow-up. The possibility of repeated observations on the same subject drastically decreases the number of experiments needed to reach a statistical significance, with a consequent reduction in the number of animals and in the quantity of drug used, providing economic and ethical benefits.

In this chapter, we describe representative experimental approaches used in our laboratory in studying and characterizing animal models of representative pathologies, namely, models of experimental infectious, ischemic, neoplastic, and metabolic-degenerative diseases.

III. Bacterial Infections

In antibacterial research, animal models of bacterial infection are used to test the efficacy of novel compounds. Systemic or localized microbial infections are traditionally monitored by measuring the bacterial load (i.e., the number of bacterial colonies/organ, and/or the survival of the infected animals). The assessment of the chronologic evolution of infection, and drug efficacy, consequently requires the sacrifice of a large number of animals and suffers from the intrinsic interindividual variability of data. With the aim to establish if and at what extent *in vivo* MRI can substitute or complement traditional assays, we have investigated, using MRI, two experimental models of bacterial infections, namely, thigh infection (Marzola *et al.*, 1999b) and pneumonia (Marzola *et al.*, 2005). To this purpose, thigh infection was induced in three groups of animals: the first group was used for histologic examination, the second group was used for bacterial viable count examination, and the third group was used for MRI examination. Experiments on lung infection were conducted on a single group of animals that were sacrificed, after MRI, for histology. Although the presence of infection in the thigh muscle was detectable by standard T_2-weighted (T_2W) spin-echo (SE) images, detection of pneumonia was more critical. In general, lung imaging is particularly challenging for standard MRI, being the lung parenchyma characterized by a very low ^{1}H MRI signal intensity. Low signal is due to the low proton density of the lung tissue (roughly 20% less than that of other tissues (Johnson and Hedlund, 1996)) and to the peculiar morphologic architecture constituted by microscopic arrangement of air-tissue interfaces that produces relevant susceptibility artifact and strongly decreases the T_2* relaxation time. New experimental approaches based on the use of hyperpolarized Xe and He gases have been proposed (Albert *et al.*, 1994; Middleton *et al.*, 1995) for lung imaging; although extremely promising, these techniques are not widely available at present and are not usable with standard instrumentation. Several ^{1}H MRI techniques have been also proposed and are aimed at increasing the signal-to-noise ratio (SNR) of the lung parenchyma, including projection reconstruction techniques (Gewalt *et al.*, 1993), SE or gradient-echo (GRE) sequences with short-echo time (Hatabu *et al.*, 1996), or inversion recovery preparation to the acquisition sequence with suppression of the muscle and/or the fat signal (Mai *et al.*, 1999). Recently oxygen-enhanced MRI, in which T_1W images are acquired while subjects breath normal air and pure oxygen, has been proposed to investigate pulmonary functionality in both clinical (Ohno *et al.*, 2008) and preclinical (Watt *et al.*, 2008) studies. Oxygen, being paramagnetic, increases the signal of the lung in T_1W images. A map of oxygen distribution in lungs can then be obtained by considering the difference between images acquired during air and pure oxygen breathing. The previously mentioned techniques are based on the idea that the signal from the lung parenchyma has to be increased. In the detection of pneumonia, we have exploited the high contrast between normal lung tissue and inflamed regions. In inflamed regions of the lung, where the functionality is impaired, the air content of pulmonary tissue is reduced, with a consequent increase in T_2* and in the SNR compared with the normal parenchyma.

A. Bacterial Thigh Infection

Thigh infection was induced in male Cr1:CD-1(ICR)BR mice by intramuscular (IM) injection of 0.125 ml of an overnight Mueller-Hinton broth culture of *Staphylococcus aureus* ($\approx 3 \times 10^7$ bacteria/mouse) in the left hind leg. To investigate the sensitivity of MRI to different therapeutic treatments, three groups of animals were observed: control group ($n = 5$), a group treated with imipenem-cilastatin ($n = 5$), and a group treated with vancomycin ($n = 5$). Although imipenem-cilastatin has marked bactericidal effect against *S. aureus*, vancomycin has only a bacteriostatic effect (Marzola *et al.*, 1999b). Animals were anesthetized by intraperitoneal (IP) injection of chloral hydrate (400 mg/kg) and placed in a homemade 5-cm internal diameter (i.d.) coil. SE T_1- and T_2-weighted (T_1W, T_2W) images were acquired at 4.7 T with the following parameters: repetition time (TR) and echo time (TE) amounted to 800 and 20 ms, respectively, for T_1W images and to 2000 and 70 ms, respectively for T_2W images. Other parameters were slice thickness = 2 mm, field-of-view (FOV) = 8×4 cm^2, matrix size = 256×128 (corresponding to an in-plane space resolution of 312×312 μm^2). Images were acquired in both coronal and transversal orientation; 11 and 7 contiguous slices were acquired in the two orientations, respectively. Two additional groups of animals were used for microbiologic investigations (n = 35) and for pathology (n = 14). Each group was further subdivided into three groups according to the therapeutic dosing regimen. Details about experimental protocols used for bacterial counts (BC) assessment and pathology examination can be found in Marzola *et al.* (1999b). Briefly, for BC, at the designed time points, mice were sacrificed by cervical dislocation, and the infected leg was excised and homogenized in physiologic saline. The homogenized solution was serially diluted, and the quantitative BC were performed by plating 10 μl of each dilution on agar-containing plates, which were incubated at 37 °C for 24 h. The resulting count was expressed as CFU/ml (colony-forming units/ml). For pathology, animals were sacrificed by blood withdrawal under deep carbon dioxide (CO_2) anesthesia. After skin removal, the whole body of the animals was retained in 10% buffered formalin for fixation (1-week fixation period). Afterward, the left leg sample was removed from the coxofemoral joint, decalcified in Christenson's fluid, and cut in three transversal slices; these were then processed, included in paraffin blocks and cut to obtain 5-μm-thick sections, and stained with hematoxylin eosin. Two blind investigators evaluated and graded the following parameters: fascial inflammation, inflammation of the muscle tissue (myositis), and abscess of flemmon.

In Fig. 1A and B, we show images obtained 48 h after infection for one animal belonging to the control group (no antibiotic treatment). No abnormality in the infection-bearing leg is apparent in T_1W images, apart from an increased dimension of this leg. It is interesting to note that one traditional assessment of the entity of bacterial infection was a measurement of the leg diameter performed by calliper (Acred, 1986). In T_2W images the infected leg appears strongly hyperintense compared with the normal leg; a subcutaneous edematous region is easily visible (arrow). The efficacy of the drug is clearly reflected in MR images: Fig. 1C and D shows T_1W and T_2W images acquired for one animal belonging to the group treated with imipenem-cilastatin; no hyperintensity in the infected leg muscle is detectable compared with the normal leg. In the group treated with vancomycin, the hyperintensity of the muscle in the infected leg was comparable to that observed in the control group (images not shown).

The ratio between the signal intensity (SI) of the muscle in the infected and in the normal leg obtained from T_2W images was used to quantify the lesion:

$$R_{\mathrm{i/n}} = \frac{\mathrm{SI}_{\text{infected leg}}}{\mathrm{SI}_{\text{normal leg}}}. \tag{1}$$

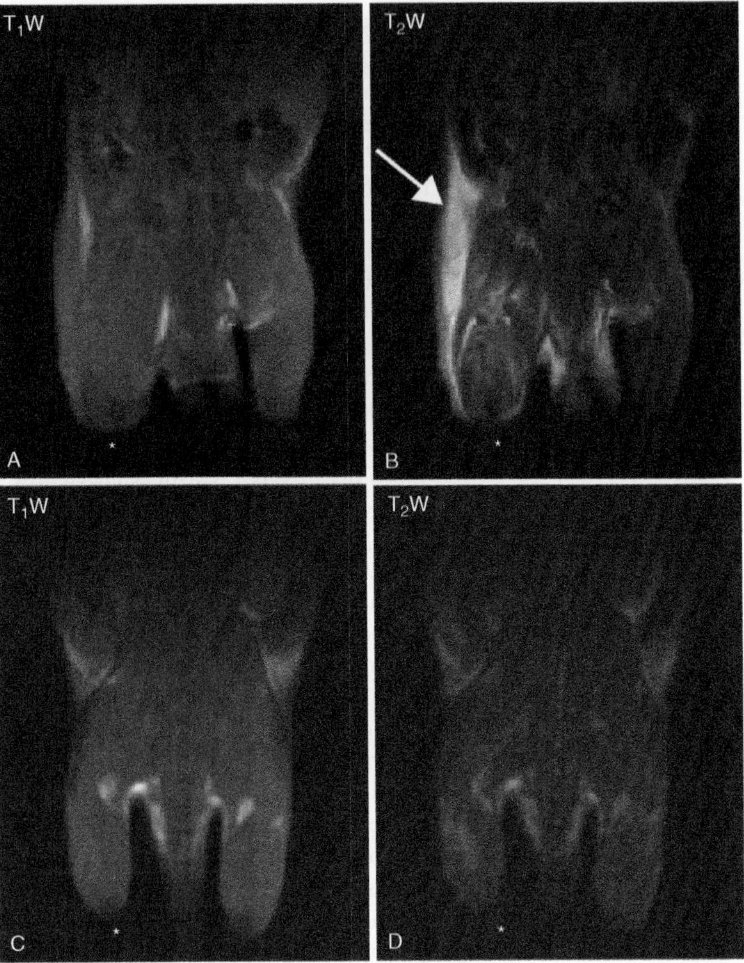

Fig. 1 Bacterial thigh infection. (A) T_1W and (B) T_2W coronal slices obtained 48 h after infection from an animal belonging to the control group. The dimension of the lesioned leg (*) is clearly increased, and strong alteration in the signal intensity of T_2W image is detected. (C) T_1W and (D) T_2W coronal slices obtained 48 h after infection from an animal belonging to the group treated with imipenem-cilastatin. No hyperintensity in the infected leg muscle (*) is detectable (adapted from Marzola *et al.* (1999b) with permission).

The signal intensities were obtained by the region-of-interest (ROI) analysis. Five transversal contiguous slices were selected across the lesion with the criterion to cover the whole thigh. An operator-defined ROI was manually traced on the muscle of both the infected and the normal leg, avoiding the bone, as well as the subcutaneous edema, which appears strongly hyperintense. Figure 2A reports

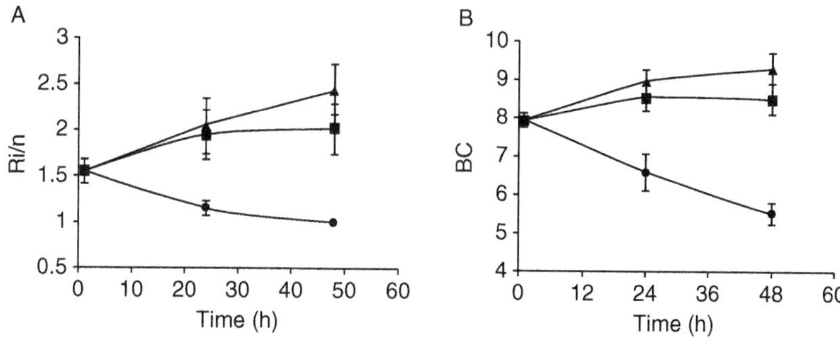

Fig. 2 Bacterial thigh infection. (A) Dependence of $R_{i/n}$ and (B) BC on time elapsed after infection induction. (Triangles) control group; (squares) group treated with vancomicin; (circles) group treated with imipenem-cilastatin (adapted from Marzola *et al.* (1999b) with permission).

the time dependence of the ratio $R_{i/n}$ for the three groups. $R_{i/n} = 1$ indicates absence of abnormality, whereas higher values of $R_{i/n}$ indicate more marked abnormality.

Figure 2B reports the time dependence of BC. In the untreated group of animals, $R_{i/n}$ increases with time, indicating a progressive worsening of the infection; a qualitative similar trend has been obtained for BC. In the group treated with vancomycin, an antibiotic characterized by a bacteriostatic effect against *S. aureus*, the increase in $R_{i/n}$ is less pronounced than in the control group and the value of $R_{i/n}$ remains substantially constant between 24 and 48 h; this trend is similar to that observed for BC. In the group treated with imipenem-cilastatin, an antibiotic characterized by a marked bactericidal effect, $R_{i/n}$ continuously decreases, reaching a value close to 1, 48 h after infection induction. A similar decreasing trend was observed for BC in this treatment group. A good correlation was also found with histologic data.

B. Pneumonia

Infection was induced in a group of mice ($n = 5$) weighing 18–22 g by intranasal administration of about 1×10^6 CFU/mouse of *Streptococcus pneumoniae*. A group of noninfected animals ($n = 5$) was used as the control group. Animals were anesthetized by IP injection of pentobarbital (at a 60 mg/kg dose) and placed in the prone position in a 35-mm i.d. birdcage coil. Three copper electrocardiogram (ECG) electrodes were subcutaneously implanted in the chest of the animals for ECG monitoring. The ECG signal was filtered and transformed in a square wave that was used as triggering for the acquisition sequence. Axial, ECG-gated, spoiled GRE images were acquired at each heartbeat in the systolic phase with the following parameters: TE = 5 ms, slice thickness = 1.2 mm, FOV = 6×6 cm^2, and matrix size = 256×256 (corresponding to in-plane space resolution of 234×234 μm^2). To obtain a reasonable SNR, four averages were used, resulting in an acquisition time of about 200 s. Images were acquired 48 h after infection induction. Immediately after imaging, animals were sacrificed by anesthetic overdose and the lungs were excised, inflated with 10% buffered formalin, and prepared for histology. For each animal, transversal sections (5 μm thick), 1.2 mm apart, were obtained and stained with hematoxylin and eosin. In each slice the area of the lesion was obtained by standard image analysis software. Quantification of lesion volume from MR images was obtained by manually delineating a ROI to cover the whole lung surface in each acquired slice. A second ROI was taken on the background noise. The number of pixels belonging to the lung surface and having signal intensities greater than five times the standard deviation of the noise was counted for each slice containing lung tissue. This analysis was performed in pathologic and normal animals; the average value obtained for normal animals was subtracted as a baseline.

Bacterial lesions in lung were evident in MR images as relatively high-intensity pixels compared with the normal lung parenchyma, whose signal was at the noise level. Figure 3 shows two images acquired for mice belonging to the infected (A) and control (B) group at approximately the same anatomic position. In the control mouse, lungs are characterized by SI at the level of the background noise, whereas vessels and heart ventricles show very high SI; heart and skeletal muscle have similar SIs. In Fig. 3A, relevant alterations of the SI in localized areas of the lung parenchyma can be observed compared with the normal lung parenchyma (see arrows). In this model of infection, lesions are generally localized in the perivascular and pericardiac regions. In Fig. 4, we compare MRI with histologic slices obtained at a similar anatomic position in the same animal.

At histology, foci of pneumonia, characterized by perivascular-peribronchiolar and alveolar inflammatory cell infiltrates, and pleuritis are observed. Figure 4 indicates that the regions that appear lesioned at histology (arrows), specifically the apical and pericardial regions of the lung, roughly correspond to regions of

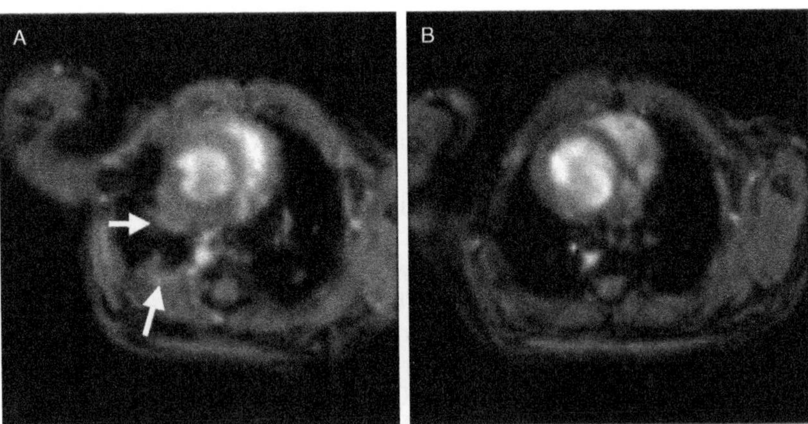

Fig. 3 Pneumonia. Comparison between transversal images obtained at similar anatomic position for mice belonging to the infected (A) and control (B) group. Arrows indicate regions of infection.

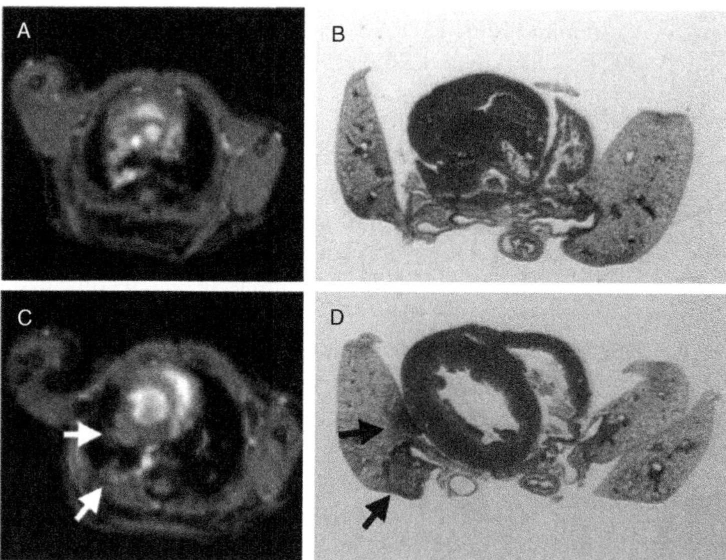

Fig. 4 Pneumonia. Comparison between (A, C) MRI and (B, D) histological slices obtained at a similar anatomic position in the same animal. Arrows indicate regions of infection. (See Plate no. 10 in the Color Plate Section.)

high SI in the MRI slices. However, a quantitative comparison between MRI and histology slices cannot be obtained, since the well-known alteration in tissue shape and morphology is caused by histologic processing of animal tissues. A quantitative comparison between histology and MRI could be obtained by comparing the volume of the lesion with the two techniques. The results showed that there is a good correlation ($r^2 = 0.8478$) between MRI and histologic determined volumes.

IV. Ischemic Pathologies

Although useful in different anatomic districts, MRI has found major applications in brain imaging. The development of diffusion-weighted MRI (DW-MRI) has revolutionized research in cerebral ischemia because it is sensitive to the hyperacute phase (Hoehn *et al.*, 2001). After the pioneer work by Moseley *et al.* (1990), several papers have shown that a decrease in water apparent diffusion coefficient (ADC) occurs within minutes from the occlusion of the middle cerebral artery (see Hoehn *et al.*, 2001 for a review), whereas abnormalities in T_2 occur only after hours. The increase in ADC in the early phase of ischemic insult is mainly due to cytotoxic cell swelling that causes a massive transfer of water from extracellular to intracellular space. The assessment of regional impairment in cerebral blood perfusion also plays an important role in ischemic lesion characterization. Cerebral blood perfusion can be assessed by MRI by acquiring fast images (weighted by the T_2* relaxation time) during the first passage of a bolus of contrast agent, typically gadolinium (Gd)-DTPA (Rosen *et al.*, 1990) or iron oxide particles (Fabene *et al.*, 2007; Loubeyre *et al.*, 1999). Other methods are based on the arterial spin labeling technique, which consists in acquiring images made sensitive to the inflowing spins (Hoehn *et al.*, 2001; Weber *et al.*, 2006). fMRI, in which the cerebral functional response to a given stimulus is investigated by MRI techniques, is increasingly used in experimental cerebral ischemia (Weber *et al.*, 2006). fMRI provides information about cerebral activity and spatial and temporal reorganization processes also in response to specific therapeutic treatments. We have implemented an experimental protocol aimed at studying cerebral ischemia, its time evolution, and also the effect of an experimental drug (Reggiani *et al.*, 2001) by using DW-MRI on the experimental model of permanent middle cerebral artery occlusion (MCAO).

A. Permanent MCAO

Permanent MCAO was performed in male Sprague-Dawley rats according to the method published by Tamura *et al.* (1981) with minor modifications (Reggiani *et al.*, 2001; Sbarbati *et al.*, 2000). A group of $n = 24$ rats weighing 300–400 g was used. After completion of MRI experiments, animals were sacrificed for histology and electron microscopy. The study was based on T_2W and DW images, acquired 6, 24, and 144 h after MCAO. Animals were anesthetized with fentanyldroperidol at 2.5 ± 0.5 mg/kg IP (Leptofen, Farmitalia, Carlo Erba, Italy) and placed in a homemade 5-cm i.d. radiofrequency (RF) coil. Transversal images were acquired at 4.7 T with the following parameters: TR = 1000 ms; TE = 70 ms; *b*-factor = 500 s/mm^2, diffusion-sensitive gradient pulses applied along the z direction (slice direction). Eleven transversal slices with 0.5-mm slice thickness and 1-mm slice separation were acquired. T_2W images were acquired with the same parameters as DW images, but without diffusion-sensitive gradient pulses. The drug, GV150526, a selective glycine receptor antagonist of the *N*-methyl-D-aspartate (NMDA) receptor (Ratti *et al.*, 1995; Reggiani *et al.*, 2001) was administered through the tail vein at a dose of 3 mg/kg, 5 min before MCAO.

T_2W and DW images are characterized by different sensitivity windows during the evolution of ischemic lesion. Table I reports ischemic lesion volumes as determined by either T_2W or DW images. Six hours after MCAO, the lesion volumes were greatly underestimated by T_2W; this was observed in both vehicle and drug-treated animals. On the contrary, at later time points (144 h) no lesion was detectable in DW images while still clearly detected in T_2W images. The effect of treatment with GV150526 was clearly assessed by MRI. At each time point investigated, the infarct volume was smaller in treated than in control animals ($p < 0.001$). Results reported here are referred to an experimental protocol in which the drug is administered before MCAO. The complete study showed that MRI is sensitive to the effect of the treatment also when administered after MCAO (Reggiani *et al.*, 2001).

Table I
Permanent MCAO

Time elapsed after MCAO (h)	Drug (preischemia administration)		Vehicle	
	T_2W	DW	T_2W	DW
6	1.1 ± 0.5	8.4 ± 3.7	10.3 ± 5.1	43.5 ± 14.5
24	14.7 ± 5.9	28.2 ± 12.2	93.1 ± 18.5	100.8 ± 20.3
144	16.4 ± 6.5	nd[a]	87.6 ± 19.6	nd[a]

[a]No data available.
Infarct volumes (expressed in mm^3) measured from MRI (T_2W and DW).

V. Neoplastic Pathologies

MRI plays a crucial role both in diagnosis of tumors and in monitoring of their response to therapies in both clinical and preclinical environments. Experimental tumor tissues are generally characterized by a long T_2 relaxation time (compared with neighboring healthy tissues) and consequently are easily detected and delineated by T_2W images. Standard T_2W images allow for noninvasive, *in vivo* measurement of tumor volume and its time evolution, although in the presence of irregular or infiltrating lesions, such evaluation can be difficult. Tumor size has been used for a long time as a standard endpoint for experimental drug screening, and as a prospective endpoint for planning clinical trials, and it is widely used in clinical practice for making decisions in tumor treatments (Padhani, 2002). However, there are several recognized limitations to the use of tumor size changes as a marker of therapeutic efficacy. Such limitations are particularly evident when evaluating the effect of antiangiogenic drugs, which selectively inhibit tumor vasculature before any effect on tumor size can be visible (Brindle, 2002). Functional techniques sensitive to tumor vascularization have been developed based on dynamic acquisition of images at high time resolution during the arrival of contrast agents in the tumor tissue (Bhujwalla *et al.*, 1999). These techniques, known as dynamic contrast-enhanced MRI (DCE-MRI) can be divided into (i) techniques that use low molecular weight contrast agents and that rapidly distribute in the extracellular space and (ii) techniques that use high molecular weight contrast agents designed for prolonged intravascular retention. Preclinical studies have indicated that DCE-MRI with macromolecular contrast agents is more specific (compared with low molecular weight contrast agents) for detection of tumor microvessel features. This is due to the peculiar characteristic of tumor vasculature of being hyperpermeable to macromolecules. Gd-DTPA-albumin is a prototype contrast agent obtained by covalent binding of several Gd-DTPA moieties to albumin (Ogan, 1988), resulting in a molecule with 90 kDa molecular weight. Recently, small molecular weight contrast agents that, thanks to their ability to reversibly binds to plasma proteins, behave similar to intravascular macromolecular contrast agents have been proposed for DCE-MRI studies (Marzola *et al.*, 2005;

Preda *et al.*, 2004). Interestingly it has been reported that DCE-MRI experiments performed with these contrast agents can be more sensitive to alteration induced by antiangiogenic drugs compared to experiments performed by using standard macromolecular or low molecular weight contrast agents (Boschi *et al.*, 2008; Marzola *et al.*, 2005; Preda *et al.*, 2004).

We have implemented an experimental protocol exploiting DCE-MRI with Gd-DTPA-albumin for the characterization of tumor vasculature in an experimental model of colon carcinoma and for the assessment of an antiangiogenic efficacy of an experimental drug.

A. Colon Carcinoma

HT-29 human colon carcinoma fragments were implanted subcutaneously in the flank of 10 nude mice weighing approximately 25 g. Animals were inserted in the study when the tumors reached a weight of approximately 500 mg. The experimental drug (SU6668) is a small molecule inhibitor of the angiogenic receptor tyrosine kinases (RTKs) Flk-1/KDR (VEGFR-2), PFGFRβ, and FGFR (Laird *et al.*, 2000). Animals were divided in two groups; one group received the drug and the other group received the vehicle. Tumor volumes were obtained by caliper measurement of tumor diameters (d and D), according to the formula $d^2 \times D/2$. Gd-DTPA-albumin, synthesized according to Ogan (1988), was obtained from R. Brasch (Contrast Media Laboratory, University of California, San Francisco) and is characterized by an average molecular weight of 94,000 Da, corresponding to approximately 45 molecules of Gd-DTPA covalently bound to each albumin molecule. Mice were anesthetized by inhalation of a mixture of air and O_2 containing 0.5–1% halothane and placed in prone position into a 3.5-cm i.d. transmitter-receiver birdcage coil. Images were acquired using a Biospec tomograph (Bruker, Karlsruhe, Germany) equipped with a 4.7-T, 33-cm-bore horizontal magnet (Oxford Ltd., Oxford, UK). Coronal SE and transversal multislice, fast SE T_2W (RARE, $TE_{eff} = 70$ ms) images were acquired for tumor localization and good visualization of extratumoral tissues. Afterward, a dynamic series of 3D, transversal spoiled-gradient-echo (SPGR) images were acquired with the following parameters: TR/TE = 50/3.5 ms, flip angle (α) = 90°, matrix size = 128 × 64 × 32, FOV = 5 × 2.5 × 3 cm^3 (corresponding to 0.39 × 0.39 mm^2 in-plane resolution and 0.94 mm slice thickness), and number of averages (NEX) = 1. The acquisition time for a single 3D image was 104 s; a dynamic scan of 24 images was acquired with 30-s time intervals between each image (total acquisition time 53 min). A bolus of Gd-DTPA-albumin was injected into the tail vein at a dose of 30 μmol of Gd/kg (26 ml/kg, typically 60 μl for mouse) during the time interval between the first and the second scan. A phantom containing 1 mM Gd-DTPA in saline was inserted in the field of view and used as an external reference standard. The MRI protocol was derived from that reported in Daldrup *et al.* (1998), with some modifications (Marzola *et al.*, 2003).

Briefly, precontrast T_1 values were measured using the IR-snapshot flash technique (Haase *et al.*, 1989), a series of 12 consecutive snapshot flash images were acquired after a 5000-ms inversion pulse with the following parameters: FOV = 5 × 2.5 cm^2, slice thickness = 2 mm, matrix size 128 × 64, TR/TE = 10/2.8 ms, $\alpha = 7°$, and a centric phase-encoding scheme. Some images were obtained at lower space resolution (matrix size 64 × 32) in order to verify that the T_1 values obtained were not affected by the relatively long acquisition time of the single image. In our experience, when working with mice, it is not possible to measure the signal directly from the blood vessels because the signal of the blood is hyperintense due to flow effects. Consequently, the plasma kinetics of the contrast medium was determined *ex vivo* by withdrawing blood samples from a different group of mice before and 5, 15, 30, and 60 min after Gd-DTPA-albumin administration. A total of 15 animals were used, corresponding to three animals for each time point. The blood samples were examined using the same sequences as performed in animals (see Marzola *et al.*, 2003 for details).

From the SI of MR images, it is possible to calculate the longitudinal relaxation time of the different tissues (after $T_{1\text{pre}}$ has been independently measured), according to Daldrup *et al.* (1998),

$$\frac{\text{SI}(t)_{\text{post}}}{\text{SI}_{\text{pre}}} = \frac{1 - e^{(-\text{TR}/T_1(t)_{\text{post}})}}{1 - e^{(-\text{TR}/T_1(t)_{\text{pre}})}}. \tag{2}$$

Longitudinal relaxation rates are correlated to contrast agent concentration through

$$\Delta R_1(t) = [R_1(t) - R_1(0)] = \frac{1}{T_1(t)_{\text{post}}} - \frac{1}{T_1(t)_{\text{pre}}} = [Gd(t)]\cdot r_1, \tag{3}$$

where $T_1(t)_{\text{pre}}$ and $T_1(t)_{\text{post}}$ represent, respectively, the longitudinal relaxation times of the tissue before and at different time points after contrast agent injection. [Gd(t)] indicates the molar concentration and r_1 (expressed in Mm^{-1} s^{-1}) the relaxivity of Gd ion in the tissue. Assuming that r_1 is constant in the different tissues examined, the parameter $\Delta R_1(t)$ is directly proportional to the Gd concentration. This assumption represents an inherent approximation in DCE-MRI techniques. In fact, relaxivity of contrast agents is strictly dependent on the microviscosity of the medium, and can change in different tissues. We have performed *in vitro* measurements of Gd-DTPA-albumin relaxivity in pure water and in a protein-rich aqueous solution (Marzola *et al.*, 2003), and we have observed a 68% increase of the Gd-DTPA-albumin relaxivity. However, the increase was more pronounced (200%) for Gd-DTPA, thus enforcing the use of macromolecules against small molecules contrast agents in this specific application. The time dependence of $\Delta R_1(t)$ was analyzed in terms of a two-compartment tissue model composed of plasma and interstitial water-equilibrating pools (Daldrup *et al.*, 1998; Marzola *et al.*, 2003).

In this model it is assumed that the exchange is due to passive diffusion of the contrast agent. As explained in detail previously (Marzola *et al.*, 2003), the time dependence of $\Delta R_1(t)$ can be expressed by

$$\Delta R_1(t) \propto \mathrm{CT}(t) = \mathrm{kPS}\int_0^t C_0\exp(-\vartheta(a))\mathrm{d}(\vartheta) + \mathrm{fPV}C_0\exp(-\mathrm{A}(t)), \qquad (4)$$

where CT(t) is the total concentration of Gd in both interstitial water and plasma space, $C_0\exp(-A(t))$ is the experimentally *ex vivo* measured concentration of Gd in plasma, fPV is the fractional plasma volume of the tissue, and kPS is the transendothelial permeability. This expression was fitted to the $\Delta R_1(t)$ values extracted from the experimental signal intensity using a two-parameter best-fit nonlinear algorithm.

After acquisition, data were transferred onto a personal computer (PC) for analysis. The fitting routine was written in Matlab 5.2 (The MathWorks Inc., Natick, MA). Images were analyzed on a pixel-by-pixel basis to obtain parametric maps of kPS and fPV, or on a ROI basis to obtain the average value of kPS and fPV in the selected ROI; in each animal, the central five slices of the 3D dataset were analyzed. For each considered slice, ROIs were manually tracked to cover the tumor rim and the tumor core. A band approximately 2 mm wide at the periphery, on the external side of the tumor, was considered as the rim. The signal in the rim (and in the core) was averaged and analyzed to obtain the mean kPS and fPV values in the rim (or in the core) of the selected slice.

After the last MRI examination, mice were sacrificed and tumoral tissue removed and prepared for histology. The experimental protocol used for histology and immunohistochemistry has been reported in detail (Marzola *et al.*, 2004). The mean number of vessels and vessel area was obtained from CD31 immunohistochemical staining of tumor tissue. Animals were examined at MRI before and 24 h after receiving a single administration of SU6668 or vehicle. Figure 5 shows axial T_2W and T_1W precontrast and T_1W postcontrast images obtained for one animal bearing a subcutaneous tumor. The T_2W image clearly delineates the tumor tissue as an area of strongly hyperintense signal. In the precontrast T_1W image, the SI of the tumor, skeletal muscle, blood, and myocardium is very similar. After contrast medium administration (the image shown was acquired about 50 min after injection), the signal from blood and vascularized regions of the tumor is greatly enhanced. As described earlier, from the time dependence of the signal intensity, it is possible to extract the time dependence of the enhancement in longitudinal relaxation rate (ΔR_1) of the different tissues that is proportional to the contrast agent concentration. Figure 5D shows the time dependence of ΔR_1 (or Gd-concentration) in pixels belonging to the periphery or the core of the tumor; the best fitting to experimental data is also shown. The intercept of the fitting curve with the y-axis measures the blood volume, whereas its rate of rising measures the vascular permeability. In this experimental model, and, in general, in xenografts, the periphery of the tumor is well vascularized, whereas the core is

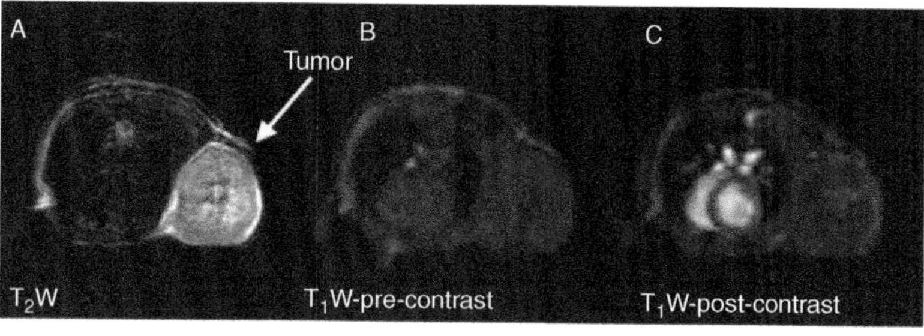

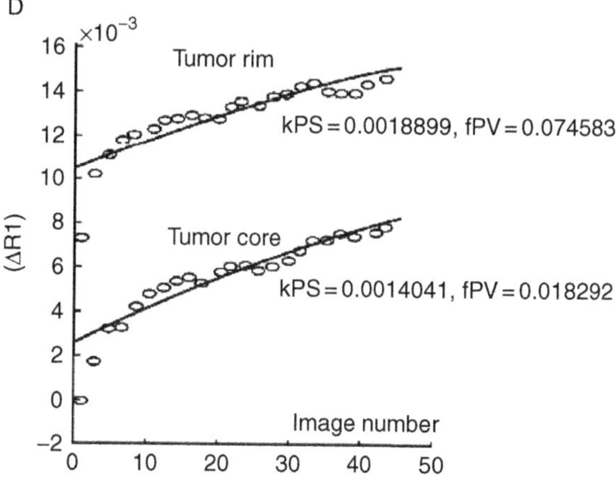

Fig. 5 Colon carcinoma. T_2W, T_1W-precontrast, and T_1W-postcontrast images acquired approximately at the tumor center for one animal belonging to the group treated with SU6668, before treatment. (A) Axial T_2W RARE image; (B) axial T_1W gradient-echo images acquired before, and (C) 50 min after injection of Gd-DTPA-albumin. (D) Time dependence of ΔR_1 (or Gd-concentration) in pixels belonging to the periphery or the core of the tumor; the best fitting to experimental data is also shown. fPV and kPS are expressed in ml/cm^3 of tissue and ml/min/cm^3 of tissue, respectively. (adapted from Marzola *et al.* (2004) with permission).

mainly necrotic. The fitting of theoretical equation to experimental data can be performed also pixel-by-pixel, providing a parametric map of fractional plasma volume and transendothelial permeability. The maps relative to the slice shown in Fig. 5A are reported in Fig. 6 (upper line). In this particular slice, regions with high plasma volume correspond to regions with high vascular permeability, but this is not always true; in some tumors, we have found areas of high vascular permeability in mostly necrotic regions (Marzola *et al.*, 2003) in agreement with other investigators (Bhujwalla *et al.*, 2003). Twenty-four hours after receiving a single-dose treatment of SU6668, the fPV and kPS maps were strongly altered with a strong decrease in both parameters, as apparent in Fig. 6 (lower line). From quantitative analysis on the group of treated animals, we observed a decrease in kPS of 51% ($p < 0.0001$) and 26% ($p < 0.05$) in the tumor rim and core, respectively. The decrease in fPV amounted to 58% and 35%in the tumor rim and core, respectively.

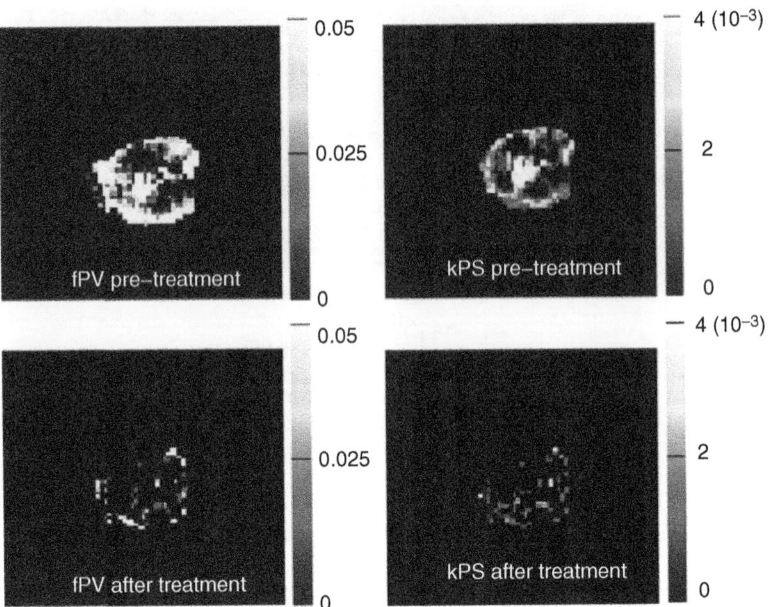

Fig. 6 Colon carcinoma. Upper line: fPV and kPS maps obtained for the slice shown in Fig. 5 (i.e., before treatment). Lower line: fPV and kPS maps obtained for the same animal but 24 h after treatment (adapted from Marzola *et al.* (2004) with permission). (See Plate no. 11 in the Color Plate Section.)

No statistically significant alteration was observed in the control group. By DCE-MRI, it was possible to assess the effect of SU6668 on blood vessels, after only 24 h of treatment (single-dose administration), well before any effect on tumor size was detectable.

VI. Lipid Accumulation in Metabolic-Degenerative Disorders

Lipid accumulation represents a common feature of several pathological degenerative states (e.g., obesity and age-induced atrophy of organs; Marzola *et al.*, 1999a). Obesity is a health problem widely diffused in industrialized countries that causes complications such as hypertension, diabetes (type 2 diabetes), and atherosclerosis. Today at least 30% of adult Americans are obese (Lonnqvist *et al.*, 1999). The causes of obesity are still under investigation. Overeating and/or scarce physical activity play an important role, but some hereditary factors also seem to be relevant. In 1950, a genetic defect was identified in obese mice (Ingalls *et al.*, 1950), the sequencing of the mouse obese gene was later identified and sequenced (Zhang *et al.*, 1994), and it was demonstrated that the ob gene is expressed in white and brown adipose tissue and encodes a protein called leptin (Lonnqvist *et al.*, 1999). In the ob-ob mice, two mutations have been demonstrated: extinguished leptin mRNA expression and a nonsense mutation leading to the production of an inactive form of leptin that results in a compensatory 20-fold increase in leptin mRNA (Lonnqvist *et al.*, 1999). Obesity in the mutant ob-ob mice can be consequently attributed to a deficiency in the active leptin. Ob-ob mutant mice have been used in a number of studies aimed at clarifying the role of leptin in obesity and in development of antiobesity drugs. MRI and localized magnetic resonance spectroscopy (MRS) can be exploited to characterize these mice *in vivo*. In ^{1}H MRI, the signal is derived from water and lipids that occur as fatty droplets in the cytoplasm of adipocytes. Lipid protons have longitudinal relaxation times shorter than those of other nonlipid tissues; a well-known consequence of this is the fact that fat tissues appear as very bright structures disturbing identification of other organs and requiring selective suppression of fat signal. The fat signal originates mainly from the CH_2-CH_3 groups of the lipidic chain, which resonate 3.3 ppm apart from water. This frequency shift, which is responsible for the chemical shift artifact, allows for selective excitation (or suppression) of fat or water protons. Several techniques have been proposed in biomedical MRI to obtain separate images of water and fat protons in tissues and to evaluate the ratio between these two components (Kaldoudi and Williams, 1992).

At low magnetic fields, the Dixon method (Dixon, 1984), based upon the dephasing of fat and water signals, may be applied. At high magnetic fields, where the Dixon method is limited by susceptibility effects, the chemical shift between water and fat protons yields frequency separations large enough to permit selective excitation of fat or water protons. The excitation pulse in a single-slice excitation SE experiment can be designed to be frequency selective in such a way that only one of the two signals is excited. We have used this technique in characterization of brown adipose tissue (BAT) and thymus (Lunati *et al.*, 1999; Marzola *et al.*, 1999a). Localized spectroscopy techniques are also very useful in characterization of adipose tissues. This family of methods that encompasses single voxel or multivoxel techniques (the last known as chemical shift imaging (CSI)) exploits gradients for obtaining localization while the acquisition of the signal is performed in the absence of gradient; the chemical shift information is consequently retained. Localized spectroscopy has been used for characterizing *in vivo* BAT in terms of its content of polyunsaturated fatty acids (Lunati *et al.*, 2001; Strobel *et al.*, 2008). Here we report some experimental approaches performed by MRS aimed at phenotyping ob-ob mice.

A. Ob-ob Mice

Ob-ob animals and relative controls were obtained by Harlan, Italy. A total of $n = 10$ ($n = 5$ ob-ob and $n = 5$ controls) mice were used. For MRI, mice were anesthetized by inhalation of a mixture of oxygen and air containing 0.5–1% of isofluorane and placed in the supine position in a 3.5-cm i.d. birdcage coil. Images and localized spectra were acquired using a Biospec Avance Tomograph (Bruker, Germany) operating at 4.7 T. After a pilot acquisition, T_1W transversal and coronal slices were acquired using TR/TE = 1009/18 ms, slice thickness = 2 mm, and NEX = 1. Other parameters were FOV = 10 × 5 cm^2, matrix size = 256 × 128 and FOV = 4.5 × 4.5 cm^2, and matrix size = 256 × 256 for sagittal and transversal acquisition, respectively. Animals were positioned in the RF coil in such a way that the kidneys were approximately in the coil (and magnet) isocenter. Unlocalized spectra were acquired using a single RF pulse sequence with RF pulse duration of 50 μs and NEX = 16. Localized spectra were acquired using a stimulated-echo sequence with TR = 2500 ms, TM = 8.9 ms, TE = 22 ms, voxel size = 3 × 3 × 3 mm^3, and NEX = 128. The voxel was placed upon the liver.

Figure 7 shows T_1W, transversal images of the abdominal region obtained from an ob-ob animal (Fig. 7A) and normal control (Fig. 7B) at the level of the kidneys. The fat tissue appears bright and represents the most abundant tissue in the ob-ob animal, whereas it is quite scarce in the normal control. In Fig. 7C and D unlocalized spectra obtained from the abdominal region of the animals are shown; the peaks at 4.7 and 1.3 ppm are due to water and fat protons, respectively. Spectra and images were obtained using the same volume coil without moving the animal.

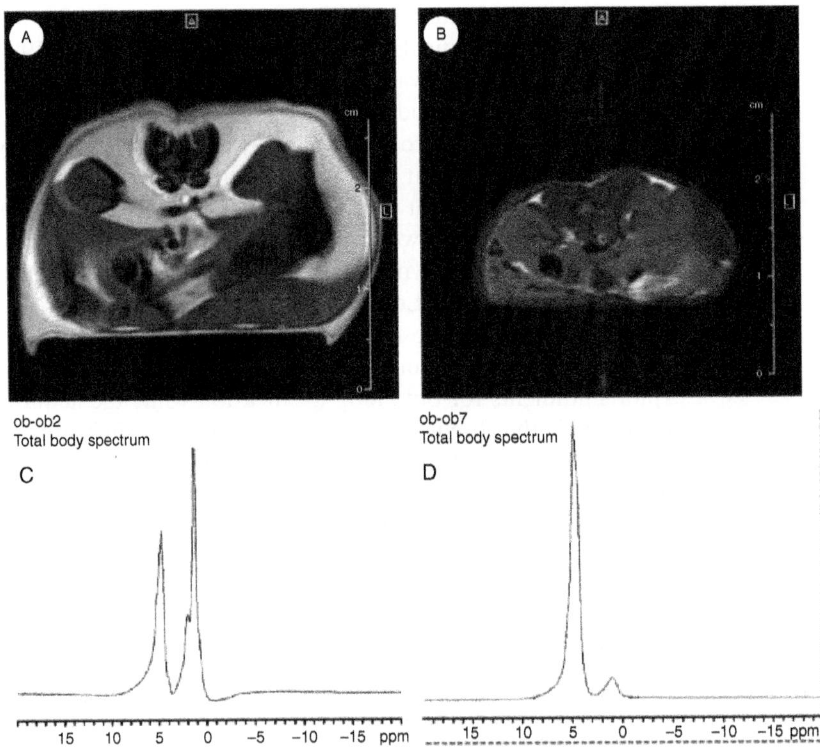

Fig. 7 Ob-ob mice. Representative SE T_1W images of the abdominal region of an ob-ob mouse (A) and control (B). Unlocalized ^1H spectra obtained from the abdominal region of an ob-ob mouse (C) and control (D).

In ob-ob animals, abdominal spectra showed two peaks of similar intensity, whereas in normal controls the water peak was greatly predominant. By indicating with W the area under the water peak and with F the area under the fat peak, the ratio F/W was calculated for each spectrum. This ratio amounted to 1.46 ± 0.44 and 0.29 ± 0.11 in ob-ob and control mice, respectively. It has been shown that the ratio between water and fat peaks obtained from proton spectra of the abdominal region is well correlated to the total body fat and represents a quantitative measure of it (Barac-Nieto and Gupta, 1996). From the calibration curve reported by Barac-Nieto and Gupta (1996), we can infer that the body fat amounts to 55% in ob-ob animals and 0.5% in control animals.

Localized spectroscopy was used to assess the liver content of fat. In Fig. 8, we show localized spectra obtained from the liver of an ob-ob mouse and normal control. These spectra qualitatively show that the liver of ob-ob animals is rich in fat, different from the liver of normal animals. The signal attributable to fat protons, in fact, accounted for about 50% and less than 1% of the total signal in ob-ob and normal control animals, respectively. Calibration of the sequence with oil phantom is required to obtain a quantification of the fat content. MRI and MRS are valuable tools in characterizing fat tissues in ob-ob animals and in assessing the effect of experimental drugs on fat deposits.

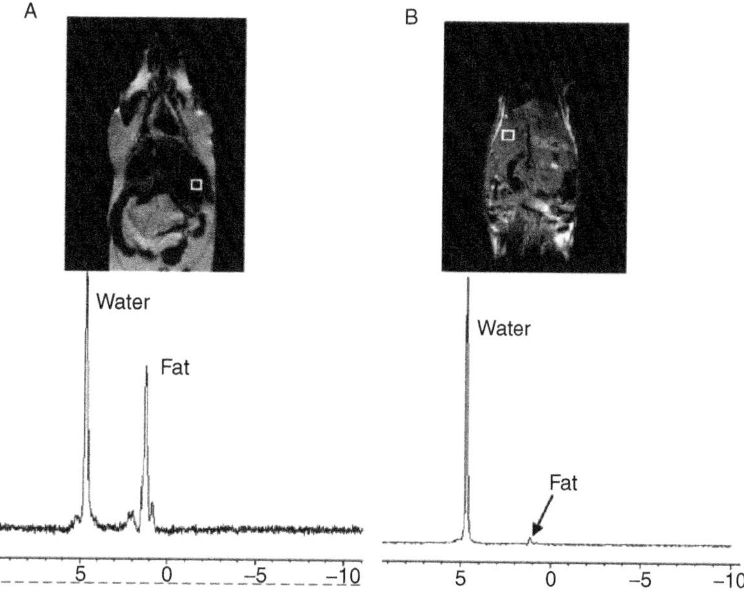

Fig. 8 Ob-ob mice. Localized spectra obtained from a 5-mm^3 pixel placed in the liver parenchyma from an ob-ob mouse (A) and a normal control (B).

VII. Conclusions

MRI has become an increasingly appreciated diagnostic tool in medicine, and it is probable that in the future, its use in preclinical research will expand. MRI has numerous advantages over conventional techniques of tissue analysis (Sbarbati and Osculati, 1996): it is harmless to tissues, the same tissue can be examined several times, several organs can be examined at the same time, and sections of relevant structures can be obtained in all planes. *In vivo* examination also results in a significant reduction of artifact due to fixation, embedding, sectioning, and staining. In addition, *in vivo* MRI examination offers the possibility to obtain functional, biochemical, and biophysical data that cannot be obtained by alternative methods. These advantages are, however, accompanied by some important drawbacks. Apart from the cost of the instrument, the main drawback is the spatial resolution, which is relatively low in comparison to conventional microscopes. Finally, the interpretation of the results is often difficult for an incomplete standardization of MRI methods and it needs interdisciplinary competence. For these reasons, to date, preclinical MRI represents a challenge to the scientist and although MRI data must be evaluated with caution, a wide use of MRI-based technologies can permit the execution of experimental paradigms that are not possible using a more traditional approach.

References

Acred, P. (1986). The selbie or thigh lesion test, experimental models in antimicrobial chemotherapy, Vol. I, p. 109. Academic Press, London.

Albert, M. S., Cates, G. D., Driehuys, B., Happer, W., Saam, B., Springer, C. S., and Wishnia, A., Jr. (1994). Biological magnetic resonance imaging using laser-polarized 129Xe. *Nature* **370**(6486), 199–201.

Barac-Nieto, M., and Gupta, R. K. (1996). Use of proton MR spectroscopy and MR imaging to assess obesity. *J. Magn. Reson. Imaging* **6**(1), 235–238.

Beckmann, N., Hof, R. P., and Rudin, M. (2000). The role of magnetic resonance imaging and spectroscopy in transplantation: From animal models to man. *NMR Biomed.* **13**(6), 329–348.

Beckmann, N., Mueggler, T., Allegrini, P. R., Laurent, D., and Rudin, M. (2001). From anatomy to the target: Contributions of magnetic resonance imaging to preclinical pharmaceutical research. *Anat. Rec.* **265**(2), 85–100.

Bhujwalla, Z. M., Artemov, D., and Glockner, J. (1999). Tumor angiogenesis, vascularization, and contrast-enhanced magnetic resonance imaging. *Top. Magn. Reson. Imaging* **10**(2), 92–103.

Bhujwalla, Z. M., Artemov, D., Nararajan, K., Solaiyappan, M., Kollars, P., and Kristjansen, P. E. G. (2003). Reduction of vascular and permeable regions in solid tumors detected by macromolecular contrast magnetic resonance imaging after treatment with antiangiogenic agent TNP-470. *Clin. Cancer Res.* **9**(1), 355–362.

Boschi, F., Marzola, P., Sandri, M., Nicolato, E., Galiè, M., Fiorini, S., Merigo, F., Lorusso, V., Chaabane, L., and Sbarbati, A. (2008). Tumor microvasculature observed using different contrast agents: A comparison between Gd-DTPA-Albumin and B-22956/1 in an experimental model of mammary carcinoma. *MAGMA* **21**(3), 169–176.

Brasch, R. C., Li, K. C., Husband, J. E., Keogan, M. T., Neeman, M., Padhani, A. R., Shames, D., and Turetschek, T. (2000). *In vivo* monitoring of tumor angiogenesis with MR imaging. *Acad. Radiol.* **7**(10), 812–823.

Brindle, K. M. (2002). Tumor therapy. *NMR Biomed.* **15**(2), 87–88.

Calamante, F., Thomas, D. L., Pell, G. S., Wiersma, J., and Turner, R. (1999). Measuring cerebral blood flow using magnetic resonance imaging techniques. *J. Cereb. Blood Flow Metab.* **19**(7), 701–735.

Daldrup, H., Shames, D. M., Wendland, M., Okuhata, Y., Link, T. M., Rosenau, W., Lu, Y., and Brasch, R. C. (1998). Correlation of dynamic contrast-enhanced magnetic resonance imaging with histologic tumor grade: Comparison of macromolecular and small-molecular contrast media. *Pediatr. Radiol.* **28**(2), 67–78.

Dixon, W. T. (1984). Simple proton spectroscopic imaging. *Radiology* **153**(1), 189–194.

Fabene, P. F., Merigo, F., Galiè, M., Benati, D., Bernardi, P., Farace, P., Nicolato, E., Marzola, P., and Sbarbati, A. (2007). Pilocarpine-induced status epilepticus in rats involves ischemic and excitotoxic mechanisms. *PLoS ONE* **2**(10), e1105.

Galiè, M., Farace, P., Nanni, C., Spinelli, A., Nicolato, E., Boschi, F., Magnani, P., Trespidi, S., Ambrosini, V., Fanti, S., Merigo, F., *et al.* (2007). Epithelial and mesenchymal tumor compartments exhibit *in vivo* complementary patterns of vascular perfusion and glucose metabolism. *Neoplasia* **9**(11), 900–908.

Gewalt, S. L., Glover, G. H., Hedlund, L. W., Cofer, G. P., MacFall, J. R., and Johnson, G. A. (1993). MR microscopy of the rat lung using projection reconstruction. *Magn. Reson. Med.* **29**(1), 99–106.

Gossmann, A., Helbich, T. H., Kuriyama, N., Ostrowitzki, M. D., Roberts, T. P. L., Shames, D. M., Van Bruggen, N., Wendland, M. F., Israel, M. A., and Brasch, R. C. (2002). Dynamic contrast-enhanced magnetic resonance imaging as a surrogate marker of tumor response to anti-angiogenic therapy in a xenograft model of glioblastoma multiforme. *J. Magn. Reson. Imaging* **15**(3), 233–240.

Haase, A., Matthaei, D., Bartkowski, R., Duhmke, E., and Leibfritz, D. (1989). Inversion recovery snapshot FLASH MR imaging. *J. Comput. Assist. Tomogr.* **13**(6), 1036–1040.

Hatabu, H., Gaa, J., Kim, D., Li, W., Prasad, P. V., and Edelman, R. R. (1996). Pulmonary perfusion: Qualitative assessment with dynamic contrast-enhanced MRI using ultra-short TE and inversion recovery turbo FLASH. *Magn. Reson. Med.* **36**(4), 503–508.

Hoehn, M., Nicolay, N., Franke, C., and Van der Sanden, B. (2001). Application of magnetic resonance to animal models of cerebral ischemia. *J. Magn. Reson. Imaging* **14**(5), 491–509.

Ingalls, A. M., Dickie, M. M., and Snell, G. D. (1950). Obese, a new mutation in the house mouse. *J. Hered.* **41**(12), 317–318.

Johnson, G. A., and Hedlund, L. W. (1996). Functional imaging of the lung. *Nat. Med.* **2**(11), 1192.

Judenhofer, M., Wehrl, H., Newport, D., Catana, C., Siegel, S., Becker, M., Thielscher, A., Kneilling, M., Lichy, M., Eichner, M., Klingel, K., Reischl, G., *et al.* (2008). Simultaneous PET-MRI: A new approach for functional and morphological imaging. *Nat. Med.* **14**(4), 459–465.

Kaldoudi, E., and Williams, S. C. R. (1992). *Concepts Magn. Reson.* **4**, 53.

Laird, A. D., Vajkoczy, P., Shawyer, L. K., Thurnher, A., Liang, C., Mohammadi, M., Schlessinger, J., Ullrich, A., Hubbard, S. R., Blake, R. A., Fong, T. A. T., Strawn, L. M., *et al.* (2000). SU6668 is a potent antiangiogenic and antitumor agent that induces regression of established tumors. *Cancer Res.* **60**(15), 4152–4160.

Lonnqvist, F., Nordfors, L., and Schalling, M. (1999). Leptin and its potential role in human obesity. *J. Intern. Med.* **245**(6), 643–652.

Loubeyre, P., De Jaegere, T., Miao, Y., Landuyt, W., and Marchal, G. (1999). Assessment of iron oxide particles (AMI 227) and a gadolinium complex (Gd-DOTA) in dynamic susceptibility contrast MR imagings (FLASH and EPI) in a tumor model implanted in rats. *Magn. Reson. Imaging* **17**(4), 627–631.

Lunati, E., Marzola, P., Nicolato, E., Fedrigo, M., Villa, M., and Sbarbati, A. (1999). *In vivo* quantitative lipidic map of brown adipose tissue by chemical shift imaging at 4.7 Tesla. *J. Lipid Res.* **40**(8), 1395–1400.

Lunati, E., Farace, P., Nicolato, E., Righetti, C., Marzola, P., Sbarbati, A., and Osculati, F. (2001). Polyunsaturated fatty acids mapping by ^{1}H MR-chemical shift imaging. *Magn. Reson. Med.* **46**(5), 879–883.

Mai, V. M., Knight-Scott, J., and Berr, S. S. (1999). Improved visualization of the human lung in 1H MRI using multiple inversion recovery for simultaneous suppression of signal contributions from fat and muscle. *Magn. Reson. Med.* **41**(5), 866–870.

Marota, J. J., Ayata, C., Moskowitz, M. A., Weisskoff, R. M., Rosen, B. R., and Mandeville, J. B. (1999). Investigation of the early response to rat forepaw stimulation. *Magn. Reson. Med.* **41**(2), 247–252.

Marota, J. J., Mandeville, J. B., Weisskoff, R. M., Moskowitz, M. A., Rosen, B. R., and Kosofsky, B. E. (2000). Cocaine activation discriminates dopaminergic projections by temporal response: An fMRI study in Rat. *Neuroimage* **11**(1), 13–23.

Marzola, P., Mocchegiani, E., Nicolato, E., Tibaldi, A., Sbarbati, A., and Osculati, F. (1999a). Chemical shift imaging at 4.7 tesla of thymus in young and old mice. *J. Magn. Reson. Imaging* **10**(1), 97–101.

Marzola, P., Nicolato, E., Di Modugno, E., Cristofori, P., Lanzoni, A., Ladel, C. H., and Sbarbati, A. (1999b). Comparison between MRI, microbiology and histology in evaluation of antibiotics in a murine model of thigh infection. *MAGMA* **9**(1-2), 21–28.

Marzola, P., Farace, P., Calderan, L., Crescimanno, C., Lunati, E., Nicolato, E., Benati, D., Degrassi, A., Terron, A., Klapwijk, J., Pesenti, E., Sbarbati, A., *et al.* (2003). *In vivo* mapping of fractional plasma volume (fpv) and endothelial transfer coefficient (Kps) in solid tumors using a macromolecular contrast agent: Correlation with histology and ultrastructure. *Int. J. Cancer* **104**(4), 462–468.

Marzola, P., Degrassi, A., Calderan, L., Farace, P., Crescimanno, C., Nicolato, E., Giusti, A., Pesenti, E., Terron, A., Sbarbati, A., Abrams, T., Murray, L., *et al.* (2004). *In vivo* assessment of antiangiogenic activity of SU6668 in an experimental colon carcinoma model. *Clin. Cancer Res.* **10**(2), 739–750.

Marzola, P., Lanzoni, A., Nicolato, E., Di Modugno, V., Cristofori, P., Osculati, F., and Sbarbati, A. (2005a). ^{1}H MRI of pneumococcal pneumonia in a murine model. *J. Magn. Reson. Imaging* **22,** 70.

Marzola, P., Ramponi, S., Nicolato, E., Lovati, E., Sandri, M., Calderan, L., Crescimanno, C., Merigo, F., Sbarbati, A., Grotti, A., Vultaggio, S., Cavagna, F., *et al.* (2005b). Effect of tamoxifen in an experimental model of breast tumor studied by dynamic contrast-enhanced magnetic resonance imaging and different contrast agents. *Invest. Radiol.* **40**(7), 421–429.

Middleton, H., Black, R. D., Saam, B., Cates, G. D., Cofer, G. P., Guenther, R., Happer, W., Hedlund, L. W., Johnson, G. A., and Juvan, K. (1995). MR imaging with hyperpolarized 3He gas. *Magn. Reson. Med.* **33**(2), 271–275.

Moseley, M. E., Cohen, Y., Mintorovitch, J., Chileuitt, L., Shimizu, H., Kucharczyk, J., Wendland, M. F., and Weinstein, P. R. (1990). Early detection of regional cerebral ischemia in cats: Comparison of diffusion- and T2-weighted MRI and spectroscopy. *Magn. Reson. Med.* **14**(2), 330–346.

Ogan, M. D. (1988). *Invest. Radiol.* **23,** 961.

Ohno, Y., Iwasawa, T., Seo, J. B., Koyama, H., Takahashi, H., Oh, Y. M., Nishimura, Y., and Sugimura, K. (2008). Oxygen-enhanced magnetic resonance imaging versus computed tomography: Multicenter study for clinical stage classification of smoking-related chronic obstructive pulmonary disease. *Am. J. Respir. Crit. Care Med.* **177**(10), 1095–1102.

Padhani, A. R. (2002). Functional MRI for anticancer therapy assessment. *Eur. J. Cancer* **38**(16), 2116–2127.

Preda, A., Novikov, V., Möglich, M., Turetschek, K., Shames, D. M., Brasch, R. C., Cavagna, F. M., and Roberts, T. P. (2004). MRI monitoring of Avastin antiangiogenesis therapy using B22956/1, a new blood pool contrast agent, in an experimental model of human cancer. *J. Magn. Reson. Imaging* **20**(5), 865–873.

Preda, A., Turetschek, K., Daldrup, H., Floyd, E., Novikov, V., Shames, D., Roberts, T., Carter, W., and Brasch, R. (2005). The choice of region of interest measures in contrast-enhanced magnetic resonance image characterization of experimental breast tumors. *Invest. Radiol.* **40**(6), 349–354.

Ratti, E., Corsi, M., Carignani, C., Cugola, A., Mugnaini, M., Gaviraghi, G., Trist, D., and Reggiani, A. (1995). *Eur. J. Neurol.* **2,** 57.

Reggiani, A., Pietra, C., Arban, R., Marzola, P., Guerrini, U., Ziviani, L., Boicelli, A., Sbarbati, A., and Osculati, F. (2001). The neuroprotective activity of the glycine receptor antagonist GV150526: An *in vivo* study by magnetic resonance imaging. *Eur. J. Pharmacol.* **419**(2-3), 147–153.

Rosen, B. R., Belliveau, J. W., Vevea, J. M., and Brady, T. J. (1990). Perfusion imaging with NMR contrast agents. *Magn. Reson. Med.* **14**(2), 249–265.

Sbarbati, A., and Osculati, F. (1996). Tissutal imaging by nuclear magnetic resonance. *Histol. Histopathol.* **11**(1), 229–235.

Sbarbati, A., Reggiani, A., Lunati, E., Arban, R., Nicolato, E., Marzola, P., Asperio, R. M., Bernardi, P., and Osculati, F. (2000). Regional cerebral blood volume mapping after ischemic lesions. *Neuroimage* **12**(4), 418–424.

Strobel, K., van den Hoff, J., and Pietzsch, J. (2008). Localized proton magnetic resonance spectroscopy of lipids in adipose tissue at high spatial resolution in mice *in vivo*. *J. Lipid Res.* **49**(2), 473–480.

Tamura, A., Graham, D. H., McCulloch, J., and Teasdale, G. M. (1981). Focal cerebral ischaemia in the rat: 1. Description of technique and early neuropathological consequences following middle cerebral artery occlusion. *J. Cereb. Blood Flow Metab.* **1**(1), 53–60.

Watt, K. N., Bishop, J., Nieman, B. J., Henkelman, R. M., and Chen, X. J. (2008). Oxygen-enhanced MR imaging of mice lungs. *Magn. Reson. Med.* **59**(6), 1412–1421.

Weber, R., Ramos-Cabrer, P., and Hoehn, M. (2006). Present status of magnetic resonance imaging and spectroscopy in animal stroke models. *J. Cereb. Blood Flow Metab.* **26**(5), 591–604.

Yuh, W. T. C. (1999). An exciting and challenging role for the advanced contrast MR imaging. *J. Magn. Reson. Imaging* **10**(3), 221–222.

Zhang, Y., Proenca, R., Maffei, M., Barone, M., Leopold, L., and Friedman, J. M. (1994). Positional cloning of the mouse obese gene and its human homologue. *Nature* **372**(6505), 425–432.

CHAPTER 15

Application of Combined Magnetic Resonance Imaging and Histopathologic and Functional Studies for Evaluation of Aminoguanidine Following Traumatic Brain Injury in Rats

Jia Lu and Shabbir Moochhala

Defence Medical Research Institute
Singapore 117510
Singapore

I. Introduction
II. Materials and Methods
  A. Animals and Chemicals
  B. Lateral Fluid-Percussive Brain Injury
  C. MRI Methods and Analysis
  D. Neurologic and Behavioral Tests
  E. Perfusion
  F. Caspase-3 Immunohistochemistry
  G. *In Situ* Terminal Transferase dUTP Nick-End Labeling (TUNEL)
III. Results and Discussion
  References

I. Introduction

Trauma brain injury (TBI) is the most common cause of brain damage and is one of the leading causes of death. It triggers a large network of morphologic and metabolic changes in the central nervous system. It has been suggested that at least two classes of injury contribute to the overall pathophysiology of TBI. The primary injury results from the initial mechanical event itself, followed by

ESSENTIAL BIOIMAGING METHODS
Reprinted from *Methods in Enzymology*, Volume 386 (Academic Press, 2004)

DOI: 10.1016/B978-0-12-375043-3.00015-9

the secondary injury, which involves a cascade of biochemical changes that contribute to delayed tissue damage and neuronal death (Faden, 1996). Magnetic resonance imaging (MRI) offers a unique window for monitoring pathophysiologic changes associated with brain injury. MRI has been used extensively in various kinds of brain lesions, both in humans and animal models (Albensi *et al.*, 2000; Bartnik *et al.*, 2001; Cihangiroglu *et al.*, 2002; Lythgoe *et al.*, 2003). It has been shown to be of great diagnostic value in terms of lesion detectability and depiction of lesion size (Palmer *et al.*, 2001). Moreover, MRI is also a powerful tool for the investigation of the time course of therapeutical approaches (e.g., MRI has been used to evaluate therapies with neuroprotective agents) (Cash *et al.*, 2001; Kalkers *et al.*, 2002). The major advantage of MRI over histologic examinations is because of its potential to noninvasively assess changes in the brain *in vivo*. It has been widely accepted that T_2-weighted (T_2W) MRI can be used to estimate the extent of cerebral lesion induced because it provides better delineation of the injured area at different time points. The areas with elevated T_2W signal intensity correlate with tissue damage as determined by established histopathologic techniques (Asanuma *et al.*, 2002; Palmer *et al.*, 2001), and hence the extent of cerebral lesion after TBI can be accurately and reproducibly estimated by *in vivo* conventional T_2W imaging. Despite numerous studies using MRI for characterizing stroke or ischemia in animal models (Dijkhuizen *et al.*, 2003; Matsumoto *et al.*, 1995; Neumann-Haefelin *et al.*, 2000; Palmer *et al.*, 2001; van Dorsten *et al.*, 2002), the utilization of MRI for TBI has been relatively limited (Albensi *et al.*, 2000; Assaf *et al.*, 1997). Currently, there is only modicum of information regarding potential correlations between MRI changes and histologic or neurologic outcome after TBI.

In this chapter, we study the temporal characterization of a lateral fluid percussion model in rats using T_2W MRI. We also compare MRI data with histologic and neurologic outcome after TBI. In addition, the neuroprotective (both prophylactic and treatment) effects of aminoguanidine (AG), a selective inducible nitric oxide synthase inhibitor, on the brain pathogenesis and neurologic performance following brain injury were evaluated. The efficacy of AG was determined by combining the serial MRI and histology for monitoring brain lesion progression over a 72-h period. We also sought to determine whether the changes in behavioral measures could be correlated with the neurologic changes after TBI.

II. Materials and Methods

A. Animals and Chemicals

Male Sprague-Dawley rats (250–350 g) were used for the study. They were acclimatized for at least a week before the experiment. The rats were subjected to the following experimental procedures: Group 1, normal; Group 2, sham-operated; Group 3, TBI + normal saline; Group 4, AG (100 mg/kg) before TBI; Group 5, AG after TBI ($n = 12$ for each group). AG was obtained from Sigma Chemical

(A-7009 Sigma, St. Louis, MO) and was dissolved in 0.9% sodium chloride solution (Sigma). Daily treatment of AG at the dosage of 100 mg/kg or normal saline was given intraperitoneally (IP) into rats starting 2 h before or 30 min after the brain injury. This dosage has been shown to be effective for traumatic brain injury and ischemia in previous studies (Cash *et al.*, 2001; Iadecola *et al.*, 1995; Stoffel *et al.*, 2000; Wada *et al.*, 1998; Zhang *et al.*, 1996). In the handling and care of all animals, the international guiding principles for animal research as stipulated by the World Health Organization (WHO) *Chronicle* (World Health Organization, 1985) and as adopted by the Laboratory Animal Centre, National University of Singapore, were followed.

B. Lateral Fluid-Percussive Brain Injury

The rats were anesthetized with sodium pentobarbital (70 mg/kg, IP) and were then ventilated and placed in a stereotaxic frame. A 1.5-cm sagittal incision from the midpoint between the ears toward the nose was made. The scalp and temporal muscle were then reflected to expose the cranium. An ~5-mm-diameter burr hole positioned 2 mm lateral to the sagittal suture and 3 mm posterior to the coronal suture was determined and drilled with a 1-mm round head drill bit. The remaining bone was then removed, and any bleeding was arrested. This positioned the burr hole parasagittally over the cerebral sensorimotor cortex. The dura was left intact. A modified head cannula from a female Luer-Loc fitting (4.5 mm) was introduced into the burr hole until it abutted the dural surface. The head cannula was then affixed rigidly to the animal's skull with dental cement. Brain injury was performed, using a lateral fluid percussion model as previously described (McIntosh *et al.*, 1989), in which brief displacement and deformation of brain resulted from the rapid epidural injection of saline into the closed cranial cavity. Animals were subjected to a 3.7-atm pressure pulse, which produces severe tissue damage in ipsilateral cerebral cortex and hippocampus (Prins *et al.*, 1996). Sham-operated animals received anesthesia and surgery, but were not subjected to trauma treatment.

C. MRI Methods and Analysis

A total of 18 animals from Group 3 (TBI, $n = 6$), Group 4 (AG before TBI, $n = 6$), and Group 5 (AG after TBI, $n = 6$) were imaged at 24, 48, and 72 h after injury (Fig. 1). MRI was performed with a Bruker 2T MRI machine with custom-made rat coil. Coronal images were collected from eight contiguous, 1.2-mm-thick slices with echo time (TE) 52.6 ms, mixing time (TM) 29.2 ms, Δ 50 ms, and b values of 300 and 30,000 s/cm^2.

Lesion measurements were performed following a direct Fourier transform (FT) of the raw time domain data. Images were displayed in the coronal plane, as collected (Fig. 2). Lesions were detected as hyperintense signals in the MRI. Selection of appropriate seed points by the operator permitted the application of

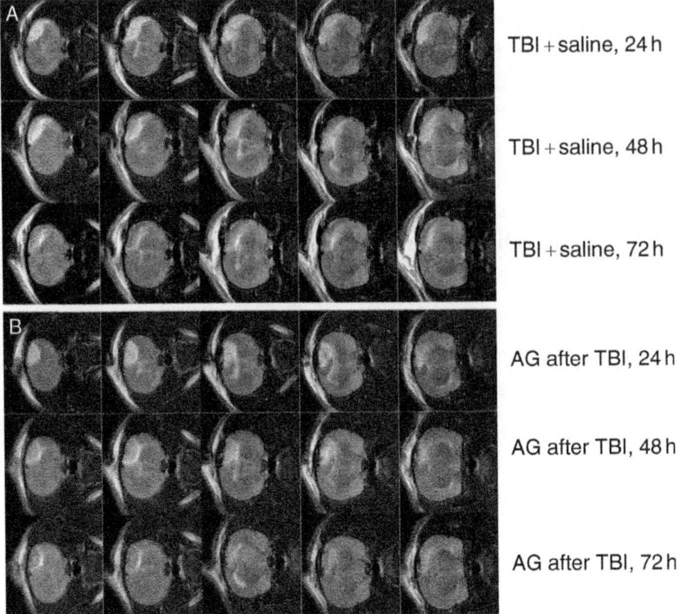

Fig. 1 An example of a series of coronal, T_2-weighted MRI of rat brain of (A) saline-treated and (B) AG after TBI at 24, 48, and 72 h. Slices shown are approximately 2.2, 1, −0.8, −2, and −3.2 mm from bregma. The region of hyperintensity in the right (top) hemisphere of each image delineates the area of injury lesion. Notice that the total area of hyperintensity appears to increase in all time intervals in the saline-treated rat (A), whereas the size is significantly reduced in the AG-treated rat (B).

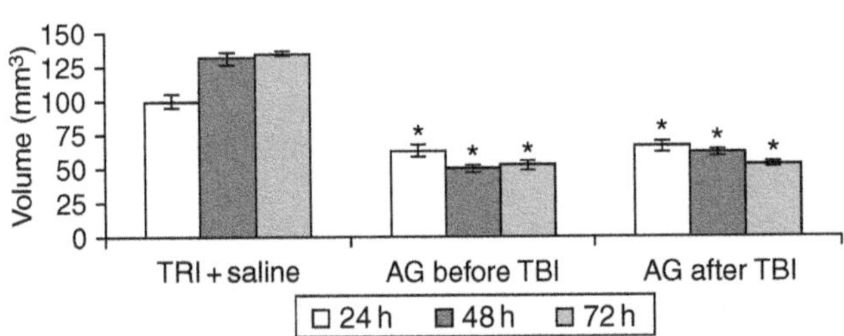

Fig. 2 Comparison of injury lesion volume, derived from the T_2-weighted MRI of saline-treated, AG before TBI and AG after TBI rats. Data are expressed as mean ± standard deviation (S.D.) ($n = 6$ in each group). Significant difference in lesion volume between the groups is revealed by one-way ANOVA. * Denotes significant difference from TBI + saline group ($p < 0.05$).

a contour-tracing algorithm to delineate the boundaries of lesions. For each selected area, in each slice, pixel counts were generated. These values were then multiplied by the slice thickness and summed to yield total volume in mm^3. To limit subjective bias, the operator was blinded to the treatment strategy. The effect of

AG on the changes in lesion volumes over time was analyzed by analysis of variance (ANOVA) with repeated measures. *P* values of <0.05 were considered significant.

D. Neurologic and Behavioral Tests

Neurologic function was evaluated at 24, 48, and 72 h after TBI. When these time points coincided with MRI scanning time points, neurologic evaluation was performed just before MRI scanning. Briefly, the performance was based on three independent tests: locomotor activity, acoustic startle response, forelimb grip-strength test, and rotametric test.

1. Locomotor Activity

The locomotor activity of the animal was recorded using Columbus Instruments (Columbus, OH) Opto-Varimex-Mini, a device that consists of a rectangular perspex container (17 in. × 17 in.) with photocell-based sensors along its length. The rat was placed at one specific corner of the container and acclimatized for a 2-min period in a sound-attenuated room with a 60-dB background noise. Any locomotor activity made by the animal was then picked up by the sensor and was recorded for 5 min (Figs. 3 and 4). Total and ambulatory locomotor activities were recorded separately using two counters. Total locomotor activity refers to any movement made by the rat that is picked up by the sensors. This can include repeated activation of a single sensor. Ambulatory locomotor activity refers to the movement made by the rat as it moves between distinct sensors, excluding repeated activation of a single sensor. By subtraction of the measure for ambulatory locomotor activity from the measure of total locomotor activity, a score of the grooming and rearing behavioral patterns of the animal can be calculated, given that no convulsive activity was observed. Locomotor activity was carried out only at 24 h after TBI.

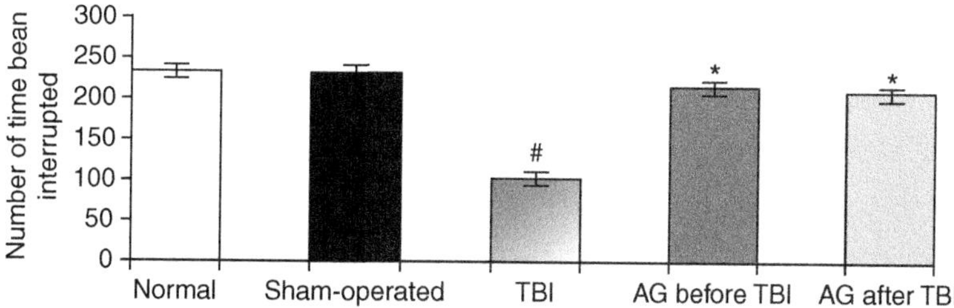

Fig. 3 Total locomotor response action in different groups of rats. Total locomotor response is reduced in rats subjected to TBI with saline injection. This adverse effect is reversed when the animals are administered with AG. # Denotes significant difference from normal and sham-operated groups ($p < 0.05$); * denotes significant difference from TBI + saline ($p < 0.05$).

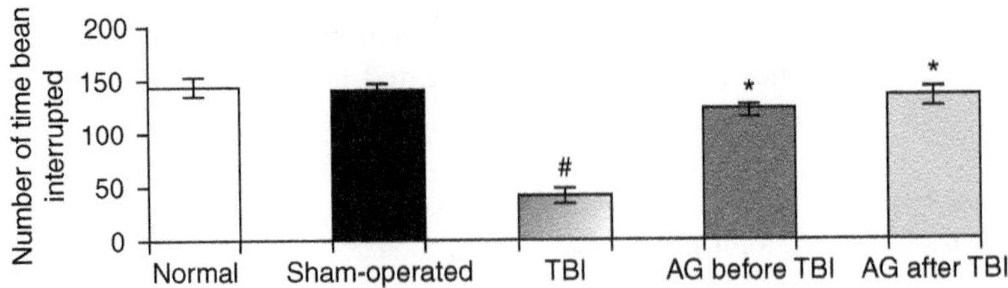

Fig. 4 Ambulatory locomotor response action in different groups of rats. Animals subjected to TBI with saline injection show significantly lower scores. Administration of AG significantly improves the locomotor performance. # Denotes significant difference from normal and sham-operated groups ($p < 0.05$); * denotes significant difference from TBI + saline ($p < 0.05$).

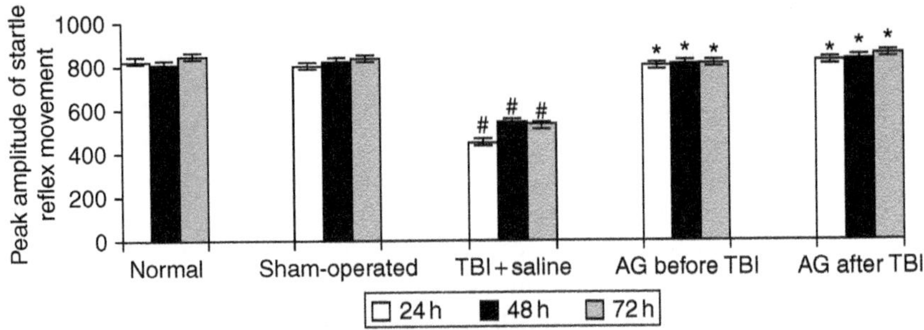

Fig. 5 Acoustic startle reflex in different groups of rats. A marked decrease in acoustic startle response was observed in rats subjected to TBI with saline injection. An improved response was observed in rats treated with AG before or after TBI. # Denotes significant difference from normal and sham-operated groups ($p < 0.05$); * denotes significant difference from TBI + saline ($p < 0.05$).

2. Acoustic Startle Response

The animal was placed inside a Plexiglas cylinder in the acoustic startle apparatus (San Diego, CA) compartment. The animal was first acclimatized for 3 min in the presence of 70 dB of broadband white noise. After this period, the animal was immediately exposed to 50-ms bursts of white noise at 120 dB with a 5-s period of 70 dB of noise between each burst (Fig. 5). The peak amplitude of each startle reflex movement was recorded using the SR-Lab Software (San Diego, CA).

3. Forelimb Grip-Strength Test

Forelimb grip strength was determined using a grip strength meter (Columbus Instruments, Columbus, OH). The animals were placed on the electronic digital force gauge that measured the peak force exerted on it by the action of the animal. While drawing along a straight line leading away from the sensor, the animal was released at some point and the maximum force attained was stored on the display. The highest reading (in Newton's) of three successive trials was taken from each animal (Fig. 6).

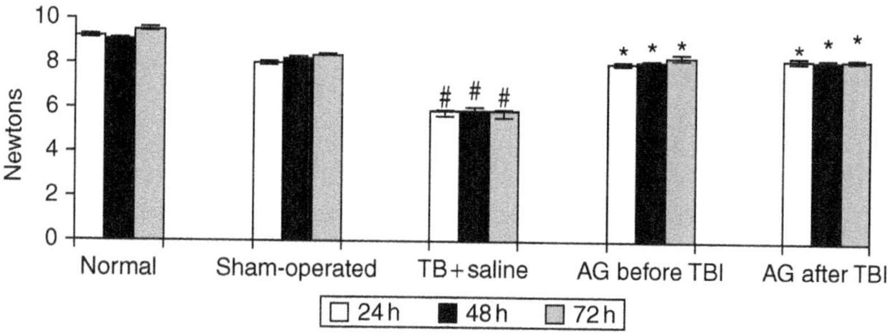

Fig. 6 Grip strength in different groups of rats. Rats subjected to TBI with saline injection show significantly lower average score, but this is significantly enhanced when the animals are administered with AG before or after TBI. # Denotes significant difference from normal and sham-operated groups ($p < 0.05$); * denotes significant difference from TBI + saline, normal and sham-operated groups ($p < 0.05$).

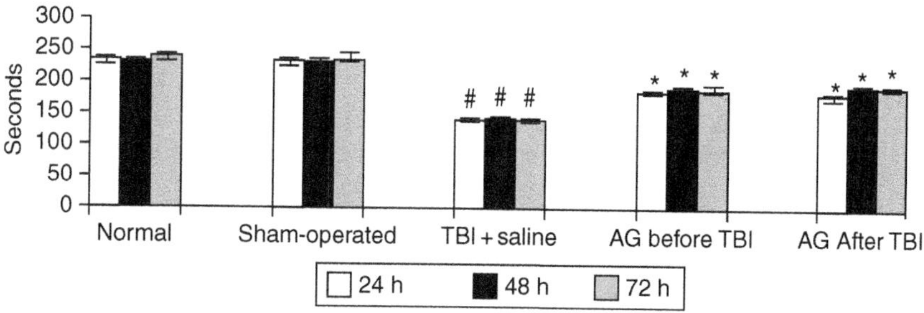

Fig. 7 Rotametric performance in different groups of rats. There is significant difference in rotameric performance among the groups. An improved rotameric performance is observed in the group with AG treatment when compared with rats subjected to TBI with saline injection. # Denotes significant difference from normal and sham-operated groups ($p < 0.05$); * denotes significant difference from TBI + saline, normal and sham-operated groups ($p < 0.05$).

4. Rotametric Test

A rotametric device (Rotamex 4/8 System, Columbus Instruments) was used to examine the ability of the animal to coordinate while being placed on a rotating rod. The rotating speed of the rod was set at 5 rpm (start speed) and 30 rpm (end speed) for a period of 240 s. An internal microcontroller was used to detect the time when a subject fell from the rod. The average reading (in seconds) of three successive trials was taken from each animal (Fig. 7).

E. Perfusion

To characterize the tissue changes as a result of TBI, animals from time points corresponding to MRI data were sacrificed after scanning. Animals were deeply anesthetized with sodium pentobarbital (70 mg/kg, IP). For frozen sections, the rats were perfused with Ringer's solution transcardially for a few minutes until the liver and lungs were clear of blood, followed by an aldehyde fixative composed of a mixture of periodate-lysine-paraformaldehyde (0.01 M $NaClO_4$, 0.075 M lysine, with a concentration of 2% paraformaldehyde, pH 7.4). After the perfusion, the brains were removed and kept in a similar fixative for 2 h. They were then kept in 0.1 M phosphate buffer containing 20% sucrose overnight at 4 °C. For paraffin sections, the rats were perfused with Ringer's solution, followed by 10% neutral formalin. The brains were then kept in a similar fixative overnight.

F. Caspase-3 Immunohistochemistry

We have tried two different methods for caspase-3 immunohistochemistry. For paraffin sections, the brains were dehydrated in an ascending series of alcohol, cleared with xylene, and embedded in paraffin wax. Ten-μm-thick coronal serial sections were cut. The sections were dewaxed in xylene and hydrated with descending series of alcohol, followed by distilled water. Slides were then microwaved in 10 mM of citrate buffer (pH 6) (NeoMarkers, AP-9003) for 10 min in the micromed oven, followed by cooling at room temperature for another 10 min. Slides were washed with 1 × transcription buffered saline (TBS) for 10 min and then incubated with 3% H_2O_2 (BDH 101284N) in methanol for 10 min. After washing in 1 × TBS for 10 min, the slides were incubated in normal goat serum (Vectastain ABC kit [Rabbit IgG], Vector Lab, PK 4001) for 20 min for blocking. Caspase-3 (CPP32) Ab-4 (NeoMarkers RB-1197) was diluted 1:100 with 0.3% bovine serum albumin (BSA) (Vector Lab, SP-5050) and applied on the sections for 1 h at room temperature. Slides were washed with 1 × TBS for 10 min, slightly blotted dry, and incubated with biotinylated goat antirabbit (Vectastain ABC kit [Rabbit IgG], Vector Lab, PK 4001) for 30 min. Slides were again washed with 1 × TBS for 10 min, followed by incubation with Vectastain ABC reagent (Vectastain ABC kit [Rabbit IgG], Vector Lab, PK 4001) for 30 min. Slides were washed with 1 × TBS for 10 min, followed by detection with 3,3′-diaminobenzidine.

For frozen sections, coronal sections of the cerebrum of 10-μm thickness were cut and air-dried for 15 min at room temperature, followed by washing in 1 × phosphate buffered saline (PBS) for 5 min. Slides were then incubated with 3% H_2O_2 (BDH 101284N) in methanol for 5 min and washed in 1 × PBS for 5 min. The slides were then incubated in normal goat serum (Vectastain ABC kit [Rabbit IgG], Vector Lab, PK 4001) for 20 min for blocking. Caspase-3 (CPP32) Ab-4 (NeoMarkers RB-1197) was diluted 1:100 with 0.3% BSA (Vector Lab, SP-5050) and applied on the sections for 1 h at room temperature. Slides were washed with 1 × PBS for 10 min, slightly blotted dry, and incubated with biotinylated goat antirabbit (Vectastain ABC kit [Rabbit IgG], Vector Lab, PK 4001) for 30 min. Slides were again washed with 1 × PBS for 10 min, followed by incubation with Vectastain ABC reagent (Vectastain ABC kit [Rabbit IgG], Vector Lab, PK 4001) for 30 min. Slides were washed with 1 × PBS for 10 min, followed by detection with 3,3′-diaminobenzidine (Fig. 8).

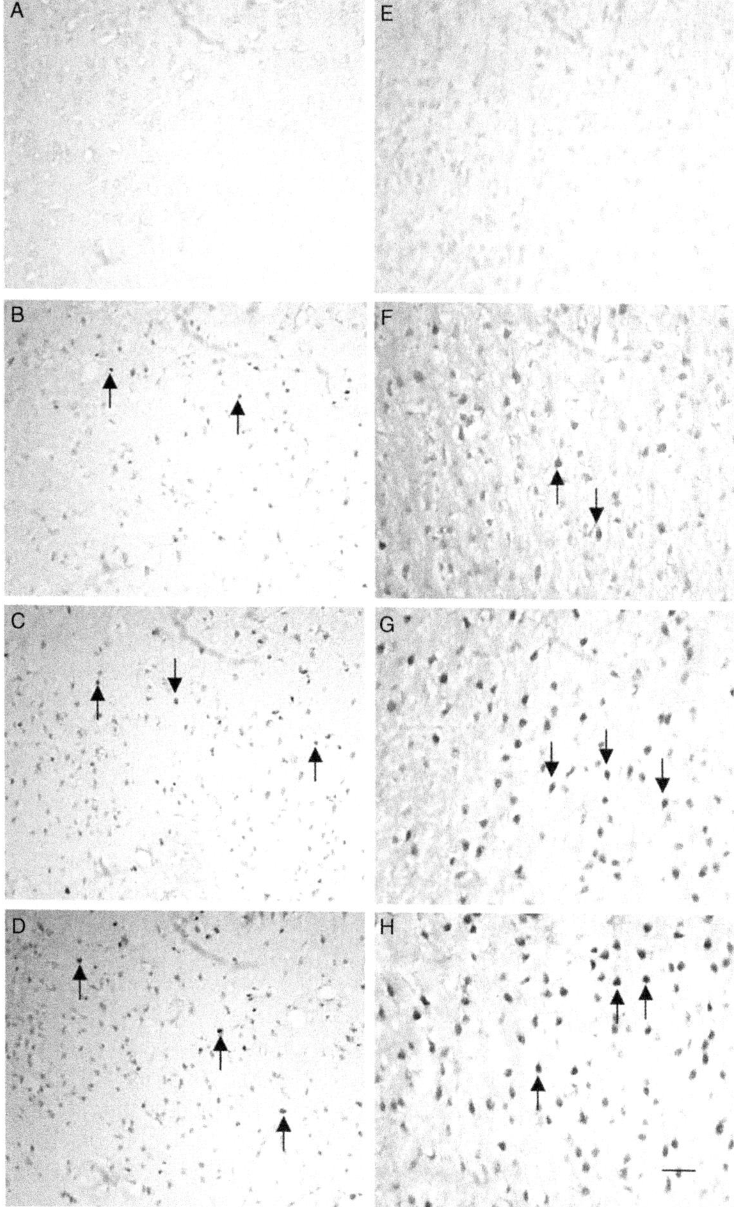

Fig. 8 Apoptotic cortical neurons after TBI by TUNEL (A-D) and caspase-3 immunohistochemistry (E-H). TUNEL positive (A) and caspase-3 immunopositive (E) neurons are absent in the contralateral cortex in rat following TBI. Many TUNEL positive (B) and caspase-3 immunopositive (F) neurons (arrows) are distributed in the ipsilateral parietotemporal cortex at 24 h after TBI. It was further increased at 48 and 72 h (C, D, G, H). Bar = 50 μm (for all).

G. *In Situ* Terminal Transferase dUTP Nick-End Labeling (TUNEL)

Degenerating neurons were identified in brain sections by *in situ* end labeling of nuclear DNA fragments using terminal deoxynucleotidyl transferase and biotin-16-dUTP as substrate (TdT-FragEL DNA Fragmentation Detection Kit, Oncogene, QIA 33). Paraffin sections were first dewaxed in xylene and hydrated with descending concentrations of alcohol, followed by washing in distilled water. Sections were slightly blotted dry and covered with 100 μl of proteinase K (2 mg/ml proteinase K diluted 1:100 in 10 mM Tris, pH 8). Slides were washed with 1 × TBS for 10 min and then covered with 100 μl of 3% H_2O_2 (BDH 101284N) in methanol for 5 min. Slides were again washed with 1 × TBS for 10 min, slightly blotted dry, and incubated with 100 μl of 1 × TdT equilibration buffer for 20 min. At the same time, the working TdT labeling reaction mixture was prepared. After carefully blotting the equilibration buffer away from the specimen, taking care not to touch the sections, 60 μl of TdT labeling reaction mixture was immediately applied on the sections and incubated at 37 °C for 1.5 h, followed by washing in two changes of 1 × TBS for 5 min each. Slides were dried around the sections and incubated with 100 μl of Stop Solution (TdT-FragEL DNA Fragmentation Detection Kit, Oncogene, QIA 33) at room temperature for 5 min. Slides were again rinsed with 1 × TBS, followed by incubation with 100 μl of blocking buffer (TdT-FragEL DNA Fragmentation Detection Kit, Oncogene, QIA 33). After blotting the blocking buffer away from the specimen, 100 μl of diluted conjugate (50 × conjugate diluted 1:300 in blocking buffer) was immediately applied to the specimen for 30 min. Slides were washed with 1 × TBS for 10 min. Incorporated biotin was detected using streptavidin-peroxidase conjugate and 3,3′-diaminobenzidine (Sigma) as chromogen (Fig. 8).

III. Results and Discussion

In this study, we used T_2W imaging to examine the temporal evolution of fluid percussion-induced TBI, and the results were then compared with histologic and neurologic evaluations. Our results showed that T_2W imaging is able to detect temporal- and region-specific changes associated with fluid percussion-induced TBI. MRI changes correlated with histologic evidence of tissue damage. Histologic examination of the brain after TBI showed apoptotic neurons in the cerebral cortex ipsilateral to the injury site, corresponding to the hyperintense area in T_2W image. The present T_2W results also showed that AG attenuated the progression of tissue damage and reduced the extent of cerebral lesion by 50% in rats following TBI when compared with those receiving saline injection. This correlates with our histologic findings, which also showed a marked reduction in the number of degenerating neurons (detected by caspase-3 immunohistochemistry and TUNEL) in the cerebrum in AG-treated rats. Moreover, neurobehavioral tests showed that administration of AG before or after TBI significantly improved rotametric performance, grip-strength score, total and ambulatory locomotor responses, and acoustic startle response. In conclusion, the utilization of T_2W MRI and histologic techniques provides important prognostic information on functional outcome. It is hoped that use of these approaches for evaluation of therapeutic strategies for head injuries will offer a chance for improved functional recovery following TBI.

Acknowledgments

Figures reprinted from Lu *et al.* (2003), with permission from Elsevier.
This study was supported by Defence Science & Technology Agency, Singapore.

References

Albensi, B. C., Knoblach, S. M., Chew, B. G., O'Reilly, M. P., Faden, A. I., and Pekar, J. J. (2000). *Exp. Neurol.* **162,** 61.

Asanuma, T., Ishibashi, H., Konno, A., Kon, Y., Inanami, O., and Kuwabara, M. (2002). *Neurosci. Lett.* **329,** 281.

Assaf, Y., Beit-Yannai, E., Shohami, E., Berman, E., and Cohen, Y. (1997). *Magn. Reson. Imaging* **15,** 77.

Bartnik, B. L., Kendall, E. J., and Obenaus, A. (2001). *Brain Res.* **915,** 133.

Cash, D., Beech, J. S., Rayne, R. C., Bath, P. M., Meldrum, B. S., and Williams, S. C. (2001). *Brain Res.* **905,** 91.

Cihangiroglu, M., Ramsey, R. G., and Dohrmann, G. J. (2002). *Neurol. Res.* **24,** 7.

Dijkhuizen, R. M., Singhal, A. B., Mandeville, J. B., Wu, O., Halpern, E. F., Finklestein, S. P., Rosen, B. R., and Lo, E. H. (2003). *J. Neurosci.* **23,** 510.

Faden, A. I. (1996). *Pharmacol. Toxicol.* **78,** 12.

Iadecola, C., Zhang, F., and Xu, X. (1995). *Am. J. Physiol.* **268,** R286.

Kalkers, N. F., Barkhof, F., Bergers, E., van Schijndel, R., and Polman, C. H. (2002). *Mult. Scler.* **8,** 532.

Lu, J., Moochhala, S., Shirhan, M., Ng, K. C., Teo, A. L., Tan, M. H., Moore, X. L., Wong, M. C., and Ling, E. A. (2003). *Neuropharmacology* **44,** 253.

Lythgoe, M. F., Sibson, N. R., and Harris, N. G. (2003). *Br. Med. Bull.* **65,** 235.

Matsumoto, K., Lo, E. H., Pierce, A. R., Wei, H., Garrido, L., and Kowall, N. W. (1995). *Am. J. Neuroradiol.* **16,** 1107.

McIntosh, T. K., Vink, R., Noble, L., Yamakami, I., Fernyak, S., Soares, H., and Faden, A. L. (1989). *Neuroscience* **28,** 233.

Neumann-Haefelin, T., Kastrup, A., de Crespigny, A., Yenari, M. A., Ringer, T., Sun, G. H., and Moseley, M. E. (2000). *Stroke* **31,** 1965.

Palmer, G. C., Peeling, J., Corbett, D., Del Bigio, M. R., and Hudzik, T. J. (2001). *Ann. NY Acad. Sci.* **939,** 283.

Prins, M. L., Lee, S. M., Cheng, C. L., Becker, D. P., and Hovda, D. A. (1996). *Brain Res. Dev. Brain Res.* **95,** 272.

Stoffel, M., Rinecker, M., Plesnila, N., Eriskat, J., and Baethmann, A. (2000). *Acta Neurochir. Suppl.* **76,** 357.

van Dorsten, F. A., Olah, L., Schwindt, W., Grune, M., Uhlenkuken, U., Pillekamp, F., Hossmann, K. A., and Hoehn, M. (2002). *Magn. Reson. Med.* **47,** 97.

Wada, K., Chatzipanteli, K., Kraydieh, S., Busto, R., and Dietrich, W. D. (1998). *Neurosurgery* **43,** 1427.

World Health Organization (1985). International guiding principles for animal research. *Chronicle* **39,** 51.

Zhang, F. Y., Casey, R. M., Ross, M. E., and Iadecola, C. (1996). *Stroke* **27,** 317.

Acknowledgments

PART IV

Preparation of Materials

CHAPTER 16

Vascular-Targeted Nanoparticles for Molecular Imaging and Therapy

Samira Guccione,* King C.P. Li,† and Mark D. Bednarski*

*Department of Radiology
Lucas MRI Research Center
Stanford University
Stanford, California 94305–5488

†Department of Radiology
Stanford University
Stanford, California 94305–5488

I. Introduction
II. Rationale Behind Choosing a Vascular Target for Molecular Imaging
 A. Facing the Vascular Permeability Problem
 B. Endothelial-Targeted Imaging of Angiogenic Vessels
 C. Integrins as Vascular Targets
 D. Nanoparticles as Molecular Imaging Agents
III. Design and Preclinical Studies of a Vascular-Targeted Molecular Imaging Agent
 A. PV Synthesis and Characterization
 B. ACPV Targeting in EAE Mice
 C. Molecular Imaging of Angiogenesis
IV. Molecular Imaging and Vascular-Targeted Therapeutics
V. Summary
References

I. Introduction

Molecular imaging involves the noninvasive real-time observation of *in vivo* biologic events at the molecular level. The opportunity to visualize targets for the development of diagnostic and pharmaceutical agents over space and time has created wide interest in this marriage of physics, biology, and chemistry. The payoff for medicine can be enormous because proposed targets arising from high

ESSENTIAL BIOIMAGING METHODS
Reprinted from *Methods in Enzymology*, Volume 386 (Academic Press, 2004)

DOI: 10.1016/B978-0-12-375043-3.00016-0

throughput screening can be validated *in vivo* and followed over both space and time. Also, pathways leading to the activity of new pharmaceutical agents can be delineated and followed before, during, and after therapy.

In nearly all cases, molecular imaging will require the delivery of a probe to the tissue site of interest. The design of probes for molecular imaging target two basic classes of biologic events: (1) alteration in metabolic processes and (2) changes in receptor expression. In the case of metabolic probes, small molecules are used that can perfuse most tissues and pathologic regions in the body (i.e., large volume of distribution). These small molecules can enter cells, get sequestered by forming compounds that are trapped in the cell, and be visible using imaging techniques. For example, ^{18}F labeled 2-deoxy-2-fluoroglucose (^{18}FDG) is a positron emitter that targets highly metabolic cells by entering the cell's glycolytic cycle and becomes trapped in the cell by enzymatic phosphorylation to form ^{18}F labeled 2-deoxy-2-fluoroglucose-6-phosphate. The initial probe is freely diffusable throughout all tissues in the body and has accessibility to pathologic regions in the body. The second class of biologic events involving changes in receptor expression has given rise to receptor target-based imaging. Here the protein of interest traditionally resides on the cell of pathologic origin. As in the first class of agents, the probe must first circulate in the bloodstream and pass through the endothelium into the target pathology, but it is retained in the region of pathology by binding to a target site in or on the surface of a cell. In some cases, binding to the receptor may induce endocytosis, but the probe usually does not enter metabolic pathways. The remaining probe materials must also clear from the body to reduce nonspecific background. This class of imaging agents has been dominated by monoclonal antibodies, antibody fragments, or large molecules labeled with technicium (^{99m}Tc) or indium (^{111}In) chelates.

Recently, new discoveries in vascular biology have focused on new targeting sites that include cells and tissues adjacent to the site of pathology. This approach has been focused primarily on the changes that have been characterized in the blood vessels. Unlike targeting parenchymal cells, to reach the target sites on the surface of the vasculature, monoclonal antibodies and ligands do not need to be transported across the microvascular wall or through the interstitial space. This dramatically reduces the chances of losing these agents to metabolism and to nonspecific binding to proteins and other tissue components. Because of the significance and accessibility of endothelial receptors, they are superb molecular targets for developing new molecular imaging agents and therapeutics.

In this chapter, we describe our approach to the design and construction of vascular receptor-targeted molecular imaging agents, with a focus on imaging the processes of inflammation and angiogenesis. Section II describes our rationale behind choosing a vascular target for molecular imaging derived from our studies on vascular permeability in tumors. Section III describes the design of our vascular-targeted probes and preclinical imaging studies. Section IV demonstrates how imaging can be incorporated into vascular-targeted delivery systems to generate highly active therapeutic agents.

II. Rationale Behind Choosing a Vascular Target for Molecular Imaging

A. Facing the Vascular Permeability Problem

Investigations into the changes during the development of pathology in human disease traditionally have focused on the cell of disease origin and not the supporting structures. For example, in cancer biology, extensive investigations on the precise genetic alterations, changes in the cancer cell, and its surface marker expression levels have been investigated for most major cancers such as colon, breast, prostate, and lung. Many molecules and a range of proteins have been developed for these targets, both as imaging and therapeutic agents. Despite intense investigations and a host of clinical trials, these materials have had only limited success, with major achievements limited to blood-borne diseases such as the lymphomas.

The poor outcome of many of these agents is primarily due to the unfavorable biodistribution of the targeting agent. There are many well-known physiologic barriers to the delivery of macromolecules, particles, and monoclonal antibodies to specific tissues *in vivo*. A blood-borne molecule that enters the circulation reaches the target cells via (1) distribution through vascular space, (2) transport across the microvascular wall, and (3) transport through the interstitial space. These materials may bind nonspecifically to proteins or other tissue components and get metabolized before reaching their target. If the probe is an antibody or antibody conjugate, it has been demonstrated that in rodent tumor models, less than 1% of injected antibody dose is distributed in the tumor. In human tumors this figure is even lower, where again less than 0.01% of the injected dose even gets to see its target (Guccione *et al.*, 2003; Herneth *et al.*, 2003; Yang *et al.*, 2003; Zhu *et al.*, 1997). Therefore, vascular permeability and transport of the agent across the endothelium is an important aspect for the successful outcome of using targets on the diseased tissues for molecular imaging. Also, it is not surprising that targeting the parenchymal cells of a disease has caused many clinical studies to fail primarily due to target accessibility and not target availability.

Therefore, the development of molecular imaging agents toward the parenchymal cells of a disease will clearly be limited by the transport of these agents through the endothelial barriers to reach their respective target. On the flip side, the discovery of new blood markers for diseases (e.g., using genomic and proteomic and other microarray methods) will also be limited by the transport of these markers through the endothelium so they can enter the bloodstream. The consequences of vascular biology for research in these vastly large, diverse, and important areas can influence the way one thinks about molecular imaging probes and the design of pharmaceutical and diagnostic agents. If, for example, one discovers the most specific target for a disease, the use of this target for diagnosis and therapy can be limited by simple accessibility due to vascular permeability. This also holds true for those who discover selective blood markers of disease, since these markers can only be detected in clinical pathology when they gain access to the bloodstream by crossing endothelial barriers. An approach to circumvent this problem is to use a vascular cell surface marker as a target for developing receptor-based molecular imaging probes.

B. Endothelial-Targeted Imaging of Angiogenic Vessels

A critical early step in any inflammatory or immune response is the promotion of leukocyte adhesion to the vascular endothelium. The first realization that unique molecules called cell adhesion molecules (CAMs) are expressed by endothelial cells during a variety of physiologic and disease processes has led to extensive research in characterizing and manipulating these molecules (Eliceiri and Cheresh, 1999; Folberg *et al.*, 1993; Ruoslahti and Engvall, 1997; Weider, 1998). Multiple endothelial ligands and receptors are now known to be upregulated during various pathologies (Folkman, 1995; Ruoslahti and Engvall, 1997) and can potentially serve as molecular targets for diagnostic and/or therapeutic agents. For example, the delivery of nutrients to tissue is a fundamental necessity to maintain life in multicellular species. To facilitate the growth of tumors, neoplastic cells are capable of elaborating a host of factors that result in the development of channels to supply these nutrients in a process called "tumor angiogenesis." Neocapillaries, as opposed to normal capillary beds, overexpress specific cell markers such as Factor V2I-related antigen, acidic and basic (heparin binding) fibroblastic growth factor (bFGF), insulin-like growth factor, platelet-derived growth factor, the CD31, CD34, Ulex endothelial antigens, vascular endothelial receptor 1 (KDR) (Flk-1), and the vascular endothelial growth factor receptor (VEGF-R2) (Folberg *et al.*, 1993; Weider, 1998). The expression of these factors is regulated by as yet not fully understood mechanisms and pathways.

C. Integrins as Vascular Targets

These and other factors result in the attraction of cells and production of proteins, including the integrins, a family of heterodimeric endothelial cell membrane proteins. These proteins serve as adhesion receptors for arginine, glycine, aspartate (RGD)-containing proteins such as laminin, fibronectin, collagens, and vitronectin (Ruoslahti and Engvall, 1997). The RGD-containing proteins are used to form the extracellular matrix of blood vessels. The integrins are one of the best characterized members of the adhesion molecule family that is upregulated in angiogenic endothelial cells found in tumors and certain inflammatory injuries. The integrins are transmembrane molecules that favor the anchorage of endothelial cells to a wide variety of extracellular matrix proteins with an exposed arginine, glycine, aspartate (single letter coding RGD) amino acid sequence. In the adult human, the specific integrin $\alpha_v\beta_3$ has a limited tissue distribution. It is not expressed on quiescent epithelial cells and appears at minimal levels on smooth muscle cells. In contrast, activated endothelial cells in tumor-associated blood vessels express high levels of $\alpha_v\beta_3$ (Eliceiri and Cheresh, 1999). In addition, other integrins such as $\alpha_1\beta_5$ have been characterized by antibody binding to tumor vessels. Staining for these antibodies has indicated the presence of this class of proteins in high concentration on the luminal side of the vessel (McDonald, 2003). Therefore, we choose the integrins as our first target for a molecular imaging agent targeted to the vasculature.

D. Nanoparticles as Molecular Imaging Agents

The ideal vehicle for targeted delivery to vascular receptors should have the following properties: (1) biocompatibility, (2) sufficiently long intravascular half-life to allow for repeated passage through and interactions with the activated endothelium, (3) the ability to have ligands and proteins conjugated on the surface in multivalent configuration to increase the affinity and avidity of interactions with endothelial receptors, (4) the ability to have functional groups for high-affinity surface metal chelation or radiolabeling for imaging, (5) the ability to encapsulate drugs, and (6) the capability to have both imaging and therapeutic agents loaded on the same vehicle. Liposomes have been extensively studied as drug delivery vehicles, and stealth liposome-encapsulated doxorubicin (Doxil) is now commercially available (Brandl, 2001; Harrington, 2001; Lasic *et al.*, 1999; Park, 2002). A major drawback of conventional liposomal particles, however, is their lack of stability. It is difficult for these particles to withstand the chemical modifications needed to attach antibodies, ligands, and imaging probes to their surface. Therefore, despite their attractiveness, we feel that the use of conventional liposomes in vascular receptor-targeted imaging would be problematic.

We have chosen to develop polymerized nanoparticles rather than conventional liposomes as our targeting vehicle because they are rigid and therefore do not easily fuse with cell membranes, and they possess surface functional groups that can be used to attach to other targeting molecules and sufficient numbers of metal ions. Polymerized nanoparticles are composed of amphiphilic lipid molecules with polar head groups and hydrophobic tails that form aggregated bilayer-type structures in aqueous solution (Storrs *et al.*, 1995a,b). A functional group (diacetylene) can be incorporated into the tail portion of the lipids, which upon irradiation with ultraviolet (UV) light, will cross-link, polymerizing the lipids into structurally stable particles. These particles then serve as a scaffold for the attachment of antibodies, ligands, contrast agents, radiopharmaceuticals, and therapeutic agents for imaging and therapy (Sipkins *et al.*, 1998, 2000). Moreover, the size distribution and rigidity of these particles can be chosen to avoid rapid clearance by the reticuloendothelial system, and the particle surface can be modified with ethylene glycol to further increase intravascular recirculation times (Storrs *et al.*, 1995a,b).

III. Design and Preclinical Studies of a Vascular-Targeted Molecular Imaging Agent

To reduce delivery to nonrelevant tissues and increase delivery to the tumor endothelium, a novel vasculature-confined versatile imaging agent that targets the surface of tumor-associated vessels needs to be developed. Delivery to healthy tissue may be reduced by confinement of the agent to the vasculature using macromolecules, and targeting of chemotherapeutic agents has been demonstrated using macromolecular immunoconjugates. Therefore, a new approach to imaging vascular targets is to utilize the changes in vascular endothelium to target imaging agents. In this section, we describe in detail a recently developed molecular-based imaging technology targeted toward the integrins that can be used to noninvasively detect and monitor vascular changes in disease such as angiogenesis and inflammation.

We have developed a lipid-based, biocompatible polymerized vesicle (PV) specifically engineered to be labeled with metals and targeted to specific vascular endothelial cell surface receptors. Endothelial cell receptors are ideal targets for this class of materials because of the material's pharmacokinetic properties and persistence in the intravascular compartment due to their size (~60–80 nm in diameter). The PVs are readily produced, inexpensive, and show no signs of toxicity *in vivo*. Contrast-enhanced magnetic resonance imaging (MRI) and scintigraphy have also been used to study the biodistribution of these nanoparticles for transition to the development of therapeutics.

Specifically, in this section we describe (1) the synthesis and characterization of these polymerized vesicles (PVs) and show that they have prolonged recirculation time, (2) demonstrate that PVs have good *in vivo* molecular imaging properties using MRI and gamma scintigraphy, and (3) give examples of how *in vivo* endothelial targeting can be achieved using an experimental autoimmune encephalitis (EAE) animal model and a rabbit V2 carcinoma model (Folkman, 1992; Sipkins *et al.*, 1998, 2000; Storrs *et al.*, 1995b).

A. PV Synthesis and Characterization

To form antibody-conjugated paramagnetic polymerized vesicles (ACPVs), we initially constructed a particle containing biotinylated lipids. Via biotin molecules on the particle surface, an avidin bridge was used to attach biotinylated antibodies (Sipkins *et al.*, 1998; Storrs *et al.*, 1995b).

Paramagnetic polymerized vesicles (PPVs) containing 0.5% biotinylated lipid, 29.5% Gd^{3+} chelator lipid, 10% amine-terminated lipid, and 60% filler lipid (PDA) were formed. The resulting PPVs are red (absorption maxima at 498 and 538 nm) and stable at room temperature even in the presence of serum. ACPVs are formed by addition of biotinylated antibody and avidin in a ratio of 2.7–1 to the PPVs (Scheme 1).

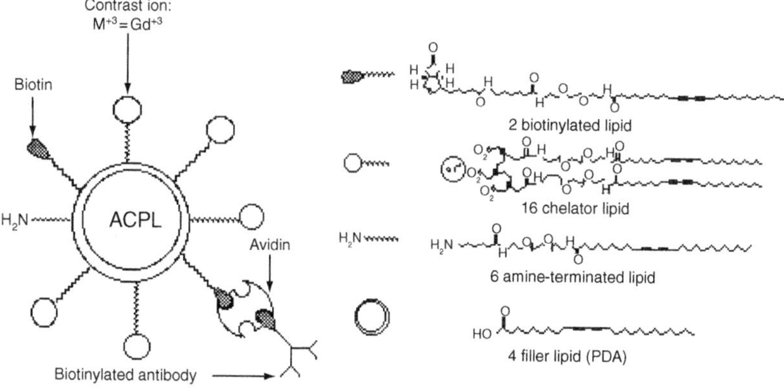

Scheme 1 Schematic representation of an antibody-conjugated polymerized vesicle (ACPV).

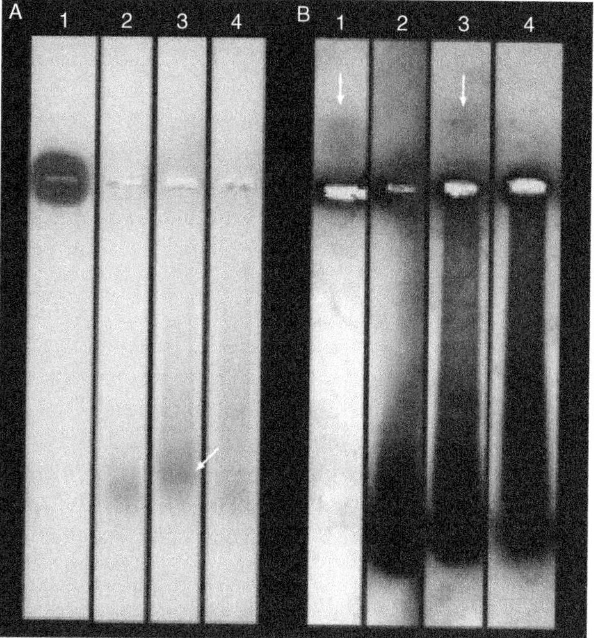

Fig. 1 Demonstration of anti-VCAM antibody-avidin conjugation to biotinylated vesicles by immunodetection.

Figure 1 demonstrates the attachment of avidin and antibody to ACPV using immunodetection. Lane 1 in Fig. 1 (panel A) shows intense staining of 0.5 μg avidin, which, at its isoelectric point, moves slowly from the loading well. Lane

2 (panel A) is a 5-μl sample of PPVs, which move as a discrete band toward the positive pole. Lane 3 (panel A) is a 5-μl sample of PPVs, preincubated with avidin and unbiotinylated antivascular cell adhesion molecule (VCAM) antibody. Avidin now comigrates with the vesicle band (arrow), indicating that it has bound to the surface of the PPV; no free avidin is detected near the loading well. Lane 4 (panel A) represents a 5-μl sample of ACPVs. This preparation is similar to that described in Lane 3 (panel A); however, the anti-VCAM antibody is now biotinylated, allowing conjugation of antibody to the avidin-PPV complex to form the ACPV. As in Lane 3 (panel A), no free avidin is detected, indicating that avidin is now bound to the PPV. Interestingly, no avidin band appears with the liposomes, suggesting that antibody conjugation to the particle surface sterically hinders binding of the antiavidin alkaline phosphatase immunodetection antibody to the complex.

Figure 1 (panel B) shows the results of immunodetection by anti-immunoglobulin G (IgG) alkaline phosphatase to assess antibody binding to PPVs. PPV preparations and antibody-avidin incubations were performed as described earlier. Lane 1 (panel B) shows a 2.5-μg aliquot of biotinylated anti-VCAM antibody that moves as a distinct band toward the negative pole (arrow). Lane 2 in Fig. 1 (panel B), as Lane 2 in Fig. 1 (panel A), is a 5-μl PPV sample that travels toward the positive pole; Lane 3 (panel B) is a 5-μl sample of PPVs, preincubated with avidin and unbiotinylated antibody, which contains 2.2 μg total antibody. As in Lane 1 (panel B), a free antibody band is detected (arrow), indicating that unbiotinylated antibody does not bind to the avidin-PPV complex. Finally, Lane 4 (panel B) is, 5-μl sample of PPVs, preincubated with avidin and biotinylated antibody, which again contains 2.2 μg total antibody. Note that the free antibody band is no longer detectable, demonstrating conjugation of biotinylated antibody to the avidin-coated liposome and formation of the ACPV. We have also shown that the ACPV is functional in a competitive inhibition assay.

For these studies, anti-intercellular cell adhesion molecule-1 (ICAM-1) ACPVs incubated on enzyme-linked immunosorbent assay (ELISA) plates coated with soluble ICAM-1 demonstrated inhibition of free monoclonal anti-ICAM-1 antibody binding. Further evidence that the anti-ICAM-1 antibody-conjugated paramagnetic vesicles could recognize antigens *in vitro* was provided by cell-binding assays using fluorescently tagged ACPVs. PPVs containing the same ratios of lipids as described previously were coupled to Texas Red fluorophore (Pierce, Rockford, IL) according to a standard protocol. The fluorescent PPVs were then conjugated to anti-ICAM-1 antibodies as described earlier. Endothelial cells (bEnd 3) were plated onto 100-mm plastic SPECTri dishes and grown until confluent. Cells were stimulated with 1 μg/ml bacterial lipopolysaccharide approximately 24–48 h before use to elicit expression of ICAM-1 and other cell adhesion molecules. Unstimulated cells constitutively expressing only low levels of CAMS were designated as controls. ACPVs were incubated with the cells for 2 h at room temperature. Using fluorescence microscopy, anti-ICAM-1 ACPVs can be seen bound to the stimulated cells, outlining the morphology of individual cell membranes (Fig. 2). Minimal binding to unstimulated cells occurred.

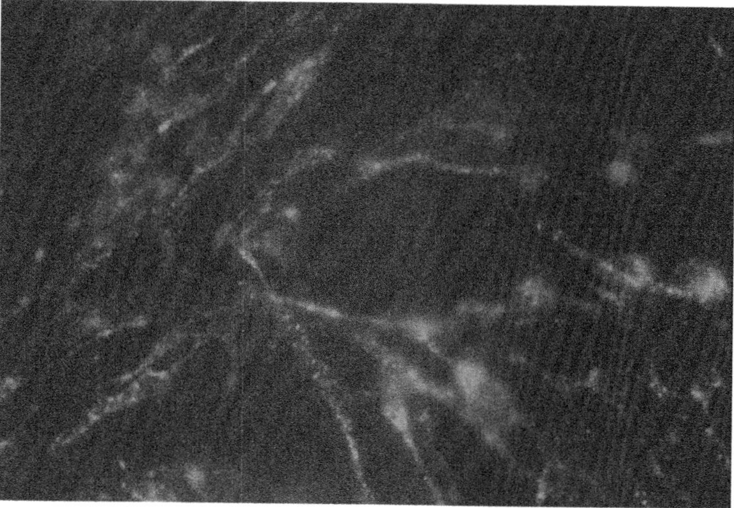

Fig. 2 Fluorescent ACPV labeling of stimulated endothelial cells expressing ICAM-1 cell adhesion molecules. (See Plate no. 12 in the Color Plate Section.)

B. ACPV Targeting in EAE Mice

To visualize CAM expression using a clinical imaging technique, a particle must carry a sufficient number of contrast materials for enhancement, recirculate in the blood pool, maintain its integrity *in vivo*, and be easily attached to a monoclonal antibody for specific receptor targeting. Fluorescently labeled anti-ICAM-1 ACPVs were next used in *in vivo* experiments so that the localization of the particle, as seen in contrast changes in imaging, could be confirmed with fluorescence microscopy. EAE was induced in SJL/J mice according to a proteolipid protein (PLP) immunization protocol (animals were cared for in accordance with institutional guidelines). When clinical signs of grade 2 disease were apparent (tail paralysis and limb weakness), the anti-ICAM-1 ACPVs (prepared as described earlier) were injected via a tail vein (10 μl/g representing 100 mg/kg Gd^{3+} and 15 μg total antibody) and allowed to recirculate for 24 h. Mice were then sacrificed and perfused with phosphate buffered saline (PBS). The brains were removed and cut in half sagittally, one half frozen for direct fluorescence-microscope analysis of thin sections and the other half fixed in paraformaldehyde and used for fluorescence and gamma imaging.

Fluorescence microscopy was used to examine areas of cerebellum in which fluorescent anti-ICAM-1 ACPVs were observed attached to the endothelium of small vessels (Fig. 3). Two controls, an anti-V β11 T-cell receptor ACPV (targeted to an antigen not expressed in the SJL/J mouse) injected in diseased animals and an anti-ICAM-1 ACPV injected in healthy animals, showed no ACPV binding. In Fig. 3, a fluorescent micrograph of cerebellum counterstained with hematoxylin shows three vessels in cross-section. Small vessels (sv) are bound by fluorescent

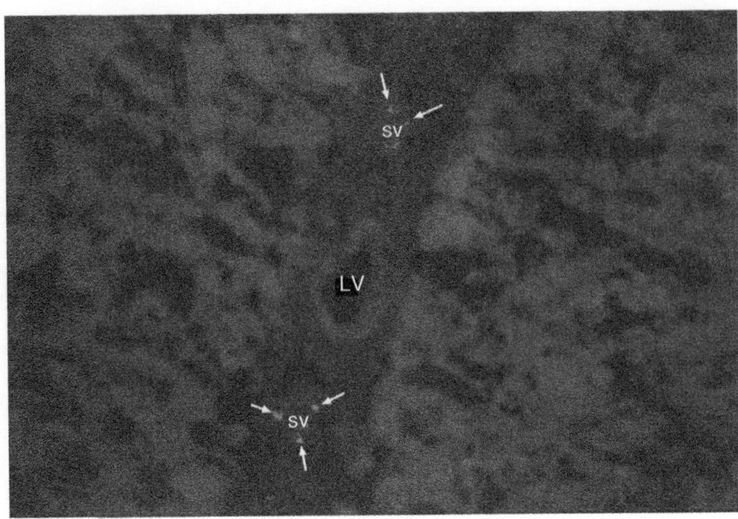

Fig. 3 Fluorescent anti-ICAM-1 ACPVs bind *in vivo* to cerebellar vasculature of a mouse with grade 2 EAE. Anti-ICAM-1 ACPVs (arrows) are shown bound to small vessels (sv), but not to the central large vessel (LV). (See Plate no. 13 in the Color Plate Section.)

anti-ICAM-1 ACPVs (arrows) while a central arteriole (LV) is negative for fluorescence. This is consistent with the pattern of expression of ICAM-1, which is upregulated on endothelium of venules and capillaries, but is not expressed on arterioles or larger vessels.

High-resolution T_1-weighted (T_1W) and T_2-weighted (T_2W) images of the intact brains were obtained on a 9.4-T MR scanner General Electric (Waukesha, WI) using 3DFT spin-echo pulse sequences. Parameters for T_1-weighted images were repetition time (TR) = 200 ms, echo time (TE) = 4 ms, number of excitations (NEX) = 1, and matrix = 256 × 256 × 256, resulting in a voxel size of approximately 50 μ^3. T_2-weighted parameters were TR = 1000 ms, TE = 20 ms, NEX = 8, and matrix = 256 × 256 × 256. Coronal and axial images are shown in Fig. 4. Figure 4A shows a T_2-weighted scan of the EAE mouse cerebrum (rostral) and cerebellum (caudal) to define the normal anatomy. Figure 4B shows a T_1-weighted scan of the same EAE mouse injected with anti-ICAM-1 ACPVs. Diffuse enhancement is present throughout the brain, lending particularly significant contrast between white and gray matter in the cerebellum. Small punctate lesions are observed throughout the image, but seem to be concentrated in the cerebellum (lower part of Fig. 4B). Figure 4C is a T_1-weighted scan of an EAE mouse injected with control anti-V β11 ACPVs. No significant enhancement is observed. Similarly, a scan of a healthy mouse injected with anti-ICAM-1 ACPVs showed no enhancement (Fig. 4D).

We have demonstrated that ACPVs, a new target-specific molecular imaging agent, can be successfully delivered to CAMs upregulated in disease. This result

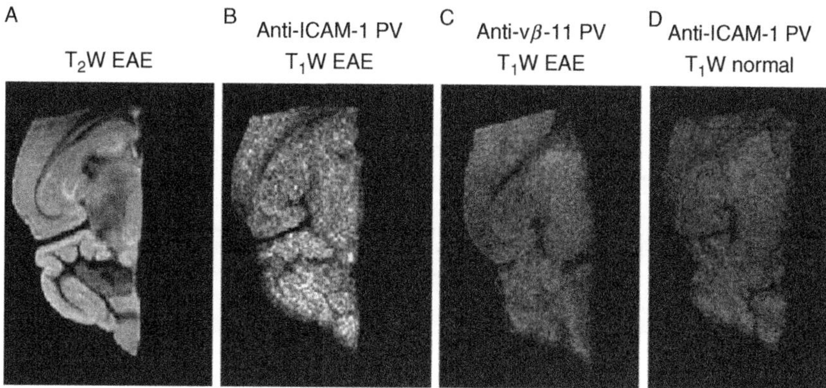

Fig. 4 High-resolution MR images of the EAE mouse brain with anti-ICAM-1 PV contrast enhancement versus controls.

lays the groundwork for *in vivo* imaging studies of other endothelial antigens, particularly those related to angiogenesis.

C. Molecular Imaging of Angiogenesis

Murine antibodies against the $\alpha_V\beta_3$ integrin (LM609) were conjugated to PVs and evaluated in a rabbit tumor model (V2 carcinoma) that has previously shown upregulation of the integrin on the vasculature. Rabbit tumor models were used because antibodies against the $\alpha_V\beta_3$ integrin do not cross-react with murine models. V2 carcinoma cells were inoculated into the thigh muscle or placed subcutaneously in New Zealand white rabbits. The rabbits were closely monitored until a palpable tumor was established. For *in vivo* MR studies, rabbits with palpable tumors (approximately 1–3 cm in diameter) were injected intravenously with either 5 ml/kg anti-$\alpha_V\beta_3$ (LM609)-labeled ACPVs (1 mg antibody/kg, 0.005 mmol Gd^{3+}/kg) or control ACPVs with isotype-matched control antibodies. MRI was performed using a 1.5-T GE Signa MR imager using an extremity coil and the following imaging parameters: TR = 300 ms, TE = 18 ms, NEX = 2, field of view (FOV) = 16 cm, 256 × 256 matrix, slice thickness = 3 mm. MR images were obtained immediately before contrast injection and at immediate, 30 min, 1 h, and 24 h postcontrast injection in the coronal plane. The rabbits were euthanized immediately after the last MRI experiment, and the tumor tissues were harvested for immunohistochemical studies. Figure 5 illustrates the MR findings of a V2 carcinoma-carrying rabbit injected with LM609-labeled ACPVs. At immediate, 30 min, and 1 h postcontrast injection, no noticeable enhancement of the tumor or tumor margin occurs as compared with the precontrast image (Fig. 5A, 1), whereas at 24 h postcontrast injection (Fig. 5A, 2), enhancement of the tumor margin is clearly visible. Isotype-matched controls showed low contrast enhancement in 24-h postcontrast injection in both tumor models (compare images 1 and 2 in Fig. 5B).

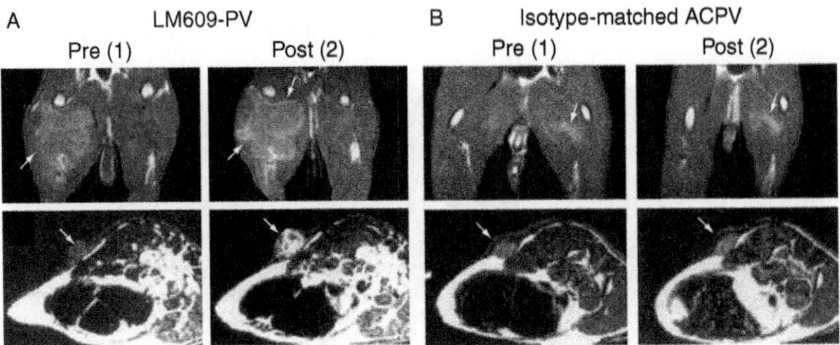

Fig. 5 (A) MR images of V2 carcinoma in the thigh muscle of a rabbit and subcutaneously before (1), and at 24 h (2) after anti-$\alpha_v\beta_3$-labeled ACPV injection. (B) MR images of isotype-matched controls.

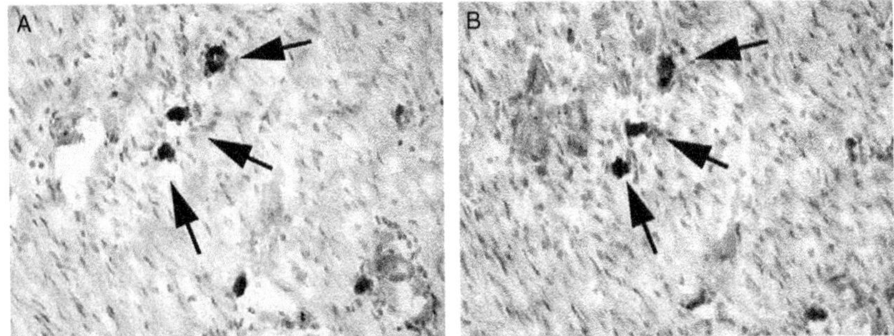

Fig. 6 Immunohistochemical slides taken at the tumor margin of the same rabbit shown in Fig. 5. (A) Stained using anti-$\alpha_v\beta_3$ antibodies, and (B) stained using polyclonal antimouse antibodies, which should bind to the LM609 antibodies on the ACPVs. Arrows indicate the most prominently stained areas.

Figure 6 illustrates immunohistochemical slides taken at the tumor margin of the same rabbit shown in Fig. 5. Figure 6A was stained using anti-$\alpha_v\beta_3$ antibodies, and Fig. 6B was stained using polyclonal antimouse antibodies, which should bind to the LM609 antibodies on the ACPVs. Notice that the locations of the stained regions in Fig. 6A and B are identical, illustrating that the LM609-labeled ACPVs have indeed localized to the sites of $\alpha_v\beta_3$ upregulation. Our results also show that the zone of $\alpha_v\beta_3$ upregulation seen on immunohistochemistry corresponds to the zone of enhancement seen on LM609-labeled ACPVs enhanced MRI. Also note that the stain is localized to the vessels and is not distributed throughout the tumor cells.

We have also recently reported the imaging and therapy of a solid tumor with LM609-ACPVs labeled with indium 111 (^{111}In). Targeting of LM609-ACPVs was demonstrated by parenteral injection in the V2 carcinoma rabbit model by scintographic imaging of the tumor with LM609-^{111}In ACPVs. Scintographic imaging of

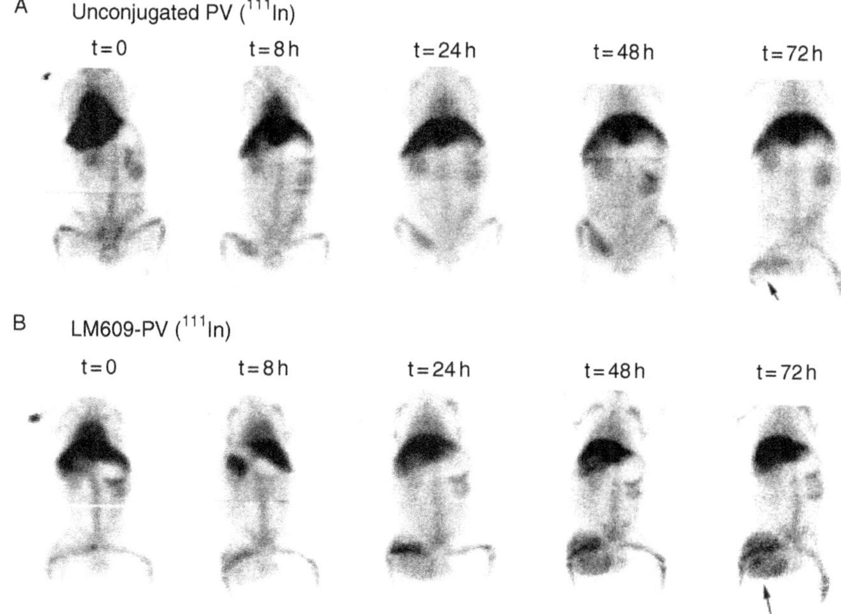

Fig. 7 Imaging of a solid tumor with LM609-ACPVs labeled with indium-111 (^{111}In).

the V2 carcinoma implanted in the rabbit thigh was performed using 100 nm LM609-^{111}In PVs after a single IV injection. Before imaging, the tumor volume was approximately 3 cm^3. Gamma emission was monitored over a 72-h period and showed accumulation of 22% of the total injected radiation in the tumor at 72 h relative to 3% for the ^{111}In ACPVs, which lacks the anti-$\alpha_v\beta_3$ integrin antibody LM609 (Fig. 7). The accumulation of the targeted vesicle represents approximately 1% of the injected dose per gram of tumor tissue. However, this dose is a severe underestimation of the dose to the tumor vasculature because of the confinement of the vesicle to the tumor vasculature, which represents a small fraction of the total tumor mass. The blood pool half-life was 18 h for the LM609-^{111}In ACPVs and was similar to the complex without antibody.

IV. Molecular Imaging and Vascular-Targeted Therapeutics

Since the seminal work by Folkman and coworkers, there has been tremendous interest in using changes in tumor vasculature as target for therapy (Passe *et al.*, 1997). We have recently developed a cationic form of the targeted nanoparticle (NP) based on the previously described PV format that can bind tumor vasculature with high specificity, transport genetic material into the tumor endothelium, and be followed using molecular imaging techniques (Fig. 8). In this application, we

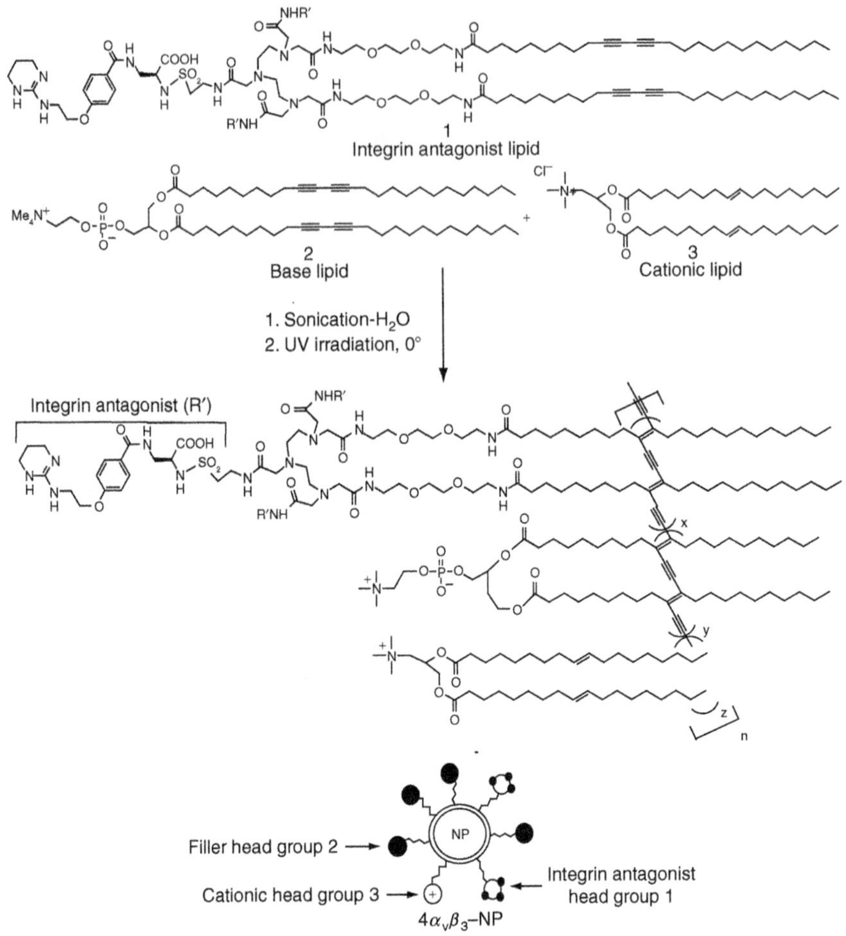

Fig. 8 Formation of targeted NPs for gene delivery to the tumor endothelium. Modified with permission from fig. 1 of Hood *et al.* (2002).

used an integrin antagonist (IA) that binds the integrin $\alpha_v\beta_3$ (Hulka and Edmister *et al.*, 1997) with high specificity as the targeting moiety. We first imaged these materials to screen for a highly selective targeting system and then turned our attention to delivering therapeutic genes to the vasculature. For therapy, a plasmid with the mutant form of *Raf-1* was used as the therapeutic agent. This was used because the disruption of the Ras-Raf-MEK-ERK pathway suppresses angiogenesis *in vivo*, and suppression of *Raf-1* activity has been reported to promote apoptosis (Hawighorst *et al.*, 1997; Mayr *et al.*, 1996). The mutant form of *Raf-1* that we use fails to bind adenosine triphosphate (ATP) (ATP^{μ}-Raf), and it has a dominant negative effect. To evaluate the therapeutic efficacy of this targeted NP-plasmid complex [IA-NP-Raf(−)], systemic injection of the complex in six mice bearing established 400-mm^3 M21-L tumors was performed. The M21-L tumors do not express the integrin $\alpha_v\beta_3$, so any observed therapeutic effect should be from the effect on endothelial cells alone. Control groups received systemic injections of the nontargeted complex [nt-NP-Raf(−)], or PBS (six mice with established 400-mm^3 M21-L tumors per group). A blocking experiment was also performed with the coinjected of IA-NP-Raf(−) and a 20-fold molar excess of the soluble IA. Our results demonstrated that control mice injected with PBS or nt-NP-Raf(−) formed large tumors (>1200 mm^3) within 25 days and were euthanized. In contrast, mice injected with a single injection of IA-NP-Raf(−) showed rapid tumor regression (Figs. 9 and 10), with four of the six mice showing no evidence of tumor 6 days after NP-Raf treatment.

The two remaining mice showed a >95% reduction in tumor mass. It is important to note that the tumor regressions were sustained for >250 days, suggesting that the indirect effect of this approach may be widespread. It is also significant that injection of excess soluble $\alpha_v\beta_3$ ligand completely blocked the antitumor effect of IA-NP-Raf(−), demonstrating that this is a specific effect based on the ability of the IA-NP-plasmid complex to promote apoptosis of the angiogenic endothelium (Stomper *et al.*, 1997).

Established syngeneic pulmonary and hepatic metastases of colon carcinoma were used for further evaluation of this therapeutic approach. Murine CT-26 carcinoma cells were injected either intravenously to induce pulmonary metastases or intrasplenically into Balb/C mice to induce hepatic metastases. NP-gene complexes were given after these metastases were allowed to establish for 10 days. Control groups included mice treated with PBS, IA-NP complexed to a control

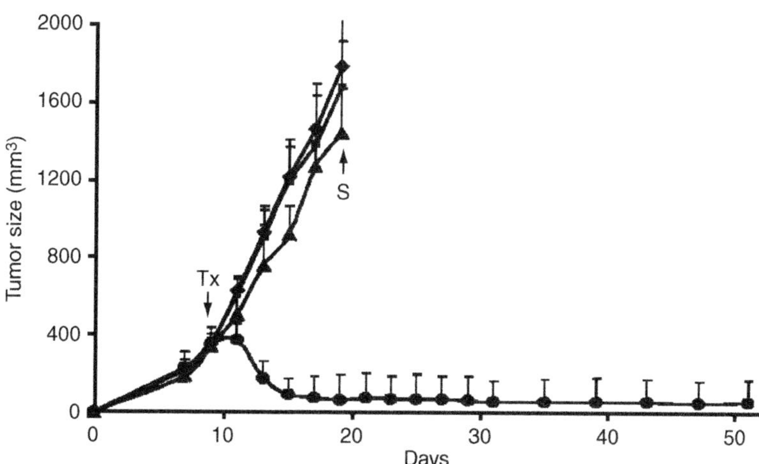

Fig. 9 Tumor size measurements as a function of time. (◆), PBS; (●), NP-plasmid; (▲), blocking experiment; (■), targeted NP-Raf(−) plasmid; Tx, treatment; S, sacrifice.Modified with permission from fig. 4 of Hood *et al.* (2002).

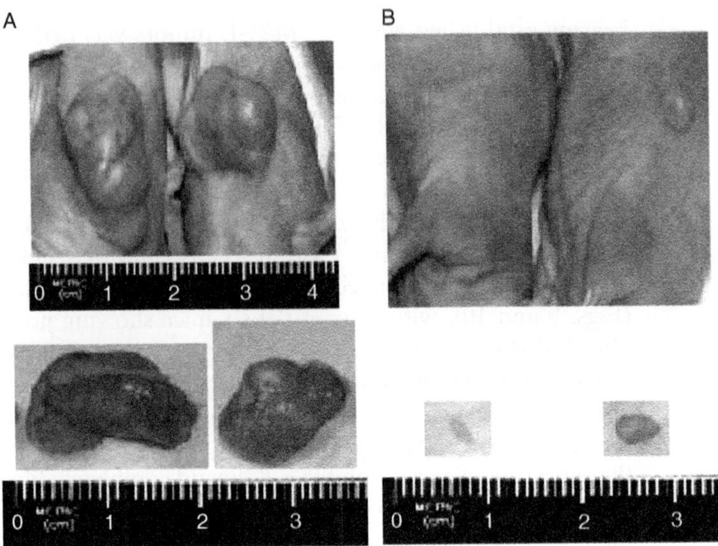

Fig. 10 M21-L murine melanoma tumors in control animals (A), and animals treated with a single injection of IA-NP-Raf(−) complex (B).Modified with permission from supplemental fig. 2 of Hood *et al.* (2002).

vector, or a nt-NP-Raf(−). Our results showed that in the control mice, extensive tumor burden in their lungs or livers were observed, whereas in mice treated with IA-NP-Raf(−), little or no visible tumor metastasis was present, resulting in a drastic reduction of the wet lung or liver weight. Blocking experiments in which mice received a coinjection of IA-NP-Raf(−), along with a 20-fold molar excess of the soluble targeting ligand, showed tumor burden similar to that in control mice (Stomper *et al.*, 1997).

V. Summary

In summary, we have shown *in vivo* imaging of angiogenic tumors using anti-avb3-targeted polymerized vesicles comprised the murine antibody LM609 attached to PVs labeled with the MR contrast agent gadolinium (Gd) in the V2 carcinoma model in rabbits. MRI studies using this targeted contrast agent revealed large areas of avb3 integrin expression in tumor-associated vasculature that conventional MRI failed to show. Immunohistochemical staining of the tumors showed colocalization of the ACPVs with the avb3 integrin in the tumor blood vessels without penetration into the surrounding tumor tissue. Other investigators have used microemulsions conjugated to an antibody targeted against avb3 as imaging agents. These materials also show contrast enhancement of tumor vasculature undergoing angiogenesis (Wickline and Lanza, 2003). Other markers such as the PECAM-1 (CD-31), VCAM-1 (CD54), and VEGF receptor (flk-1) have been shown to be upregulated on tumor endothelium and associated with angiogenesis, but have not been used in imaging studies.

References

Brandl, M. (2001). *Biotechnol. Annu. Rev.* **7,** 59.

Eliceiri, B. P., and Cheresh, D. A. (1999). *J. Clin. Invest.* **103,** 1227.

Folberg, R., Rummelt, V., Parys-Van Ginderdeuren, R., Hwang, T., Woolson, R. F., Pe'er, J., and Gruman, L. M. (1993). *Opthalmology* **100,** 1389.

Folkman, J. (1992). *Semin. Cancer Biol.* **3,** 65.

Folkman, J. (1995). *N. Engl. J. Med.* **333,** 1757.

Guccione, S., Yang, Y. S., Shi, G. Y., Lee, D. Y., Li, K. C. P., and Bednarski, M. D. (2003). *Radiology* **228,** 560.

Harrington, K. J. (2001). *Expert Opin. Investig. Drugs* **10,** 1045.

Hawighorst, H., Knapstein, P. G., Weike, W., *et al.* (1997). *Cancer Res.* **57,** 4777.

Herneth, A. M., Guccione, S., and Bednarski, M. (2003). *Eur. J. Radiol.* **45,** 208.

Hood, J. D., Bednarski, M. D., Frausto, R., Guccione, S., Reisfeld, R. A., Xiang, R., and Cheresh, D. A. (2002). *Science* **296,** 404.

Hulka, C. A., Edmister, W. B., Smith, B. L., *et al.* (1997). *Radiology* **205,** 837.

Lasic, D. D., Vallner, J. J., and Working, P. K. (1999). *Curr. Opin. Mol. Ther.* **1,** 177.

Mayr, N. A., Yuh, W. T., Magnotta, V. A., *et al.* (1996). *Int. J. Radiat. Oncol. Biol. Phys.* **36,** 623.

McDonald, D. (2003). New targets and novel strategies. "Proceedings of the Second Annual Meeting of the Society of Molecular Imaging," p. 220. San Francisco.

Park, J. W. (2002). *Breast Cancer Res.* **4,** 95.

Passe, T. J., Bluemke, D. A., and Siegelman, S. S. (1997). *Radiology* **203,** 593.

Ruoslahti, E., and Engvall, E. (1997). *J. Clin. Invest.* **100,** S53.

Sipkins, D. A., Cheresh, D. A., Kazemi, M. R., Nevin, L. M., Bednarski, M. D., and Li, K. C. P. (1998). *Nat. Med.* **4,** 623.

Sipkins, D. A., Gijbels, K., Tropper, F. D., Bednarski, M., Li, K. C. P., and Steinman, L. (2000). *J. Neuroimmunol.* **104,** 1.

Stomper, P. C., Winston, J. S., Herman, S., *et al.* (1997). *Breast Cancer Res. Treat.* **45,** 39.

Storrs, R. W., Tropper, F. D., Li, H. Y., *et al.* (1995a). *J. Am. Chem. Soc.* **117,** 7301.

Storrs, R. W., Tropper, F. D., Li, H. Y., *et al.* (1995b). *J. Magn. Reson. Imaging* **5,** 719.

Weider, N. (1998). *J. Pathol.* **184,** 119.

Wickline, S. A., and Lanza, G. M. (2003). *Circulation* **107,** 1092.

Yang, Y., Guccione, S., Li, K. C., and Bednarski, M. D. (2003). *Acad. Radiol.* **10,** 1165.

Zhu, H., Baxter, L. T., and Jain, R. K. (1997). *J. Nucl. Med.* **38,** 731.

CHAPTER 17

Generation of DOTA-Conjugated Antibody Fragments for Radioimmunoimaging

Peter M. Smith-Jones* and David B. Solit†

*Nuclear Medicine Service
Department of Radiology
Memorial Sloan-Kettering Cancer Center
New York, New York 10021

†Department of Medicine
Memorial Sloan-Kettering Cancer Center
New York, New York 10021

I. Introduction
II. Selection of a Radionuclide and Chelating Agent
III. Generation of Antibody Fragments
  A. Reagents
  B. Method
IV. Conjugation of DOTA to Intact Antibodies or Fragments
  A. Reagents
  B. Method
V. Radiolabeling of DOTA Conjugates
  A. Reagents
  B. Method
VI. Characterization of DOTA-F(ab′)$_2$ Conjugates
  A. Reagents
  B. Method for Number of Sites
  C. Method for Immunoreactivity
VII. PET Imaging
VIII. Conclusion
References

ESSENTIAL BIOIMAGING METHODS
Reprinted from *Methods in Enzymology*, Volume 386 (Academic Press, 2004).

DOI: 10.1016/B978-0-12-375043-3.00017-2

I. Introduction

Since the identification of antibodies as mediators of the immune response to foreign antigens, efforts have been made to harness the specificity and cytotoxicity of these proteins as targeted cancer agents. Technological advances, in particular hybridoma technology, which allows for the efficient generation of large quantities of epitope-specific monoclonal antibodies (Kohler and Milstein, 1975), have led to the realization of this promise, and several monoclonal antibodies are now approved for use as molecular imaging probes or as therapeutic agents (Table I). Full-length immunoglobulin G (IgG) antibodies, which consist of two identical heavy and light chains, are used for most clinical applications. Unconjugated ("naked") antibodies such as Herceptin (traztuzumab) (Baselga *et al.*, 1996) and Rituxan (rituximab) (Coiffier *et al.*, 1998) have modest activity in patients with breast cancer and lymphoma. These antibodies kill cancer cells by enhancing complement fixation or initiating antibody-dependent cell-mediated cytotoxicity (Sliwkowski *et al.*, 1999). They may also exert antitumor activity by modulating intracellular signaling pathways activated by the cell surface target to which they bind.

To improve on the promising results achieved with naked antibodies, several conjugated monoclonal antibodies have been generated. In this strategy, the antibodies are used as a delivery vehicle to target drugs, immunotoxins, or radiation directly to the tumor cells (Kaminski *et al.*, 2001; Sievers *et al.*, 2001; Witzig *et al.*, 1999). Antibodies labeled with gamma- and positron-emitting radionuclides can also be imaged. This technology allows for the identification of distant sites of cancer spread and has found clinical application in prostate, ovarian, and colorectal cancers (Table I). Radioimmunoimaging may also have a role in cancer therapy selection by allowing for real-time noninvasive quantitation of target expression at

Table I
Selected FDA-Approved Monoclonal Antibodies in Clinical Use

	Disease	Target	Conjugate
Cold antibodies			
Rituximab (Rituxan)	Lymphoma	CD20	–
Traztuzumab (Herceptin)	Breast cancer	HER2	–
Alemtuzumab (Campath)	CLL	CD52	–
Conjugated antibodies			
Ibritumomab tiuxetan (Zevalin)	Lymphoma	CD20	^{111}In, ^{90}Y
Tositumomab (Bexxar)	Lymphoma	CD20	^{131}I
Radioimmunoimaging reagents			
Capromab pendetide (ProstaScint)	Prostate cancer	PSMA	^{111}In
Satumomab pendetide (OncoScint)	Colorectal/ovarian	TAG-72	^{111}In
Arcitumomab (CEA-Scan)	Colorectal/ovarian	CEA	^{99m}Tc

CLL, chronic lymphocytic leukemia.

metastatic tumor sites. A critical challenge in the development of novel biologic therapies that inhibit single transduction pathways in patients with solid tumors has been the difficulty in identifying the subset of patients whose tumors express a particular molecular target. The identification of such patients is particularly challenging when the expression pattern of the target changes during the course of a patient's disease, as has been observed with transmembrane tyrosine kinases such as epidermal growth factor receptor (EGFR) and HER2/neu (Scher *et al.*, 1995; Signoretti *et al.*, 2000). Radioimmunoimaging technology, therefore, may provide an advantage in this setting over the use of traditional immunohistochemical techniques, which require an invasive procedure to obtain tissue for analysis.

This chapter outlines the methods used for generation of radiolabeled monoclonal antibodies for use as imaging probes. The radionuclides most commonly used are reviewed, and the methods for the generation and conjugation of full-length and $F(ab')_2$ antibody fragments are outlined.

II. Selection of a Radionuclide and Chelating Agent

Tables II and III list some of the more commonly used positron- and gamma-emitting metallic radionuclides. Positron-emitting isotopes are typically produced in a cyclotron and have relatively short half-lives (Table II). Therefore,

Table II
Properties of Commonly Used Positron-Emitting Isotopes

Isotope	Half-life (h)	Decay energy (MeV)	Positron abundance (%)	Positron energy (%)	Gamma-ray energy (%)
^{68}Ga	67.6 min	2.91	89	0.82 MeV (1.2) 1.89 MeV (88)	1.08 MeV (3)
^{66}Ga	9.5	5.18	55	0.92 MeV (3.8) 4.15 MeV (50)	
^{64}Cu	12.7	1.68	19	0.65 MeV (17.4) 1.67 MeV (43.1)	1.35 MeV (0.5)
^{86}Y	14.7	5.27	26	0.9 MeV (1.1) 1.03 MeV (1.9) 1.13 MeV (1.3) 1.22 MeV (11.9) 1.55 MeV (5.6) 1.74 MeV (1.7) 1.99 MeV (3.6) 3.14 MeV (2.0)	0.44 MeV (16.9) 0.52 MeV (4.9) 0.58 MeV (94.8) 0.63 MeV (32.6) 0.65 MeV (9.2) 0.70 MeV (15.4) 0.78 MeV (22.4) 1.08 MeV (83) 1.15 MeV (30.5) 1.85 MeV (17.2) 1.92 MeV (20.8)

Reference: http://ie.lbl.gov/education/isotopes.htm.

Table III
Properties of Selected Commercially Available Metallic Radionuclides Suitable for Gamma Camera Imaging

Isotope	Half-life (h)	Decay mode (%)	Gamma-ray energy (%)
^{99m}Tc	6.01	Isomeric transition (100)	140.5 keV (89)
^{111}In	67.3	Electron capture (100)	171.3 keV (90)
			245.4 keV (94)
^{67}Ga	78.3	Electron capture (100)	93.3 keV (39.2)
			184.6 keV (21.2)
			300.2 keV (16.8)
			393.5 keV (4.7)

Reference: http://ie.lbl.gov/education/isotopes.htm.

incorporation of the radioisotope into the imaging probe must be performed shortly before its injection into the subject.

For dynamic imaging in which the goal is to noninvasively monitor changes in a cell surface protein over time in response to a novel drug or other intervention, we prefer the use of the positron emitter ^{68}Ga. It has a short 68-min half-life and a high abundance of positrons (89%) (Table II). When designing a dynamic molecular probe for detecting treatment-induced changes in a cell surface protein, several criteria must be fulfilled. The molecular probe must have a high affinity for the imaging target and a short biologic half-life. It must cause no change in the imaging target. Furthermore, the pharmacokinetics of the imaging probe must not be altered by the targeted agent being studied. The antibody portion of the probe may be based upon a murine, chimeric, humanized, or human antibody. Because the goal of such preclinical studies is often the generation of molecular probes for repetitive human use, the use of murine monoclonal antibodies is potentially problematic. The formation of human antimouse antibodies could significantly alter the biodistribution of an antibody-derived molecular probe and thus significantly limit its clinical use. Therefore, although murine monoclonal antibodies may suffice for preclinical studies, the use of human, humanized, or chimeric antibodies is theoretically preferable.

In our experience, the short half-life of ^{68}Ga allows repetitive daily imaging when conjugated to $F(ab')_2$ antibody fragments, and such probes have been used by our group to dynamically and noninvasively monitor drug-induced changes in cell surface receptor proteins. For example, we have used ^{68}Ga-labeled fragments of Herceptin, a monoclonal antibody that binds to the transmembrane tyrosine kinase HER2/neu (Baselga *et al.*, 1996), to noninvasively image changes in HER2/neu expression following treatment with the Hsp90 inhibitor, 17-allylamino-geldanamycin (17-AAG) (Smith-Jones *et al.*, 2003). Hsp90 is a cellular chaperone protein required for the maturation and stability of a subset of signaling proteins, including tyrosine kinases and steroid receptors (Pratt and Welch, 1994). Inhibition of Hsp90 by 17-AAG causes the proteasomal degradation of HER2 and other Hsp90-dependent client proteins (Mimnaugh *et al.*, 1996). We found that ^{68}Ga-DOTA-F(ab′)$_2$ Herceptin was able to image HER2-expressing tumors and that adequate contrast between tumor and normal tissues was apparent within 3 h of tracer administration (Fig. 1) (Smith-Jones *et al.*, 2003). A linear correlation was observed between the data obtained by micropositron emission tomography (microPET) and direct assessment of tissues by gamma counter. The short half-life of ^{68}Ga and the rapid clearance of the F(ab′)$_2$ fragments allowed for daily imaging. Furthermore, the tracer amount of the ^{68}Ga-DOTA-F(ab′)$_2$ Herceptin probe had no effect on HER2 expression in the tumor as confirmed by immunoblot analysis. This is a critical finding because antibodies to other cell surface tyrosine kinases have been reported to induce receptor downregulation (Kasprzyk *et al.*, 1992).

^{68}Ga can be generated from the decay of ^{68}Ge ($T_{1/2} = 271$ days), and therefore an onsite cyclotron is not required. Several generator systems have been proposed to produce ^{68}Ga (Ehrhardt and Welch, 1978; Loc'h *et al.*, 1980). We are currently

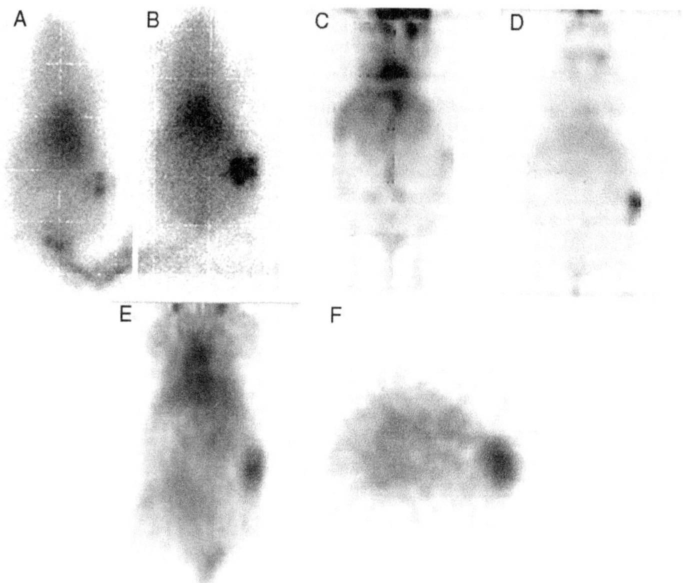

Fig. 1 (A, B) Planar gamma camera images of a BT-474 xenograft-bearing mouse 6 h (A) and 30 h (B) after injection with ^{111}In-Herceptin. (C, D) MicroPET images of a BT-474 xenograft-bearing mouse 2 h (C) and 28 h (D) after injection with ^{64}Cu-Herceptin. (E) Coronal and (F) transverse microPET images of a BT-474 xenograft-bearing mouse 3 h after injection with ^{68}Ga-F(ab′)$_2$ Herceptin. The greatest contrast between tumor and normal tissue is observed with intact Herceptin labeled with ^{64}Cu ($T_{1/2}$ = 12.7 h). The use of intact antibody results in limited tumor-specific uptake at early time points (C). ^{68}Ga-F(ab′)$_2$ Herceptin provides adequate contrast between normal and tumor tissues at early time points (E, F), and the short half-lives of both ^{68}Ga and the F(ab′)$_2$ antibody fragements allow for daily imaging of dynamic changes in HER2/neu expression. Tumors are implanted within the right flank.

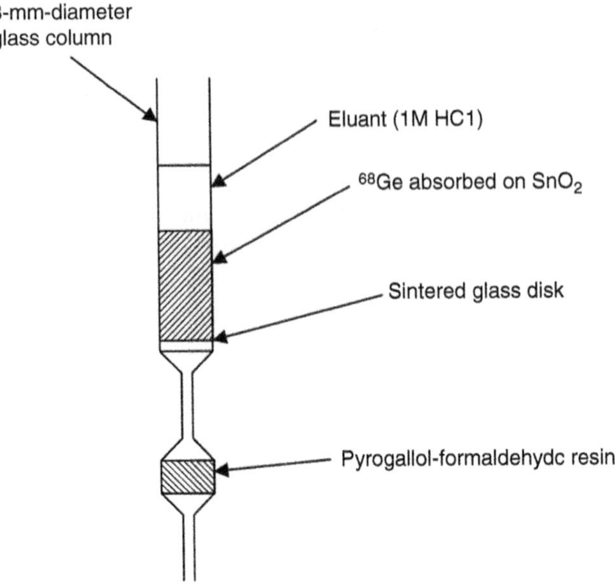

Fig. 2 ^{68}Ga can be produced without the use of a cyclotron using a ^{68}Ge generator. ^{68}Ge is absorbed on a SnO_2 solid support, and ^{68}Ga is eluted using 1 M HCl. A pyrogallol-formaldehyde resin is used to purify the product by removing traces of ^{68}Ge.

using a SnO_2-based system (Ehrhardt and Welch, 1978) (4-ml column) with an inline pyrogallol-formaldehyde resin column (Schumacher and Maier-Borst, 1980) (0.5 ml) to remove any eluted ^{68}Ge (Fig. 2). The ^{68}Ga is eluted in 5 ml of 1 M HCl and has a contamination of 10^{-6}% of ^{68}Ge.

For intact antibody biodistribution studies, we prefer a longer half-life isotope such as ^{64}Cu. For this application, repetitive imaging is not required and the longer half-life of ^{64}Cu (12.7 h) allows for imaging at later time points. After 24 h, most full-length antibodies have been cleared from the blood pool and antigen-negative normal tissues but are still retained within antigen-expressing tumor tissues, providing the greatest contrast between tumor and normal tissue (see Fig. 1). ^{66}Ga is another positron-emitting isotope with a long half-life (9.5 h), but its use is less desirable in imaging applications than ^{64}Cu due to emission of high-energy beta particles that lower image resolution. Similarly, ^{86}Y ($T_{1/2}$ of 14.7 h) can be used for antibody biodistribution studies, but its high-energy gamma emissions interfere with the characteristic 511-keV gamma rays, which are characteristic of the positron annihilation that forms the basis for PET scanning technology, thus degrading image quality.

Gamma-emitting isotopes (^{99m}Tc, ^{111}In, ^{131}I) can also be used for *in vivo* imaging, but are not detected by PET and require the use of a planar gamma camera or a SPECT (single photon emission computed tomography) camera (Table III).

Both PET and SPECT are able to generate three-dimensional images. Although gamma camera technology may be preferable for some applications due to its lower cost and greater availability in the clinic, PET imaging currently delivers the highest resolution. For imaging purposes, ^{99m}Tc is preferable to other gamma-emitting isotopes due to its generation of an optimal monoenergetic gamma ray (Table III). ^{111}In is limited by its high abundance of moderate-energy gamma rays, and ^{67}Ga is the least desirable choice for imaging applications due to its low abundance of higher energy gamma rays.

Numerous chelators have been proposed to coordinate radioactive metal ions. Systems based on 1,4,7,10-tetraazacyclododecane-*N*,*N*′,*N*″,*N*‴-tetraacetic acid (DOTA) (Chappell *et al.*, 2003; Deshpande*et al.*, 1990; Smith-Jones *et al.*, 2000) and diethylenetriaminepentaacetic acid (DTPA) (Nikula *et al.*, 1995; Wagner and Welch, 1979; Westerberg *et al.*, 1989) have been shown to be the most versatile (Fig. 3). The primary advantage of DOTA over DTPA is that it produces a more stable chelate, but it has the disadvantage of slightly slower reaction kinetics. Bifunctional conjugates have more donor groups to chelate the metal ions and are therefore more stable than standard DOTA and DTPA chelators. DOTA generally produces a sufficiently stable metal chelate and is commercially available,

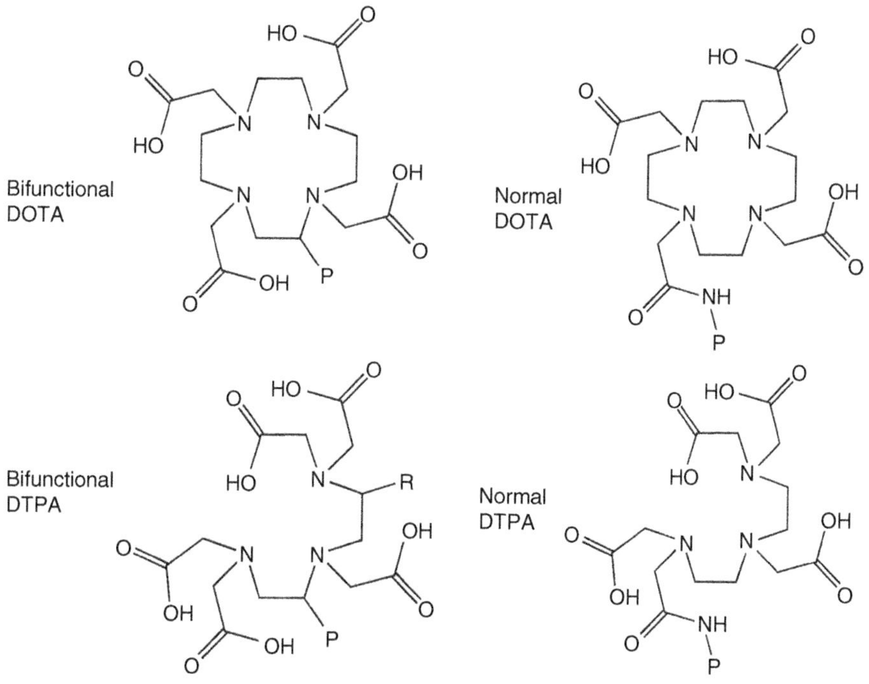

Fig. 3 Chemical structures of DOTA and DTPA conjugates. P is the site of conjugation to the protein structure. The DOTA and DTPA chelating agents normally attach to lysine residues.

whereas other bifunctional forms of these two agents have to be synthesized. All of the radionuclides listed in Table II form a stable chelate with DOTA.

III. Generation of Antibody Fragments

As discussed earlier, antibody fragments may be preferable to intact antibodies as dynamic imaging probes due to their shorter biologic half-lives. As a result of their smaller size, they are cleared more quickly from nonantigen-expressing tissues and therefore provide greater tumor to normal tissue contrast at early time points (Fig. 1) (Harrison and Tempero, 1995). Furthermore, they may migrate more efficiently through the extravascular space into the interior of poorly vascularized tumors than intact antibodies and may be less immunogenic due to the removal of the Fc region. In this section, we outline a method for generating antibody fragments that retain the ability to specifically bind to their antigen target. The method involves selective digestion of the antibody with pepsin, followed by purification of the product using a protein A column to remove residual undigested intact antibody. The product is then purified by high-performance liquid chromatography (HPLC) to resolve the $F(ab')_2$ fragments from the digested Fc portions. During fragmentation, the reaction must be closely monitored by HPLC to prevent overdigestion, which may reduce immunoreactivity.

A. Reagents

- 20 mM sodium acetate (pH 4.5)
- 10 mM Tris-HCl (pH 8.0)
- 0.1 M glycine (pH 2.8)
- 50 mM sodium phosphate (pH 7.1)
- Immobilized pepsin (Pierce Biotechnology Inc., Rockford, IL)
- Immobilized protein A (Pierce Biotechnology Inc.)
- 30 kDa centrifugal filters (Amicon, Millipore, Bedford, MA)

B. Method

1. Suspend 0.25 ml immobilized pepsin with 5 ml of 20 mM sodium acetate buffer. Centrifuge and remove supernatant. Repeat washing step five times.
2. Add 10 mg of IgG to 3 ml of 20 mM sodium acetate buffer and concentrate to 1 ml in a 30-kDa centrifugal filter. Remove filtrate and repeat washing step five times.
3. Add IgG in 1 ml of sodium acetate to immobilized pepsin and mix slurry on a shaker at 37 °C for 6–48 h.

4. At various times, remove a 5-μl fraction of the solution and analyze by size-exclusion HPLC (TSK 3000 column) to see the amount of intact IgG.
5. When the amount of intact IgG is <5%, add 3 ml of 10 mM Tris-HCl and separate the gel by centrifugation.
6. Pour a 2-ml protein A column and equilibrate it with 5 × 2 ml of 10 mM Tris-HCl.
7. Load digested IgG onto column and wash column with 10 mM Tris-HCl.
8. Collect the first eluted protein peak (measure absorbance at 280 nM) and concentrate this eluate with a 30-kDa centrifugal filter.
9. Undigested IgG Fc, and Fc fragments may be recovered by washing the column further with 0.1 M glycine.
10. Purify crude $F(ab')_2$ fraction by size-exclusion HPLC using a TSK 3000 column and an eluant of 50 mM sodium phosphate.
11. Concentrate HPLC purified $F(ab')_2$ with a 30-kDa centrifugal filter and then sterilize by filtration through a 0.22-μm filter. This product, when stored at 4 °C, may remain stable for up to several years.

IV. Conjugation of DOTA to Intact Antibodies or Fragments

Conjugation of DOTA to intact antibodies or fragments involves first generation of the active ester of DOTA, which is then reacted with lysine residues on the protein. The conjugated antibody is then purified by ultrafiltration prior to radiolabeling.

A. Reagents

- 1,4,7,10-Tetraazacyclododecane-*N*,*N*′,*N*″,*N*‴-tetraacetic acid (DOTA; Strem Chemical, Newburyport, MA)
- *N*-Hydroxysuccinimide
- 1-Ethyl-3-(3-dimethylaminopropyl)carbodiimide
- 0.25 M Ammonium acetate
- Chelex 100 resin, 100–200 mesh (Bio-Rad, Hercules, CA)

B. Method

1. Pour a 10-ml column of Chelex 100 resin and wash with 5 × 10 ml of 0.25 M ammonium acetate. Pass remaining buffer through column and collect metal-free buffer in a plastic bottle.

2. Dissolve 146 mg DOTA (0.361 mM) and 36 mg *N*-hydroxysuccinimide (0.313 mM) in 1 ml of water and adjust the pH to 7.3 with NaOH. Dilute solution to 2 ml and cool in an ice bath for 30 min before adding 10 mg of 1-ethyl-3-(3-dimethylaminopropyl)carbodiimide. Let reaction proceed for 1 h on ice to form the active ester.
3. For each mg of $F(ab')_2$, add 80 μl of active ester solution and allow to react overnight at 4 °C.
4. Concentrate reaction mixture in a 30-kDa centrifugal filter to about 10 mg/ml. Add an equal volume of 0.25 M ammonium acetate and concentrate to 10 mg/ml. Repeat washing step 20 times.

V. Radiolabeling of DOTA Conjugates

To radiolabel DOTA-conjugated antibodies with ^{68}Ga, ^{68}Ga eluted from the ^{68}Ge generator is concentrated by extracting with ether and then back extracting to a small volume of water. The ^{68}Ga or an alternative isotope is then reacted with antibody in an ammonium acetate buffer. Finally, the reaction is quenched with DTPA, with the product run over a size-exclusion column to remove unchelated isotope.

A. Reagents

- 1–5 mCi of ^{68}Ga in 5 ml of 1 M HCl
- 12 M HCl
- Diethyl ether
- 1 M metal-free ammonium acetate
- *General*: All apparatus used should be plastic and free of any metal contamination. In particular, colored plastic tubes and pipette tips should be avoided, since metals are sometimes used to achieve the colored effect.

B. Method

1. In a glass tube place ^{68}Ga, an equal volume of 12 M HCl, and 1 ml of diethyl ether. Shake the tube and allow layers to separate.
2. Add 50 μl of deionized water to a 1.5-ml conical polypropylene centrifuge tube and add ether layer containing ^{68}Ga. Place tube in a heating block and remove ether under a gentle stream of air.
3. Repeat ether extraction and repeat evaporation step.
4. Add 10 μl of 1 M ammonium acetate to back-extracted ^{68}Ga and spot-test 0.5 μl onto a pH indicator strip. The pH should be >5.

5. Add 10 μl of a 10-mg/ml solution of the DOTA-F(ab′)$_2$ conjugate and incubate at 37 °C for 10 min.
6. Add 50 μl of 5 mM DTPA to quench reaction and load solution onto a 10-ml P6 column equilibrated with 0.5% bovine serum albumin in phosphate buffered saline (BSA-PBS).
7. Elute column with BSA-PBS and collect the ^{68}Ga-DOTA-F(ab′)$_2$ fraction, which elutes after about 3 ml.

All the other metals listed in Table II may be used in an analogous manner to label the DOTA-F(ab′)$_2$ conjugate as long as the labeling is performed within the pH range of 5–7 in the presence of 0.25–1.0 M ammonium acetate.

VI. Characterization of DOTA-F(ab′)$_2$ Conjugates

Upon initial generation of the DOTA-antibody conjugate, the quality of the product must be verified. This involves determining the number of DOTAs per antibody by labeling the antibody with a known quantity of nonradioactive indium spiked with ^{111}In and then examining the two species formed. The immunoreactivity of the antibody conjugate is also determined to confirm that the conjugation process has not disrupted binding of the antibody to its antigen target. This may result from overdigestion at the time of fragment generation. Alternately, it may occur with DOTA conjugation if a large number of lysine residues are present in or around the antigen-binding site.

For most antibodies the immunoreactivity should be >90% and the number of DOTAs bound/F(ab′)$_2$ should be 3–6. If the immunoreactivity is too low and the number of DOTAs attached is less than 4, then the conjugation procedure should be repeated using fresh F(ab′)$_2$ and a lower volume of the active ester solution. Conversely, if the immunoreactivity is preserved and the number of DOTAs bound is less than 1, then the conjugation step should be repeated using the same F(ab′)$_2$, but with the volume of the active ester solution of DOTA increased. Once prepared and characterized, the conjugate may be stored in a plastic vial at 4 °C for up to several years. The immunoreactivity test should be repeated prior to radiolabeling each batch of DOTA-F(ab′)$_2$ to confirm that the conjugate is stable. We have several conjugates that are still >90% immunoreactive after storage for >18 months at 4 °C.

A. Reagents

- ^{111}In (0.05 M HCl)
- 1 M metal-free ammonium acetate
- 1 mM $InCl_3$ (0.05 M HCl)
- 5 mM DTPA (pH 7.0)

- 5 mM DTPA (pH 5.0)
- Silica gel-impregnated glass fiber (ITLC-SG; 1 × 10 cm, Gelman, Ann Arbor, MI)
- DOTA-F(ab′)$_2$
- 0.5% BSA-PBS

B. Method for Number of Sites

1. Add 1 μl of ^{111}In (ca. 200–500 μCi) to 100 μl of 1 mM $InCl_3$ and add 10, 20, and 30 μl portions of this solution to three 20-μl samples of DOTA-F(ab′)$_2$. Incubate solutions at 37 °C for 16 h.
2. Add 50 μl of 5 mM DTPA to the three reaction mixtures and reincubate at 37 °C for 6 h.
3. Spot-test 5 μl of the solutions onto a 10-cm ITLC-SG strip. Develop strip in 5 mM DTPA (pH 5.0).
4. Cut strip at an R_f of 0.5 and count both parts in an gamma counter. F(ab′)$_2$ activity remains at the origin and [In-DTPA] moves with the solvent front.
5. Calculate the number of DOTAs attached to each F(ab′)$_2$ according to the following formula:

$$\text{Number attached} = \frac{(\text{activity in lower strip}) \times (\text{in concentration (in mol)})}{(\text{total activity}) \times (\text{antibody concentration (in mol)})}$$

C. Method for Immunoreactivity (Lindmo *et al.*, 1984)

1. Add 1 μCi of ^{111}In-DOTA-F(ab′)$_2$ to 3 ml of 0.5% BSA-PBS and add 50 μl of this solution to 18 × 1.5 ml centrifuge tubes. Place three of these tubes to one side.
2. Prepare ca. 20 × 10^6 cells expressing the correct antigen expression in 3.5 ml of PBS.
3. To three tubes, add 0.5 ml of suspended cells.
4. To three tubes, add 0.25 ml cells and 0.25 ml PBS.
5. To three tubes, add 0.15 ml cells and 0.35 ml PBS.
6. To three tubes, add 0.10 ml cells and 0.40 ml PBS.
7. To three tubes, add 0.50 ml PBS.
8. Briefly vortex all 15 samples and place on a rocker for 1 h so that the cells remain in suspension.
9. Centrifuge all 15 tubes and aspirate supernatant.
10. Add 1 ml of ice-cold PBS, centrifuge tubes, and aspirate supernatant.
11. Count all 18 tubes in a gamma counter.

12. Subtract the mean of the nonspecific binding from the 12 test samples and plot a reciprocal of the number of cells added (x-axis) to the total/bound ratio. The intercept gives the immunoreactive fraction, which binds at an infinite excess of antigen.

VII. PET Imaging

As an example, outlined as follows is our standard procedure for imaging mice with the ^{68}Ga-DOTA-F(ab′)$_2$ Herceptin probe using the Concorde Microsystems microPET scanner. This is a commercially available, dedicated small animal PET scanner. Flood phantom measurements are performed on a daily basis with a cylindrical ^{68}Ge phantom to ensure detector linearity and uniformity.

1. Animals are injected with 100–500 μCi of the ^{68}Ga-DOTA-F(ab′)$_2$ Herceptin and returned to their cages, where they are fed and watered *ad libertum*.
2. 2–3 h after injection, the animals are anesthetized using an isoflurane-oxygen (Baxter Healthcare, Deerfield, IL) gas mixture and placed in the microPET camera.
3. Coincident data are collected for the 511 keV gamma rays with a 250–750-keV window for 5–10 min.
4. After imaging, the data are reconstructed using back projection filtering.
5. Regions of interest (ROI) are drawn around the organs expressing the antigen (i.e., tumor), as well as major organs such as the heart, liver, and kidneys.
6. An average is taken of the maximum activity per voxel in the three consecutive slices that have the highest uptake of activity. This number is then corrected for the size of the organ-tumor, the efficiency of the microPET camera, and the time difference between injection and imaging before the uptake is expressed as a percentage of the injected dose per gram.

Upon generation of a novel antibody-based molecular probe, we identify the pattern of nonspecific tracer uptake by preinjecting animals with a large quantity of cold antibody (or fragment) to saturate all antigen sites. The radiolabeled antibody probe is then injected to determine the pattern of nonspecific renal and hepatobiliary excretion of the probe.

VIII. Conclusion

The previous procedures outline a method for the generation of radiolabeled F(ab′)$_2$ fragments for *in vivo* imaging applications. The recent dramatic advance in our understanding of the pathophysiology of cancer has led to the identification of targets expressed preferentially on transformed cells. Using molecular imaging probes based upon conjugated antibody fragments, the expression of these targets can be noninvasively quantitated. This should allow for the real-time identification of patients whose tumors express a particular molecular target, thus facilitating their inclusion in clinical trials of novel targeted agents. Furthermore, this technology may aid in the development of such agents by allowing for the noninvasive monitoring of treatment-induced changes in target protein expression (Smith-Jones *et al.*, 2003). Such detailed pharmacodynamic monitoring is not currently feasible in patients with solid tumors using current technologies and will likely be critical for the successful development of novel targeted therapies.

References

Baselga, J., Tripathy, D., *et al.* (1996). *J. Clin. Oncol.* **14,** 737.
Chappell, L. L., Ma, D., *et al.* (2003). *Nucl. Med. Biol.* **30,** 581.
Coiffier, B., Haioun, C., *et al.* (1998). *Blood* **92,** 1927.
Deshpande, S. V., DeNardo, S. J., *et al.* (1990). *J. Nucl. Med.* **31,** 473.
Ehrhardt, G. J., and Welch, M. J. (1978). *J. Nucl. Med.* **19,** 925.
Harrison, K. A., and Tempero, M. A. (1995). *Oncology (Huntingt.)* **9,** 625.
Kaminski, M. S., Zelenetz, A. D., *et al.* (2001). *J. Clin. Oncol.* **19,** 3918.
Kasprzyk, P. G., Song, S. U., *et al.* (1992). *Cancer Res.* **52,** 2771.
Kohler, G., and Milstein, C. (1975). *Nature* **256,** 495.
Lindmo, T., Boven, E., *et al.* (1984). *J. Immunol. Methods* **72,** 77.
Loc'h, C., Maziere, B., *et al.* (1980). *J. Nucl. Med.* **21,** 171.
Mimnaugh, E. G., Chavany, C., *et al.* (1996). *J. Biol. Chem.* **271,** 22796.
Nikula, T. K., Curcio, M. J., *et al.* (1995). *Nucl. Med. Biol.* **22,** 387.
Pratt, W. B., and Welch, M. J. (1994). *Semin. Cell Biol.* **5,** 83.
Scher, H. I., Sarkis, A., *et al.* (1995). *Clin. Cancer Res.* **1,** 545.
Schumacher, J., and Maier-Borst, W. (1980). *Int. J. Appl. Radiat. Isot.* **31,** 31.
Sievers, E. L., Larson, R. A., *et al.* (2001). *J. Clin. Oncol.* **19,** 3244.
Signoretti, S., Montironi, R., *et al.* (2000). *J. Natl. Cancer Inst.* **92,** 1918.
Sliwkowski, M. X., Lofgren, J. A., *et al.* (1999). *Semin. Oncol.* **26,** 60.
Smith-Jones, P. M., Vallabahajosula, S., *et al.* (2000). *Cancer Res.* **60,** 5237.
Smith-Jones, P. M., Solit, D., *et al.* (2003). *J. Nucl. Med.* **44,** 361.
Wagner, S. J., and Welch, M. J. (1979). *J. Nucl. Med.* **20,** 428.
Westerberg, D. A., Carney, P. L., *et al.* (1989). *J. Med. Chem.* **32,** 236.
Witzig, T. E., White, C. A., *et al.* (1999). *J. Clin. Oncol.* **17,** 3793.

PART V

General Methods

CHAPTER 18

The Application of Magnetic Resonance Imaging and Spectroscopy to Gene Therapy

Po-Wah So,[*] Kishore K. Bhakoo,[†] I. Jane Cox,[‡] Simon D. Taylor-Robinson,[§] and Jimmy D. Bell[¶]

[*]Preclinical Imaging Unit
Department of Clinical Neuroscience
King's College London
Institute of Psychiatry
James Black Centre
London SE4 9NU, United Kingdom

[†]Translational Molecular Imaging Group
Singapore Bioimaging Consortium
Agency for Science
Technology and Research (ASTAR)
#02–02 Helios, Singapore 138667
Singapore

[‡]Imaging Sciences Department
Division of Clinical Sciences
Imperial College London
London W12 0HS, United Kingdom

[§]Department of Hepatology and Gastroenterology
Division of Medicine
Faculty of Medicine
Imperial College London
St Mary's Hospital
London W2 1NY, United Kingdom

[¶]Metabolic and Molecular Imaging Group
MRC Clinical Sciences Centre
Imperial College London
Hammersmith Hospital
London W12 0HS, United Kingdom

DOI: 10.1016/B978-0-12-375043-3.00018-4

I. Introduction
II. Magnetic Resonance Techniques
III. MR Overview
IV. MR Imaging (MRI)
V. MR Spectroscopy (MRS)
VI. Role of Magnetic Resonance Methods in GT
  A. Monitoring Gene Delivery
  B. MR-Guided and Enhanced GT
  C. Imaging Gene Expression
VII. MRI-Based Systems
VIII. MRS-Based Systems
  A. Monitoring Therapeutic Response
IX. Conclusions
References

I. Introduction

Gene therapy (GT) is defined as the genetic modification of cells to produce a therapeutic effect (Mulligan, 1993). One approach is to genetically modify cells *in vivo* and the other is to genetically modify patient cells *ex vivo* and then their subsequent readministration back to the patient. GT can replace defective genes with a normal copy in monogenetic disorders, such as in cystic fibrosis (Knowles *et al.*, 1995). However, disorders are commonly polygenic in origin and GT is used to affect a therapeutic effect, such as enhancing tumor cell death in cancer (Vile *et al.*, 2000). Successful GT is often limited by the inefficient delivery of genes, because of short *in vivo* half-lives, lack of cell-specific targeting, and low-transfection efficiencies. Quite simply, genes can be incorporated and delivered in the form of naked DNA plasmids (Li and Huang, 2000). However, while relatively effective *in vitro*, the low-transfection delivery of plasmids *in vivo* has led to the development of other gene delivery systems for subsequent application in man and has been categorized into viral (Walther and Stein, 2000) and nonviral GT (Brown *et al.*, 2001) vectors. A feature of all viruses is their ability to introduce their genetic material into the host cells on infection; genetic modification of viruses and exploitation of this capability, allows the introduction of therapeutic genes into infected cells. Viral vectors include adenoviruses (Ko *et al.*, 1996; Nguyen *et al.*, 1997), adenoassociated adenovirus (Carter and Samulski, 2000; Tal, 2000), retroviruses (Hanania *et al.*, 1994; Wiznerowicz *et al.*, 1997), and the *Herpes simplex* virus (HSV; Blasberg and Tjuvajev, 1999; Ross *et al.*, 1995; Schellingerhout *et al.*, 1998). The major problems with viral GT vectors are difficulties in large-scale production and host immunogenicity, hence the proposal for nonviral GT vectors, including oligonucleotides (Fichou and Férec, 2006), lipoplexes, and polyplexes (Li and Huang, 2000) and for synthetic oligonucleotides including antisense or siRNA to inactivate genes involved in pathological processes (Aigner, 2006). Lipoplexes include micellar or liposomal formulations, consisting of DNA covered with lipid in an organized structure, and have been used in several clinical trials, including cancer (Nabel *et al.*, 1993). Complexes of polymers and DNA are known as polyplexes. Although less efficient than viral vectors in terms of the amount of gene required for cell transfection, nonviral vectors have a reduced risk of eliciting an immune response. Physical methods have also been developed, such as the gene gun and electroporation to assist gene delivery (Bonnekoh *et al.*, 1996; Suzuki *et al.*, 1998; Wagner *et al.*, 1992). However, although many of these strategies are relatively effective within the confines of a laboratory environment, clinical trials have been less promising.

To increase safety and efficacy, GT vectors need to be targeted. Some viruses exhibit a preference for certain tissues, such as the HSV, which is neurotropic. Otherwise, targeting can be programmed via surface moieties, including conjugation of GT vectors to targeting ligands (Peng, 1999; Russell and Cosset, 1999; Varga *et al.*, 2000), or employment of tissue selective promoters (Beck *et al.*, 2004; Gunther *et al.*, 2005; Sadeghi and Hitt, 2005; Saukkonen and Hemminki, 2004).

In an attempt to overcome the multifold challenges in GT, protocols need to be devised to aid development and monitoring of GT in a preclinical setting, and also to be readily translatable to the clinic. Moreover, because of the possibility that only transient expression of the therapeutic gene may be achieved (Ye *et al.*, 1999), these methods need to be noninvasive, nontoxic, and capable of temporally monitoring gene expression. The products of gene expression are its specific mRNA and protein. Commonly, the latter product is measured as there can be ~2–20,000-fold more protein molecules per molecule of mRNA. Furthermore, it is rare for the protein to be directly visualizable, and reporter systems need to be employed. A reporter system consists of a reporter gene that undergoes expression, usually under the same genetic control as the gene of interest, to produce a reporter protein that can be visualized: levels of reporter protein correlating to levels of the protein produced. An ideal reporter gene *in vivo* must satisfy a number of criteria: the capability to provide a unique signal, so that reporter gene expression can be monitored *in vivo* against a background of natively expressed genes; small enough to be incorporated into bicistronic constructs along with therapeutic genes and the ability to serve as a direct marker for the entire delivery system; and not interfere with normal tissue function.

At present a number of imaging methods are currently under development that will allow gene delivery, uptake, expression and subsequent therapeutic changes to be mapped out *in vivo*, with a view to tailoring GTs to individual patient requirements. These include clinical imaging techniques such as ultrasound; computerized tomography (CT); magnetic resonance (MR); and nuclear techniques, positron emission tomography (PET) and single photon emission tomography (SPECT) (Theodore *et al.*, 1999). New technologies, such as electric source imaging (using electroencephalographic or electrocardigraphic techniques; Grimm *et al.*, 1998; Huppertz *et al.*, 1998), electrical impedance mapping (Morucci and Rigaud, 1996), magnetic field gradient measurements (magnetoencephalography or magnetocardiography; Nakaya and Mori, 1992; Roberts *et al.*, 1998), and microwave scattering tomography (Caorsi *et al.*, 1994), are also under assessment for use in man. Optical modalities such as bioluminescence (Pasini *et al.*, 1998), fluorescence (Chaudhuri *et al.*, 2001), and near-infrared fluorescence (NIRF; Weissleder *et al.*, 1999) imaging have become significantly more established, especially in rodent models. However, application of these latter methods are limited in the clinic as the signal from tissues can be scattered by tissues prior to detection, rendering these technologies only applicable to small rodents or following surgical exposure of tissues. Uniquely, MR techniques bridge the gap between technologies that have gained everyday acceptance in the clinical arena (magnetic resonance imaging, MRI) and those that still are relatively research tools (magnetic resonance spectroscopy, MRS). Here, we review the application of MRI and MRS to the study of GT and their potential role in defining and refining future GT development strategies.

II. Magnetic Resonance Techniques

The last two decades have seen an increasing interest in the utilization of nuclear magnetic resonance (NMR) techniques, MRI and MRS, to biological and clinical problems. Indeed, since its first human applications in the early 1980s, MRI has become one of the main clinical imaging modalities, while MRS, which provides direct biochemical information on the function of animal and human organs *in vivo* and *in vitro*, has become the technique of choice for much clinical and biological *in vivo* research. Indeed, it is the application of NMR in the clinical setting that has led to the convention of dropping "nuclear" and its negative connotations from NMR to use the term, MRS. A great advantage of both MRI and MRS is that they are noninvasive, safe and reproducible modalities, allowing serial information to be collected, or in the case of MRS, dynamic biochemical changes to be observed. Furthermore, MR techniques can encompass both laboratory and clinical needs.

In vivo MR studies are normally carried out using large, whole body superconducting magnets. The strength of magnetic fields is usually measured in Tesla (T) with most clinical MRI systems operating between 0.5 and 3 T, usually 1.5 T; although there are clinical research systems that operate at 4.7 T and some at 8 T. With increasing magnetic field strengths, improved sensitivity and resolution is achieved but the cost of high field whole body systems (>3 T) can be prohibitive. Animal systems range from 2 to 11.7 T, with most modern systems ranging from 4.7 to 9.4 T. Higher field strengths are needed to compensate for the comparatively higher resolutions needed to image rodents. *In vitro* MRS and MRI of cell suspensions and tissue samples are often performed at up to 11.7 T, well beyond the range of most clinical systems.

III. MR Overview

There are a number of MR sensitive nuclei available for biological and clinical investigations, including hydrogen-1 (^{1}H), carbon-13 (^{13}C), nitrogen-15 (^{15}N), fluorine-19 (^{19}F), sodium-23 (^{23}Na), and phosphorus-31 (^{31}P). These nuclei allow the production of either an image (MRI) providing anatomical information (principally ^{1}H, although ^{31}P images can be obtained under some very specific conditions); or a frequency spectrum, providing biochemical information (MRS). By MRS, biochemical and pharmacological information can thus be obtained from endogenous and/or exogenous low-molecular-weight metabolites, containing ^{1}H (signal from amino acids, organic acids, lipids, sugars, cell-membrane components), ^{31}P (signal from nucleoside triphosphates such as ATP and from phosphocreatine, inorganic phosphate [Pi] and phosphorylated intermediates in the cell membrane synthetic [phosphomonoesters] and degradation pathways [phosphodiesters]), ^{13}C (glycogen, sugars, amino acids, and lipids), and ^{19}F (fluorinated drug products).

IV. MR Imaging (MRI)

The ability to generate images of intact living objects noninvasively and nondestructively has made MRI one of the leading clinical and biological imaging modalities. In general, MR images consist of high-resolution maps of intracellular tissue water. The contrast normally observed in an MR image therefore corresponds to differences in content and or MR characteristics of the water molecules within different regions of a given organ or tissue. The clinical information (anatomic and/or dynamic), obtained from MRI examinations can be modified either by tailoring the MR pulse sequences to highlight or nullify signal from different water-containing or fat compartments in the body, or by the use of MR contrast agents. Thus, excellent tissue contrast, and therefore discrimination of areas of interest, can be obtained by proper choice of experimental parameters. Amongst many applications, MRI techniques are being used to determine organ development and/or atrophy, angiography, functional imaging (fMRI), dynamic changes in arterial blood flow or biliary drainage, for example.

Recent advances in high-field magnets have permitted an expansion of the MRI modality into previously unforeseen areas of research (Bowtell *et al.*, 1995). This area of application, which has led to the imaging of isolates within cells, has been termed "MRI microscopy." The resolution is about 1 μm and in combination with contrast agents, which highlight physiological changes in the cell, has opened up exciting possibilities.

The use of intravenously injected contrast agents is a well-established method for improving the conspicuity of certain body tissues and therefore improve diagnostic yield in clinical and research arenas (Mathur de Vre and Lemort, 1995).

MR contrast agents are usually biologically inert chelates of gadolinium or other paramagnetic elements such as iron and exert their action by altering proton relaxation times (Kirsch, 1991; Tweedle *et al.*, 1991). The MRI (proton) signal can undergo relaxation back to equilibrium by either longitudinal (T_1) or transverse (T_2) relaxation mechanisms. Contrast agents enhance either predominantly T_1 or T_2 relaxation. Low-molecular-weight gadolinium chelates, such as gadolinium diethylenetriamine-pentaacetic acid (Gd-DTPA), are common T_1 contrast agents, and lead to areas of hyperintensity by employment of appropriate MRI parameters (T_1-weighted MRI). Whilst T_2 contrast agents such as superparamagnetic iron oxides (SPIOs) cause hypointense areas (due to signal loss) by T_2-weighted MRI (Watson *et al.*, 1992). However, the ability of a particular contrast agent to highlight a tissue depends on sufficient accumulation, its specificity and molecular weight if it is not freely diffusible (Bañez-Coronel *et al.*, 2008). Individual contrast agents have particular affinity for certain body compartments such as the blood, bile, the hepatic parenchyma, or the reticuloendothelial system (Earls and Bluemke, 1999). For example, in the liver, Gd-DTPA and manganese dipyridoxyl diphosphate are concentrated in hepatic parenchymal tissue and subsequently in the bile, producing a brightening of the liver, whereas SPIOs are taken up by Kupffer cells and other reticuloendothelial cells and produce hepatic darkening (Clement *et al.*, 1998). This is important in improving the conspicuity of focal lesions, especially in the context of a cirrhotic liver where tumors develop on the background of nodular regeneration (Low, 1997).

In general, commercially available contrast agents are nonspecific and adequately serve the needs of clinical imaging as classically, MRI has been performed to assess the extent and progression of pathology, noninvasively. However, such anatomical and/or functional changes occur distal to the primary pathological process. Studying or monitoring early events that cause disease may lead to novel interventional strategies to prevent/alleviate disease, and the possibility of "personalized" medicine. The "*in vivo* characterization and measurement of biological processes at the cellular or molecular level" is defined by the term, "molecular imaging." The nature of molecular imaging is such so as to require contrast agents specific for the molecule or biological process being studied. Such contrast agents, commonly referred to as imaging probes, ideally, should be specific, exert no biological effects, should possess high relaxivity (i.e., effective at modulating relaxation) and favorable pharmacokinetics. Thus, an imaging probe consists of two components, one that provides specificity and the other, a contrast agent. Specificity/targeting are commonly achieved by exploitation of the specificity of the antigen-antibody interaction. Targeting will, of course, partly render favorable pharmacokinetic properties to the probe, by enhancing its accumulation at the target site. However, the imaging probe needs to distribute to the target at sufficient levels, this is only possible if the imaging probe can persist in the vasculature long enough to accumulate at target sites, that is, not rapidly excreted from the body and/or accumulate in nontarget sites, commonly the liver.

Sensitivity is often the issue in molecular imaging since the molecule or target, to be imaged in biological processes, tends to be present at low quantities (10^{-9}-10^{-13} mol/g) and sufficient imaging probe needs to be present to effectively modulate the proton signal in the vicinity to generate contrast. In the case of low-molecular-weight gadolinium chelates, mM concentrations are required for detection and hence, the popularity of SPIO-based imaging probes in molecular imaging, requiring only nM-μM concentrations. Also, if small enough (10–50 nm diameter), SPIOs will substantially affect T_1 rather than T_2-relaxation generating positive contrast (Moore *et al.*, 2000), and certain formulation, such as Endorem™, are in common clinical usage. SPIOs are nanoparticles consisting of a crystalline iron oxide core surrounded by a polymer coating. The various types of SPIOs differ from each other, in terms of size and coating. The size, charge, and nature of the coating determine the stability, biodistribution, and metabolism of SPIOs (Chouly *et al.*, 1996). The coating is usually carbohydrate in nature, such as dextran, or consists of synthetic polymers, polycations, or polyamines. Furthermore, the coating can provide functional groups for chemical modification and allow targeting of the nanoparticles in molecular imaging. Not only do SPIOs significantly enhance T_2 relaxation of surrounding protons, they also induce local susceptibilities, thereby augmenting T_2*; rendering SPIOs readily visible by both T_2- and T_2*-weighted MRI. However, SPIO-based agents usually generate signal loss (negative contrast) which is difficult to quantify and, also, indistinguishable from hemorrhage and air-tissue interfaces by conventional MRI. Thus, the drive toward development of new sequences, for example, off-resonance (Cunningham *et al.*, 2005), "white marker" (Seppenwoolde *et al.*, 2003), and ultra-short-echo (UTE) time methods. Of these, only UTE methods appear to be capable of distinguishing signal voids arising from SPIOs from that generated by air-tissue interfaces and hemorrhage (Protti *et al.*, 2009).

As mentioned earlier, SPIOs are the preferred contrast agent in molecular imaging due to relatively high sensitivity compared to gadolinium chelates. However, local gadolinium chelate concentrations can be elevated for improved MRI sensitivity by their incorporation into nanoparticles, such as liposomes (Kamaly *et al.*, 2009; Winter *et al.*, 2003). Gadolinium chelates have been incorporated into lipid bilayers and for some liposomes, filled with perfluorocarbons (PFC; Winter *et al.*, 2003). Gadolinium chelate-loaded liposomes may be visualized by T_1-weighted MRI, and in the case of PFC-filled liposomes also by ^{19}F MRI. The ^{19}F nucleus has 80%, the sensitivity of the ^{1}H nucleus and the absence of endogenous ^{19}F signals in the body confers advantages to the use of ^{19}F MRI to image PFC nanoparticles *in vivo*, both quantitatively and qualitatively (Morawski *et al.*, 2004).

Another less common mode of generating contrast is by the use of chemical exchange saturation transfer (CEST) agents (Ward *et al.*, 2000). Such agents have exchangeable protons, for example, –NH and –OH, which resonate at specific chemical shifts distinct from that of bulk water. Application of an appropriate radiofrequency pulse saturates the exchangeable protons, transfer of their magnetization to protons of bulk water, leading to attenuation of the water signal.

The advantage of using CEST agents is that contrast can be switched "on" and "off" by simple application of the appropriate radiofrequency pulse. Also, as there are more than one exchangeable resonance, CEST agents raise the possibility of multispectral imaging, comparable to that possible in optical-based imaging with the availability of a number of green fluorescent protein (GFP) variants (Heim *et al.*, 1994). However, the closeness of the chemical shifts of the exchangeable protons and bulk water renders specific saturation of the former difficult. This may be overcome by the use of paramagnetic chelates with exchangeable protons (PARACEST effect). The presence of paramagnetic ions shifts the chemical shift of the bound water away from bulk water, allowing distinct saturation of the exchangeable protons (Terrano *et al.*, 2004).

V. MR Spectroscopy (MRS)

Information from MRS is normally presented in the form of a spectrum. Whatever the chosen nucleus under MRS examination, the nuclei from individual metabolites resonate at a given frequency, depending on the chemical environment of each nucleus. This phenomenon is known as chemical shift. The intensity of each metabolite signal is related to the concentration of the metabolite. Analysis of the MR spectrum allows noninvasive insight into metabolite concentrations, intracellular pH and the metabolic state of pathological tissue, as well as dynamic changes in the metabolism of living tissue in both health and disease. However, only compounds present at millimolar concentrations are normally detectable utilizing the clinical MR systems currently available (Cady, 1990).

The readout from MRS is in the form of a spectrum and does not provide spatial information. However, an extension of MRS is spectroscopic imaging or chemical shift imaging (CSI) which provides information regarding metabolite location within a volume of interest (Brateman, 1986).

VI. Role of Magnetic Resonance Methods in GT

The roles of MR methods in GT can be summarized as

(i) monitoring delivery of GT vectors and cells to the target site;
(ii) targeting and enhancement of GT;
(iii) imaging expression of the therapeutic gene;
(iv) monitoring therapeutic response.

A. Monitoring Gene Delivery

Tissue-selectivity in GT is essential to minimize the toxicity and increase gene transfer to target organs *in vivo*. Monitoring of GT vectors to target tissues may be achieved by "tagging" of GT vectors with contrast agents, to allow vizualization by MRI. Kayyem *et al.* (1995) conjugated human transferrin to poly-L-lysine (PLL, a cationic polymer that can form ionic complexes with negatively charged DNA), which in turn was attached to Gd-DTPA. Gene delivery particles were then formed by complex formation of varying amounts of conjugated PLL to plasmid DNA, followed by the addition of Gd-DTPA-PDL to neutralize the negative DNA charge. K562 leukemia cells were transfected *in vitro* with the polymer/DNA complexes and T_1-weighted MRI showed greater signal intensity of cells transfected with the gadolinium complexes. Similarly, SPIOs can be used, complexed to DNA by PLL: 293 embryonic kidney cells transfected with such particles have been visualized by MRI *in vitro* and *in vivo* (de Marco *et al.*, 1998). Transfection agents including PLL are now commonly used to form complexes with SPIOs to aid SPIO transport into cells *in vitro*/*ex vivo* for cellular imaging by MRI in cell-based GT. There are many excellent reviews on the labeling of cells for MRI detection *in vivo* and the reader is advised to refer to such texts (Bulte and Kraitchman, 2004; Frank *et al.*, 2004; Modo *et al.*, 2005; Rogers *et al.*, 2006).

Viral particles are commonly used as GT vectors (Walter and Stein, 2000). Räty *et al.* (2006) developed an avidin-displaying baculovirus, which can be labeled with biotinylated SPIOs, exploiting the known affinity between avidin and biotin, for MRI visualization. The protein cage of Cowpea chlorotic mottle virus (CCMV) and MS2 capsids have been conjugated to gadolinium chelate molecules to allow tracking by MRI *in vivo* (Allen *et al.*, 2005; Anderson *et al.*, 2006). Gadolinium chelates have also been incorporated into a lentiviral vector to allow MRI monitoring of delivery of a marker gene *in vivo* (Yang *et al.*, 2001).

Liposomes have also been proposed as GT vectors and have the advantage of being nonimmunogenic compared to their viral counterparts (Douglas, 2008). Such GT vectors may be simply modified for MRI tracking by entrapment of MRI contrast agents within aqueous lumen, for example, manganese chloride (Magin *et al.*, 1986) and Gd-DTPA (Unger *et al.*, 1988). Gadodiamide- and doxorubicin-containing liposomes have been used to enable MRI monitoring of liposomal distribution after delivery to brain tumors in rats (Saito *et al.*, 2004) and mice. SPIO-encapsulated liposomes have been used to monitor siRNA delivery in a breast cancer xenograft model in mice following systemic administration (Mikhaylova *et al.*, 2009). The use of such liposomes can be limited as the relaxivity of enclosed contrast agents may be attenuated by the limited exchange between bulk water with the enclosed contrast agents, or the liposomes are degraded with the release of the contrast agents. Hence, the development of liposomes in which gadolinium-chelates have been conjugated to lipids and incorporated into the liposomal lipid bilayer (Kabalka *et al.*, 1988). The biodistribution of cationic liposomes bound to DNA has been evaluated over time by MRI (Leclercq *et al.*, 2003). As well as being readily monitored *in vivo* by MRI, Gadolinium-liposomes have been shown to be able to transfect cells *in vitro*, indicating their promise as GT vectors (Kamaly *et al.*, 2009).

Recently, MRI has been used to monitor siRNA delivery *in vivo* (Medrova *et al.*, 2007). Using a SPIO, labeled with a near-infrared dye, and covalently linked to siRNA and membrane-translocating peptides, siRNA delivery to two different tumor models was observed. Conjugation to tumor-targeting ligands was unnecessary due the enhanced permeability and retention effect of hyperpermeable tumor vasculature.

Alternatively, GT vectors and cells can be imaged *in vivo* by imaging gene expression specific to them (strategies to do so are detailed below).

B. MR-Guided and Enhanced GT

The delivery of GT vectors can be guided by MRI by either labeling of the GT vectors with MRI contrast agents. Alternatively, delivery of GT vectors by non-systemic administration, for example, an MRI-compatible biopsy needle, can also be guided by MRI by inclusion of gadolinium chelates in the GT vector formulation (Susil *et al.,* 2003).

Currently, a limitation of GT protocols is the low efficiency of gene transfer at the target site. For example, *in vivo* gene transfer in the vasculature can be <1% and 5%, for nonviral and viral vectors, respectively. Controlled heating has been shown *in vitro* studies to enhance gene transfer by increasing plasma permeability and cell metabolism and/or increased activity of heat-shock proteins (Madio *et al.*, 1998; Tang *et al.*, 1996). Practically, heating needs to be performed locally at the target site rather than over the whole body and a loopless MR antenna can be used as a small internal heating device, allowing MR thermal mapping (Qiu *et al.*, 2004) and enhancement of GT (Gao *et al.*, 2006).

Local heating and/or increased cell porosity can also be induced by ultrasound, enhancing gene/GT vector delivery into cells and gene expression under the control of heat-sensitive promoters (Deckers *et al.*, 2009). In tandem with MRI, the latter modality providing mapping of tissue temperatures to enable controlled heating (Cline *et al.,* 1992), ultrasound has been shown to enhance heat-sensitive promoter-driven gene expression (Guilhon *et al.,* 2003; Huang *et al.*, 2000; Smith *et al.*, 2002).

C. Imaging Gene Expression

The success or failure of GT is judged by whether the therapeutic gene is expressed and performs its function at the target location. Conventional methods of assessing gene expression include use of microarrays, proteomics and use of reporter genes in both immunohistochemistry and histochemical staining, and *in situ* hybridization. However, such methods are *in vitro*-based, requiring death of the organism or invasive sampling and so, of limited use in serial (and interventional) studies and transfer to the clinical arena. Also, such methods do not allow for monitoring of dynamic cellular processes and prevents simultaneous monitoring of a number of tissues. *In vivo* assessment would allow phenomena such as tolerance, complementation and redundancies in biological pathways to be studied

(Gassman and Hennet, 1998). Hence, the necessity of noninvasive imaging modalities such as MRI to determine spatiotemporal expression of genes *in vivo*, essential for development of GT protocols.

Strategies for imaging gene expression can be categorized into direct and indirect. The former involves detection of the therapeutic gene directly or following interaction with an imaging probe. Rarely, can the therapeutic gene be visualized or detected by MRI and MRS, respectively and hence, the requirements of an MR probe to associate specifically and allow MR detection of the therapeutic protein. For indirect methods, reporter technologies need to be employed, compared to that used in conventional methods of assessing gene expression. In reporter technologies, reporter genes are fused to the gene of interest, commonly under the same genetic regulation. As the therapeutic gene is expressed, that is, production of its protein, the reporter gene also expresses its protein. A fixed relationship needs to exist between the levels of the therapeutic and reporter proteins, to allow quantitative determination of gene expression. For MR detection of gene expression, the reporter protein may be either directly observed by MR methods or following interaction with a specific MR probe.

Irrespective of whether direct or indirect imaging strategies are used, MR serves to detect a specific protein, that is, the therapeutic protein or the reporter protein, respectively. The protein can either be a cell-surface protein or a receptor, and interaction with an MR probe leads to its retention on the cell surface or internalization into the cell. Alternatively, the protein can be an intracellular protein and/or an enzyme. The MR probe will enter the cell and associate with the protein and be retained by the cell for detection by MR methods. If the protein is an enzyme, "smart" probes are used, such probes are only MR detectable are only activated, that is, MR detectable, in the presence of the protein.

VII. MRI-Based Systems

The simplest method of imaging a protein (therapeutic or reporter) is to use an imaging probe consisting of an antibody (to confer specificity) and a contrast agent (for MRI detection). Thus, the protein would need to be a cell surface entity. Although this method has not been adopted to assess gene expression in GT, it has been used to image endogenously expressed proteins for diagnostic and cell-labeling applications. For example, SPIOs conjugated to $F(ab)_2$ fragments of an E-selectin antibody has been used to image E-selectin *in vitro* (Kang *et al.*, 2002) and *in vivo* (Kang *et al.*, 2006). Artemov and colleagues have used a biotinylated antibody to the HER-2/neu receptor, and visualized the tagged receptor with avidin conjugated to Gd-DTPA (Artemov *et al.*, 2003a) or SPIO (Artemov *et al.*, 2003b). A number of publications have shown the imaging of other tumor specific antigens by antibodies conjugated to contrast agents (Cerdan *et al.*, 1989; Funovics *et al.*, 2004; Moore *et al.*, 2004; Remsen *et al.*, 1996; Renshaw *et al.*, 1986; To *et al.*, 1992; Suzuki *et al.*, 1996). As well as imaging the therapeutic protein in this way, the same method can be used to image the reporter protein, for example, the truncated H2k antigen, recently proposed by our group (So *et al.*, 2005). By transfection of human cervical carcinoma (HeLa) cells with the plasmid for the gene expressing this protein, we were able to visualize signal loss from the transfected cells by T_2-weighted MRI following labeling with anti-H2k-SPIOs. Similarly, Tannous *et al.* (2006) proposed the expression of biotin on the cell surface as a tag to allow labeling with avidin-conjugated contrast agents for MRI visualization. The disadvantage to imaging cell surface entities is whether their expression is high enough for sufficient binding and accumulation of contrast agent at the cell. Also, commonly, conjugation to antibodies are used to provide specificity to imaging probes but use of antibodies can be problematic due to their size, rendering extravasation difficult, except in instances of enhanced permeability of blood vessels, as may be seen in tumors. This issue may be overcome by the use of engineered antibody fragments.

Aside from direct visualization of the protein by antibodies conjugated to contrast agents, the other methods to image gene expression are based on use of reporter technologies. A number of the reporter systems proposed to capitalize on cellular mechanisms of regulating and storing iron (Ganz and Nemeth, 2006). Since iron is paramagnetic and capable of enhancing T_2-relaxation, cellular accumulation of iron would allow detection by MRI. Transferrin (Tf) carries two iron ions (becoming halo-Tf) in the blood, and is transported into the cell following binding with the transferrin receptor (TfR) on the cell surface. The complex is internalized into an endosome, and then iron is released from the endosomes to be stored in association with ferritin. Storage in this form prevents the possible toxic consequences of increased iron concentrations in the cell, resulting from the Fenton reaction. Ferritin consists of two types of subunits, heavy and light, and can store $<$4500 atoms of iron, and enhance both T_1 and T_2 relaxation. Genove *et al.* (2005) and Cohen *et al.* (2005) proposed the use of ferritin genes as reporter genes for MRI. The overexpression of ferritin leads to increased cellular iron sequestration by ferritin and upregulation of TfR and so, increased cellular uptake of iron. The increased levels of iron in the cells render them visible by T_2-weighted MRI. The advantage of this reporter system is that exogenous administration of an imaging probe is not required. Genove *et al.* (2005) genetically modified adenoviridae to carry genes encoding either the heavy or light chain subunits of ferritin. Transfection with such adenoviridae leads to signal loss in transfected cells *in vitro*. Injection of such viruses *in vivo*, resulted in negative enhancement of areas where ferritin gene transfer had occurred, for up to five weeks postinoculation. Cohen and colleagues fused the gene encoding the heavy subunit of ferritin with that of GFP and hemaglutinin, to enable correlation of MRI, fluorescence and histochemical data, respectively. Expression was controlled by the standard tetracycline-off gene control system (Gossen and Bujard, 1992). This reporter system was shown to allow visualization of transfected cells *in vitro* and *in vivo* by MRI and correlated well with the other imaging systems. The advantage of the ferritin-based reporter system is that no exogenous administration of an imaging probe is required.

Another reporter system that exploits cellular mechanisms of handling iron is the engineered human TfR (ETR) and Tf-SPIO (transferrin conjugation to SPIOs) system (Weissleder *et al.*, 2000). As with the ferritin methods, the strategy is to increase cellular accumulation of iron, by increasing iron transport into the cell. However, TfR expression decreases with increasing cellular iron concentrations, and so the researchers modified the TfR gene to produce a TfR that is insensitive to cellular iron concentrations, ETR. Amplification of MRI contrast was achieved by the administration of Tf-SPIO rather than using the endogenous receptor ligand, halo-Tf, SPIOs contain 2064 iron atoms as compared to only two iron atoms as carried by halo-Tf: indeed, contrast was not achieved with halo-Tf (Weissleder *et al.*, 2000). The sensitivity of this technique was estimated to be able to detect a minimum of one labeled cell per 50 μm^3 *in vivo* (Moore *et al.*, 2001). Using a HSV-based amplicon vector carrying the ETR, lacZ and CYP2B1 (rat cytochrome c P450 2B1) genes (Ichikawa *et al.*, 2002), the expression of all three genes were shown to be closely correlated, supporting the use of ETR as a reporter gene in therapeutic GT protocols.

More recently, Deans *et al.* (2006) adopted a twin approach, employing both upregulation of ETR and ferritin. Further work needs to be performed to determine the relative effectiveness of using either ETR or ferritin alone, or in combination with other.

As with the ferritin reporter systems, the tyrosinase reporter system proposed by Enochs *et al.* (1997) does not require the administration of exogenous imaging probes. Tyrosinase catalyzes the rate-limiting step in the cellular synthesis of melanin, and increased tyrosinase expression leads to increased melanin concentrations (Alfke *et al.*, 2003). Melanin is a biopolymer pigment, conferring color to tissues, such as skin. It has a high affinity for a variety of paramagnetic metal ions, including iron, and explains the high-signal intensity seen in melanotic melanomas by T_1-weighted MRI (Atlas *et al.*, 1990). Cell lines transfected with the tyrosinase gene were shown to bind iron in particular, and the binding to vary with DNA dose (Enochs *et al.*, 1997), and give rise to high-signal intensity by T_1-weighted MRI. Similar findings were observed by Yuan *et al.* (2003) following transfection of HepG2 cells with the tyrosinase gene. Melanogenesis, however, leads to the formation of toxic intermediates. Normally, this potential toxicity is attenuated by the reactions occurring in specialized organelles, melanosomes (Riley, 2003). Thus, Alfke *et al.* (2003) modified the technology to employ tetracycline to regulate expression of the tyrosinase gene, to decrease potential toxicological effects. Melanin is very stable and persists in the body for long periods of time, and so this methodology requires refinement to allow higher temporal imaging.

The reporter gene, lacZ, which encodes β-galactosidase, is commonly used for assessment of gene expression. Gene expression can be assessed by assaying for β-galactosidase activity using chromogenic substrates, for example,

5-bromo-4-indolyl β-D-galactopyranoside (X-gal) which is hydrolyzed by β-galactosidase to form an intense blue precipitate. This methodology has been adapted for MRI detection of gene expression by exchanging the chromogenic substrate with a "smart" MR probe. The "smart" MR probe is also a substrate for β-galactosidase and following enzymatic action, leads to the formation of an MR detectable product. EgadME is one such MR probe, proposed by Louie *et al.* (2000). EgadME consists of a chelator that binds gadolinium with high affinity and occupies eight of the nine coordination sites of gadolinium. A galactopyranose residue is positioned so as to block the access of a water molecule to the remaining gadolinium coordination site. This water-inaccessible conformation is not MR active and only becomes MR visible when the galactopyranose residue is cleaved off by β-galactosidase. The removal of the galactose cap allows water access to the gadolinium ion and hence, enhancement of T_1-relaxation. Employing the *Xenopus laevis* embryo model, Louie and colleagues showed the MRI visualization of lacZ expression in the intact embryo. At the two cell stage, both cells were injected with EgadME, but only one cell received either the mRNA or the DNA coding for β-galactosidase (Louie *et al.*, 2000). The embryo was allowed to develop and then imaged live by MRI. Following MRI, the embryo was chemically fixed and stained with X-gal for histochemical analysis. It is known that at the two-cell stage, one cell divides to produce the cell population on one side of the embryo and the other, the cell population on the other side. Thus, positive X-gal staining observed predominantly on one side of the embryo, correlated with high-intensity regions of the MR image. While imaging gene expression was possible with this methodology, the technology requires the cellular entry of EgadMe in all cells. This was achieved by the microinjection into cells, but this is unlikely to be possible for most applications. Subsequently, enhanced cell penetration by imaging probes have been facilitated by conjugation to membrane translocating peptides such as the tat peptide from human immunodeficiency virus (Bhorade *et al.*, 2000; Josephson *et al.*, 1999; Lewin *et al.*, 2000; Zhao and Weissleder, 2004). We have recently shown bifunctionalization of EgadMe to allow binding to such cell translocation carrier systems, as well as to other ligands (Wardle *et al.*, 2007). Employment of smart probes have a distinct advantage over nonsmart MR probes as contrast will only be observed in the vicinity of the therapeutic/reporter protein rather than also due to its nonspecific presence in that area.

Recently, a new reporter protein (lysine-rich protein, LRP) was proposed, based on employment of CEST contrast (Gilad *et al.*, 2007). Since LRP is rich in lysine residues with amide protons capable of CEST, this system was able to generate significant contrast of cells transfected with the LRP gene. CEST-MRI was able to detect the xenografts generated from inoculation of the LRP-expressing cells into the brain. A caveat to employment of this reporter system is that as amide exchange is strongly pH-dependent, contrast can be decreased by ischaemia or cell death (Zhou *et al.*, 2003).

VIII. MRS-Based Systems

An MRS-based method of assessing gene expression is dependent on generation of a metabolite with a unique chemical shift value as a result of gene expression. Thus, commonly, the therapeutic or reporter gene encodes an enzyme. Therapeutic genes include cytosine deaminase from yeast (yCD), absent in mammalian cells and converts 5-fluorocytosine (5-FC) to 5-fluorouracil (5-FU). 5-FU is an antimetabolite and its incorporation into DNA leads to cell death by cell cycle arrest and apoptosis. Used in cancer chemotherapy, the dosage is limited by its systemic toxicity which can be overcome by the transduction of CD only in cancer tissues and the use of 5-FC rather than 5-FU (Crystal *et al.*, 1997). 5-FC and 5-FU have different chemical shift values in the ^{19}F MR spectrum (Aboagye *et al.*, 1998), and *in vivo* ^{19}F MRS has been used to monitor the metabolism of 5-FC and quantify CD expression in a yCD-expressing tumor cells implanted in a mouse model (Stegman *et al.*, 1999).

Proposed reporter genes include arginine kinase (AK) which is nonendogenous to mammalian tissues. AK phosphorylates arginine to form phosphoarginine (PArg) providing a unique signature in the ^{31}P MR spectrum of muscle. A recombinant adenovirus coding for arginine kinase (rAdCMVAK) was injected into the right hindlimbs of neonatal mice. Two weeks after injection of rAdCMVAK, a unique ^{31}P-MRS resonance was observed. It was observable in all rAdCMVAK-injected hindlimbs and was not present in the contralateral control or the vehicle-injected limb (Walter *et al.*, 2000). AK activity persisted for at least eight months after injection, providing a useful reporter gene that allows noninvasive and repeated monitoring of gene expression after viral mediated gene transfer to muscle. Similarly, creatine kinase (CrK) can be used as a reporter protein in tissues such as the liver which does not express endogenous CrK, by monitoring the production of phosphocreatine (Auricchio *et al.*, 2001; Koretsky *et al.*, 1990). Recently, CrK has been used as a reporter gene to monitor hepatic expression of the low-density lipoprotein receptor (LDLr) following transduction in mice using a genetically modified adenovirus (Li *et al.*, 2005). An excellent correlation was observed between CrK and LDLr expression in hepatocytes *in vitro*. The use of CrK as a reporter gene allows accurately measurement of CrK activity by magnetization transfer (Askenasy and Koretsky, 2002). However, both kinase reporter genes would be dependent on cellular energy metabolism which may change over time.

Choline kinase (CK) is over expressed in some cancer types including breast cancer, and shown to be activated by oncogenes and mitogenic signals, with inhibitors shown to have potential antitumor activity in human xenograft models *in vivo* (Bañez-Coronel *et al.*, 2008). Suppression of CK activity in breast cancer cells was achieved by siRNA and its activity measured by analyzing methanol-chloroform-water extracts of cells by ^{1}H MRS. The use of ^{1}H MRS in this study illustrates the potential of *in vivo* ^{1}H MRS to assess efficacy of siRNA treatment.

The *Escherichia coli ppk* gene has been the latest MRS-reporter gene proposed (Ki *et al.*, 2007). This gene encodes polyphosphate (PolyP) kinase which catalyzes the formation of polyP, linear polymers of orthophosphate residues linked by high-energy phosphoanhydride bonds. (Endogenous levels of polyP in mammalian cells are below that detectable by ^{31}P MR methods.) Ki *et al.* (2007) demonstrate the expression of the bacterial reporter gene in a number of mammalian cell lines, prior to detecting polyP production using both ^{31}P MRS and CSI in HEK 293T cells. They show that *ppk* expression does not affect cell growth or alter ATP levels but its effect *in vivo* has not been tested. The advantage of this reporting system is that exogenous administration of a probe is not required.

β-Galactosidase can also be used as a reporter protein for MRS. These MR probes are substrates for this enzyme that generates a product with a distinctive chemical shift. Probes include 4-fluoro-2-nitrophenol-β-D-galactopyranoside (Cui *et al.*, 2004) and its less toxic isomer 2-fluoro-4-nitrophenol-β-D-galactopyranoside (Kodibagkar *et al.*, 2006), and used to differentiate between lacZ and non-LacZ expressing human xenografts in nude mice by ^{19}F MRS and CSI (Yu *et al.*, 2008).

Finally, a fast although less specific method to detect transgene expression could be achieved by the use of *in vitro* MRS (Bell *et al.*, 1994; Nicholson *et al.*, 1999). This would be accomplished by measuring the level of "marker metabolites" in body fluids such as urine, blood, CSF and bile, instead of transfected cells. This method would be limited to a binomial form of detecting gene expression, (on/off), and would depend on the ability of the "marker metabolites" to cross the cell membrane and accumulate in body fluids. Nevertheless, this method could be relatively effective as a broad way of detecting transgene expression. One could envisage it as a fast and inexpensive first-pass approach to detect gene expression in human subjects, before more sophisticated *in vivo* methods are applied.

The application of MR methods to quantitatively image gene expression remains very much in its infancy despite the creative approaches adopted. Specifically regarding MR-based gene reporter systems, key papers for the use of MRS was published in 1990 (CrK, Koretsky *et al.*, 1990) and for MRI, in 1997 (tyrosinase, Weissleder *et al.*, 1997), 2000 (ETR, Weissleder *et al.*, 2000; EgadME, Louie *et al.*, 2000), and 2005 (ferritin, Cohen *et al.*, 2005; Genove *et al.*, 2005). One notes the sparsity of subsequent papers for each approach, with only a few of the methods reproduced in other laboratories, suggesting questions still remain over these strategies. Whether imaging the therapeutic or reporter protein, the major obstacle to the use of MR is its insensitivity as compared to other translatable techniques, especially PET. Molecular targets needs to be expressed at high levels and the imaging probes, as well as being specific, needs to accumulate at sufficient levels at target sites for detection. Detection is dependent both on their relaxivities and adequate accumulation at the target site: accumulation being determined by both pharmacokinetic and targeting properties. Thus, aside from enhancing MR hardware and software capabilities to provide greater sensitivity per experiment, many efforts are required to significantly improve relaxivities of imaging probes and their targeted distribution in the body.

A. Monitoring Therapeutic Response

MRI has been included in the diagnostic armoury of outcome measures in assessing the efficacy of GT. One of the main advantages of MRI, over other imaging methods, is its ability to not only detect gene transfer and expression *in vivo* but to also produce high-resolution anatomical and functional images. In neurological and musculoskeletal diseases, a combination of tissue perfusion, morphological measurements, MR angiography, vascular remodeling and metabolic measurements would be invaluable tools for the long-term assessment of the efficacy of GT (Walter *et al.*, 2005). For example, MR angiography provided qualitative evidence of improved distal flow in a study investigating the safety and efficacy of intramuscular GT with vascular endothelial growth factor (VEGF) in patients with chronic critical leg ischemia (Shyu *et al.*, 2003).

MRI is commonly used to monitor longitudinal changes in tumor size and perfusion, and MRS may be used to measure bioenergetics and metabolism, associated with GT (Kettunen and Gröhn, 2005). In a study of the efficacy of adv/tk/GCV GT in a syngeneic BT4C rat malignant glioma model, MRI was one of the measures used to assess treatment effect and tissue responses by comparison of signal intensities and tumor volume (Tyynela *et al.*, 2002). In a study of the antitumor efficacy of the gene encoding HSV thymidine kinase (HSVtk) to activate the prodrug ganciclovir (GCV) in a model of rat prostate cancer MRS studies, serial *in vivo* MRS of the tk-transfected MATLyLu tumors demonstrated a decreased ATP/Pi ratio during growth and an increase in the ATP/Pi ratio during regression initiated by treatment with GCV. Also significant differences were found in the phosphomonester (PME) to total phosphate ratios in treated, compared with untreated tumors (Eaton *et al.*, 2001).

MRI and MRS uniquely allow researchers and clinicians to be used to directly assess morphological, functional and metabolic changes directly and longitudinally throughout the lifetime of the patient, if necessary.

IX. Conclusions

Analysis of gene delivery and expression in the clinical setting currently involves molecular assays of histological biopsy material, but MR techniques hold the promise of noninvasive and dynamic assessment of the location, magnitude and duration of transgene expression. With the continued impetus to employ GT protocols to treat disease, there will be a great demand for accurate *in vivo* methodologies to determine the long-term consequences and benefits of GT. Furthermore, both MR modalities are uniquely equipped to extend the monitoring role from the laboratory bench into the patient.

Acknowledgments

Some of the work described in this chapter has been supported by the British Medical Research Council (MRC). The authors are grateful to the UK NIHR Biomedical Facility at Imperial College London, the Wellcome Trust for infrastructure support and Alberto Segundo Kruteler Quijada *por inspiratio*.

References

Aboagye, E. O., Artemov, D., Senter, P. D., and Bjujwalla, Z. M. (1998). Intratumoral conversion of 5-fluorocytosine to 5-fluorouracil by monoclonal antibody-cytosine deaminase conjugates: Non-invasive detection of prodrug activation by magnetic resonance spectroscopy and spectroscopic imaging. *Cancer Res.* **58,** 4075–4078.

Aigner, A. (2006). Gene silencing through RNA interference (RNAi) *in vivo*: Strategies based on the direct application of siRNAs. *J. Biotechnol.* **124**(1), 12–25.

Alfke, H., Stoppler, H., Nockern, F., Heverhagen, J. T., Kleb, B., Czybayko, F., and Klose, K. J. (2003). *In vitro* MR imaging of regulated gene expression. *Radiology* **228,** 488–492.

Allen, M., Bulte, J. W. M., Liepold, L., Basu, G., Zywicke, H. A., Frank, J. A., Young, M., and Douglas, T. (2005). Paramagnetic viral nanoparticles as potential high-relaxivity magnetic resonance contrast agents. *Magn. Reson. Med.* **54,** 807–812.

Anderson, E. A., Isaacman, S., Peabody, D. S., Wang, E. Y., Canary, J. W., and Kirshenbaum, K. (2006). Viral nanoparticles donning a paramagnetic coat: Conjugation of MRI contrast agents to the MS2 capsid. *Nano Lett.* **6,** 1160–1164.

Artemov, D., Mori, N., Ravi, R., and Bhujwalla, Z. M. (2003a). Magnetic resonance molecular imaging of the HER-2/neu receptor. *Cancer Res.* **63,** 2723–2727.

Artemov, D., Mori, N., Okollie, B., and Bhujwalla, Z. M. (2003b). MR molecular imaging of the Her-2/neu receptor in breast cancer cells using targeted iron oxide nanoparticles. *Magn. Reson. Med.* **49,** 403–408.

Askenasy, N., and Koretsky, A. P. (2002). Transgenic livers expressing mitochondrial and cytosolic CK: Mitochondrial CK modulates free ADP levels. *Am. J. Physiol. Cell. Physiol.* **282,** C338–C346.

Atlas, S., Braffman, B., LoBrutto, R., Elder, D., and Herlyn, D. J. (1990). Human malignant melanomas with varying degrees of melanin content in nude mice: MR imaging, histopathology, and electron paramagnetic resonance. *Comput. Assist. Tomogr.* **14,** 547–554.

Auricchio, A., Zhou, R., Wilson, J. M., and Glickson, J. D. (2001). *In vivo* detection of gene expression in liver by ^{31}P nuclear magnetic resonance spectroscopy employing creatine kinase as a marker gene. *Proc. Natl. Acad. Sci.* **98,** 5205–5210.

Bañez-Coronel, M., de Molina, A. R., Rodríguez-González, A., Sarmentero, J., Ramos, M. A., García-Cabezas, M. A., García-Oroz, L., and Lacal, J. C. (2008). Choline kinase alpha depletion selectively kills tumoral cells.. *Curr. Cancer Drug Targets* **8,** 709–719.

Beck, C., Uramoto, H., Boren, J., and Akyurek, L. M. (2004). Tissue-specific targeting for cardiovascular gene transfer. Potential vectors and future challenges. *Curr. Gene Ther.* **4,** 457–467.

Bell, J. D., Preece, N. E., and Parkes, H. G. (1994). NMR of body fluids and tissue extracts. *In* "NMR in Physiology and Biomedicine," (R. J. Gillies, ed.), pp. 221–236. Academic Press, London.

Bhorade, R., Weissleder, R., Nakakoshi, T., Moore, A., and Tung, C. H. (2000). Macrocyclic chelators with paramagnetic cations are internalised into mammalian cells via a HIV-tat derived membrane translocation peptide. *Bioconjug. Chem.* **11,** 301–305.

Blasberg, R., and Tjuvajev, J. (1999). Herpes simplex virus thymidine kinase as a marker/reporter gene for PET imaging of gene therapy. *Q. J. Nucl. Med.* **43,** 163–169.

Bonnekoh, B., Greenhalgh, D. A., Bundman, D. S., Kosai, K., Chen, S. H., Finegold, M. J., Krieg, T., Woo, S. L., and Roop, R. (1996). Adenoviral-mediated herpes simplex virus-thymidine kinase gene transfer *in vivo* for treatment of experimental human melanoma. *J. Invest. Dermatol.* **106,** 1163–1168.

Bowtell, R. W., Peters, A., Sharp, J. C., Mansfield, P., Hsu, E. W., Aiken, N., Horsman, A., and Blackband, S. J. (1995). NMR microscopy of single neurons using spin echo and line narrowed 2DFT imaging. *Magn. Reson. Med.* **33,** 790–794.

Brateman, L. (1986). Chemical shift imaging: A review. *Am. J. Roentgenol.* **146,** 971–980.

Brown, M. D., Schätzlein, A. G., and Ljeoma, F. (2001). Gene delivery with synthetic (non viral) carriers. *Int. J. Pharm.* **229,** 1–21.

Bulte, J. W., and Kraitchman, D. L. (2004). Iron oxide MR contrast agents for molecular and cellular imaging. *NMR Biomed.* **17,** 484–499.

Bulte, J. W., de Jonge, M. W., de Leij, L., The, T. H., Kamman, R. L., Blaauw, E., Zuiderveen, F., and Go, K. G. (1990). Passage of DMP across a disrupted BBB in the context of antibody-mediated MR imaging of brain metastases. *Acta Neurochir. Suppl.* **51,** 43–45.

Cady, E. B. (1990). "Clinical Magnetic Resonance Spectroscopy." Plenum Press, New York.

Caorsi, S., Gragnani, G. L., and Pastorino, M. (1994). An electromagnetic imaging approach using a multi-illumination technique. *IEEE Trans. Biomed. Eng.* **41,** 406–409.

Carter, P. J., and Samulski, R. J. (2000). Adeno-associated viral vectors as gene delivery vehicles. *Int. J. Mol. Med.* **6**(1), 17–27.

Cerdan, S., Lotscher, H. R., Kunnecke, B., and Seelig, J. (1989). Monoclonal antibody-coated magnetite particles as contrast agents in magnetic resonance imaging of tumors. *Magn. Reson. Med.* **12,** 151–163.

Chaudhuri, T. R., Mountz, J. M., Rogers, B. E., Partridge, E. E., and Zinn, K. R. (2001). Light-based imaging of green fluorescent protein-positive ovarian cancer xenografts during therapy. *Gynecol. Oncol.* **83,** 432–438.

Chouly, C., Pouliquen, D., Lucet, I., Jeune, J. J., and Jallet, P. (1996). Development of superparamagnetic iron oxide nanoparticles for MRI: Effect of size, charge and surface nature on biodistribution. *J. Microencapsul.* **13,** 245–255.

Clement, O., Siauve, N., Lewin, M., de Kerviler, E., Cuenod, C. A., and Frija, G. (1998). Contrast agents in magnetic resonance imaging of the liver: Present and future. *Biomed. Pharmacother.* **52,** 51–58.

Cline, H. E., Schenck, J. F., Hynynen, K., Watkins, R. D., Souza, S. P., and Jolesz, F. A. (1992). MR-guided focused ultrasound surgery. *J. Comput. Assist. Tomogr.* **16,** 956–965.

Cohen, B., Dafni, H., Meir, G., Harmelin, A., and Neeman, M. (2005). Ferritin as an endogenous MRI reporter for non-invasive imaging of gene expression in C6 glioma tumors. *Neoplasia* **7,** 109–117.

Crystal, R. G., Hirschowitz, E., Lieberman, M., Daly, J., Kazam, E., Henschke, C., Yankelevitz, D., Kennedy, N., Silverstein, R., Ohwada, A., Russi, T., Mastrangeli, A., *et al.* (1997). Phase I study of direct administration of a replication deficient adenovirus vector containing the *E. coli* cytosine deaminase gene to metastatic colon carcinoma of the liver in association with the oral administration of the pro-drug 5-fluorocytosine. *Hum. Gene Ther.* **8,** 985–1001.

Cui, W., Otten, P., Li, Y., Koeneman, K., Yu, J., and Mason, R. P. (2004). Novel NMR approach to assessing gene transfection: 4-Fluoro-2-nitrophenyl-beta-D-galactopyranose as a prototype reporter molecular for beta-galactosidase. *Magn. Reson. Med.* **51,** 616–620.

Cunningham, C. H., Arai, T., Yang, P. C., McConell, M. V., Pauly, J. M., and Conolly, S. M. (2005). Positive contrast magnetic resonance imaging of cells labelled with magnetic nanoparticles. *Magn. Reson. Med.* **53,** 999–1005.

Dean, A. E., Wadghiri, Y. Z., Bernas, L. M., Yu, X., and Rutt, B. K. (2006). Cellular MRI contrast via coexpression of transferrin receptor and ferritin. *Magn. Reson. Med.* **56,** 51–59.

Deckers, R., Quesson, B., Arsaut, J., Eimer, S., Couillaud, F., and Moonen, C. T. (2009). Image-guided, non-invasive, spatiotemporal control of gene expression. *Proc. Natl. Acad. Sci. USA* **106,** 1175–1180.

de Marco, G., Bogdanov, A., Marecos, E., Moore, A., Simonova, M., and Weissleder, R. (1998). MR imaging of gene delivery to the central nervous system with an artificial vector. *Radiology* **208,** 65–71.

Desser, T. S., Rubin, D. L., Muller, H. H., Qing, F., Khodor, S., Zanazzi, G., Young, S. W., Ladd, D. L., Wellons, J. A., and Kellar, K. E. (1994). Dynamics of tumour imaging with Gd-DTPA-polyethylene glycol: Dependence on molecular weight. *J. Magn. Reson. Imag.* **4,** 467–472.

Douglas, K. L. (2008). Toward development of artificial viruses for gene therapy: A comparative evaluation of viral and non-viral transfection. *Biotechnol. Prog.* **24,** 871–883.

Earls, J. P., and Bluemke, D. A. (1999). New MR imaging contrast agents. *Magn. Reson. Imag. Clin. N. Am.* **7,** 255–273.

Eaton, J. D., Perry, M. J., Todryk, S. M., Mazucco, R. A., Kirby, R. S., Griffiths, J. R., and Dalgleish, A. G. (2001). Genetic prodrug activation therapy (GPAT) in two rat prostate models generates an immune bystander effect and can be monitored by magnetic resonance techniques. *Gene Ther.* **8,** 557–567.

Enochs, W., Petherick, P., Bogdanova, A., Mohr, U., and Weissleder, R. (1997). Paramagnetic metal scavenging by melanin: MR imaging. *Radiology* **204,** 417–423.

Fichou, Y., and Férec, C. (2006). The potential of oligonucleotides for therapeutic applications. *TIB* **24,** 563–570.

Frank, J. A., Anderson, S. A., Kalsih, H., Jordon, E. K., Lewis, B. K., Yocum, G. T., and Arhab, A. S. (2004). Methods for magnetically labeling stem and other cells for detection by *in vivo* magnetic resonance imaging. *Cytotherapy* **6,** 621–625.

Funovics, M. A., Kapeller, B., Hoeller, C., Su, H. S., Kuntsfield, R., Puig, S., and Macfelda, K. (2004). MR imaging of the her2/neu and 9.2.27 tumor antigens using immunospecific contrast agents. *Magn. Reson. Imag.* **22,** 843–850.

Ganz, T., and Nemeth, E. (2006). Regulation of iron acquisition and iron distribution in mammals. *Biochim. Biophys. Acta* **1763,** 690–699.

Gao, F., Qiu, B., Kar, S., Zhan, X., Hoffman, L., and Yang, X. M. (2006). Intravascular magnetic resonance/radiofrequency may enhance gene therapy of atherosclerotic in-stent stenosis. *Acad. Radiol.* **13,** 526–530.

Gassman, M., and Hennet, T. (1998). From genetically altered mice to integrative physiology. *News Physiol. Sci.* **13,** 53–57.

Genove, G., DeMarco, U., Xu, H., Goins, W. F., and Ahrens, E. T. (2005). A new transgene reporter for *in vivo* magnetic resonance imaging. *Nat. Med.* **11,** 450–454.

Gilad, A. A., McMahon, M. T., Walczak, P., Winnard, P. T., Jr., Raman, V., van Laarhoven, H. W., Skoglund, C. M., Bulte, J. W., and van Zijl, P. C. (2007). Artificial reporter gene providing MRI contrast based on proton exchange. *Nat. Biotechnol.* **25,** 217–219.

Gossen, A., and Bujard, H. (1992). Tight control of gene expression in mammalian cells by tetracycline-responsive promoters. *Proc. Natl. Acad. Sci. USA* **89,** 5547–5551.

Grimm, C., Schreiber, A., Kristeva-Feige, R., Mergner, T., Hennig, J., and Lucking, C. H. (1998). A comparison between electric source localisation and fMRI during somatosensory stimulation. *Electroencephalogr. Clin. Neurophysiol.* **106,** 22–29.

Guilhon, E., Quesson, B., Maraud-Gaudry, F., de Verneuil, H., Canioni, P., Salomir, R., Voisin, P., and Moonen, C. T. (2003). Image-guided control of transgene expression based on local hyperthermia. *Mol. Imag.* **2,** 11–17.

Gunther, M., Wagner, E., and Ogris, E. M. (2005). Specific targets in tumor tissue for the delivery of therapeutic genes. *Curr. Med. Chem. Anticancer Agents* **9,** 157.

Hanania, E. G., and Deisseroth, A. B. (1994). Serial transplantation shows that early hematopoietic precursor cells are transduced by MDR-1 retroviral vector in a mouse gene therapy model. *Cancer Gene Ther.* **1,** 21–25.

Heim, R., Prasher, D. C., and Tsien, R. Y. (1994). Wavelength mutations and posttranslational autoxidation of green fluorescent protein. *Proc. Natl. Acad. Sci. USA* **91,** 12501–12504.

Huang, Q., Hu, J. K., Lohr, F., Zhang, L., Braun, R., Lanzen, J., Little, J. B., Dewhirst, M. W., and Li, C. Y. (2000). Heat-induced gene expression as a novel targeted cancer gene therapy strategy. *Cancer Res.* **60,** 3435–3439.

Huppertz, H. J., Otte, M., Grimm, C., Kristeva-Feige, R., Mergner, T., and Lucking, C. H. (1998). Estimation of the accuracy of a surface matching technique for registration of EEG and MRI data. *Electroencephalogr. Clin. Neurophysiol.* **106,** 409–415.

Ichikawa, T., Högemann, D., Saeki, Y., Tyminski, E., Terada, K., Weissleder, R., Chiocca, E. A., and Basilion, J. P. (2002). MRI of transgene expression: Correlation to therapeutic gene expression. *Neoplasia* **4,** 523–530.

Josephson, L., Tung, C. H., Moore, A., and Weissleder, R. (1999). High-efficiency intracellular magnetic labelling with novel superparamagnetic-Tat peptide conjugates. *Bioconjug. Chem.* **10,** 186–191.

Kalbalka, G. W., Buonocore, E., Hubner, K., Davis, M., and Huang, L. (1988). Gadolinium-labeled liposomes containing paramagnetic amphipathic agents: Targeted MRI contrast agents for the liver. *Magn. Reson. Med.* **8,** 89–95.

Kamaly, N., Kalber, T., Ahmad, A., Oliver, M. H., So, P.-W., Herlihy, A. H., Bell, J. D., Jorgensen, M. R., and Miller, A. D. (2009). Biomodal paramagnetic and fluorescent liposomes for cellular and tumor magnetic resonance imaging. *Bioconjug. Chem.* **19,** 118–129.

Kang, H. W., Josephsen, L., Petrovsky, A., Weissleder, R., and Bogdanov, A., Jr (2002). Magnetic resonance imaging of inducible E-selectin expression in human endothelial cell culture. *Bioconjug. Chem.* **13,** 122–127.

Kang, H. W., Torres, D., Wald, L., Weissleder, R., and Bogdanov, A., Jr (2006). Targeted imaging of human endothelial-specific marker in a model of adoptive cell transfer. *Lab. Invest.* **86,** 599–609.

Kayyem, J., Kumar, R., Fraser, S., and Meade, T. (1995). Receptor-targeted co-transport of DNA and magnetic resonance contrast agents. *Chem. Biol.* **2,** 615–620.

Kettunen, M. I., and Gröhn, O. H. J. (2005). Tumour gene therapy monitoring using magnetic resonance imaging and spectroscopy. *Current Gene Ther.* **5,** 685–696.

Ki, S., Sugihara, F., Kasahara, K., Tochio, H., Okada-Marubayashi, A., Tomita, S., Morita, M., Ikeguchi, M., Shirakawa, M., and Kokubo, T. (2007). Magnetic resonance-based visualization of gene expression in mammalian cells using a bacterial polyphosphate kinase reporter gene. *Biotechniques* **42,** 209–215.

Kirsch, J. E. (1991). Basic principles of magnetic resonance contrast agents. *Top Magn. Reson. Imag.* **2,** 1–18.

Knowles, M. R., Hohneker, K. W., Zhou, Z., Olsen, J. C., Noah, T. L., Hu, P. C., Leigh, M. W., Engelhardt, J. F., Edwards, L. J., Jones, K. R., Grossman, M., Wilson, J. M., *et al.* (1995). A controlled study of adenoviral-vector-mediated gene transfer in the nasal epithelium of patients with cystic fibrosis. *N. Engl. J. Med.* **333,** 823–831.

Ko, S. C., Gotoh, A., Thalmann, G. N., Zhau, H. E., Johnston, D. A., Zhang, W. W., Kao, C., and Chung, L. W. (1996). Molecular therapy with recombinant p53 adenovirus in an androgen-independent, metastatic human prostate cancer model. *Hum. Gene Ther.* **7,** 1683–1691.

Kodibagkar, V. D., Yu, J., Liu, L., Hetherington, H. P., and Mason, R. P. (2006). Imaging beta-galactosidase activity using 19F chemical shift imaging of lacZ gene-reporter molecule 2-fluoro-4-nitrophenol-beta-D-galactopyranoside. *Magn. Reson. Imag.* **24,** 959–962.

Koretsky, A. P., Bronsan, M. J., Chen, L. H., Chem, J. D., and Van Dyke, T. (1990). NMR detection of creatine kinase expressed in liver of transgenic mice: Determination of free ADP levels. *Proc. Natl. Acad. Sci. USA* **87,** 3112–3116.

Leclercq, F., Cohen-Ohana, M., Mignet, N., Sbarbati, A., Herscovici, J., Scherman, D., and Byk, G. (2003). Design, synthesis, and evaluation of gadolinium cationic lipids as tools for biodistribution studies of gene delivery complexes. *Bioconjug. Chem.* **14,** 112–129.

Lewin, M., Carlesso, N., Tung, C. H., Tang, X. W., Cory, D., Scadden, D. T., and Weissleder, R. (2000). Tat peptide-derivatized magnetic nanoparticles allow *in vivo* tracking and recovery of progenitor cells. *Nat. Biotechnol.* **18,** 410–414.

Li, S., and Huang, L. (2000). Nonviral gene therapy: Promises and challenges. *Gene Ther.* **7,** 31–34.

Li, Z., Qiao, H., Lebherz, C., Choi, S. R., Zhou, X., Gao, G., Kung, H. F., Rader, D. J., Wilson, J. M., Glickson, J. D., and Zhou, R. (2005). Creatine kinase, a magnetic resonance-detectable marker gene for quantification of liver-directed gene transfer. *Hum. Gene Ther.* **16,** 1429–1438.

Louie, A. Y., Huber, M. M., Ahrens, E. T., Rothbacher, U., Moats, R., Jacobs, R. E., Fraser, S. E., and Meade, T. J. (2000). *In vivo* visualization of gene expression using magnetic resonance imaging. *Nat. Biotechnol.* **18,** 321–325.

Low, R. N. (1997). Contrast agents for MR imaging of the liver. *J. Magn. Reson. Imag.* **7,** 56–67.

Madio, D. P., Van-Gelderen, P., DesPres, D., Olson, A., de-Zwart, J., Fawcett, T., Holbrook, N. J., Mandel, M., and Moonen, C. T. (1998). On the feasibility of MRI-guided focused ultrasound for local induction of gene expression. *JMRI* **8,** 101–104.

Magin, R. L., Wright, S. M., Niesman, M. R., Chan, H. C., and Swartz, H. M. (1986). Liposome delivery of NMR contrast agents for improved tissue imaging. *Magn. Reson. Med.* **3,** 440–447.

Mathur de Vre, R., and Lemort, M. (1995). Biophysical properties and clinical applications of magnetic resonance imaging contrast agents. *Br. J. Radiol.* **68,** 225–247.

Medrova, Z., Pham, W., Farrar, C., Petkova, V., and Moore, A. (2007). *In vivo* imaging of siRNA delivery and silencing in tumors. *Nat. Med.* **13,** 372–377.

Mikhaylova, M., Stasinopoulos, I., Kato, Y., Artemov, D., and Bhujwalla, Z. M. (2009). Imaging of cationic multifunctional liposome-mediated delivery of COX-2 siRNA. *Cancer Gene Ther.* **16,** 217–226.

Modo, M., Hoehn, J. W., and Bulte, J. W. (2005). Cellular MR imaging. *Mol. Imag.* **4,** 143–164.

Moore, A., Marecos, E., Bogdanov, J. A., and Weissleder, R. (2000). Tumoral distribution of long-circulating dextran-coated iron oxide nanoparticles in a rodent model. *Radiology* **214,** 568–574.

Moore, A., Josephson, L., Bhorade, R. M., and Basilion, J. P. (2001). Human transferrin receptor gene as a marker gene for MR imaging. *Radiology* **221,** 244–250.

Moore, A., Medarova, Z., Potthast, A., and Dai, G. (2004). *In vivo* targeting of underglycosylated MUC-1 tumor antigen using a multimodal imaging probe. *Cancer Res.* **64,** 1821–1827.

Morawski, A. M., Winter, P. M., Crowder, K. C., Caruthers, S. D., Fuhrhop, R. W., Scott, M. J., Robertson, J. D., Abendschein, D. R., Lanza, G. M., and Wickline, S. A. (2004). Targeted nanoparticles for quantitative imaging of sparse molecular epitopes with MRI. *Magn. Reson. Med.* **51,** 480–486.

Morucci, J. P., and Rigaud, B. (1996). Bioelectrical impedance techniques in medicine. Part III: Impedance imaging. Third section: Medical applications. *Crit. Rev. Biomed. Eng.* **24,** 655–677.

Mulligan, R. C. (1993). The basic science of gene therapy. *Science* **260,** 926–932.

Nabel, G. J., Nabel, E. G., Yang, Z., Fox, B. A., Plautz, G. E., Gao, X., Huang, L., Shu, S., Gordon, D., and Chang, A. E. (1993). Direct gene transfer with DNA-liposome complexes in melanoma: Expression biological activity, and lack of toxicity in humans. *PNAS* **90,** 11307.

Nakaya, Y., and Mori, H. (1992). Magnetocardiography. *Clin. Phys. Physiol. Meas.* **13,** 191–229.

Nguyen, D. M., Wiehle, S. A., Koch, P. E., Branch, C., Yen, N., Roth, J. A., and Cristiano, R. J. (1997). Delivery of the p53 tumor suppressor gene into lung cancer cells by an adenovirus/DNA complex. *Cancer Gene Ther.* **4,** 191–198.

Nicholson, J. K., Lindon, J. C., and Holmes, E. (1999). Metabonomics': Understanding the metabolic responses of living systems to pathophysiological stimuli via multivariate statistical analysis of biological NMR spectroscopic data. *Xenobiotica* **29,** 1181–1189.

Pasini, P., Musiani, M., Russo, C., Valenti, P., Aicardi, G., Crabtree, J. E., Baraldini, M., and Roda, A. (1998). Chemiluminescence imaging in bioanalysis. *J. Pharm. Biomed. Anal.* **18,** 555–564.

Peng, K. W. (1999). Strategies for targeting therapeutic gene delivery. *Mol. Med. Today* **5,** 448–453.

Protti, A., Herlihy, A., Tessier, J., So, P.-W., Kalber, T., and Bell, J. D. (2009). Diagonal-SPRITE and its applications for *in vivo* imaging at high field. *Open Magn. Reson. J.* **2,** 1–7.

Qiu, B., El-Sharkawy, A. M., Paliwal, V., Gao, F., Karmarkar, P., Atalar, E., and Yang, X. (2004). Simultaneous radiofrequency (RF) heating and magnetic resonance (MR) thermal mapping using an intravascular MR imaging/RF heating system. *Magn. Reson. Med.* **54,** 226–230.

Räty, J. R., Liimatainen, T., Wirth, T., Airenne, K. J., Ihalaninen, T. O., Huhtala, T., Hamerlynck, E., Vihinen-Ranta, M., Närvänen, A., Ylä-Herttuala, S., and Hakumäki, J. M. (2006). Magnetic resonance imaging of viral particle distribution *in vivo*. *Gene Ther.* **13,** 1440–1446.

Remsen, L. G., McCormick, C. I., Roman-Goldstein, S., Nilaver, G., Weissleder, R., Bogdanov, A., Hellstrom, K. E., Kroll, R. A., and Neuwelt, E. A. (1996). MR of carcinoma-specific monoclonal antibody conjugated to monocrystalline iron oxide nanoparticles: The potential for non-invasive diagnosis. *Am. J. Neuroradiol.* **17,** 411–418.

Renshaw, P. F., Owen, C. S., Evans, A. E., and Leigh, J. S., Jr (1986). Immunospecific NMR contrast agents. *Magn. Reson. Imag.* **4,** 351–357.

Riley, P. A. (2003). Melanogenesis and melanoma. *Pigment Cell Res.* **16,** 548–552.

Roberts, T. P., Poeppel, D., and Rowley, H. A. (1998). Magnetoencephalography and magnetic source imaging. *Neuropsychiatry Neuropsychol. Behav. Neurol.* **11,** 49–64.

Rogers, W. J., Meyer, C. H., and Kramer, C. M. (2006). Technology insight: *In vivo* cell tracking by use of MRI. *Nat. Clin. Pract. Cardiovasc. Med.* **3,** 554–562.

Ross, D., Kim, B., and Davidson, B. (1995). Assessment of ganciclovir toxicity to experimental intracranial gliomas following recombinant adenoviral-mediated transfer of the herpes simplex virus thymidine kinase gene by magnetic resonance imaging and proton magnetic resonance imaging. *Clin. Cancer Res.* **1,** 651–657.

Russell, S. J., and Cosset, F. L. (1999). Modifying the host range properties of retroviral vectors. *J. Gene Med.* **1,** 300–311.

Sadeghi, H., and Hitt, M. M. (2005). Transcriptionally targeted adenovirus vectors. *Curr. Gene Ther.* **5,** 411–427.

Saito, R., Bringas, J. R., McKnight, T. R., Wendland, M. F., Mamot, C., Drummond, D. C., Kirpotin, D. B., Park, J.W., Berger, M. S., and Bankiewicz, K. S. (2004). Distribution of liposomes into brain and rat brain tumor models by convection-enhanced delivery monitored with magnetic resonance imaging. *Cancer Res.* **64,** 2572–2579.

Saukkonen, K., and Hemminki, A. (2004). Tissue-specific promoters for cancer gene therapy. *Expert Opin. Biol. Ther.* **4,** 683–693.

Schellingerhout, D., Bogdanov, A., Marecos, E., Spear, M., Breakefield, X., and Weissleder, R. (1998). Mapping the *in vivo* distribution of herpes simplex virions. *Hum. Gene Ther.* **9,** 1543–1549.

Seppenwoolde, J.-H., Viergever, M. A., and Bakker, C. J. G. (2003). Passive tracking exploiting local signal conservation: The white matter phenomena. *Magn. Reson. Imag.* **50,** 784–790.

Shyu, K. G., Chang, H., Wang, B. W., and Kuan, P. (2003). Intramuscular vascular endothelial growth factor gene therapy in patients with chronic critical leg ischemia. *Am. J. Med.* **114,** 85–92.

Smith, R. C., Machluf, M., Bromley, P., Atala, A., and Walsh, K. (2002). Spatial and temporal control of transgene expression through ultrasound-mediated induction of the heat protein 70B promoter *in vivo*. *Hum. Gene Ther.* **13,** 697–706.

So, P.-W., Hotee, S., Herlihy, A. H., and Bell, J. D. (2005). Genetic method for imaging transgene expression. *Magn. Reson. Med.* **54,** 218–221.

Stegman, L. D., Themetulla, A., Beattie, B., Kievit, E., Lawrence, T. S., Blasberg, R. G., Tjuvajev, J. G., and Ross, B. D. (1999). Non-invasive quantitation of cytosine deaminase transgene expression in human tumor xenografts with *in vivo* magnetic resonance spectroscopy. *Proc. Natl. Acad. Sci. USA* **96,** 9821–9826.

Susil, R. C., Krieger, A., Derbyshire, J. A., Tanacs, A., Whitcomb, L. L., Fichtinger, G., and Atalar, E. (2003). System for MR image-guided prostate interventions: Canine study. *Radiology* **228,** 886–894.

Suzuki, M., Honda, H., Kobayashi, T., Wakabayashi, T., Yoshida, J., and Taka, M. (1996). Development of a target-directed magnetic resonance contrast agent using monoclonal antibody-conjugated magnetic particles. *Noshuyo Byori* **13,** 27–32.

Suzuki, T., Shin, B. C., Fujikura, K., Matsuzaki, T., and Takata, K. (1998). Direct gene transfer into rat liver cells by *in vivo* electroporation. *FEBS Lett.* **425,** 436–440.

Tal, J. (2000). Adeno-associated virus-based vectors in gene therapy. *J. Biomed. Sci.* **7**(4), 279–291.

Tang, M., Redemann, C., and Szoka, F. (1996). *In vitro* gene delivery by degraded polyamidoamine dendrimers. *Bioconjug. Chem.* **7,** 703–714.

Tannous, B. A., Grimm, J., Perry, K. F., Chen, J. W., Weissleder, R., and Breakefield, X. O. (2006). Metabolic biotinylation of cell surface receptors for *in vivo* imaging. *Nat. Methods* **3,** 391–396.

Terreno, E., Castelli, D. D., Cravotto, G., Milone, L., and Aime, S. (2004). Ln(III)-DOTAMGly complexes: A versatile series to assess the determinants of the efficacy of paramagnetic chemical exchange saturation transfer agents for magnetic resonance imaging applications. *Invest. Radiol.* **39,** 235–243.

Theodore, W. H., Delgado-Escueta, A. V., and Porter, R. J. (1999). Frontiers in brain imaging and therapeutics. Introduction. *Adv. Neurol.* **79,** 865–871.

To, S. Y., Castro, D. J., Luftkin, R. B., Soudant, J., and Saxton, R. E. (1992). Monoclonal antibody-coated magnetite particles as contrast agents for MR imaging and laser therapy of human tomors. *J. Clin. Laser Med. Surg.* **10,** 159–169.

Tweedle, M. F., Hagan, J. J., Kumar, K., Mantha, S., and Chang, C. A. (1991). Reaction of gadolinium chelates with endogenously available ions. *Magn. Reson. Imag.* **9,** 409–415.

Tyynela, K., Sandmair, A. M., Turunen, M., Vanninen, R., Vainio, P., Kauppinen, R., Johansson, R., Vapalahti, M., and Yla-Herttuala, S. (2002). Adenovirus-mediated herpes simplex virus thymidine kinase gene therapy in BT4C rat glioma model. *Cancer Gene Ther.* **9,** 917–924.

Unger, E., Needleman, P., Cullis, P., and Tilcock, C. (1988). Gadolinium-DTPA liposomes as a potential MRI contrast agent.Work in progress *Invest. Radiol.* **23,** 928–932.

Varga, C. M., Wickham, T. J., and Lauffenburger, D. A. (2000). Receptor-mediated targeting of gene delivery vectors: Insights from molecular mechanisms for improved vehicle design. *Biotechnol. Bioeng.* **70,** 593.

Vile, R. G., Russel, S. J., and Lemoine, N. R. (2000). Cancer gene therapy: Hard lessons and new courses. *Gene Ther.* **7,** 2.

Wagner, E., Zatloukal, K., Cotten, M., Kirlappos, H., Mechtler, K., Curiel, D. T., and Birnstiel, M. L. (1992). Coupling of adenovirus to transferrinpolylysine/DNA complexes greatly enhances receptor-mediated gene delivery and expression of transfected genes. *Proc. Natl. Acad. Sci. USA* **89,** 6099–6103.

Walter, G., Barton, E. R., and Sweeney, H.L (2000). Non-invasive measurement of gene expression in skeletal muscle. *Proc. Natl. Acad. Sci. USA* **97,** 5151–5155.

Walter, G., Cordier, L., Bloy, D., and Sweeney, H. L. (2005). Noninvasive monitoring of gene correction in dystrophic muscle. *Magn. Reson. Med.* **54,** 1369–1370.

Walther, W., and Stein, U. (2000). Viral vectors for gene transfer: A review of their use in the treatment of human diseases. *Drugs* **60,** 249–271.

Ward, K. M., Aletras, A. H., and Balaban, R. S. (2000). A new class of contrast agents for MRI based on proton chemical exchange dependent saturation transfer (CEST). *J. Magn. Reson.* **143,** 79–87.

Wardle, N. J., Herlihy, A. H., So, P.-W., Bell, J. D., and Bligh, S. W. (2007). Synthesis of a novel 'smart' bifunctional chelating agent 1-(2-[beta-D-galactopyranosyl-oxyl]ethyl)[7-(1-carboxy-3-[4-aminophenylpropyl)-4,10-bis(carboxymethyl)-1,4,7,10-tetraazacyclododecane (Gal-PA-DO3A-NH2) and its Gd(III) complexes. *Bioorg. Med. Chem.* **15,** 4714–4721.

Watson, A. D., Rocklage, S. M., and Carvlin, M. J. (1992). Contrast agents. *In* "Magnetic Resonance Imaging," (D. Stark, and W. G. Bradley, eds.), pp. 372–437. Mosby-Year Book, Missouri.

Weissleder, R., Simonova, M., Bogdanova, A., Bredow, S., Enochs, W., and Bogdanov, A. (1997). MR imaging and scintigraphy of gene expression through melanin induction. *Radiology* **204,** 425–429.

Weissleder, R., Tung, C. H., Mahmood, U., and Bogdanov, A., Jr (1999). *In vivo* imaging of tumors with protease-activated near-infrared fluorescent probes. *Nat. Biotechnol.* **17,** 375–378.

Weissleder, R., Moore, A., Mahmood, U., Bhorade, R., Benveniste, H., Chiocca, E. A., and Basilion, J. P. (2000). *In vivo* magnetic resonance imaging of transgene expression. *Nat. Med.* **6,** 351–355.

Winter, P. M., Morawski, A. M., Caruthers, S. D., Fuhrhop, R. W., Zhang, H., Williams, T. A., Allen, J. S., Lacy, E. K., Robertson, J. D., Lanza, G. M., and Wickline, S. A. (2003). Molecular imaging of angiogenesis of early-stage atherosclerosis with alpha(v)beta3-integrin-targeted nanoparticles. *Circulation* **108,** 2270–2274.

Wiznerowicz, M., Fong, A. Z. C., Mackiewicz, A., and Hawley, R. G. (1997). Double-copy bicistronic retroviral vector platform for gene therapy and tissue engineering: Application to melanoma vaccine development. *Gene Ther.* **4,** 1061–1068.

Yang, X., Atalar, E., Li, D., Serfaty, J- M., Wang, D., Kumar, A., and Cheng, L. (2001). Magnetic resonance imaging permits *in vivo* monitoring of catheter-based vascular gene delivery. *Circulation* **104,** 1588–1590.

Ye, X., Rivera, V. M., Zoltick, P., Cerasoli, F., Jr., Schnell, M. A., Gao, G., Hughes, J. V., Gilman, M., and Wilson, J. M. (1999). Regulated delivery of therapeutic proteins after *in vivo* somatic cell gene transfer. *Science* **283,** 88–91.

Yu, J. X., Kodibagkar, V. D., Liu, L., and Mason, R. P. (2008). A 19F-NMR approach using reporter molecule pairs to assess beta-galactosidase in human xenografts tumors *in vivo*. *NMR Biomed.* **21,** 704–712.

Yuan, J. P., Liang, B. L., Xie, B. K., and Zhong, J. L. (2003). Magnetic Resonance Imaging (MRI) in evaluation of tyrosinase gene expression in HepG2 Cell. *Ai Zheng* **22,** 156–159[Article in Chinese].

Zhao, M., and Weissleder, R. (2004). Intracellular cargo delivery using tat peptide and derivatives. *Med. Res. Rev.* **24,** 1–12.

Zhou, J., Payen, J. F., Wilson, D. A., Traystman, R. J., and van Zijl, P. C. M. (2003). Using the amide proton signals of intracellular proteins and peptides to detect pH effects in MRI. *Nat. Med.* **9,** 1085–1090.

CHAPTER 19

Voxelation Methods for Genome Scale Imaging of Brain Gene Expression

Daniel M. Sforza and Desmond J. Smith

Department of Molecular and Medical Pharmacology
Geffen School of Medicine
UCLA
23-120 CHS, Box 951735
Los Angeles, California 90095-1735

I. Update
  A. Significant Points
II. Introduction
III. Methods
  A. Sample Preparation
  B. Histologic Staining
  C. Physical Voxelation
  D. RNA Isolation and Quality Check
  E. Microarrays, RNA Labeling, and Hybridization
IV. Data Analysis
  A. Low-Level Analysis
  B. High-Level Analysis
  C. Image Reconstruction
References

I. Update

In the original chapter, we described methods for constructing brain expression maps of the mouse and human brain using voxelation. We focused on the use of a voxelation instrument to create expression images for single genes at 1 mm^3 resolution employing real-time polymerase chain reaction (PCR). The voxelation device has since been used in combination with microarrays to create expression maps for a section of the mouse brain at the level of the striatum for nearly all known genes

ESSENTIAL BIOIMAGING METHODS

DOI: 10.1016/B978-0-12-375043-3.00019-6

(Chin *et al.*, 2007). Gene clusters expressed in cortex, corpus callosum and hypothalamus were identified. In addition, a gene cluster with a dorsal/ventral expression gradient was found. One member of the cluster was cystathionine β-synthase, a gene previously implicated in dorsal neural tube defects in humans, suggesting that the cluster may be involved in specifying the dorsal/ventral axis in the mammalian brain. We have also developed methodologies for creation of proteomic maps of expression at 1 mm^3 resolution using voxelation and mass spectrometry (Petyuk *et al.*, 2007). Expression maps for 1000 proteins were constructed from a brain slice possessing the same coordinates as the transcriptomic atlas. There was good agreement between the protein maps and the corresponding transcript maps. We are currently working on using voxelation to create 3D maps of protein expression in the mouse brain at 1 mm^3 resolution. On the bioinformatics front, combinatorial optimization methods have been developed for analysis of voxelation data, allowing robust identification of discriminative groups of genes in Alzheimer's and Parkinson's disease (Berretta *et al.*, 2008; Hourani *et al.*, 2008). As array methods continue to drop in price and are ultimately supplanted by next generation sequencing technologies, voxelation will continue to find useful applications in neuroscience. Plans for building a voxelation device, as well as expression maps and data are available from our web site (http://labs.pharmacology.ucla.edu/smithlab/).

A. Significant Points

- Pooling multiple replicates of voxelation array data yields improved data quality.
- Expression patterns of individual genes of particular interest can be confirmed using real-time PCR.
- Voxelation can be used to map expression patterns of transcripts, proteins, and metabolites.
- A cost-effective alterative to the 1 mm resolution voxelation device is to replace the lithographically constructed blades with stainless steel razor blades.

II. Introduction

Imaging techniques have granted access to significant results on structure and function in the central nervous system. In addition, the completion of the human genome sequence promises to accelerate even further the already extraordinary developments of molecular biology. Therefore, it is a natural step to seek an integration of both fields for a better understanding of the molecular basis of the brain. One strategy employs reporter genes, and this has been a major advance in molecular imaging. However, although this approach has important advantages, such as *in vivo* imaging, it does not provide convenient access to genome-wide information but only the examination of one, or at most, a few genes at a time (Gambhir *et al.*, 1999a,b; Herschman *et al.*, 2000; Louie *et al.*, 2000; Zacharias *et al.*, 2000). One recently developed approach for genome-scale acquisition of brain gene expression patterns employs microarray analysis of spatially registered voxels (cubes) harvested from the brain (Liu and Smith, 2003; Singh and Smith, 2003). This method is called voxelation and provides a mapping of gene expression analogous to the images reconstructed in biomedical imaging techniques, such as X-ray computerized tomography (CT), positron emission tomography (PET), and magnetic resonance imaging (MRI).

Voxelation has permitted high-throughput gene expression reconstructions in human and rodent brains (Brown *et al.*, 2002a,b; Ossadtchi *et al.*, 2002; Singh *et al.*, 2003). One study using human brains compared gene expression between brains from normal individuals and brains from individuals with Alzheimer's disease (Brown *et al.*, 2002a). The mouse studies investigated global gene expression patterns in brains of a Parkinson's disease model induced by toxic doses of methamphetamine compared with controls (Brown *et al.*, 2002b).

The previously mentioned voxelation studies used fresh tissue slabs, but a weakness of this approach is the deformation of the tissue during the process of physical voxelation, which can make problematic the registration of gene expression analysis results to the neuroanatomy. Although this is not a major problem for low-resolution studies, it becomes a significant factor at higher resolution. Therefore, we have developed a new voxelation protocol to overcome this drawback and make feasible higher-resolution studies (Sforza *et al.*, 2004). The new procedure involves the use of a fixation process to avoid tissue deformation and to allow histologic staining (Annese and Toga, 2002), as well as cryoprotection to allow harvesting of slabs from frozen specimens (Rosene and Rhodes, 1990). These protocols have been shown to preserve RNA quality and yield at excellent levels, and allow the use of quality demanding downstream applications such as real-time PCR or DNA microarrays (Sforza *et al.*, 2004).

In the following sections, we review the complete protocols and methods for high-resolution voxelation, from samples preparation to data analysis and image reconstruction.

III. Methods

The following protocol can be applied to rodent or monkey studies and requires the use of intercardiac perfusion. Here, we provide the times and volumes of the solutions used for adult C57BL/6J male mice (10–24 weeks, 25–31 g) for which the protocol was developed (Sforza *et al.*, 2004), but it can be easily adapted to the other cases. For all perfusions, a small mechanical pump was used that allowed a flux of 1.5 ml/min. To easily switch among the different solutions and avoid the formation of bubbles, a serial connection of three-way stopcocks with swivel male luer lock was used (MX231–1L; Medex, Hilliard, OH) and carefully filled with the solutions before starting the procedure.

A. Sample Preparation

1. Mice must undergo intracardiac perfusion under deep halothane anesthesia. For each animal the vasculature is cleared with 11–22 ml of ice-cold phosphate buffered saline solution (PBS).
2. Fixation: 67 ml of 4% paraformaldehyde in PBS (pH 7.4) is perfused for a period of 45 min.
3. Cryoprotection: mice are additionally perfused with 67 ml of 10%, 20%, and 30% ice-cold phosphate buffered sucrose solutions (pH 7.4). The sucrose solutions are each perfused for 45 min.
4. After perfusion, brains are removed from the skull and immediately frozen in chilled isopentane or liquid nitrogen. Tissue blocks are kept at −70 °C until RNA testing and histologic processing.

This complete protocol lasts approximately 190 min.

B. Histologic Staining

As voxelation studies are pushed to higher resolution, registration between the harvested voxels and the neuroanatomy becomes increasingly important. At lower levels of resolution, visual inspection and digital photographs of fresh sections are sufficient for registration. However, the inherent low contrast of fresh specimens makes it difficult to identify boundaries between structures of small size or subtly different microscopic anatomy, and this hinders image reconstruction at high resolution. Proper use of the described fixation and cryoprotection protocol allows the use of histologic stains to improve contrast in the voxelated section and facilitate image registration. There are methods available for histologic staining of tissue compatible with the recovery of good quality RNA for gene expression studies (Bonaventure *et al.*, 2002).

C. Physical Voxelation

The equipment required for voxelation depends on the specimen under study and on the desired resolution. A detailed description of voxelation devices and procedures for human and rodent species can be found by Liu and Smith (2003). Furthermore, supplementary information on the design and construction of these pieces of equipment (including blueprints) is given at our web site (http://labs.pharmacology.ucla.edu/smithlab/). The devices essentially consist of two-dimensional arrays of blades, together with supporting and guiding mechanisms to facilitate registered harvesting of voxels. Voxelation devices have been constructed that harvest square voxels of size 3.3 mm (used in the human studies, a 425-voxel template, consisting of 25 voxels in length and 17 voxels in width) to 1 mm (used in the rodent studies, a 400-voxel template, 20 × 20 voxels) (Singh *et al.*, 2003).

The selection of the actual section for voxelation obviously depends on the nature of the investigation. At the moment all voxelation studies have investigated coronal sections. Human studies on Alzheimer's disease focused on left coronal hemisections that included the hippocampus, corresponding to section 17 of the University of Maryland Brain and Tissue Bank protocol, method 2 (http://medschool.umaryland.edu/BTBank/) (Brown *et al.*, 2002a). The thickness of the slab is also an important factor in order to obtain enough RNA for microarray hybridization, as well as for the accuracy of the regions identified on the section. In the human studies, the slice thickness was 8 mm. In the study of the mouse model of Parkinson's disease (Brown *et al.*, 2002b), a different strategy was applied. The whole brain was divided into slices of thickness 1 mm using a brain matrix (Harvard Apparatus, Inc., Holliston, MA). Each slice was then divided into four voxels, giving a total of 40 voxels, and an average volumetric resolution of 7.5 μl. The existence of voxelation instruments for the rodent brain will allow acquisition of expression images at 1 mm (1 μl) resolution (Singh *et al.*, 2003).

It is important to obtain digital pictures of the selected slab before and after voxelation in order to evaluate possible deformation induced by the procedure, as we already mentioned, this is more likely to be a problem as resolution is increased. In addition, digital pictures are required for image registration and reconstruction (see Section IV).

D. RNA Isolation and Quality Check

There are many commercially available RNA isolation kits. Lately, we have obtained excellent yields and quality using the RNeasy Lipid Tissue Mini Kit column (Qiagen, Hilden, Germany). Frozen samples are placed in QIAzol Lysis Reagent (Qiagen) and homogenized using a Tissue-Tearor homogenizer (BioSpec Products, Bartlesville, OK). Subsequent steps are done according to the instructions provided by the manufacturer of the RNeasy kit. Total RNA quality is assessed by microcapillary electrophoresis using the Agilent BioAnalyzer 2100 (Agilent Technologies, Palo Alto, CA). Evaluation of 18-s and 28-s RNA peaks and background noise are employed for this purpose.

The cryoprotection step is very important to achieve good RNA quality and recovery. It is well known that paraformaldehyde fixation results in an apparent decrease in both the recovery and quality of RNA extracted from brain (Goldsworthy *et al.*, 1999; Parlato *et al.*, 2002; Scheidl *et al.*, 2002). However, we have shown that sucrose perfusion following fixation helps preserve the RNA (Sforza *et al.*, 2004).

The long time required for the complete protocol might raise doubts about RNA quality, but these are unfounded. Our experience is consistent with published work in the sense that the quality of RNA from human brains depends on brain pH, a measure of premortem condition, rather than postmortem interval (Harrison *et al.*, 1995).

E. Microarrays, RNA Labeling, and Hybridization

High-resolution voxelation requires the use of a large number of microarrays, so the use of spotted cDNA arrays is the natural option due to their relatively low cost. The list of clones used in published voxelation investigations can be obtained at our web site (http://labs.pharmacology.ucla.edu/smithlab/). To produce targets for hybridization to the cDNA microarrays, 10 μg of total RNA is labeled with fluorescent nucleotides by chemical coupling following reverse transcription. The total RNA is mixed with 6μg of anchored oligo-dT (5′-TTTTTTTTTTTTT-TTTTT VN-3′) and hybridization achieved by incubation at 70 °C for 10 min, followed by 10 min at 4 °C in a total volume of 18 μl. The annealed RNA is then reverse-transcribed in a 30-μl reaction mix containing reaction buffer (50 mM Tris-HCl, 75 mM KCl, 3 mM $MgCl_2$, pH 8.3); 10 mM dithiothreitol; 200 μM dATP, dGTP, and dCTP; 51μM dTTP; 149 μM amino-allyl-UTP (Sigma, St. Louis, MO); and 200U SuperScript II reverse transcriptase (Life Technologies, Gaithersburg, MD). The reactions are incubated at 42 °C for 2 h. Following incubation, 10 μl of 1 M NaOH and 10 μl of 0.5 M EDTA are added to degrade the template RNA, and the samples are incubated at 70 °C for 10 min. The reaction is neutralized by the addition of 10 μl of 1 M HCl, followed by 300 μl of Qiagen Buffer PB (PCR Cleanup kit; Qiagen, Valencia, CA). Reactions are purified using Qiagen's PCR cleanup kit following the manufacturer's directions with the substitution of 80% ethanol for Qiagen's PE buffer and water for Qiagen's EB buffer.

Following purification, individual samples are desiccated, resuspended in 7 μl 0.1 M sodium bicarbonate buffer, and chemically coupled to monofunctional reactive cyanine dyes (Amersham Biosciences, Buckinghamshire, England). Unbound cyanine dyes are removed by purification with Qiagen's PCR cleanup kit as described earlier. Following purification, the labeled samples are combined in Cy3-Cy5 pairs, desiccated, and resuspended in 100 μl hybridization buffer (25% formamide, 5× SSC, 0.1% sodium dodecyl sulfate (SDS), 10 μg yeast tRNA, 10 μg poly-A-RNA, 1 μg human COT-1 DNA). Immediately prior to hybridization, the microarrays are prehybridized in a solution of 5× SSC, 1% SDS, and 1% bovine serum albumin (BSA) at 55 °C for 45 min. Following prehybridization, the arrays are vigorously washed in ddH_2O to remove all traces of the prehybridization solution, rinsed in isopropanol, and dried at room temperature (RT).

The labeled RNA samples are denatured at 95 °C for 2 min and placed on the prehybridized arrays, covered with Lifterslip coverslips (25 mm × 60 mm; Erie Scientific, Inc., Portsmouth, NH), placed in a hybridization chamber (Corning, Acton, MA) with 30 μl hybridization buffer to maintain humidity, and incubated at 42 °C for 16 h in a standard hybridization oven. After hybridization, the arrays are washed in 2× SSC to remove the coverslips, placed in 2× SSC, 0.1% SDS at 55 °C with agitation for 5 min then washed with two successive 5 min washes with 1× SSC and 0.1× SSC at RT. The washed arrays are dried by centrifugation at 50 × *g* for 5 min and immediately scanned using a GenePix 4000A microarray scanner (Axon Instruments, Union City, CA).

IV. Data Analysis

Voxelation studies yield large amounts of data, and a variety of different analytical techniques can be employed for data mining. There are low- and high-level analyses of the microarray data, described in Sections IV.A and IV.B. Also important is how to display the large amount of information retrieved from microarrays in a meaningful and appealing manner. This is discussed in Section IV.C. Unless otherwise specified, all computational algorithms described are written in Matlab scripting language (Matlab 5.3 or later required) and can be retrieved from the lab web site (http://labs.pharmacology.ucla.edu/smithlab/). The algorithms are run on a personal computer and are not highly demanding of resources, so a workstation is not required.

A. Low-Level Analysis

Low-level analysis refers to image processing of scanned microarray images and normalization (within array and interarrays). Images are usually processed by the software bundle included with the scanner, and they allow automatic spot segmentation and acquisition of intensity values in both channels. In our case the microarray scanner is a GenePix 4000A (Axon Instruments) with GenePix Pro 3.0 software. An important step is the normalization of the data to correct the multiple sources of systematic variation in cDNA microarray experiments that affect measured gene expression levels (Yang *et al.*, 2002). The normalization procedure we have applied in our studies consists of the removal of spatial trends due to array printing by a nonlinear transformation of the data set and the compensation for differences in the labeling of Cy3 and Cy5 dyes by aligning the histograms of the dye signals both within, as well as between, microarrays. The normalization method relies on the assumption that most of the genes do not change significantly between different experimental conditions.

B. High-Level Analysis

After the data have been properly normalized, calculated gene expression values can be subjected to further analysis in the search of relevant biologic information. The most common first step in the analysis of the data is the identification of significantly changing expression values; this singles out genes that are upregulated or downregulated in the comparison between control and experimental conditions. Even more interesting is the identification of clusters of coregulated and antiregulated genes, which can potentially identify regulatory networks (Brown *et al.*, 2002a,b).

There are also exploratory techniques that do not rely on a priori hypotheses or assumptions concerning the data, such as singular value decomposition. This method can identify clusters of genes (gene “vectors”) that most efficiently explain the variance in the data. It has been shown that these gene vectors display interesting regional patterns of expression, and their associated genes may play an important role in differentiation of the mouse and human brain (Brown *et al.*, 2002a,b). In addition, a gene vector has been identified that shows a significant spatial shift away from the striatum in the normal mouse brain toward the hippocampus in the Parkinson's brain (Brown *et al.*, 2002b). These results suggest that high-throughput acquisition of gene expression patterns in combination with singular value decomposition has the potential to identify functionally abnormal neuroanatomic regions in neurologic disease states. This is especially relevant given the fact that for many neuropsychiatric disorders, such as schizophrenia, Down syndrome, and autism, the location of functionally abnormal brain regions associated with the diseases remains enigmatic. The higher resolution gene expression images that can be obtained following the protocols described here would potentially allow the precise identification of such important regions, given that they exist.

Another technique that has proved powerful in modeling microarray data from voxelation is the analysis of variance (ANOVA) (Kerr and Churchill, 2001; Kerr *et al.*, 2000; Ossadtchi *et al.*, 2002). With microarray data analysis, there is always an underlying question: how to calculate valid estimates of gene expression values that take into account potential sources of variation, both from experimental design and error. ANOVA can provide corrected estimates of change in gene expression with the estimation of potential confounding effects. The use of ANOVA to analyze voxelation data was found to produce results consistent with those from singular value decomposition (Ossadtchi *et al.*, 2002).

C. Image Reconstruction

High-resolution voxelation can result in demanding data sets for image reconstruction. The addition of a staining step in the protocol can help greatly, especially at high resolution, as we have already discussed. The basic problem is to align an actual voxelated slab to a corresponding atlas image. The final image represents the overlapping of an anatomic image and gene expression levels converted into pseudocolor. The registration between the picture of the actual voxelated section and the atlas image is accomplished using an implementation of the thin-plate splines warping method (Bookstein, 1989). This method interpolates surfaces between scattered fiducial landmarks, and its name refers to a physical analogy involving the bending of a thin sheet of metal subject to point constraints (the landmarks that relate both images). The manual selection of corresponding fiducial landmarks on both images allows the algorithm to warp the desired image onto the atlas reference. Gene expression images are further improved using interpolation and smoothing functions. For the high-resolution human expression images, the smoothing used about 2–4 voxels and for the high-resolution rodent images, only 1 voxel. Examples of final images obtained from voxelation are displayed in Fig. 1.

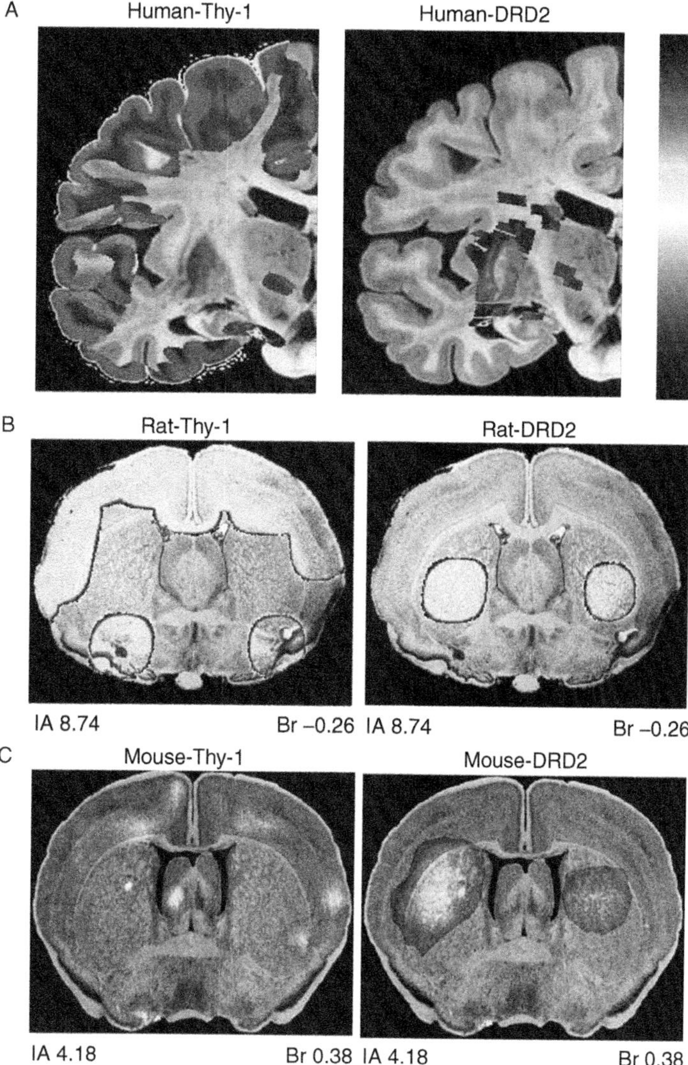

Fig. 1 Human and rodent brain voxelation gene expression images for Thy-1 and DRD2 (dopamine D2 receptor) genes. Images are the result of the methods explained in the text. Gene expression patterns are shown in pseudocolor and smoothed across voxels. Thy-1 is expressed in the cortex, DRD2 in the striatum (caudate/putamen). (A) Human brain, atlas section from Virtual Hospital: The Human Brain (http://www.vh.org). The voxel size was 3.3 mm. (B) Rat brain, coronal atlas section from Paxinos and Watson (Paxinos and Watson, 1986). The voxel size was 1 mm. Coordinates in mm: IA, interacural; Br, bregma. (C) Mouse brain, coronal atlas section from the Mouse Brain Library (http://www.mbl.org) (Williams, 2000). The voxel size was 1 mm. (See Plate no. 14 in the Color Plate Section.)

Acknowledgments

This work was supported by the NIH/NIDA (DA015802, DA05010) NARSAD Young Investigator Award, Tobacco-Related Disease Research Program (11RT-0172), and Alzheimer's Association (IIRG-02–3609).

References

Annese, J., and Toga, A. W. (2002). Postmortem Anatomy. *In* "Brain Mapping: The Methods," (A. W. Toga, and J. C. Mazziotta, eds.), p. 537. Academic Press, New York.

Berretta, R., Costa, W., and Moscato, P. (2008). Combinatorial optimization models for finding genetic signatures from gene expression datasets. *Methods Mol. Biol.* **453,** 363.

Bonaventure, P., Guo, H., Tian, B., Liu, X., Bittner, A., Roland, B., Salunga, R., Ma, X. J., Kamme, F., Meurers, B., Bakker, M., Jurzak, M., *et al.* (2002). Nuclei and subnuclei gene expression profiling in mammalian brain. *Brain Res.* **943,** 38.

Bookstein, F. L. (1989). Principal warps: Thin-plate splines and decomposition of deformations. *IEEE Trans. Pattern Anal. Mach. Intell.* **11,** 567.

Brown, V. M., Ossadtchi, A., Khan, A. H., Cherry, S. R., Leahy, R. M., and Smith, D. J. (2002a). High-throughput imaging of brain gene expression. *Genome Res.* **12,** 244.

Brown, V. M., Ossadtchi, A., Khan, A. H., Yee, S., Lacan, G., Melega, W. P., Cherry, S. R., Leahy, R. M., and Smith, D. J. (2002b). Multiplex three-dimensional brain gene expression mapping in a mouse model of Parkinson's disease. *Genome Res.* **12,** 868.

Chin, M. H., Geng, A. B., Khan, A. H., Qian, W. J., Petyuk, V. A., Boline, J., Levy, S., Toga, A. W., Smith, R. D., Leahy, R. M., and Smith, D. J. (2007). A genome-scale map of expression for a mouse brain section obtained using voxelation. *Physiol. Genomics* **30,** 313.

Gambhir, S. S., Barrio, J. R., Herschman, H. R., and Phelps, M. E. (1999a). Assays for noninvasive imaging of reporter gene expression. *Nucl. Med. Biol.* **26,** 481.

Gambhir, S. S., Barrio, J. R., Herschman, H. R., and Phelps, M. E. (1999b). Imaging gene expression: Principles and assays. *J. Nucl. Cardiol.* **6,** 219.

Goldsworthy, S. M., Stockton, P. S., Trempus, C. S., Foley, J. F., and Maronpot, R. R. (1999). Effects of fixation on RNA extraction and amplification from laser capture microdissected tissue. *Mol. Carcinog.* **25,** 86.

Harrison, P. J., Heath, P. R., Eastwood, S. L., Burnet, P. W., McDonald, B., and Pearson, R. C. (1995). The relative importance of premortem acidosis and postmortem interval for human brain gene expression studies: Selective mRNA vulnerability and comparison with their encoded proteins. *Neurosci. Lett.* **200,** 151.

Herschman, H. R., MacLaren, D. C., Iyer, M., Namavari, M., Bobinski, K., Green, L. A., Wu, L., Berk, A. J., Toyokuni, T., Barrio, J. R., Cherry, S. R., Phelps, M. E., *et al.* (2000). Seeing is believing: Non-invasive, quantitative and repetitive imaging of reporter gene expression in living animals, using positron emission tomography. *J. Neurosci. Res.* **59,** 699.

Hourani, M., Mendes, A., and Moscato, P. (2008). Genetic signatures for a rodent model of Parkinson's disease using combinatorial optimization methods. *Methods Mol. Biol.* **453,** 379.

Kerr, M. K., and Churchill, G. A. (2001). Statistical design and the analysis of gene expression microarray data. *Genet. Res.* **77,** 123.

Kerr, M. K., Martin, M., and Churchill, G. A. (2000). Analysis of variance for gene expression microarray data. *J. Comput. Biol.* **7,** 819.

Liu, D., and Smith, D. J. (2003). Voxelation and gene expression tomography for the acquisition of 3-D gene expression maps in the brain. *Methods* **31,** 317.

Louie, A. Y., Huber, M. M., Ahrens, E. T., Rothbacher, U., Moats, R., Jacobs, R. E., Fraser, S. E., and Meade, T. J. (2000). *In vivo* visualization of gene expression using magnetic resonance imaging. *Nat. Biotechnol.* **18,** 321.

Ossadtchi, A., Brown, V. M., Khan, A. H., Cherry, S. R., Nichols, T. E., Leahy, R. M., and Smith, D. J. (2002). Statistical analysis of multiplex brain gene expression images. *Neurochem. Res.* **27,** 1113.

Parlato, R., Rosica, A., Cuccurullo, V., Mansi, L., Macchia, P., Owens, J. D., Mushinski, J. F., De Felice, M., Bonner, R. F., and Di Lauro, R. (2002). A preservation method that allows recovery of intact RNA from tissues dissected by laser capture microdissection. *Anal. Biochem.* **300,** 139.

Paxinos, G., and Watson, C. (1986). "The Rat Brain in Stereotaxic Coordinates." Academic Press, Orlando, FL.

Petyuk, V. A., Qian, W. J., Chin, M. H., Wang, H., Livesay, E. A., Monroe, M. E., Adkins, J. N., Jaitly, N., Anderson, D. J., Camp, D. G., 2nd, Smith, D. J., and Smith, R. D. (2007). Spatial mapping of protein abundances in the mouse brain by voxelation integrated with high-throughput liquid chromatography-mass spectrometry. *Genome Res.* **17,** 328.

Rosene, D. L., and Rhodes, K. J. (1990). Cryoprotection and freezing methods that control ice crystal artifact and frozen sections from fixed and unfixed blocks of monkey and human brain tissue. *In* "Methods in Neuroscience, Vol. 3: Quantitative and Qualitative Microscopy," (P. M. Conn, ed.), p. 360. Academic Press, New York.

Scheidl, S. J., Nilsson, S., Kalen, M., Hellstrom, M., Takemoto, M., Hakansson, J., and Lindahl, P. (2002). mRNA expression profiling of laser microbeam microdissected cells from slender embryonic structures. *Am. J. Pathol.* **160,** 801.

Sforza, D. M., Annese, J., Liu, D., Levy, S., Toga, A. W., and Smith, D. J. (2004). Anatomical methods for voxelation of the mammalian brain. *Neurochem. Res.* **29,** 1299.

Singh, R. P., and Smith, D. J. (2003). Genome scale mapping of brain gene expression. *Biol. Psychiatry* **53,** 1069.

Singh, R. P., Brown, V. M., Chaudhari, A., Khan, A. H., Ossadtchi, A., Sforza, D. M., Meadors, A. K., Cherry, S. R., Leahy, R. M., and Smith, D. J. (2003). High-resolution voxelation mapping of human and rodent brain gene expression. *J. Neurosci. Methods* **125,** 93.

Williams, R. W. (2000). Mapping genes that modulate mouse brain development: A quantitative genetic approach. *Results Probl. Cell Differ.* **30,** 21.

Yang, Y. H., Dudoit, S., Luu, P., Lin, D. M., Peng, V., Ngai, J., and Speed, T. P. (2002). Normalization for cDNA microarray data: A robust composite method addressing single and multiple slide systematic variation. *Nucleic Acids Res.* **30,** e15.

Zacharias, D. A., Baird, G. S., and Tsien, R. Y. (2000). Recent advances in technology for measuring and manipulating cell signals. *Curr. Opin. Neurobiol.* **10,** 416.

INDEX

Page numbers followed by f indicate figures

A

1-[^{11}C]Acetate synthesis. *See also* Carbon-11 radiotracers
  [^{11}C]CO_2 gas trap and purification method, 161–162
  chemistry synthesizer, CTI acetate module, 162–163, 162f
  Hudson robotic system, 160–161, 161f
Alzheimer's disease (AD)
  MRI applications, 290–291
  PET, 13–14
Aminoguanidine evaluation, TBI
  caspase-3 immunohistochemistry, 332–333
  in situ TUNEL, 334
  lateral fluid-percussive brain injury, 327
  MRI methods and analysis, 327–329
  neurologic and behavioral test
    acoustic startle response, 330
    forelimb grip-strength test, 330
    locomotor activity, 329
    rotametric test, 331
  perfusion, 331–332
β-Amyloid (Aβ) plaques, 292f
Aneurysm, stroke, 244f
Angiogenesis, optical imaging
  antibody-conjugated paramagnetic polymerized vesicles (ACPVs), 349–351
  arthritis study, 260
  dorsal skin window chamber model, 253
  endothelial-targeted imaging, 342
  fluorescent protein-labeled tumor cells, 256–260
  intravascular fluorescent probes, markers
    BF velocity measurement, 264–266
    capillary perfusion and permeability, 263–264
  multiphoton laser-scanning microscope (MPLSM), 259–260
  PET quantitation, 16–17
  transgenic mouse model
    arthritis synovium, 261f
    conjunctiva capillary, Tie2-GFP mouse, 261f
    corneal angiogenesis assay, 262–263
    laser-scanning confocal microscopy (LSCM), Tie2-GFP mouse, 261–262
  tumor development imaging
    blood flow, 255
    hypoxia, 256
    tortuosity, 255
    tumor size, 256
    tumor vascular length density, 254
    vascular permeability (VP), 255
    vessel dilation, 255
  tumor-host interaction
    antivascular endothelial growth model (VEGF), 258
    green fluorescent protein (GFP), 256–260
    vascular response, 257–258
    window chamber model images, 257f
Antibody-conjugated paramagnetic polymerized vesicles (ACPVs), 344, 345f
Anti-intercellular cell adhesion molecule (ICAM), 346, 347f
Antivascular endothelial growth model (VEGF), 258
Anti-VCAM antibody-avidin conjugation, 345f
Apoptosis, PET, 17
Apparent diffusion coefficient (ADC), 276, 309–310
Arterial spin labeling (ASL)
  continuous (CASL), 280
  MR relaxation, 188–189
  pulsed (PASL), 280–282
Atlas space
  b2k and b2kf baboon atlas development
    animal age, 57
    image acquisition and registration, 57–58, 60–61
    sagittal section image, 59f
    template image development, 58–60, 61
    validation, 60, 61
  n2k and n2kf macaque template images, 61–62

B

Bacterial infections, MRI
pneumonia
histological slices comparison, 309f
Streptococcus pneumoniae, 307–308
transversal images comparison, 308f
thigh infections
region-of-interest (ROI) analysis, 306–307
signal intensity (SI), 305
Staphylococcus aureus, 304–305
Blood oxygenation level-dependent (BOLD) effect, 33–34, 188–189
Blood velocity measurements, LSCM, 264–266, 265f
Brain disease, MRI
cerebral ischemia
ADC changes, stroke, 284–286
BOLD, 288
brain reorganization, stroke, 287–288
CBF, stroke, 286
diffusion/perfusion mismatch region, 285f
intraluminal suture occlusion, 285f
penumbra, 286–287
spreading depression, 287
CNS inflammation
experimental allergic encephalopathy (EAE), 293
magnetization transfer ratio (MTR), 294
multiple sclerosis, 293–294
epilepsy
long-term changes, 289–290
short-term changes, 289
gene expression, voxelation methods
data analysis, 405–407
histologic staining, 402
microarrays, RNA labeling, hybridization, 404
physical voxelation method, 402–403
RNA isolation, quality check, 403
sample preparation, 402
magnetization transfer contrast (MTC)
measurements, 282–284
origin of, 283f
neurodegenerative disorders
Alzheimer's disease, 290–291
Huntington's disease, 291
Parkinson's disease, 290
perfusion, CBF measurement
arterial spin labeling, 279–282
arterial spin labeling (ASL), 279–282
bolus tracking, 278
flow-sensitive alternating inversion recovery (FAIR), 281f
sample diffusion measurement
apparent diffusion coefficient (ADC), 276
diffusion tensor imaging (DTI), 276
pulsed filed gradient (PFG) experiment, 276–277
water diffusion, 277f
spin relaxation
nuclear magnetic resonance principle, 272f
T_1 (*See* spin-lattice relaxation time)
T_2 and T_2* (*See* Spin-spin relaxation time)
Brownian motion, MRI, 34–35

C

Cancer imaging technique
cellular and molecular imaging
target detection, 200–208
technical strategy, 209–214
^{13}C MRS, 216–218
^{1}H MRS, 214–216
MR metabolic Boyden chamber
ECM cell region, 225f
invasive index, 227f
MBC assay demonstration, 226f
oxygen tension characterization, 224f
^{31}P MRS, 219–221
preclinical models, 226–229
spin-lattice relaxation time (T_1), 221–222
T_2* and T_2 relaxation, 221
tumor pH, 221–222
vascular imaging, tumors
extrinsic/exogenous contrast, 190–200
intrinsic/endogenous contrast, 188–190
MR relaxation mechanisms, 186–187
Carbon-11 radiotracers
1-[^{11}C]acetate synthesis
[^{11}C]CO_2 gas trap and purification method, 161–162
chemistry synthesizer, CTI acetate module, 162–163, 162f
Hudson robotic system, 160–161, 161f
dosimetry calculations
biological clearance data, 166
cumulative activity, 166
medical internal radiation dose (MIRD), 165
GAP studies
[^{11}C]CO_2 determination, 169
^{11}C fate, glycolytic pathway, 173f
effective dose equivalent (EDE), 168
kinetic modeling, 169–177

regional perfusion and metabolism measurement, 166–168
total acidic metabolites analysis, 169
1-[^{11}C]D-glucose synthesis
ammonia addition, 158
[^{11}C]CO_2 gas trap, 158
end of bombardment (EOB), 158
gantry system, 157f
purification, 159
reaction vessel, 158
scheme 1 radiosynthesis, 154f
sugar-borate complex, 156
1-[^{11}C]palmitate synthesis
[^{11}C]CO_2 gas trap, 159–160
filtration method, 160
gantry system, 160f
reaction vessel, 159
quality assurance
chemical purity, 164–165
radioactivity balance, 164
radiochemical purity, 163–164
radionuclidic identity and purity, 163
sterility, apyrogenicity, isotonicity, and acidity, 165
specific activity (SA)
definition, 155–156
improvement concerns, 156
Cell adhesion molecules (CAMs), 342
Cellular and molecular imaging, MRI and MRS
target detection
MR spectroscopy and water exchange, 206–208
sensitivity and typical concentration, 200–202
T_1 contrast agents, 202–203
T_2 contrast agents, 204–206
technical strategy, MR microscopy
RF sensitivity, 210–211
signal-to-noise ratio, 209–210
surface microcoils, 212–214
volume microcoils, 211–212
Central nervous system (CNS) inflammation, MRI applications
experimental allergic encephalopathy (EAE), 293
magnetization transfer ratio (MTR), 294
multiple sclerosis, 293–294
Cerebral blood flow (CBF) measurement
laser Doppler flowmetry, 244
motor evoked potential (MEP) monitoring, 246–247
Cerebral ischemia, MRI applications
ADC changes, stroke, 284–286
BOLD, 288
brain reorganization, stroke, 287–288
CBF, stroke, 286
diffusion/perfusion mismatch region, 285f
intraluminal suture occlusion, 285f
penumbra, 286–287
spreading depression, 287
Chemical exchange, protons, 32
Chemical shift, MRS, 380
^{13}C MRS, 216–218
Colon carcinoma, 312–316
Continuous arterial spin labeling (CASL) measurement, 280
Contrast agents (CA), tumor imaging
high molecular weight agents, 197–200
low molecular weight agents, 190–197
clearance model, 192
dynamic rCBV map generation, 196f
fast exchange regime, 193
intermediate exchange regime, 194
Kety model, 191
Larmor frequency, 193–194
magnetic field heterogeneity, 192–193
mixed flow model, 192
PS-limited model, 191
slow exchange regime, 194
susceptibility-induced relaxation effects, 194f

D

Densitometric analysis, drug efficacy, 141
Diethylenetriaminepentaacetic acid (DTPA), 363f
Diffusion tensor imaging (DTI), 276
DOTA-conjugated antibody imaging
characterization
immunoreactivity, 368–369
number of sites, 368
reagents, 367–368
conjugation
methods, 365–366
reagents, 365
FDA-approved monoclonal antibodies, 358
fragments generation
method, 364–365
reagents, 364
PET imaging, 369
radiolabeling technique, 366–367
radionuclide and chelating agent selection
chemical structures, 363f
gamma-emitting isotopes, 362–363

DOTA-conjugated antibody imaging (*cont.*)
^{68}Ge generator, 362f
herceptin, 360–361
Hsp90, 360–361
metallic radionuclides, gamma camera imaging, 360
microPET, 360–361
planar gamma camera images, 361f
positron-emitting isotopes, 359–360
Drug imaging, MRI/Magnetic resonance spectroscopy (MRS)
biomarkers
degenerative joint disease, 147
neurodegenerative disorders, 146
neurotransmitter systems, 146
oncology, 146–147
chemical shift dispersion, 137
fluorine sensitivity, 137
limitations, 137, 138
noninvasive assessment and pharmacodynamic studies
densitometric analysis, 141
in vivo morphometry, 139–141, 140f
interanimal variability, 144f
qualitative characterization, 138–139
time dependence, 139f
tissue perfusion and oxygenation, 135–136
vascular permeability, 136
voxel range, 136–137
Dynamic contrast-enhanced MRI (DCE-MRI), 311–312

E

Echo planar imaging (EPI)
drawback, 72–73
rapid MRI, 72
signal loss susceptibililty, 73
Endothelial-targeted imaging, angiogenic vessels, 342
Epilepsy, MRI applications
long-term changes, 289–290
short-term changes, 289
Epilepsy, PET, 13

F

Functional magnetic resonance imaging (fMRI). *See* Magnetic resonance imaging (MRI)

G

Gadolinium diethylenetriamine-pentaacetic acid (Gd-DTPA), 383–384
Gallium scintigraphy, 13
Gamma-emitting isotopes, 362–363
General linear model (GLM) analysis, brain, 77, 80–81
Gene therapy
imaging gene expression, 382–383
monitoring gene delivery, 380–382
MRI-based systems
Gd-DTPA, 383–384
melanogenesis, 385
reporter gene, 385–386
transferrin receptor (TfR), 384–385
MRS-based systems
β-Galactosidase, 388
choline kinase (CK), 387
5-fluorouracil (5-FU), 387
vector formulation, 382
Genome scale imaging, voxelation methods
data analysis
high-level analysis, 405–406
image reconstruction, 406–407
low-level analysis, 405
histologic staining, 402
microarrays, RNA labeling, hybridization, 404
physical voxelation method, 402–403
RNA isolation, quality check, 403
sample preparation, 402
1-[^{11}C]D-Glucose, 1-[^{11}C]acetate, and 1-[^{11}C] palmitate (GAP) studies
gantry system, 157f, 160f
Hudson robotic system, 161f
kinetic modeling, myocardium
blood flow, 171–172
compartmental model method, 169,170f, 169–170, 175f
fatty acid metabolism, 175–177
glucose utilization, 172–174
oxidative metabolism, 174–175
metabolite analysis
[^{11}C]CO_2 determination, 169
total acidic metabolites (TAM) analysis, 169
regional perfusion and metabolism measurement
data acquisition, 166–167
data reconstruction and time-activity curve generation, 168
specific activity (SA), 155–156

synthesis modules, 156–163
1-[^{11}C]D-Glucose synthesis. *See also* Carbon-11 radiotracers
ammonia addition, 158
[^{11}C]CO_2 gas trap, 158
end of bombardment (EOB), 158
gantry system, 157f
purification, 159
reaction vessel, 158
scheme 1 radiosynthesis, 154f
sugar-borate complex, 156

H

Herceptin, monoclonal antibody, 360–361
^{1}H MRS, 214–216, 222
HuEP5C7, stroke, 249
Huntington's disease, MRI applications, 291

I

(+/-)2-Imidazole-1-yl-3-ethoxycarbonylpropionic acid (IEPA), 222
Integrins, vascular targets, 342–343
Intracranial pressure (ICP) monitoring. *See* Stroke
Inversion recovery (IR) sequence, 275
Ischemic pathology, MRI
apparent diffusion coefficient (ADC), 309–310
permanent MCAO, 310

K

Kety model, Contrast agent (CA), 191

L

Larmor frequency, 193–194
Laser Doppler flowmetry. *See* Stroke
Laser-scanning confocal microscopy (LSCM) imaging technique
blood velocity measurement, 264–266, 265f
corneal angiogenesis assay, 262–263
vascular imaging, 261–262
Ligand-binding assay. *See* Multiple ligand concentration receptor assay (MLCRA) method

M

Magnetic resonance imaging (MRI)
aminoguanidine evaluation, TBI
caspase-3 immunohistochemistry, 332–333
in situ TUNEL, 334
lateral fluid-percussive brain injury, 327
MRI methods and analysis, 327–329
neurologic and behavioral test, 329–331
perfusion, 331–332
blood oxygenation level-dependent (BOLD) effect, 33–34
brain disease, animal models
cerebral ischemia, 284–288
CNS inflammation, 291–294
epilepsy, 289–290
magnetization transfer contrast (MTC), 282–284
neurodegenerative disorders, 290–291
perfusion, cerebral blood flow (CBF), 277–282
sample diffusion, 276–277
spin-relaxation, 271–275
brain function, fMRI
activity detection, 74
block design paradigm, 75–76
blood oxygenation signal, 70–72
BOLD response pattern, 78f
data preparation, 77
echo planar imaging (EPI), 72–73
event-related designs, 76
group comparisons, 80
injury and stroke, 80
intensity detection, 69
model-based detection, BOLD signal, 77
response recording method, 75
software assistance, 75
statistical inference and activation threshold, 78–79, 79f
time-locked stimulus response, 69
visual cortex stimulation, 74
cancer
arterial spin labeling (ASL), 188–189
BOLD effect, 189f
high molecular weight contrast agents, 197–200
low molecular weight contrast agents, 190–197
MR contrast agents (CA), 190
MR relaxation mechanisms, vascular imaging, 186–187
compartmentation effects, water, 32

Magnetic resonance imaging (MRI) (*cont.*)
drug imaging and pharmacokinetic (PK) studies, MRS
advantage and disadvantages, 147–148
biomarkers, 145–147
chemical shift dispersion, 137
fluorine sensitivity, 137
interanimal variability, 144f
limitations, 137, 138
physiological parameters, 141
qualitative characterization, disease phenotype, 138–139
quantitative analysis, *in vivo* morphometry, 139–145, 140f
time dependence, parameters, 139f
tissue perfusion and oxygenation, 141–143
vascular permeability, 143–145
voxel range, 136–137
exchange effects, water, 31–32
exercising skeletal muscle
metabolic and hemodynamic responses, 44
NMR relaxation, 38–41, 42–43
small animal experiments, 44–45
T_1 and T_2 relaxation times, 36
water compartmentation, 36–38
functional imaging (fMRI), macaque monkeys
anesthetic procedures, 50–51
animal experiments, 50
apparatus required, 51
in awake monkeys, 51
brain mechanism analysis, 48
cognitive neuroscience, 49
data analyses, 52
history, 49
human brain comparison, 50f
macroscopic neuronal information, 48–49
neuron electrical activity analysis, 48
scan procedures, 52
gene therapy
Gd-DTPA, 383–384
melanogenesis, 385
reporter gene, 385–386
transferrin receptor (TfR), 384–385
magnetization transfer mechanism, 32
paramagnetic relaxation, 33
pathologies, animal models
bacterial infections, 303–309
ischemic pathology, 309–310
metabolic-degenerative disorders, 316–319
neoplastic pathologies, 311–316
spin motion effects, water
apparent diffusion coefficient (ADC), 34–35
blood motion analysis, 35
Brownian motion, 34–35
spin relaxation
dipole-dipole interaction, 30–31
macromolecules and biological tissues, 31
magnetization, 28–29
motional averaging, 31
relaxation times (T_1 and T_2), 28–29
simple liquids, 31
spin-lattice relaxation rate, 29–30
spin-spin relaxation rate (R_2), 30
tissue properties, 28
Magnetic resonance spectroscopy (MRS)
drug imaging (*See* Drug imaging, MRI/ Magnetic resonance spectroscopy (MRS))
gene therapy
β-Galactosidase, 388
choline kinase (CK), 387
5-fluorouracil (5-FU), 387
Magnetization prepared rapid gradient echo (MPRAGE)
baboon template image, 57–60
macaque template image, 61–62
Magnetization transfer contrast (MTC), 282–284
Melanogenesis, 385
Metabolic Boyden chamber (MBC) assay, cancer
demonstration model, 226f
ECM cell region, 225f
invasive index, 227f
oxygen tension characterization, 224f
Metabolic-degenerative disorders, MRI
lipid accumulation, 316–317
localized spectra, 319f
ob-ob mice, 317–319
single voxel/multivoxel techniques, 317
T_1W images, 318f
Microcoils, 211
Micro-PET, 6–7, 360–361
Morphometry, drug efficacy, 139–141, 140f
Motor evoked potential (MEP) monitoring, CBF, 246–247
MPRAGE. *See* Magnetization prepared rapid gradient echo (MPRAGE)
Multiphoton laser-scanning microscopic (MPLSM) technique, 259–260
Multiple-injection positron emission tomography (M-I PET)
compartmental models
arterial plasma concentration, 110–111
ordinary differential equations (ODEs), 110
experimental protocol and considerations
animal preparation, 116

blood activity measurement, 116–118
regional time-activity curve (TACs) generation, 118–120
experiments designing procedure
design variables, 131
D-optimal criterion, 130–131
Hessian matrix, 131
sensitivity functions, 128–130, 129f
history and concepts, kinetic characterization, 106–107
identifiability, parameter, 108
models and data fitting
equation implementations, 120
numerical solution, differential equations, 122–123
parameter estimation, 120–122
parameter estimation considerations, 123–124
time-activity curve, 125f
results and interpretation
model selection/goodness of fit, 128
parameter precision, 126–127
residual examination, 125–126
specialized applications, 109
standard model equations
association rate constant, 112
free tracer binding, 112
time-varying plasma radioactivity, 111–112
three parallel, coupled models, 112–115, 113f
Multiple ligand concentration receptor assay (MLCRA) method
applications
density distinction, 98
sequential *vs.* nonsequential studies, 98–100
two-point studies, 100–101
blood sampling avoidance, 92
data analysis
distribution volume ratios (DVRs) evaluation, 95–96
parameter optimization, 96–98, 97f
scanning procedure, 94
sequential acquisition method, 94–95
equilibrium administration, 92
in vivo and *in vitro* methods, 90
mathematical considerations, 91
nonsequential studies, 92–93
pharmacological effect and interventions, 86–87, 92
potential confounds, 90–91
principles, 89–90
radiation dosimetry, 91
radiochemistry and specific activity (SA) determination, 93–94
receptor saturation, 91
Myocardium enzymatic pathway imaging
GAP study
blood flow quatification, 171–172
$[^{11}C]CO_2$ determination, 169
compartmental model method, 169–170, 170f
effective dose equivalent (EDE), 168
fatty acid metabolism, 175–177
glucose utilization (MGU), 172–174
oxidative metabolism, 174–175
regional perfusion and metabolism measurement, 166–168
total acidic metabolites analysis, 169
Kitagawa gas detector solid-phase system, 156
positron annihilation and coincidence detection, 154f
radiotracer synthesis, 155f
short-lived isotopes, 153, 153–154

N

Nanoparticles. *See* Vascular-targeted nanoparticles
Neoplastic pathology, MRI
dynamic contrast-enhanced MRI (DCE-MRI), 311–312
Gd-DTPA-albumin, 312
HT-29 human colon carcinoma, 312
longitudinal relaxation rates, 313
maps, colon carcinoma, 316f
pre and post contrast images, 313
Neurodegenerative disorders, MRI applications
Alzheimer's disease, 290–291
Huntington's disease, 291
Parkinson's disease, 290
Neuroimaging techniques
advantages, 56
anatomic interpretation, statistical images, 63–64
b2k and b2kf baboon atlas development
animal age, 57
image acquisition and registration, 57–58, 60–61
sagittal section image, 59f
template image development, 58–60, 61
validation, 60, 61
functional imaging data analysis
PET image registration, 62–63
SPM analysis, 63

Neuroimaging techniques (*cont.*)
human atlas space studies, 56
n2k and n2kf macaque template images, 61–62
three-dimensional atlas template image, 56–57
trauma brain injury
acoustic startle response, 330
forelimb grip-strength test, 330
locomotor activity, 329, 329f, 330f
rotametric test, 331
Neuropathology, MRI applications
cerebral ischemia
ADC changes, stroke, 284–286
BOLD, 288
brain reorganization, stroke, 287–288
CBF, stroke, 286
diffusion/perfusion mismatch region, 285f
intraluminal suture occlusion, 285f
penumbra, 286–287
spreading depression, 287
CNS inflammation
experimental allergic encephalopathy (EAE), 293
magnetization transfer ratio (MTR), 294
multiple sclerosis, 293–294
epilepsy
long-term changes, 289–290
short-term changes, 289
neurodegenerative disorders
Alzheimer's disease, 290–291
Huntington's disease, 291
Parkinson's disease (PD), 290
Nuclear magnetic resonance (NMR) technique, exercising skeletal muscle
interstitial space, 42
intracellular space, 38–41
vascular space, 42–43

O

Oncology
biomarker, MRI/MRS, 146–147
PET, 8–13
Optical imaging technique, angiogenesis
angiogenesis and development, tumor
blood flow, 255
hypoxia, 256
tortuosity, 255
tumor size and density, 255, 256
vascular permeability (VP), 255
vessel dilation, 255
arthritis angiogenesis study, 260
dorsal skin window chamber model, 253
intravascular fluorescent probes, markers
BF velocity measurement, 264–266
capillary perfusion and permeability, 263–264
multiphoton laser-scanning microscope (MPLSM), 259–260
transgenic mouse model
arthritis synovium, 261f
conjunctiva capillary, Tie2-GFP mouse, 261f
corneal angiogenesis assay, 262–263
laser-scanning confocal microscopy (LSCM), Tie2-GFP mouse, 261–262
tumor-host interaction
antivascular endothelial growth model (VEGF), 258
green fluorescent protein (GFP), 256–260
vascular response, 257–258
window chamber model images, 257f
Osteomyelitis, PET, 15
Oxygenation, MRI, 141–143

P

1-[^{11}C]Palmitate synthesis. *See also* Carbon-11 radiotracers
[^{11}C]CO_2 gas trap, 159–160
filtration method, 160
gantry system, 160f
reaction vessel, 159
Paramagnetic polymerized vesicle (PPV), 344
Paramagnetic relaxation, MRI, 33
Parkinson's disease (PD), MRI applications, 290
PET. *See* Positron emission tomography (PET)
Pharmacodynamic studies. *See* Drug imaging, MRI/Magnetic resonance spectroscopy (MRS)
^{31}P MRS, 219–221
Pneumonia, MRI, 307–309
Positron emission tomography (PET)
angiogenesis quantitation, 16–17
apoptosis, 17
biological function evaluation, 7–8
cardiology
cardiac neurotransmission, 15
myocardial viability, 14–15
DOTA-conjugated antibody, 369
drug evaluation
dynamic data collection, 5–6
pharmacokinetic studies, 6
gene expression, 18
infectious and inflammatory diseases
fever, unknown origin, 16

osteomyelitis, 15
prosthetic joint infections, 15–16
local receptor density estimation, multiple-injection (M-I) paradigms
compartmental models, 110–111
experimental protocol and considerations, 115–120
experiments designing procedure, 128–130
history and concepts, kinetic characterization, 106–107
identifiability, parameter, 108
models and data fitting, 120–124
model selection/goodness of fit, 128
parameter precision, 126–127
residual examination, 125–126
specialized applications, 109
standard model equations, 111–112
three parallel, coupled models, 112–115, 113f
multidrug resistance (MDR) assessment, 16
multiple ligand concentration receptor assay (MLCRA) method
applications, 98–101
blood sampling avoidance, 92
data analysis, 95–96
equilibrium administration, 92
experimental procedure, 94–95
in vivo and *in vitro* methods, 90
mathematical considerations, 91
nonsequential studies, 92–93
pharmacological effect and interventions, 86–87, 92
potential confounds, 90–91
principles, 89–90
radiation dosimetry, 91
radiochemistry and specific activity (SA) determination, 93–94
receptor saturation, 91
neurology
Alzheimer's disease (AD), 13–14
epilepsy, 13
l-[methyle-11C]methionine (MET), 13
movement disorders, 14
oncology
breast cancer detection, 11
colorectal carcinoma, 10
differential diagnosis, 9
^{18}F-FDG radiotracer, 8
localization, unknown origin, 9–10
metastasis detection, 11
nonsmall cell lung cancer (NSLC), 10
recurrence/restaging, 12–13
staging accuracy, 10–11
treatment response analysis, 11–12
small animal imaging
applications, 6–7
limitations, 7
tracers, 4–5
tumor hypoxia, 17
Proton transfer enhancement factor (PTE), 207
Pulsed arterial spin labeling (PASL) measurement, 280–282

R

Raclopride
binding potential, 86–87
equilibrium administration, 92
two-point Scatchard plots, 87f
Radio frequency (RF) sensitivity, 210–211
Radioimmunoimaging, DOTA-conjugated antibody. *See also* DOTA-conjugated antibody imaging
characterization, 367–369
labeling
method, 366–367
reagents, 366
Rapid MRI. *See* Echo planar imaging (EPI)
Receptor imaging. *See* Multiple ligand concentration receptor assay (MLCRA) method
Region-of-interest (ROI) analysis, 306–307

S

Spin-echo (SE) sequence, 273
Spin-lattice relaxation time
magnetization changes, 275f
paramagnetic contrast agents, 274–275
T_1 measurements, 275
Spin-spin relaxation time
BOLD imaging, 273
spin-echo sequence, 274f
T_2 and T_2* plain measurements, 273
Spreading depression, 287
Stroke, 80
animal models, 239–240
data collection and analysis
HuEP5C7, model application, 249
infarct volume, 248–249
neurologic evaluation, 246–247
radiographic imaging, 247–248
operative technique

Stroke (*cont.*)
ICP monitor and laser Doppler probe placement, 243
positioning, 243
transorbital approach, 243
vessel occlusion, 244–245
physiologic monitor, 242
postoperative care
clinical examination, 246
monitoring, 246
preoperative care
anesthesia and preparation, 240–242
animal and supplies requirement, 240
materials and manufactures, 241f
primate models, 240
Superparamagnetic iron oxides (SPIOs), 377–378

T

T_1 contrast agents, cancer, 202–203
Template image development, brain
baboon atlas, 58–60, 58f, 61
functional imaging data analysis, 62–63
macaque atlas, 61–62
Terminal transferase dUTP nick-end labeling (TUNEL), TBI, 334
1,4,7,10-Tetraazacyclododecane-N,N′,N″,N‴-tetraacetic acid (DOTA), 363f
Transferrin receptor (TfR), MRI, 384–385
Transverse (T_1 and T_2) relaxation times, 28–29
Trauma brain injury (TBI), MRI
caspase-3 immunohistochemistry, 332–333
imaging methods and analysis, 327–329
in situ TUNEL, 334
lateral fluid-percussive brain injury, 327
neurologic and behavioral test
acoustic startle response, 330
forelimb grip-strength test, 330
locomotor activity, 329
rotametric test, 331
perfusion, 331–332
T_2* relaxation, cancer, 221
Tumors, MRI vascular imaging
extrinsic/exogenous contrast
contrast agents (CA), 190
high molecular weight contrast agents, 197–200
low molecular weight contrast agents, 190–197
intrinsic/endogenous contrast
arterial spin labeling (ASL), 188–189
BOLD effect, 189f
tissue relaxation mechanisms, 186–187
TUNEL. *See* Terminal transferase dUTP nick-end labeling

V

Vascular-targeted nanoparticles
amphiphilic lipid molecule, 343
angiogenic vessels, 342
design and preclinical studies
ACPV targeting, 347–349
molecular imaging, 349–351
PV synthesis and characterization, 344–346
integrins, 342–343
permeability problem, 341–342
therapeutics, molecular imaging, 351–354
Voxelation methods, brain gene expression
data analysis
high-level analysis, 405–406
image reconstruction, 406–407
low-level analysis, 405
histologic staining, 402
microarrays, RNA labeling, hybridization, 404
physical voxelation method, 402–403
RNA isolation, quality check, 403
sample preparation, 402

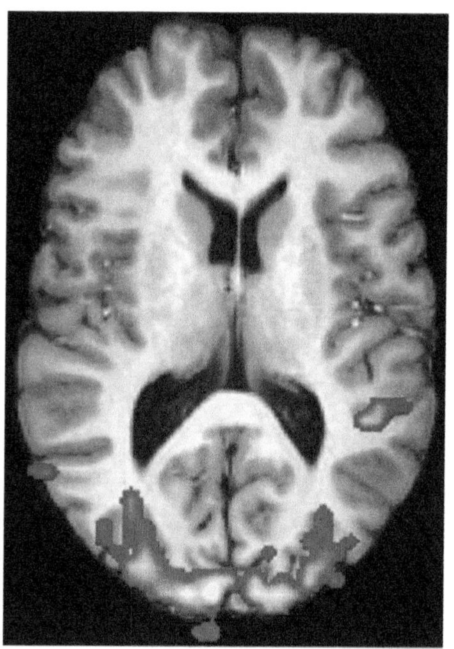

Plate 1 (Figure 5.1 on page 70 of this volume)

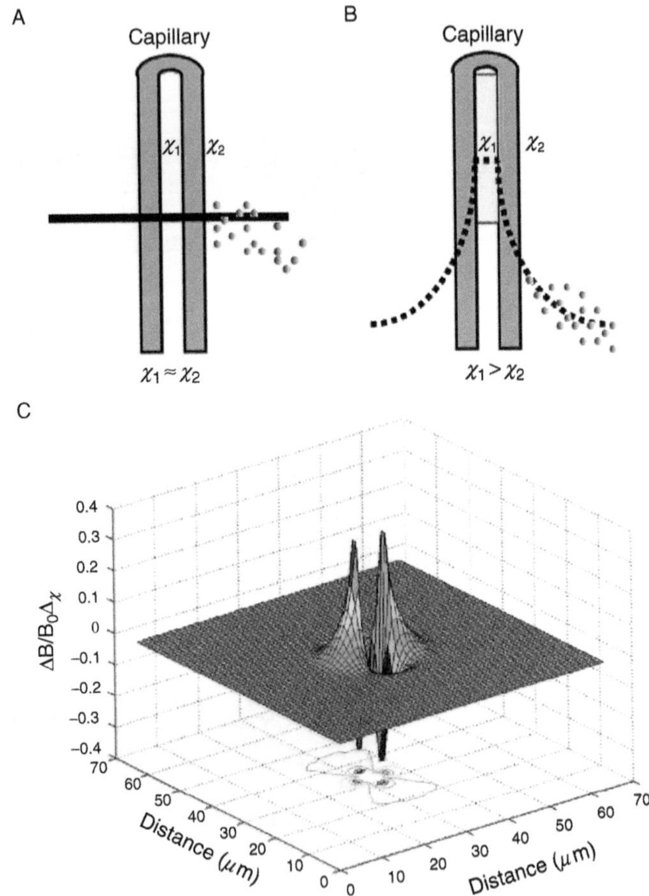

Plate 2 (Figure 10.1 on page 189 of this volume)

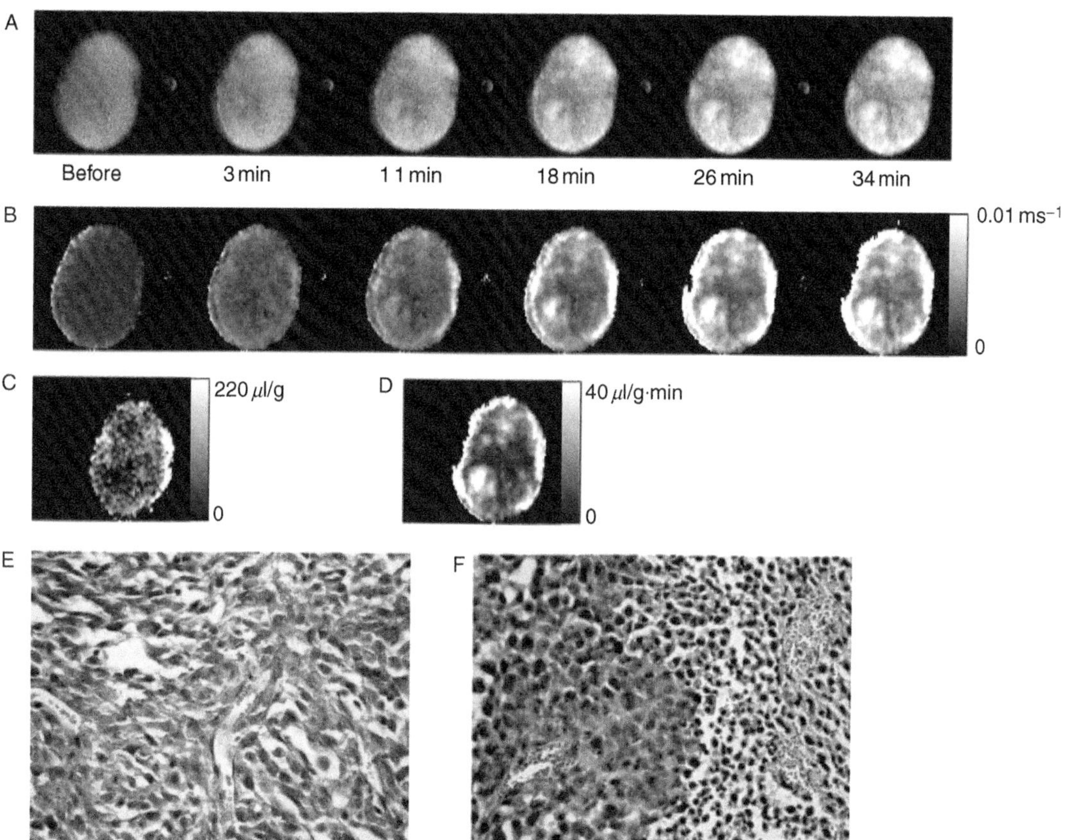

Plate 3 (Figure 10.5 on page 199 of this volume)

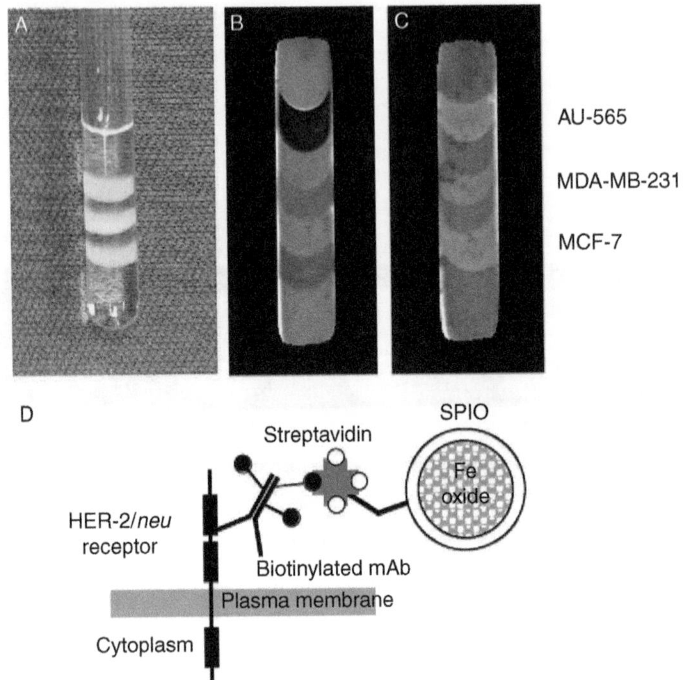

Plate 4 (Figure 10.6 on page 205 of this volume)

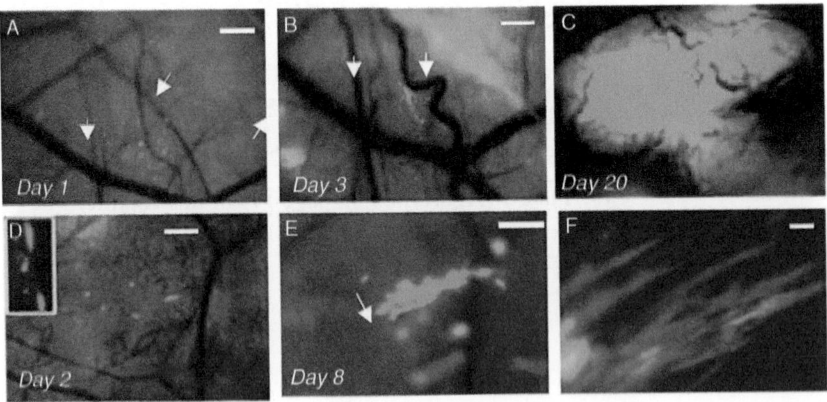

Plate 5 (Figure 12.2 on page 257 of this volume)

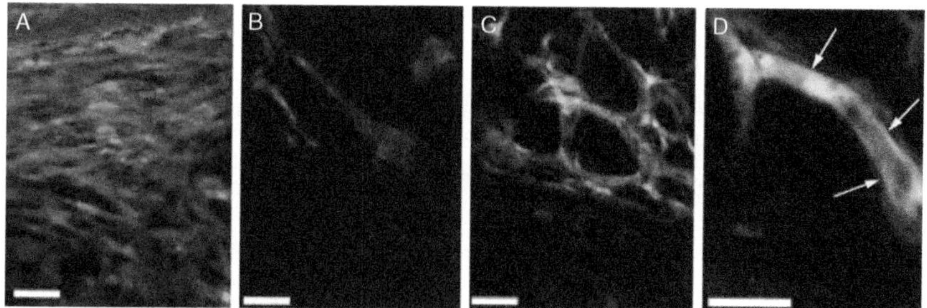

Plate 6 (Figure 12.4 on page 259 of this volume)

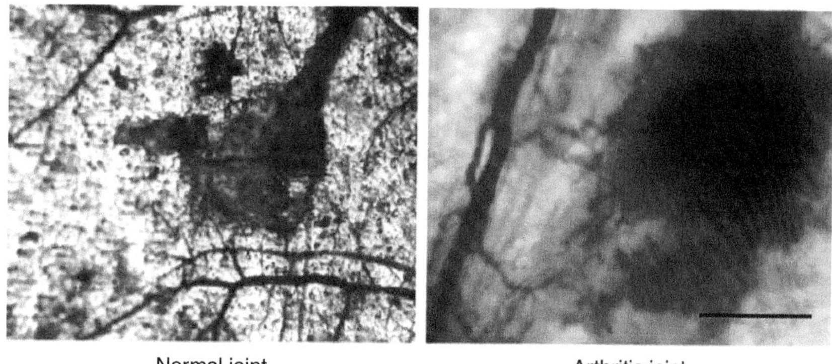

Plate 7 (Figure 12.5 on page 261 of this volume)

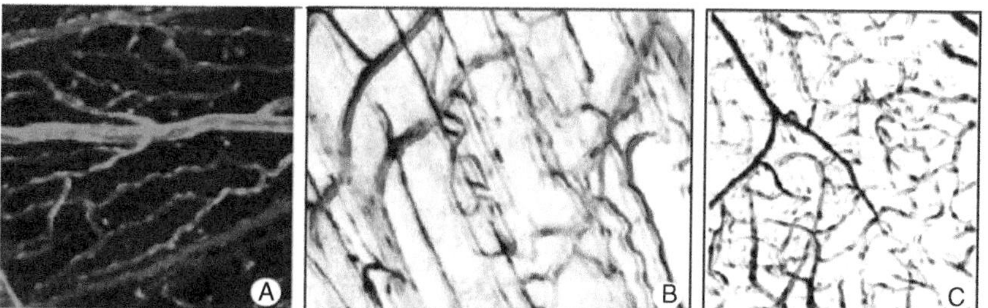

Plate 8 (Figure 12.6 on page 261 of this volume)

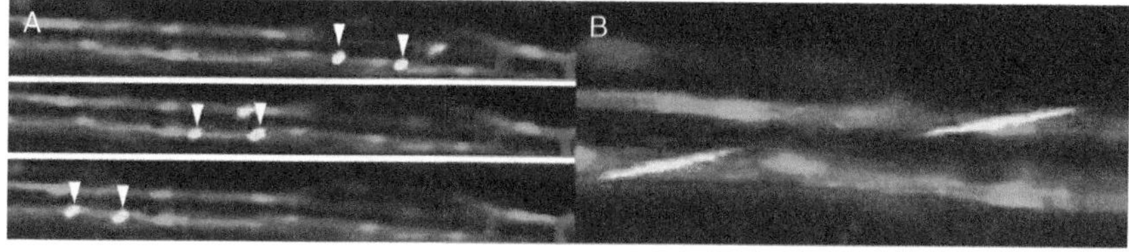

Plate 9 (Figure 12.8 on page 265 of this volume)

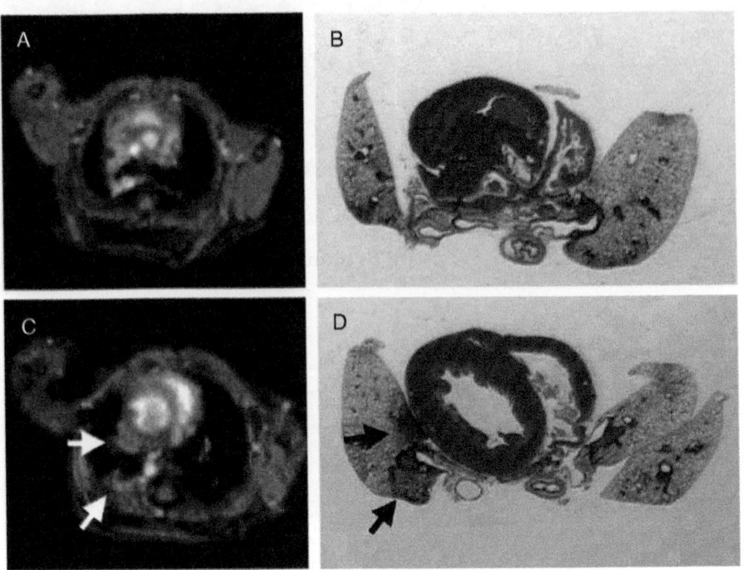

Plate 10 (Figure 14.4 on page 309 of this volume)

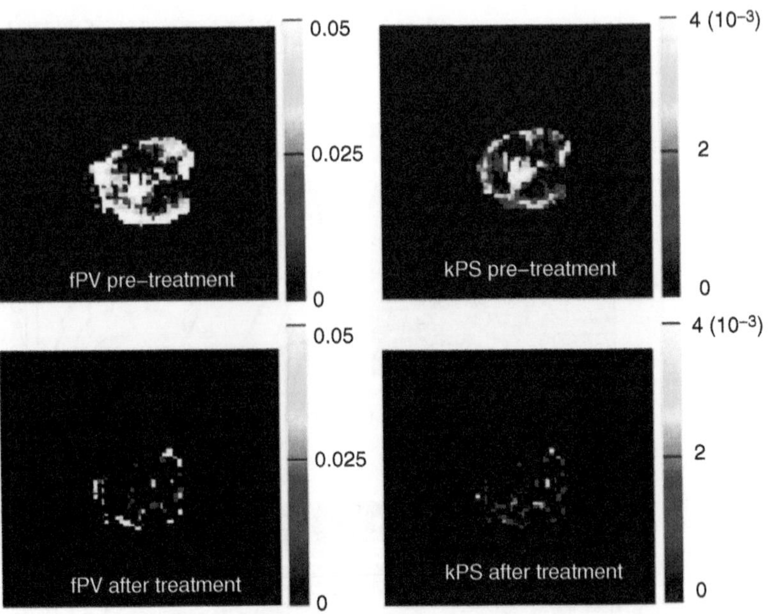

Plate 11 (Figure 14.6 on page 316 of this volume)

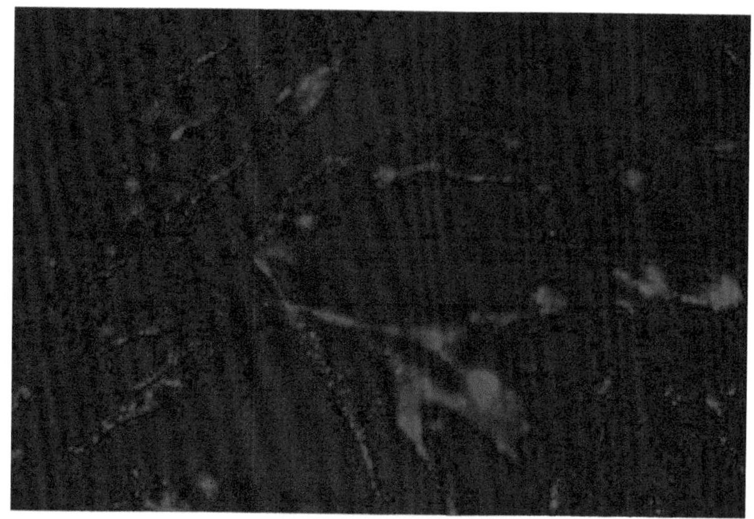

Plate 12 (Figure 16.2 on page 347 of this volume)

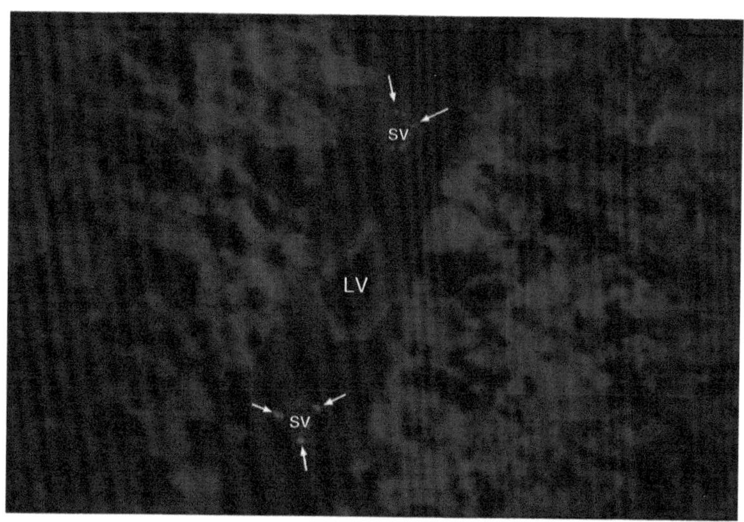

Plate 13 (Figure 16.3 on page 348 of this volume)

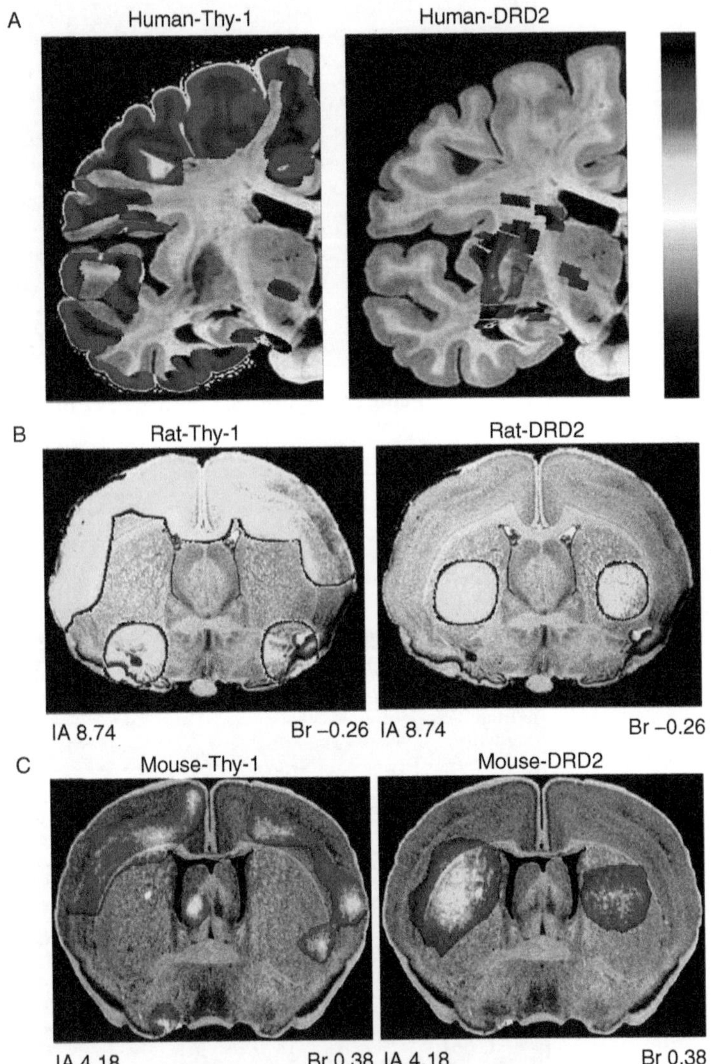

Plate 14 (Figure 19.1 on page 407 of this volume)

Printed and bound by CPI Group (UK) Ltd, Croydon, CR0 4YY
08/06/2025
01896869-0015